History of the
Basel Institute for Immunology

History of the **Basel Institute for Immunology**

Compiled and narrated by Ivan Lefkovits
Founding Member of the Basel Institute for Immunology

339 figures, 183 in color, 2017

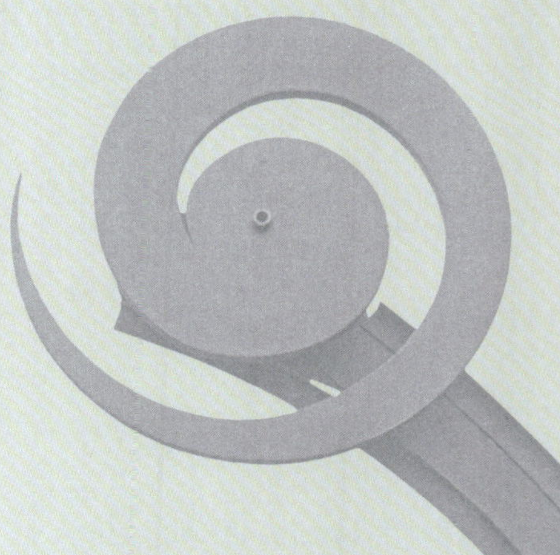

Basel · Freiburg · Paris · London · New York · New Delhi ·
Bangkok · Singapore · Tokyo · Sydney

KARGER

Prof. Dr. Ivan Lefkovits

Founding Member of the
Basel Institute for Immunology

Library of Congress Cataloging-in-Publication Data

CIP data available from the publisher upon request.

Graphic Design and Typesetting: Gerri Schmid
Production Editing: Patrick Näf
Copy Editing: Elisabeth Stöcklin
Proof Reading: Herbert Wäckerlin
Image Processing: Alice Hauenstein
Graphic Production Manager: Patrik Brunner

www.karger.com
Printed in Switzerland on acid-free and non-aging paper (ISO 9706)
by Werner Druck & Medien AG, Basel
ISBN 978–3–318–05934–2
e-ISBN 978–3–318–05935–9

Cover illustration: *Double Helix* (Jean Tinguely)

Contents

The History of Scientific Achievements and of the Social Impact of the Basel Institute for Immunology	XVIII
Preface	XVIII
The Storyteller's Dilemma	XIX

Book 1: 1969–1985

Recounting the Years 1968–1969	2
A New Institute	2
Finding a Director	4
Searching for Scientists	7
Planning the Building	8
Floor Plans	10
The Rheinfelden Meetings	13
Recruitment from Round the World	16
Rheinfelden Two	18

Adolf Jann discussed with Alfred Pletscher the long-term strategies for pharmaceutical research. A decision was made to establish a Basel Institute for Immunology. Niels K. Jerne was chosen as director. Jerne and Jann sealed the agreement with a handshake. Planning the building started, and floor plans were drawn up. On April 29th, 1968, the foundation stone was laid. Jerne left for a recruitment round-the-world journey.

The Year 1970	20
First Contracts Signed	20
The 1st Krafft Meeting	21
Countdown to the Opening	23
Advisors and Consultants	25
The 2nd Krafft Meeting	26
The Opening, October 1970	27
Research Interests in Brief	27
Preparing for Scientific Endeavors	29
First Internal Seminar – *Ruggero Ceppellini*: Human Histocompatibility System	33
First Formal Seminar – *Klaus Rajewsky*	33

First contracts were signed. Jerne called a foundation meeting, later referred to as "the first Krafft meeting". An advisory board and a board of consultants were established. On October 1st, 1970, the institute opened. In 7 laboratories 25 scientists started to work (A. Kelus, I. Lefkovits, T. Staehelin, S. Fazekas, E. Jacobson, T.-W. Tao-Wiedmann, C. Steinberg, L. Du Pasquier, F. Loor, D. Braun, J.-C. Jaton, H. Pohlit, G. Roelants, B. Askonas, D. Dresser, J. Andersson, O. Sjöberg, J. Hay, J. Obel, V. Miggiano, D. Bernoco, S. Shin, A. Falvey, W. McKeehan, M. Schreier).

Six months after the "partial" opening, the remaining areas were completed. On June 17th the official inauguration of the institute took place. Tinguely's Double Helix (a present from Maja and Paul Sacher) was installed. Niels Jerne delivered at the conference "The Challenge of Life", organized by Roche, a lecture entitled "Newer Knowledge of Immunobiology". Monday lunch seminars were initiated. Several courses were held including the EMBO course on homogeneous antibodies. Tonegawa started to work on the project of generation of antibody diversity. By the end of the year, 17 papers had been published. The Santa Lucia celebration completed the year.

The Year 1971 35

The Machine Is Switched On 36

The Monday Lunch Seminar 13.07 38

Inauguration of the BII, June 1971 38

Tinguely's Double Helix 40

Gerry Edelman at the BII Lab Bench 43

The Challenge of Life 43

EMBO Advanced Study Course 44

Balance Sheet 44

Continuous Colloquium throughout the Year 45

Science in the Seminar Room 45

Science at the Bench 46

Research Directions Outlined 49

Published Papers and Submitted Manuscripts 55

First International Congress of Immunology 55

BII List of Scientists 56

BII List of Technicians 56

The BII Facilities 59

Reception 60

Workshop 60

Radioisotopes 61

Cell Sorter Facility 61

Animal Facilities 61

Media Kitchen 62

Laboratory and Institute Cleaning 63

Purchasing / Budgets / Travel 63

Secretarial Facilities 63

Library 63

Artwork and Photography 64

Computer Infrastructure 64

Transport 64

Cafeteria 65

Electron Microscopy 65

Other Facilities 66

Political Issue: Women in Switzerland, 1971 66

The BII became fully functional. The scientific activities were matched by contributions at meetings, symposia and workshops. Several members took up teaching responsibilities at various universities in Switzerland and abroad. The institute established several boards to ensure that the high standards of the institute were achieved and then maintained. These boards were: the International Advisory Board, the Swiss Board of Consultants and the Board of Trustees.

The Year 1972 68

Visiting Research Workers 68

Research Directions 70

Extramural Lecturing 74

Contributions at Meetings, Symposia and Workshops 74

Venia Legendi 75

Roche Nutley Creates the V.D. Mattia Award 76

Adolf Jann and the English-Language Kindergarten 76

Yellow Submarine 77

Self-Service in Affluent Settings 77
The Advisory Structures 78
Members of the International Advisory Board (IAB) 78
Members of the Swiss Board of Consultants (SBC) 78
Members of the Board of Trustees (BT-BII) 79
From Niels Jerne's Notes 81
Gerald M. Edelman, Member of the BII Advisory Board, Nobel Prize Winner 85
Erna Möller and Göran Möller Visiting the BII at the Early Stage 85

The Year 1973 86

The Director in His Office 86
Conferences and Symposia 87
Demonstrations at the BII for the 6th Postgraduate Course in Experimental Medicine, University of Zurich 88
Lectures at Hoffmann-La Roche Research Department, Basel 89
Roche Conflicts 89
Jerne's Quote on the 1973 Research Projects 90
New Projects Added 90

Most of the new scientists joined existing groups. Jerne's office became the place for discussing the state of knowledge and future projects. Besides publications in prestigious journals, institute members participated in a number of workshops and conferences. Roche became involved in conflicts regarding the pricing policy of their drugs in the UK. The BII Annual Reports became an invaluable source of information worldwide – with 123 reports for 1973.

The Year 1974 96

The Teaching Laboratory and the Blackboard 96
Visiting Scientists 97
Course I: Advanced Course on Protein Biosynthesis 97
Course II: Advanced Study Course on Lymphocytes 98
From Basel to Brighton 98
Georges Köhler's Doctoral Thesis 99
Werner Haas Joins the BII 99
Tommy Meo to Ann Arbor, Then to St. Louis and Back to Basel 100
Jon Sprent to London 100
Graham Mitchell and Melbourne Zoo 100
Roche Successes 101
Nobel Prize for Christian de Duve, a Long-Standing Friend of the BII 101
Reporting and Disseminating Results 103

A new category of "visiting scientists" was established (in order to comply with the strict cantonal quota for foreigners). A major innovation in the building was the conversion of laboratory 011 into a teaching laboratory. Two courses were given there: Advanced Course on Protein Biosynthesis and Advanced Study Course on Lymphocytes. In Brighton, at the Second International Congress of Immununology, 14 members delivered lectures. Tonegawa and colleagues published 4 papers on the generation of antibody diversity. Georges Köhler completed his doctoral thesis.

The Year 1975 105

Procedure for Selecting New Members 105
The Terrarium Becomes a Vivarium for Cold-Blooded Species 106
Who Joined Who 108
Twenty Categories 109
Workshops and Conferences 110
Jerne on the Endocrine System and on the Nervous System 110
Coutinho on Protein A Plaque Assay at Christmas 111
Nobel Prize 1975 for Renato Dulbecco, Advisory Board Member 111

The turnover of scientists balanced out: 7 scientists left, and 18 scientists replaced them. The terrarium was converted into a vivarium to accommodate additional species of amphibians. Eighteen BII members participated at workshops and conferences in Basel, Aarhus, Amsterdam and Mainz.

Ben Pernis, a founding member of the BII, accepted a call to Columbia University, New York. An EMBO course on lymphocyte physiology was held at the BII. Niels Jerne called for an extramural conference on idiotypes (Baumanière, France). At the 41st Cold Spring Harbor Symposium, 8 members presented their results, among them Susumu Tonegawa with work that led to his Nobel Prize. Georges Köhler returned to Basel to establish a hybridoma technology research group. In a factory belonging to Roche, Italy, an explosion occurred, releasing dioxin into the air.

The Year 1976 112
Turnover of Scientists at the BII Creates an Alumni Network 112
The 64 Scientists Who Left the BII up until the End of 1975 113
Ben Pernis Leaves for Columbia University, New York 115
Katherine Knight to Chicago 115
Zoltan Nagy to Hungary, Then (with a Delay) to Canada 116
EMBO Course on Lymphocyte Physiology 116
Conference on Idiotypes in Les-Baux-de-Provence, April 1976 117
An Excerpt from Jerne's Introduction to the Annual Report 119
41st Cold Spring Harbor Symposium 119
Tommy Meo's Move to Munich and the Final One to Paris 120
Georges Köhler Returns to the BII 121
The Seveso Disaster and Its Implications 121

Theo Staehelin, a permanent member of the BII, accepted the position of head of the "Applied Immunology Project" at Roche. Berenice Kindred and Wulf Droege left for Heidelberg and Jonathan Sprent for London. The Roche Institute of Molecular Biology in Nutley celebrated its 10th anniversary. Several BII members participated as speakers or chairpersons at the 3rd International Congress of Immunology in Melbourne. Niels Jerne hinted that he had health problems and started discussing his succession.

The Year 1977 123
Scientific Concepts by Niels Jerne 123
Clonal Selection in Jerne's Words 124
Joghem van Loghem, Lucien Aarden and the CLB 125
Charley Steinberg and Manuscripts 126
Mel Cohn's Seminar Series 127
Alcohol and Spirit 128
Theo Staehelin Leaves for Roche 128
Roche Recruits Scientists from the BII 129
Roberto Poljak and the 3D Structure of Proteins 130
Scott Rodkey Joins Dietmar Braun 131
Berenice Kindred Leaves for Heidelberg and Tübingen 132
Wulf Droege Leaves for Heidelberg 132
Jonathan Sprent Leaves for London 132
Andreas Ziegler to Charité, Berlin 133
Sister Institute in Nutley, 10th Anniversary 133
From Basel to Sydney, 3rd International Congress of Immunology 134
Roche Research Institute of Marine Pharmacology, Dee Why, Australia 134
Jerne on Retiring – Health Problems, Not Serious, but... 134
BTA 1: Jerne and 65 + 1 136
BTA 2: "Snow-White", the Second Performance of the Basel Theater for the Arts 137

Georges Köhler organized the first workshop on hybridoma technology. The emphasis was on B lymphocyte fusions in the mouse system. Two permanent positions became vacant after Ben Pernis and Theo Staehelin had left the BII. They were filled by Georges Köhler and Harald von Boehmer. Susumu Tonegawa was awarded the Max Cloëtta Prize, the ▶

The Year 1978 140
T Cell Factors 140
The Antibody Repertoire 140
The BII Workshop 141
EMBO Laboratory Course on B Lymphocyte Fusion 143
Matthias Wabl Leaves for the Max Planck Institute, Tübingen 143
Dietmar Braun to Ciba-Geigy 144

John W. Stocker to Roche 144
Again Ten Permanent Members 145
Max Cloëtta Prize for Susumu Tonegawa 147
Nobel Prize for Basel in 1978, but Not Yet for the BII 147

▶ highest scientific recognition in Switzerland. Matthias Wabl (a close collaborator of Louis Du Pasquier and Charley Steinberg) left for the Max Planck Institute, Tübingen.

The Year 1979 148
By Indirections Find Directions Out (Jerne Quoting Polonius) 148
Preparations for the Festschrift for Niels Jerne 148
The Manuscript of Linus Pauling 149
Immunological Methods Volume 1 Published 150
Sefik Alkan to Novartis and Alba Therapeutics 151
Werner Haas on His Scientific Alter Ego Harald von Boehmer 152
Antonio Coutinho Moves to Umeå and Then Paris 152
Mathematical Model of the Immune Network Theory 153
Niels Jerne's Resolution to Resign 154

Niels Jerne presented at the Advisory Board meeting his intention to retire in the foreseeable future. The Advisory Board and permanent members recommended that he continue holding the office. The Introduction to the Annual Report 1979 was the last one written by Jerne. It was his legacy, with issues close to his heart, such as "repertoire" and "idiotypic network". Antonio Coutinho moved from Basel to Umeå and then to Paris.

The Year 1980 155
Georg Wick on a Sabbatical from Innsbruck 155
Hans Hengartner Moves to the University Hospital, Zurich 155
Gianni Garotta to Roche, Basel 156
From Basel to Paris 156
How to Behave at Meetings and Seminars 157
The Mary Jane Potash Memorial Seminars 157
The Search for a New Director 158
Fritz Melchers: Primus inter Pares 159
New Director with a Supervisory Council 160
Farewell Party for Niels Jerne, October 1980 161
A Letter from Provence 162
Nobel Prize to Former Members of the Advisory Board 163

Several scientists, Salvatore Cammisuli, Jacques Chiller, Gianni Garotta, Sarah Howie and Hans Hengartner, completed their BII assignment and moved to other places: Jacques Chiller back to California, Hans Hengartner to University Hospital, Zurich. The president of Roche, Fritz Gerber, thanked Niels Jerne for his services and appointed Fritz Melchers as the new BII director. Roche established a tighter supervision over the institute by creating a supervisory council.

The Year 1981 164
10th Anniversary of the BII 164
Anniversary Celebration Continued at the BII 165
Haute Cuisine at the Anniversary Party 166
BTA3: The Stem Cell Ballet 166
The Origin of the Basel Theater for the Arts, BTA 168
RIMB, Nutley, Honors the BII's 10th Anniversary 170
Festschrift and Glazed Cake 171
University of Basel Paid Reverence to Jerne 171
Idiotypes 171
Immunological Methods Volume 2 by Academic Press 173
Russian Translations: Методы исследований 173

The celebration of the 10th anniversary of the institute was accompanied by a scientific symposium and by a major ballet performance of the BTA. The ballet was written and choreographed by Chris and Colleen Paige, Maria Leptin, Norman Iscove and others. A two-volume Festschrift on the occasion of Niels Jerne's 70th birthday was handed over to the septuagenarian. A conference on idiotypes was organized by Claudia Berek, Howard Etlinger and Michael Julius.

Ruggero Ceppellini, a founding member of the BII, retired at the age of 65 years. A symposium on the major histocompatibility complex in man was organized in his honor. Theo Staehelin (former permanent member, affiliated with Roche since 1977) arranged a hybridoma course at the BII in order to spread hybridoma technology across the Swiss community. A course on B lymphocyte differentiation was organized by Chris Paige and Richard Pink. Kirsten Fischer Lindahl ran a workshop on class-I-like antigens.

The Year 1982 174

Ruggero Ceppellini's Retirement 174
The Roche "Monoclonal Antibodies" Project Continues 175
A Work Permit for the Head of the Cell Sorter Facility 175
The Basel Population and the Chauffeur of Bus 34 176
Roaccutane, Bollag and Pletscher 176
The BII Research Environment Forms Geniuses 177
The Horizontal Structure and "Laissez-Faire" 177
The Role of Gender 178
Irreproducible Results and Improper Scientific Conduct 178
B Hybridoma Course by Theo Staehelin's Group at Roche 180
Course and Workshop on B Lymphocyte Differentiation 180
Monograph on T Cell Hybridomas 181
Kirsten Fischer Lindahl's Workshop on Class-I-Like Antigens 181
Don Bellgrau's Work on Cytotoxic T Cell Precursors 182
Proteomic Laboratory 182

Antonio Lanzavecchia established a human immunology laboratory focusing on T and B cell biology. Klaus Karjalainen initiated a molecular biology group, related mainly to (soluble) TCR receptors. Prior to expiration of their limited contracts, both scientists became permanent members. Fritz Melchers organized a workshop on the Mechanisms of B Cell Neoplasia. Harald von Boehmer, Bonnie Mathieson and Werner Haas held a course on T lymphocyte differentiation. Christine Brack, who decisively contributed to the success of Tonegawa, moved to University Hospital Basel.

The Year 1983 183

Antonio Lanzavecchia Starts a "Human Immunology" Laboratory 183
Polly Matzinger, the Clever Bunny, Arrives 184
Klaus Karjalainen Starts a Molecular Biology Group 186
DNA Cloning and Transfection Become a Major Experimental Approach 187
Workshop on the Mechanisms of B Cell Neoplasia 187
Course and Workshop on T Lymphocyte Differentiation 188
Human Proteome Project 188
Christine Brack Moves to University Hospital Basel 189
From Basel to Kyoto 191
Committee on Ethics and Conditions of Experimentation with Animals 191
Seveso Oak Forest Park 192

Zdenek Trnka, administrative director of the BII, retired at the age of 65 years. A symposium organized by Fritz Melchers, Roland Gisler and Bede Morris, "Sheep as an Experimental Model in Immunology", was held in his honor. Fritz Melchers and Roland Gisler organized a course on the microanatomy of the immune system. Manfred Brockhaus and Richard Pink completed their term at the BII and were hired by the Research Department of Roche. Peter Robinson left for the German Cancer Research Centre, Heidelberg; Stephen Fazekas returned to Australia. Niels Jerne and Georges Köhler were awarded the Nobel Prize for Medicine (shared with César Milstein from Cambridge).

The Year 1984 193

New Approaches: In situ Hybridization, cDNA Libraries, FACS 193
Manfred Brockhaus and Richard Pink to Roche Basel 194
Manfred Brockhaus, TNF, Alzheimer 194
Richard Pink, Chicken Immunology 194
Roche Malaria Vaccine 195
Peter Robinson, Complexity of Qa-2 Antigens 196
Advances in Monoclonal Antibodies 196
Zlatko Dembic Dropped Cells on the Floor 196
Storage of Embryos in Liquid Nitrogen 197
Seminars at the Meetings of the Board of Advisors and the Board of Swiss Consultants 197
Stephen Fazekas Returns to Australia 197

Microanatomy of the Immune System 198
Retirement of Zdenek Trnka 199
Roland Gisler, Head of Administration 199
The Nobel Prize 200
The Phone Call from Stockholm 200
Press Release from the Nobel Assembly at the Karolinska Institute: Nobel Prize for Niels K. Jerne, Georges Köhler and César Milstein 202

The Year 1985 208
BTA 4: "Reflections", the Goodbye Performance for Georges Köhler 208
The Fire, February 27th, 1985 209
Girafe en Feu/Phoenix Arises from the Ashes 210

The year started routinely and uneventfully. There was no indication that in less than 8 weeks a major disaster would hit the institute. As was the case for all previous years, new members started to arrive.

Book 2: 1985–2001

Beyond Jerne's Mind 214
Antibody Response versus Immune Response 214
Innate Immunity and Acquired Immune System 215
Antonio Coutinho on Innate Immunity and Mitogen Receptors 215
Major Histocompatibility Complex 216
Natural Killer Cells 216
Antonio Coutinho Summarizes the Dilemma 217

Spring 1985 220
Chiaroscuro, February 27th, 1985 220
Legally Speaking 224
Hundreds of Letters from all over the World 225
Special Arrival of a New Member at a Special Time 226
Kirsten Fischer Lindahl Leaves for Dallas 226
Werner Haas Accepts a Position at Roche 227
Norman N. Iscove Moves to Heidelberg and Then to Toronto 227
BTA 5: "Diary", the Goodbye Performance for Norman Iscove 228
Susan Carson Comes from Sir Walter Bodmer's Laboratory 229
Conference on the Mechanisms of B Cell Neoplasia 229
Workshop on the Role of IL-2 in B Cell Physiology 230

A major fire following an explosion in the ventilation system damaged about one third of the institute, fortunately without human casualties and without harm to the animal stock. Scientists from the damaged portion of the institute "squeezed" into the intact laboratories, and for the rest of the year restoration and reconstruction work went on. Several planned courses were postponed to the following year(s). Only the B Cell Neoplasia conference and a workshop on the Role of Interleukin-2 in B Cell Physiology were held as planned. Many contracts for new members were deferred as well. Publication success did not diminish.

The Year 1986 231
New Head of Roche Pharmaceutical Research 231
Michael Steinmetz, Permanent Member, Leaves for Roche 231
Tumor Necrosis Factor and Cachectin 232
Involvement of BII Members and Former BII Members in the TNF Project 232
Zlatko Dembic to Roche, and Then to Norway 233
Lucia Mori and Her Studies on T Cell Receptors 234

Michael Steinmetz, a permanent member of the BII, accepted an offer from Roche to become head of the Roche Biology Department. This marked an era of closer collaboration with Roche: Jürgen Drews, in his double function as head of Pharma Research and head of Roche Corporate Research, tried to attract BII members to join Roche, but without interfering with BII activities. Werner Haas, John Stocker, Michael Steinmetz and Zlatko Dembic ▶

▶ accepted the call. Theo Staehelin had gone to Roche a decade earlier. BII members became involved in the TNF project. Further, a major event was to open the reconstructed institute to the Basel public. Part of this open day was a theater play performed by the members of the BII: "La Notte della Battaglia". The Chernobyl disaster caused major concern at the institute. An EMBO course on the MHC (with practical laboratory work) was organized, as well as a major workshop on tolerance. Sensitized by the fire (with no casualties), the animal committee considered improvements on the use of animals.

Masayuki Miyasaka and Lymphocyte Circulation 234
After 12 Years in Basel Michael Julius Accepted an Appointment in Montreal 235
Members Move to Sweden, the USA and Japan 235
Festivities on Completion of the BII Restoration 236
BTA 6: "La Notte della Battaglia" 238
Monte Wetzel and the BTA 239
The BTA and Self-Aggrandizement 239
Chernobyl the Same Day 240
Another Fire in the Basel Area 240
Polly, Mel and the Model of "Danger" 241
The Danger Model – A Preview 241
6th International Congress of Immunology in Toronto 242
EMBO Practical Course on Evolution and the MHC 242
EMBO Workshop on Tolerance, the Rules, the Strategies and the Mechanisms 243
Coupling of Synthetic Antigens to Carriers for Antibody Production 245
Animal Committee 245
Seminars by BII Members during the Meetings of the Advisory Board and the Board of Consultants 246
Research Categories in the Annual Report 248
A Nobel Prize for Work on Nerve Growth Factor 248
Paul Sacher Celebrates His 80th Birthday 248

Chris Paige followed a call to Canada. During his 8 years at the BII he decisively shaped the institute. He did so not only with his scientific achievements, but also as a stage director of the "BTA" and as a member of the Rescue Committee after the fire at the BII. In his honor a BTA performance, "Linear-B", was given on the new "Christopher J. Paige Memorial Stage". The institute congratulated Alfred Pletscher on the 10th anniversary of the creation of the "Zentrum für Lehre und Forschung". Another celebrated event was the 20th anniversary of the "Roche Institute of Molecular Biology" in Nutley. The most important event for the institute's reputation in science was the Nobel Prize awarded to Susumu Tonegawa.

The Year 1987 250
Jean-Claude Weill and Claude-Agnès Reynaud, from Paris 250
Chris Paige Leaves for Canada 251
BTA 7: World Premiere of "Linear-B" Performed by the BTA, Dedicated to Chris Paige 252
Hans-Georg Rammensee Leaves for Tübingen and Heidelberg 254
Other Scientists Leave the BII 254
The Roche Institute of Molecular Biology after 20 Years 254
The 10th Anniversary of the Zentrum für Lehre und Forschung 256
The Swiss National Science Foundation and Prof. Alfred Pletscher 257
Additional Services and Facilities due to Retirements 257
What Was Studied in 1987? 257
1987 Nobel Prize for Susumu Tonegawa 258

The start of the year was marked by the preparation of a BTA performance in honor of Susumu Tonegawa with the title "Susumuli, Prince de Bâle". The play was preceded by a conference: "The Genetic Basis of Diversity of Recognition in the Immune System". It was a year when the turnover accelerated and several members who for years had shaped the research direction of the institute left.

The Year 1988 262
Most Cited Swiss Papers, 1973–1988 262
Thirteen Species and More to Come 263
Martin Flajnik Leaves for Miami and Then Baltimore, USA 263
Julia Hurwitz and Chris Coleclough Accepted Positions in Memphis 264
Gordon Keller to Denver, New York and Toronto 265
Olli Lassila to Turku 265

Gerd Pluschke Remained in Basel 265
Ralph Snodgrass to Chapel Hill, North Carolina 266
Gillian Wu Left, but Kept Ties with the BII 266
Dario Grossberger Left the BII, and Soon After Gave Up Science 266
Symposium in Honor of Susumu Tonegawa 267
BTA 8: Performance of "Susumuli, Prince de Bâle" for Susumu Tonegawa 267
Roche Started Cooperating with Amgen and Cetus 269
Ruggero Ceppellini, Ole Maaloe and Bede Morris Died in 1988 269

The Year 1989 270
Immunology Was Changing in Small but Steady Steps 270
α/β as well as γ/δ T Cell Receptor 271
Fourteen Members Left the BII in 1989 271
Chris Coleclough to Memphis 271
Polly Matzinger's New Affiliation at the NIH, Washington 271
Siegfried Weiss to the University of Oslo 271
David Nemazee to Denver and La Jolla 272
Monte Wetzel Leaves for the NIH, to Bayer, to Roche 272
Anna Erdei, Yasushi Uematsu, Andreas Strasser 273
EMBO Workshop on the SCID Mouse 273
Mechanisms of B Cell Neoplasia 274
7th International Congress of Immunology in Berlin 274
Support for the Velvet Revolution in Czechoslovakia 276
BTA 9: "Pollygon", a Goodbye Tribute to Polly Matzinger 276
Maja Sacher Died 277
Nobel Prizes 277

Several (previously neglected) research directions were emphasized, such as complement-related projects. Special aspects of T cell receptor biology (γ/δ) attracted attention. Two workshops, one on "Severe-combined immunodeficient (SCID) mice" and another on "The mechanisms of B cell neoplasia", were held. The 7th International Congress of Immunology took place in Berlin with a large cohort of participants from the BII. The Velvet Revolution started in Czechoslovakia, and it received great support from the BII that was upheld for many years. The BTA performed "Pollygon" as a tribute to Polly Matzinger, who left the BII. Maja Sacher died at the age of 100 years.

The Year 1990 278
Genentech Purchased by Roche 278
Help to Former "Socialist" Countries 278
Ed Palmer Arrives for a Sabbatical 279
Roland Gisler, a Passionate Teacher 279
Lectures for Students from Marburg and Prague 280
ENII Workshop on Retroviruses in Autoimmune Diseases 281
Gennaro De Libero Moved to the ZLF, Basel 281
John Lambris Moved to Philadelphia 282
Paola Panina to Brescia and Then to Milan 282
Luciana Forni, Special Status for a Special Technician 282
Georg Wick Cooperates with the BII 283

The turnover continued – the arrivals and departures were in a harmonious balance. Departing scientists left a mark of their activities, while the newcomers could only show their potential. Roche purchased Genentech, which had just commercialized its first breakthrough product: human insulin produced from bacteria. Interferon-α_2 became thereafter the emblem of Genentech. The ENII workshop on retroviruses in autoimmune disease took place at the BII. Instruments to the value of several millions of Swiss francs were sent to "former socialist countries".

The Year 1991 284
Generation of Antibody Diversity Solved, What Next? 284
T Cell Receptors 284
Immunology Course in Prague 285

Research projects on T cell receptors and on the major histocompatibility complex remained the focus of attention. An immunology course in Prague was organized. The cell ▶

▶ sorter facilities were refurbished and modernized. The opening of the new facilities was celebrated by a BTA performance, "A Musical Portrait of the Institute". Another play, "The Network Killers", on scientific fraud and its consequences was performed by the BTA. A workshop on B cell neoplasia took place in a similar format as in previous years. A symposium to honor the retirement of Andrew Kelus took place in the institute, and the 80th birthday of Niels Jerne was celebrated in Geneva.

Steven Bauer Left the BII to Assume a Leading Position at the FDA in the USA 288

David Gray Leaves for London and Later Moves to Edinburgh 289

Richard Scheuermann to Dallas, Later to San Diego 289

Brigitta Stockinger's Career Took Off in London 289

Reconstruction of the Cell Sorter Facility 289

BTA 10: "A Musical Portrait of the BII" Staged to Celebrate Its 20th Anniversary 290

Surgery, Note by Note: Marin Marais' «Tableau de l'opération de la taille» 291

Symposium for Andrew Kelus 292

BTA 11: Commemorating 20 Years of the BII with the BTA Performance "The Network Killers" – A Theater Performance on Scientific Fraud and Its Consequences 292

Workshop on the Mechanisms of B Cell Neoplasia 293

Niels Jerne's 80th Birthday 294

Roche Acquires a Patent for the Polymerase Chain Reaction Procedure from Cetus 294

700th Anniversary of the Foundation of Switzerland, 1991 295

Several conferences and workshops were organized; among them were "Retroviruses as Antigens and Superantigens in Auto-Immunity and Tolerance" and "EMBO Workshop on Cell-Cell Interactions in Leukocyte Homing and Differentiation". Michael Steinmetz, a former BII permanent member, became head of Roche Research in Nutley, USA. Antonio Lanzavecchia became a new permanent member. The 1st Central European Summer School of Immunology (first of 4 annually) was organized by BII members in Pieštany, Czechoslovakia.

The Year 1992 297

Antonio Lanzavecchia, New Permanent Member 297

Michael Steinmetz, a Former BII Permanent Member, Becomes Head of Roche Research in Nutley, USA 297

Lecture Series for Students from Marburg and Prague 298

The 1st Central European Summer School of Immunology 298

Una Chen to Erlangen and Giessen 299

Retroviruses as Antigens and Superantigens in Autoimmunity and Tolerance 300

EMBO Workshop on Cell-Cell Interactions in Leukocyte Homing and Differentiation 300

8th International Congress of Immunology in Budapest 301

Ed Palmer joined the institute as a permanent member. Another workshop on the Mechanisms of B Cell Neoplasia was held at the BII. An informative booklet (about new members, changes, departures), "BII News", was launched. The 2nd Central European Summer School of Immunology was held in Czechia. "Gwendolyn", a sculpture created by Niki de Saint Phalle, to partner Tinguely's "Double Helix", was inaugurated.

The Year 1993 302

Ed Palmer Joins the Institute as a Permanent Member 302

Matthias Wabl Joins Again 302

BII News Booklet 303

The 2nd Central European Summer School of Immunology 303

Optimistic and Pessimistic Views on the Immune System 304

Trends in 1993 304

Sculpture Created by Niki de Saint Phalle 304

Workshop on the Mechanisms of B Cell Neoplasia 305

Nobel Prize for the Invention of the Polymerase Chain Reaction 305

The Year 1994 307

Some Considerations on MHC and Peptide Binding 307
Danger Model 308
Ivan Lefkovits: 25 Years at the BII 309
The 3rd Central European Summer School of Immunology 309
Workshop on Immunology and Developmental Biology of the Chicken 310
Roche Acquires Syntex 310
Niels K. Jerne Dies on October 7th, 1994 311

A workshop on immunology and developmental biology of the chicken was held at the BII. The 3rd Central European Summer School of Immunology was held in Slovakia. Polly Matzinger formulated the hypothesis for the immune system dubbed "the danger model". Ivan Lefkovits celebrated 25 years at the BII. Niels K. Jerne died on October 7th, 1994.

The Year 1995 312

Perspectives and New Careers 1992–1995 312
Symposium in Memory of Niels Kaj Jerne (1st Anniversary of His Death) 319
EMBO Workshop on Lymphocyte Neoplasia and DNA Rearrangements 321
The 4th Central European Summer School of Immunology 321
The BII Establishes Strict Safety Rules 322
A New Editor of the BII Annual Reports 322
1995 Nobel Prize Awarded to a Student of Walter Gehring, Biozentrum, Basel 323
9th International Congress of Immunology in San Francisco 323
Closing Down the Roche Institute of Molecular Biology, Nutley 323
Georges Köhler Died 325

An EMBO workshop on lymphocyte neoplasia and DNA rearrangements was held at the BII. The 4th Central European Summer School of Immunology was organized by BII members in Prague. The Niels Kaj Jerne Memorial Symposium was held at the Hotel Krafft, Basel (1st anniversary of his death). The closing down of the Roche Institute of Molecular Biology in Nutley was announced. The BII established strict safety rules (not only as a learning process from the devastating fire at the BII 10 years earlier, but preempting strict Swiss regulations). The 9th International Congress of Immunology in San Francisco was attended by a large number of members.

The Year 1996 326

Harald von Boehmer, Permanent Member, Leaves 326
BTA 12: Chamber Performance, "Two Divas", by Louis Du Pasquier and Fiona McConnell 327
Lectures at the BII for Students from the Philipps University Marburg 327
25th Anniversary Celebration of the BII 328
Excerpts of the Presentations Given at the Celebration 329
Seating Plan for the Dinner on the Boat 333
BTA 13: "Close Encounters of the 25th Kind" 334
Former Members Who Settled Permanently in Switzerland 334
Nobel Prize for Two Members of the Advisory Board 335
Information Booklet on the Scientific Aims of the BII – Updated for the Occasion of the 25th Anniversary Celebration 335

Harald von Boehmer gave up his permanent BII membership, accepting a high-flying appointment in Paris (Institut Necker). The BTA prepared the play "Two Divas" to express appreciation of Harald von Boehmer's scientific achievements. The 25th anniversary of the foundation of the BII was celebrated on a cruise on the river Rhine. The festivities concluded with a theater play: "Close Encounters of the 25th Kind". An updated edition of the "Booklet on the BII" was issued on the occasion of the anniversary celebration. The Nobel Prize was awarded to two members of the Advisory Board, Rolf Zinkernagel and Peter Doherty.

The Year 1997 337

Largest Methodology Book in Immunology 337
From T Cell Stimulation to T Cell Behavior 338
EMBO Practical Course on Lymphocyte Development 338
Martin Hicklin, Dr. h.c., Writes for the *Basler Zeitung* 338
Nature Paper by Marina Cella and Antonio Lanzavecchia 339
Retirement Symposium for Charley Steinberg 340
One More Goodbye Dinner for Charley Steinberg 342

Two workshops were organized: "EMBO Course on T Cells" and "From T Cell Stimulation to T Cell Behavior". Academic Press published a 4-volume immunology methods book. A retirement symposium for Charley Steinberg was held in Prague. Martin Hicklin kept the readership of the *Basler Zeitung* informed about scientific discoveries at the BII (his service to the public was later recognized by the University of Basel, which awarded him an honorary doctorate).

A workshop on B cells was held. Marco Colonna's studies on the innate immune system showed a new emphasis of research direction at the BII. Similarly to all previous International Congresses of Immunology, the 10th congress in New Delhi attracted a strong attendance from BII members as speakers and chairpersons.

The Year 1998 343

Marco Colonna's Studies on Innate Immunity 343

Workshop on the Mechanisms of B Cell Neoplasia: Chronic Stimulation of the Immune System 343

10th International Congress of Immunology in New Delhi 344

Andrew Kelus Died 345

A course and a workshop were arranged: an "EMBO Practical Course on Lymphocyte Development" and a "Workshop on Lymphoid Organogenesis". Antonio Lanzavecchia gave up his position as permanent member and moved to Bellinzona. Charley Steinberg, ex-permanent member of the BII, died. Paul Sacher, conductor, music patron and philanthropist, died at the age of 93.

The Year 1999 346

EMBO Practical Course on Lymphocyte Development 346

Workshop on Lymphoid Organogenesis 346

Antonio Lanzavecchia Moves to Bellinzona 347

Paul Sacher and the Fate of the Institute 347

Paul Sacher and the BII Advisory Board 348

Paul Sacher Supports the Unique Research Ambiance of the BII 349

Paul Sacher Died at the Age of 93 349

Charley Steinberg Died at the Age of 67 350

Jean Pieters became the last permanent member of the BII. Roche decided to close down the institute with effect of 2001. Roche intended that the institute would be restructured into a "Roche Center of Medical Genomics". This attempt was abandoned, and what survived was integrated into the Roche Research Group on Genetics.

The Year 2000 351

Perspectives and New Careers 1996–2000 351

Jean Pieters Becomes the Last Permanent Member 358

One Year and Eight Days after Paul Sacher's Death 359

Roche Made a Decision 359

Collection of Letters and E-Mails from the World Scientific Community 360

Reaction of the BII Employees 360

Emergency Meeting of the International Advisory Board 361

Fortune Favors the Prepared Mind 362

Knowledge Gap at Roche 362

Roche Center of Medical Genomics 363

Roche's Image Was Not Affected 363

New Way(s) to Support Research 364

After the Phone Calls, Business as Usual 365

Yin and Yang One Day Later, June 6th 367

A joint symposium for Fritz Melchers and Roland Gisler on the occasion of their retirement was arranged. Jon Sprent gave the last BII seminar on 20th November. The laboratories were closed down one by one, and during the month of December the last members moved their laboratories to their new destinations. Most of the members received financial support. Several early retirements ensued. Nobody became unemployed. The ▶

The Final Year 2001 368

Scientists Leaving and Their Destinations 368

Manfred Kopf 368

Ed Palmer from Basel to Basel 368

Marco Colonna Leaves for St. Louis, Missouri 368

Symposium for Fritz Melchers and Roland Gisler 369

Retirement Dinner, Not a "Last Supper" 370

Nobel Prize for Sir Paul Nurse, Member of the Advisory Board 370

Nobel Prize for Sydney Brenner, Member of the Advisory Board 371

The Seminars Continued 371
The Last BII Seminar 372
Decommissioning Tinguely's Double Helix 373

▶ famous Double Helix that had guarded the entrance to the institute for 30 years was decommissioned and transferred to the Tinguely Museum.

Remembering the Basel Institute for Immunology

Echoes of Time, Tune, Space and Future 375

Echo of Time: Part 1 376
In the Improbable Case that... 376
Incompatibilities 376
Then the Building Became Something Else 376
Affinity, Avidity and Basel 376
Statements of Affection 377
Jerne's Centennial Celebrated in Lisbon, 2011 377

Echo of Time: Part 2 379
Maurice Zauderer and Louis Pasteur 379

Echo of Tune 381
Musicians at the BII 381
A Fancy (by Louis Du Pasquier): The Illuminated Side of the Moon 382
Commemoration of Jerne, 1995 384
Epilogue 384

Echo of Space 385
From a Horizontal Structure to a Vertical Career 385
Academia and Teaching Careers 385
Biotech Companies and Their CEOs 386
Former BII Members with Careers at Roche and Novartis 388

Echo from the Future: Message to Philanthropists 388
Waiting for the End 388
The BII Was Once the Largest Basic Immunology Institute 389
Next-Generation Institute 389
Philanthropists Choose Princeton instead of Manhattan 390
Tinguely's Double Helix Lives on Forever 390

Acknowledgements 391
Subject Index 392

The intention of the following pages is to retrieve some "mosaic stones" from the narration and give them more space. Questions can be asked and maybe answered. Even stories of suspense can be told, as in the case of Maurice Zauderer. And of course one should listen to Louis Du Pasquier, who poetically said that the birth of the BII was placed under the sign of music. The story about Anita and Maurice is one of many others (Graham Mitchell and his Volkswagen, and Polly Matzinger and her motorcycle are included in the QR database). Former members of the BII founded some two dozen biotech companies, some of which could have fitted the Roche portfolio well; whatever the case, Roche can be proud that ex-BII members have been so successful. And finally there is a philosophical note about sponsors and philanthropists, all this fitting under the "Echoes of Time, Tune, Space and Future", and is also offered in the QR database.

The History of Scientific Achievements and of the Social Impact of the Basel Institute for Immunology

As I said, the narrative form is my métier, and it offers me a structure. The story unfolds with a beginning, middle, and an end. As it is so with every story, once the end reveals itself, the beginning and the middle can be understood anew.

James Carroll, *Constantine's Sword*

Preface

QR code stands for Quick Response Code and is an emblem for a type of matrix bar code first designed for the Toyota car industry. The system has become widely used due to its fast readability and large storage capacity compared to standard bar codes. The code consists of pixel dots arranged in a square pattern.

The QR codes should remain compatible with all software innovations expected in the next 10 years. The present server of the University of Basel guarantees the availability of data in the database for that period of time. The actual information in the QR codes (400 characters) will be available far beyond then.

Scientists leave a testimony of their individual achievements in the form of research publications, and these are available for scrutiny for generations to come. There exists, however, another form of testimony, which is to describe the achievements in the wider context of the institutions in which the scientists worked, and the society in which they lived.

The aim of this book is to do exactly that – to describe a scientist's life, work, successes and failures – all that is needed to provide a comprehensive picture of modern science. No history book is definitive; nevertheless, this book will have all the features of a classic printed book "zwischen zwei Buchdeckeln". And it will have an additional feature which provides contextual information in the form of an electronic glossary.

The reader will be faced with QR codes in the margins of the book. Although these iconic images are now commonplace in print media, they possess an additional function here: a platform from which to step onto the ferryboat sailing along the river Styx to the underworld of many gigabytes of information.

From the initial reactions of colleagues, it became obvious that the older generation is not overly interested in these "additional features", they just want a plain book. The young generation – well let's wait and see.

Indeed, this history can be read and used just as any other book, and the QR codes considered no more than a medieval type of illustration in the margins. Nevertheless, those who decide to float on the Styx to enter the underworld will be rewarded. Many gigabytes of information on the Basel Institute, on Switzerland, on former members (scientists, technicians), etc., will be accessible.

As the Basel Institute was based on a horizontal structure, an effort was made to redefine the meaning of "elite" science. The history of science shows that neither an individual list of publications nor the entirety of PubMed mirrors the scientific achievements within a given field. However, a broadly conceived database – practically limitless in the amount of information it stores – can do it.

The reader, depending on circumstances and personal preferences, might decide to read the book as an unbroken narrative, without distraction, from the start of the institute to its end and beyond...

Science and life are intertwined, experiments and parties are intermixed, and reports on conferences and celebrations of anniversaries are interwoven. The reader interested in science might wish to skip the more humorous and frivolous pieces, and concentrate on the descriptions of research: the distinctive layout of these paragraphs will enable him to jump from section to section. The Basel Theater of Arts, anniversary celebrations, etc., will be distinctly marked.

Instead of describing the achievements of a few famous scientists, the book elevates to fame several hundred BII employees and friends of the BII.

The Storyteller's Dilemma

Can science be described in a manner understandable to a layman? Should a book on the history of a scientific institution be written such that everyone understands it? Obviously, it depends on the mission of the book. Was it assembled in order to reveal something about the life of an institute, or rather to describe the scientific achievements of the organization?

A history book that is concerned only with day-to-day events might fall into the category of *chronicles*, but such a treatise misses the main component, the science. Life and science at the Basel Institute for Immunology have been so intertwined that it is inconceivable not to follow both threads.

Is it possible to combine both aspects in an understandable way? Is the understandability of a book an issue? Paraphrasing Søren Kierkegaard, if you write a book that is lively and comprehensive, but misses science, you will regret it. If you write only about scientific achievements and exclude the pulse of life of the institute, you will regret it also. In Kierkegaard's words the issue is this: *"I see it all perfectly; there are two possible situations – one can either do this or that. My honest opinion and my friendly advice is this: do it or do not do it – you will regret both."*

For cognoscenti, the reason why I am quoting Kierkegaard will ring a bell, while for those who do not know, at least here is a hint: Kierkegaard was a Danish philosopher, and he was admired by the main protagonist of this book, Niels Kaj Jerne.

The storyteller might in Kierkegaardian terms regret it, but in any case he tries to perform a balancing act between the scientific and the social life. The heading *The Storyteller's Dilemma* only indirectly refers to Bernard Shaw's *The Doctor's Dilemma*. Rather it is taken from the dispute between Margaret Mead (M.M.) and Niels Kaj Jerne (N.K.J.), when M.M. says that scientists are not willing to speak in an understandable way, and N.K.J. replies that social scientists are not willing to make the effort to learn even the simplest forms of scientific communications.

Since the time of the dispute between M.M. and N.K.J., the level of communication has not changed very much. To ease the situation, this work helps – with a small trick – to keep the reader's interest alive: the "difficult stuff" is displayed in a different, two-column, layout. Depending on the reader's predilections and mood, it is thus easy to take in or skip portions of the story.

A history book such as this – covering a period of more than three decades – is certain to have omissions. However, the database provides a wealth of additional material and will continue to do so for years to come. Members and friends of the BII are invited to contribute: just enter the database through a QR code and follow the instruction for depositing documents, photographs, protocols – anything that should be preserved as part of the BII heritage.

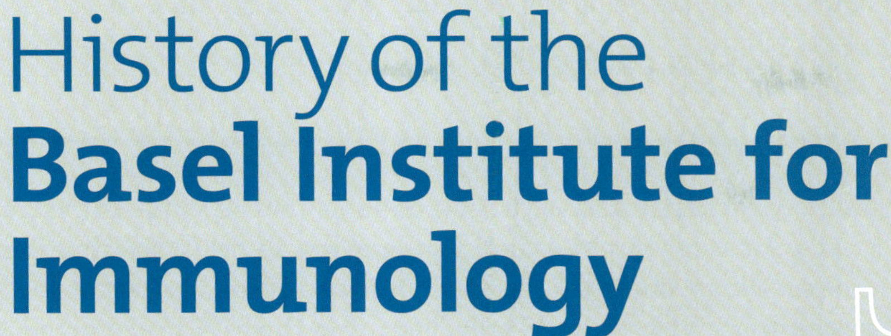

History of the **Basel Institute for Immunology**

BII

Book 1

1969–1985

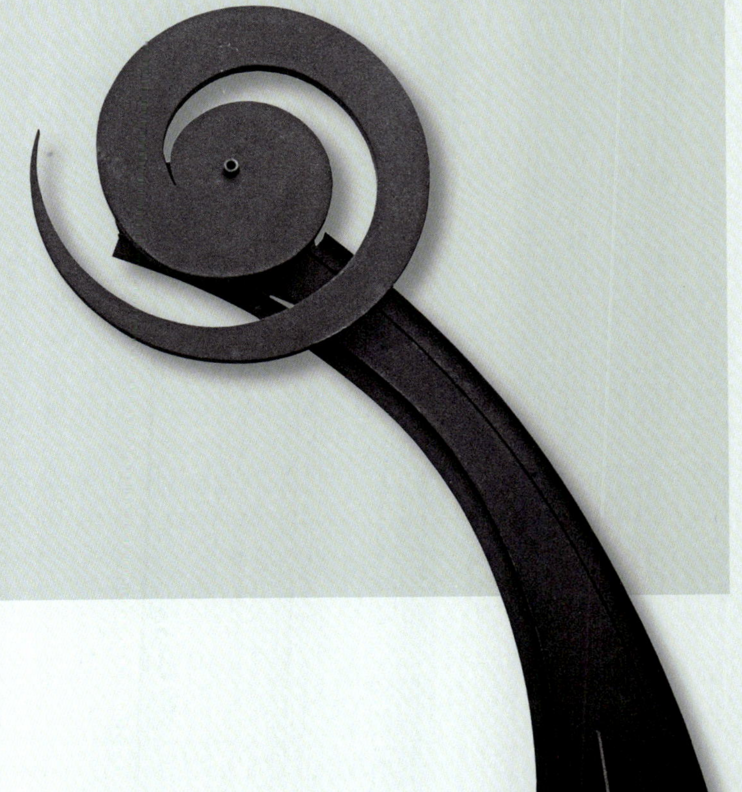

Recounting the Years 1968–1969

Adolf Jann discussed with Alfred Pletscher the long-term strategies for pharmaceutical research. A decision was made to establish a Basel Institute for Immunology. Niels K. Jerne was chosen as director. Jerne and Jann sealed the agreement with a handshake. Planning the building started, and floor plans were drawn up. On April 29th, 1968, the foundation stone was laid. In Rheinfelden a meeting with founding members was organized. Jerne left for a recruitment round-the-world journey. Upon his return, a second meeting of the starting group was held.

A New Institute

During the course of the 20th century Switzerland became very successful, both economically and culturally. Small and without natural resources, it succeeded in building up a strong industry, powerful banking and excellent services. With luck and determination it kept out of two devastating world wars and became an attractive place to live and work in, both for its own nationals and for visitors. Menial jobs were mainly done by "guest workers" and specialist jobs by "expats": Switzerland had become an increasingly desirable workplace for scientists from all over the world.

The pharmaceutical industry flourished, the banks were still considered to be respectable institutions, and the chocolate was delicious, although women still did not have the right to vote. The darkest moments of World War II were not discussed, and Paul Grüninger had not yet been rehabilitated.

The stage was set for promising things. The pressure of globalization was not yet apparent, and companies did not have to worry about results of the next quarter. The opinion leaders in industry and commerce could look ahead with farsightedness and confidence. The elite acknowledged that the only meaningful compensation for the lack of natural resources was the cultivation of human assets.

In January 1968 Adolf Jann [QR1969_01], president of the Basel pharmaceutical firm Hoffmann-La Roche, and its director general for research, Alfred Pletscher, discussed long-term strategies for pharmaceutical research and development.

Alfred Pletscher [QR1969_02] was at the peak of his successful career, both as head of research in Roche and as an opinion leader of the Swiss scientific establishment. He was aware of the fact that Roche, along with the three other major pharmaceutical companies in Basel – Ciba, Geigy and Sandoz [QR1969_03] – absorbed a large number of university graduates. And he knew that increasing numbers of them would be needed in future. Pletscher was convinced that just giving money to universities would not suffice, and the ground should be prepared to attain new knowledge through founding and financing new basic research institutes, which in turn would give rise to innovations for the benefit of society as a whole. Pletscher even went a step further and emphasized to Jann that the company's unique position in biological research carried with it the obligation to foster ground-breaking developments through such new initiatives. Jann, the most powerful man in the pharmaceutical arena, agreed with Pletscher's vision and gave the green light to start a new endeavor.

QR1969_02 BII

The headquarters of Roche were in Basel, but the company also had a strong standing in Nutley, N.J., USA. Similar discussions about the need for establishing basic research institutes were taking place in Nutley. The proponent of the idea in the USA was the President of Roche Nutley, Virginius D. Mattia [QR1969_04]. At a General Assembly meeting in 1966, V.D. Mattia (Nutley) and P.A. Plattner (Basel) presented the idea of initiating basic research institutes and providing them with full academic freedom to carry out research without the restraints of commercial success. Mattia's lecture was truly visionary. Nutley started off on its own path of setting up institutes, and there are many parallels as well as many differences between the procedures in Basel and Nutley. The path taken in Nutley is described in a later section of this book (chapter for 1987) when referring to the celebration of the 20th anniversary of the Roche Institute of Molecular Biology.

QR1969_03 BII

QR1969_04 BII

At the other two Basel pharmaceutical companies, J.R. Geigy AG and Ciba AG, similar ideas concerning the need to establish basic research institutes surfaced, with the result that the two companies made a joint decision to establish an institute to "pursue and promote basic research in the fields of biochemistry and medicine…". The new institute was named after the Basel scientist Friedrich Miescher (1844–1895) who first purified nucleic acids [QR1969_05].

QR1969_05 BII

Alfred Pletscher had a free hand to move ahead with the plan and to choose the research topics, but he hesitated over the definite choice. Johann-Rudolf Frey [QR1969_06], a dermatologist by

QR1969_06 BII

profession, who had worked at Roche for many years, suggested that immunology be chosen. Frey's opinion mattered not only because of his scientific standing, but also because he was a member of the Roche family. Pletscher agreed, and the dice started to roll.

Finding a Director

QR1969_07 BII

QR1969_08 BII

Alfred Pletscher had profound experience initiating and completing important projects, both within the Roche company and also on the nation-wide scale of Switzerland [QR1969_07]. He knew that finding a suitable person, competent at implementing a new project, was of primary importance. Several names were discussed, among others Hans Müller-Eberhard – a specialist in the field of complement. Frey suggested that Henri Isliker [QR1969_08], director of the Swiss Cancer Institute in Lausanne, should advise on the choice of director from the narrow selection of key persons. Pletscher agreed, and from the preliminary candidates that Isliker suggested, Niels Kaj Jerne turned out to be the most promising one. Accordingly, Pletscher requested Isliker to call Jerne and initiate preliminaries.

QR1969_09 BII

As Niels Jerne [QR1969_09] is the key figure in this book, many particulars will be mentioned later in the narrative. Here it suffices to say that Jerne was at that time a very well-known and highly respected immunologist, and current director of the Paul Ehrlich Institute in Frankfurt.

QR1969_10 BII

QR1969_11 BII

Henri Isliker knew Niels Jerne very well. They met in the early sixties on several occasions in Geneva at the WHO headquarters where Jerne held a top position. They became friends. The initial contact with Isliker was arranged through Eduard Kellenberger [QR1969_10], professor at the University of Geneva. Kellenberger and Jerne shared mutual interests in science (genetics of bacteriophages), and they had many friends in common (among others, Max Delbrück [QR1969_11] from Pasadena, Calif., USA). Isliker felt honored to contact Jerne, especially because he was encouraged to do so by Kellenberger, who enthusiastically endorsed Jerne's nomination. Kellenberger was an important reference point for Pletscher, for reasons which will be mentioned later on in this volume.

QR1969_12 BII

Isliker placed the call to Frankfurt in February 1968 and was fully confident of succeeding as he sensed that Jerne did not consider his current directorship of the Paul Ehrlich Institute [QR1969_12] to be the end point of his career. Furthermore, Isliker was aware that for Jerne – due to his earlier affiliation with the WHO in Geneva – Switzerland was not a *terra incognita*, and that

Also heute vor 16 Jahren bekam ich einen Anruf von meinem Freund Henry Isliker, professor in Lausanne, der mich fragte ob es mich interessieren würde in Basel ein Institut für Immunologie ~~auf~~ zu errichten und zu leiten. Hoffmann-La Roche hätte sich entschieden ein solches Institut ~~zu erstellen um~~ für Grundlagenforschung zu erstellen und zu finanzieren. Professor Pletscher hatte ihm gebeten einige Personen zu nennen die für diese Aufgabe in Frage kämen.

Years later Jerne remembers the events (translation is provided in the previous QR code)

he would enjoy living in Basel. Jerne listened carefully to Isliker's proposal, but hesitated. Indeed, he was not entirely happy at the Paul Ehrlich Institute as he realized that the research form there needed an overhaul, but the departmental structures of the once-famous institute were too rigid for a smooth and painless restructuring. Most of the research workers were very willing to adjust to potential new tasks, provided that the duties were clearly defined, with exact instructions given by the director. They hoped for a revival of the Paul Ehrlich ambiance, while Niels Jerne wanted to instigate a more modern approach to research, which he had experienced when working in the USA. Although he had his own small group at the Paul Ehrlich Institute (to be dealt with below), he had no influence on the structure and the spirit of the institute as a whole.

Jerne was very open with Isliker: he would consider a new challenge but he could not afford to make a mistake. The next step in his career must be the final one. Despite the fact that Isliker made clear-cut "promises", Jerne was worried that an institute financed by industry would not give him the freedom to develop research along the lines that he wanted. Isliker asked Jerne to meet Pletscher and Jann in Basel.

In April 1968 Jerne took the Intercity train to Basel, where he checked into the Hotel Euler and was welcomed by Alfred Pletscher. They were driven to the Roche headquarters in the Grenzacherstrasse and greeted by its president, Adolf Jann.

Jann explained his vision of establishing and funding an institute working in full academic freedom. A potential "side effect" for the sponsor would be a benefit from any scientific breakthrough achieved in the institute (the rights derived from such develop-

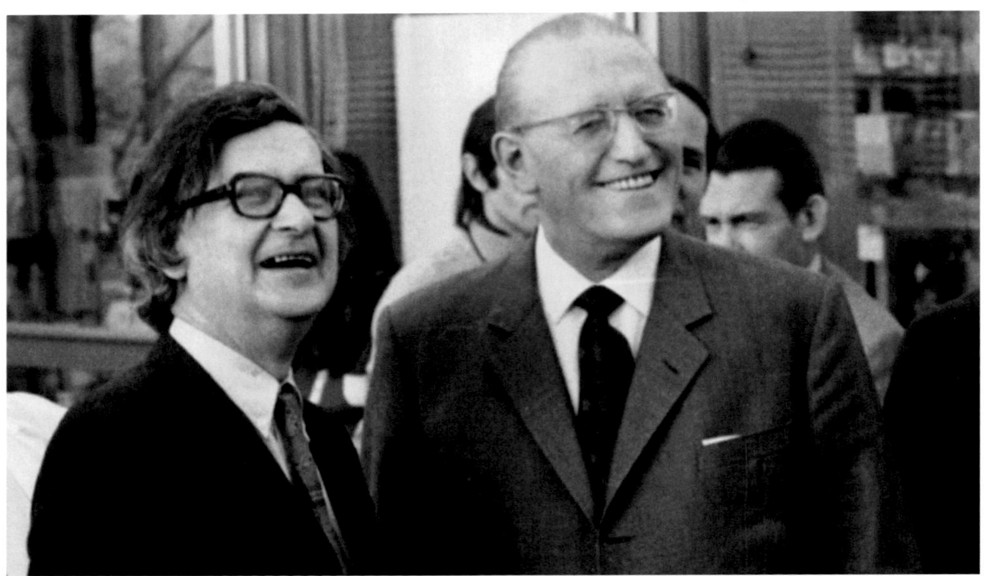

Niels Jerne and
Adolf Jann

... his [Jerne's] seminal paper on the natural selection of antibody formation had brought him worldwide prominence, fame and recognition.

ments would of course belong to the sponsoring company). Jerne presented a list of queries, which were all answered to his satisfaction, and so he realized that the proposition might work. Roche had only one single restraint, which concerned the site and size of the institute, and this was because the location for the institute had already been designated. Jerne and Pletscher were taken to inspect the site – about 1.5 km upstream the river Rhine – and Jerne liked it!

Back in Frankfurt Jerne received plans and sketches, and a few weeks later (August 15th, 1968) on a second visit to Basel, Jerne and Jann sealed the agreement with a handshake. There was no written contract between these two gentlemen. The word "gentleman" is used here to emphasize how things were done then, and Jann never broke any of his promises.

It did not take long before the Ministry of Health of the Land Hessen discovered Jerne's plans. The Hessen authorities made every effort to persuade Jerne not to leave Frankfurt. It was in Jerne's nature to conduct open and frank negotiations; thus, he explained that the offer to run a brand-new institute, built exactly to his specifications, was irresistible, and his decision to move to Basel was irrevocable. Within weeks the Ministry came up with a counterproposal that they would build a new Paul Ehrlich Institute for Jerne, if he would stay. They could start planning it immediately and in 6 years the institute would be ready. Jerne did not change his mind.

Searching for Scientists

Niels Jerne started to plan the future: he contacted Ben Pernis of Milan, Klaus Rajewsky of Cologne and Göran Möller of Stockholm and explained his plans [QR1969_13]. All three were enthusiastic: Ben spontaneously saying that Niels could count on him to join the institute; Klaus was more reserved, as he would not leave Cologne because he had good working conditions, and his family was anchored there – but in one way or another he wished to be affiliated to the new institute; Göran said bluntly that he and his wife Erna would come, but only to "warm up" the place, as they would not leave Stockholm for good.

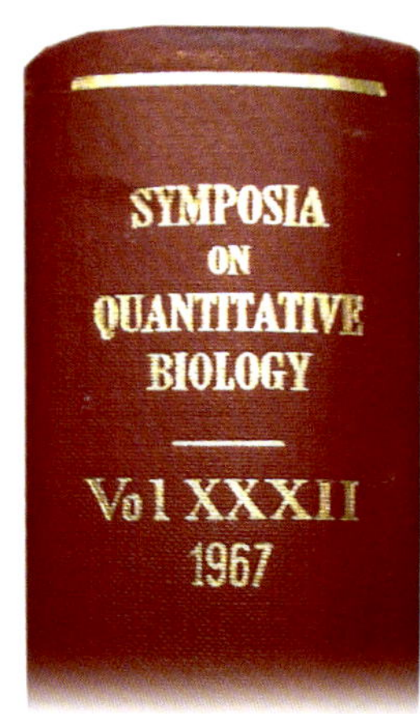

Niels Jerne was exceptionally well "connected" in the world of immunology. This was the case not only because of his previous work at the WHO (a crossroads for immunology and vaccination programs), but also through his contacts in Copenhagen, Pasadena and Pittsburgh. More than that, though, his seminal paper on the natural selection of antibody formation had brought him worldwide prominence, fame and recognition.

The annual Cold Spring Harbor Symposia [QR1969_14] have always attracted the most important scientists working in any given research field, with topics such as Human Genetics (1964), Sensory Receptors (1965), the Genetic Code (1966) and Antibodies (1967). The conference *Introductions* and the *Summaries* were always delivered by the most prominent representatives in the field. In 1967, Sir MacFarlane Burnet gave the *Introduction*, while Niels Jerne presented the *Summary*.

Thus, everybody knew Jerne, and Jerne knew everybody whose work was ground breaking. Incidentally, in 1955 Burnet was the first person to recognize the significance of Jerne's natural selection theory. Two years later in 1957, Burnet published a paper with the title *A Modification of Jerne's Theory of Antibody Production Using the Concept of Clonal Selection*.

QR1969_13 BII

Jerne made a list of people whom he intended to contact to enquire whether they would be willing to join the new institute. The list was a collage of names, grouped according to fields of interest. The "transient" nature of the list will be mentioned in more detail below. Here it suffices to say that for him the selection of people had the highest priority. In his hand was a list of names created only a few months earlier. It was the list of participants at an EMBO course held in the Paul Ehrlich Institute in November 1967, which he and Claudia Henry had organized [QR1969_15]. The European Molecular Biology Organization (with the acronym EMBO) was created in 1964 with headquarters in Heidelberg, and

QR1969_14 BII

QR1969_15 BII

it became a "quality stamp" for every major course in Europe [QR1969_16]. The course in Frankfurt was the first immunology course in Europe to teach the methodology for detecting single antibody-forming cells by the so-called plaque method and to demonstrate the induction of antibody formation in spleen cells in vitro. At this EMBO course, modern cellular immunology received a fitting international platform.

The course brought together instructors and students with a mix of age and experience. This was to Jerne's liking and had an impact on his perception of how interactions between scientists best work. He informed the former course teachers and students about the new institute and waited for an echo.

Planning the Building

Roche's architect, Mr. Altenbach, was given the responsibility for the new project: number 75 in the Roche building chronology (Building 75). Altenbach had already sent Jerne a preliminary drawing of the building and a floor plan, but Jerne requested two "competing" proposals in order to have something to compare and choose from. Although Roche thought that this was not the most efficient way to proceed, the architects obliged and produced proposals "a & b". So Jerne had two plans at hand that were not only useful when he was talking to friends and colleagues, but also helpful to create from two competing proposals a new design of the building, a kind of "c" alternative, which he considered to be optimal for realizing his vision of the institute.

The above-mentioned "competing" proposals were in fact of more intricate nature, since a Spanish architect (friend of Niels from his Geneva time) was happy to give Niels advice, but only if he submitted *several* proposals for scrutiny. The drawings made by the Roche architects arrived in Frankfurt, were unpacked by Ivan Lefkovits, spread on Niels' desk and then discussed with the said architect in Geneva.

The exchange of letters and documents between Basel and Frankfurt became more frequent, and Jerne realized that he could not deal with all the issues himself, especially as he wished to concentrate on recruiting scientific staff. And of course he still had directorial duties at the Paul Ehrlich Institute. He thus decided to delegate work relating to the actual building of the new institute, including interactions with architects and preparing the day when the *foundation stone would be laid*. In September 1968 he asked Ivan Lefkovits to take on this work; this was just 1 month after

QR1969_16 BII

Ivan's country of origin, Czechoslovakia, had been occupied by the Soviet army.

Ivan Lefkovits, along with Hiroshi Fuji and Claudia Henry, was one of the few foreigners working at the Paul Ehrlich Institute [QR1969_17]. These three scientists formed the core of Jerne's research program. For a while Lefkovits had headed Jerne's research group in Frankfurt. Fuji – with more scientific experience than Lefkovits – could not take on any leading position at the Paul Ehrlich Institute as this required proficiency in the German language, and Henry was about to leave and settle in San Francisco.

With the termination of Jerne's directorship in Frankfurt, his group was to be dismantled; thus, Lefkovits, who had no roots in Frankfurt, greatly welcomed Jerne's offer, although he fully realized that his lack of experience would make the assigned "new job" a demanding challenge. Jerne told him: "Ivan, you will make mistakes, that is unavoidable", and he added, "if I were in charge, I would make mistakes as well, perhaps different ones from yours, but still mistakes." And he concluded: "Therefore, whatever mistakes you make, I will consider as if I had made them." This gave Lefkovits the right dose of self-confidence to take up the challenge. He traveled to Basel on October 17th, 1968, and met Alfred Pletscher for the first time. He was introduced to Mr. Altenbach, and a schedule for fortnightly meetings with the team of architects was drawn up [QR1969_18]. Twelve to 15 people from various construction companies participated in these regular "Besprechungen" (8 companies were involved: Preiswerk, Selmoni, Lüftungs AG, Bogenschütz, Rosenmund, Stöcklin, WIVO and Kullmann). Although the meetings were held in "high German", some participants slipped every now and then into the colloquial "Swiss German". After the first meeting, Lefkovits returned to Frankfurt with a list of questions to discuss with Jerne.

QR1969_17 BII

On October 25th Jerne received a parcel from Basel with several drafts of *stationery* proposed for the new institute. These suggestions took Jerne by surprise, as the name of the institute on the stationery was "Roche Institute for Immunology", alongside the nicely placed Roche logo, the famous hexagon [QR1969_19]. Jerne was loyal to Roche, but in earlier discussions with Pletscher he had pointed out that having "Roche" in the name of the institute (and also the hexagon) indicated "applied research", arguing that it would make it far more difficult to recruit the particular scientists he wished to have. The issue was quickly resolved without further discussion, and the next draft, which Jerne approved on November 2nd, bore the name *Basel Institute for Immunology*, afterwards re-

QR1969_18 BII

QR1969_19 BII

The foundation stone was laid on April 12th, 1969, at a small ceremony (in Swiss German) and without much ado.

ferred to as the BII. Of course Jerne was aware that it was mainly European scientists who preferred a clear separation of "industry" and "academia", the Americans cared much less.

The new year, 1969, commenced, and the date for Lefkovits to assume his appointment in Basel drew closer. Before that, 3 major "extended" meetings with the architects in Basel took place, with Niels Jerne, Andrew Kelus, Ivan Lefkovits, Ben Pernis and Klaus Rajewsky participating. They were held on January 8th, January 27th to 29th and March 4th. On each occasion the group convened in the beautiful Hotel Euler in Basel [QR1969_20], from where they were taken to various sites, including an important visit to a specially set up exhibition of WIVO laboratory furniture that was subsequently chosen for the BII. There was one meeting with the architects at which the entire founding group had the chance to have a discussion with the people responsible for the construction of the BII. At the final meeting, there was a round-table discussion with scientists from the department Roche VI/Med. In addition, the Roche research department organized talks explaining their research aims so the two groups could get mutually acquainted and the ice between Roche researchers and BII members would be broken.

Floor Plans

Ivan Lefkovits started his assignment in Basel on April 1st, 1969. He established a "temporary laboratory of BII" [QR1969_21] on the Roche premises (in Building 7, which no longer exists), where he could continue to develop the microculture system he had started in Frankfurt 2 years earlier. His intention was to establish a method for estimating the frequency of antigen-specific precursor cells involved in the immune response.

QR1969_20 BII

QR1969_21 BII

QR1969_22 BII

Nearby, a laboratory was given to another new member, Andrew Kelus [QR1969_22], whose responsibility was to prepare everything needed to set up an animal breeding unit. Kelus also took up his appointment in Basel on April 1st, 1969. On that day Kelus and Lefkovits went out for lunch – where else than to the Euler? – and started a tradition of an annual "April 1st lunch" which continued for decades to come. Kelus' research specialty was the immunology of rabbits. From Birmingham he brought with him several breeding pairs of precious rabbits with defined allotypic and idiotypic markers of antibodies. Also in Building 7 was Dr. Johann-Rudolf Frey, the first person Pletscher had asked for advice about choosing a field of research for the planned institute. Frey

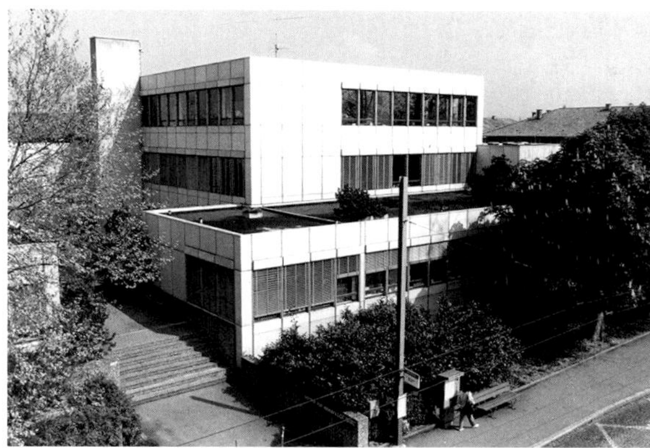

The BII building after completion

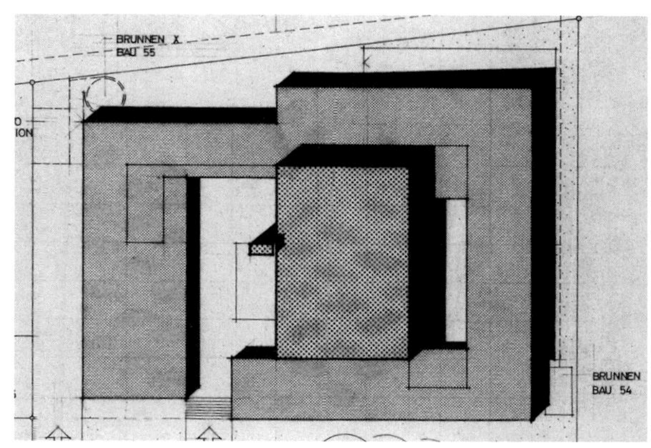

Situation plan

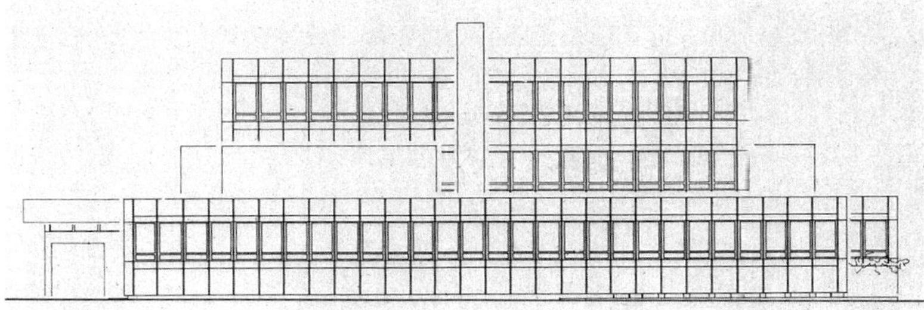

Front view

had suggested immunology and convinced Pletscher that new fundamental discoveries in this field might open new outlooks in Roche's own research and lead to the development of novel therapeutic and diagnostic approaches.

The foundation stone was laid on April 12th, 1969, at a small ceremony (in Swiss German) and without much ado.

Meetings with the architects became more frequent, and Mr. Altenbach and Mr. Wicki, an architect from the Preiswerk company, were Lefkovits' closest contacts with regard to the construction. At every meeting questions arose, and answers were expected by the next session. For a while Lefkovits and Jerne had weekly long-distance phone conferences (Basel – Frankfurt), but these ceased because Jerne really preferred *not* to be asked. His most urgent priority was a "round-the-world" journey with the purpose of meeting people whom he wished to recruit.

The floor plans had to be finalized by the end of April 1969 – this was the condition of the architects if the deadline for completion of the construction work was to be kept. Everything concern-

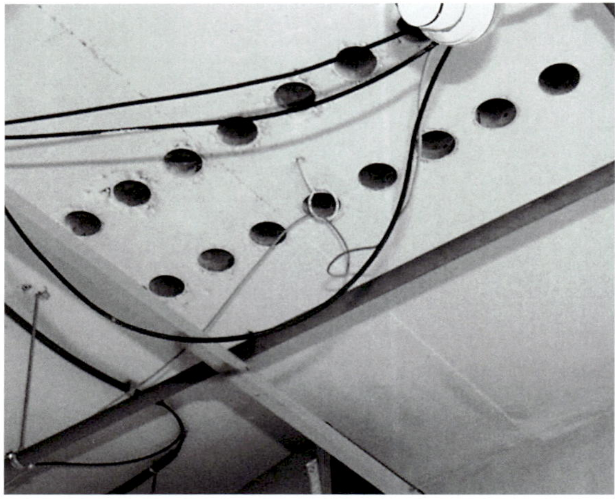

Openings through ceilings for water and gas pipes, as well as cables

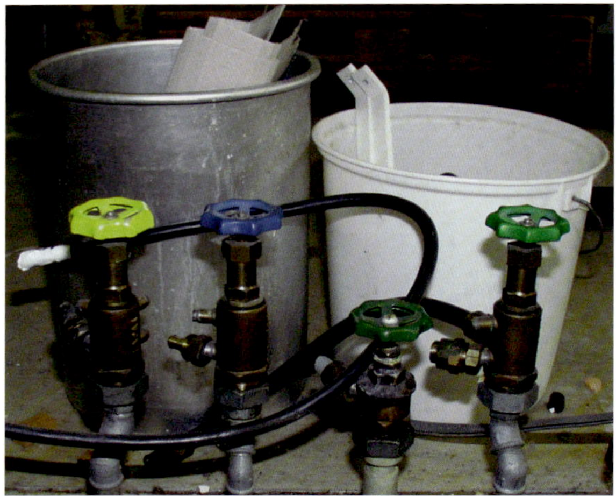

Pipes for cold, warm and deionized water

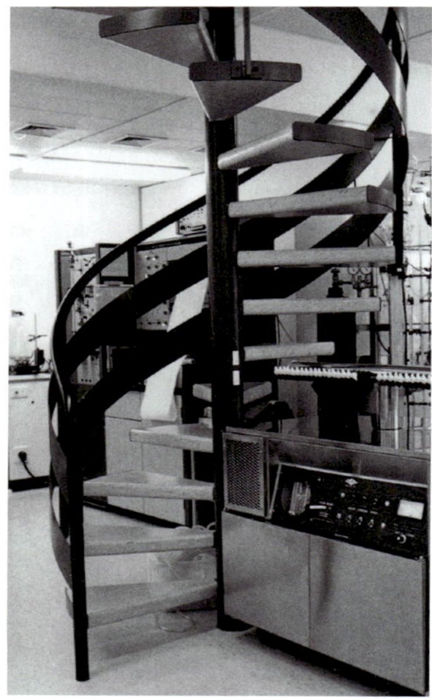

Spiral staircase connecting laboratories on two levels

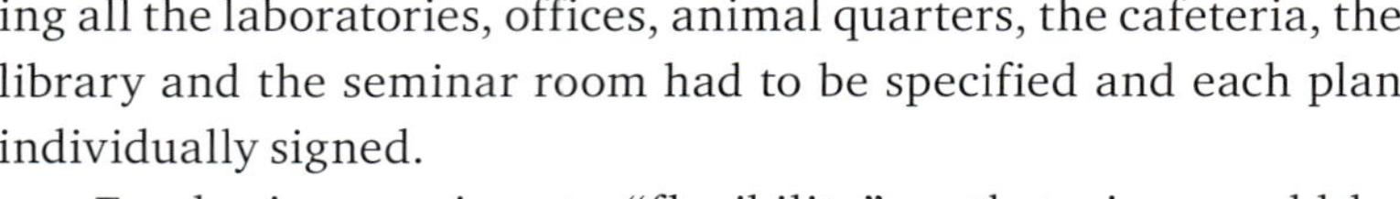

ing all the laboratories, offices, animal quarters, the cafeteria, the library and the seminar room had to be specified and each plan individually signed.

Emphasis was given to "flexibility" so that pipes could be moved and repositioned as the needs of the laboratories changed. This turned out to be very useful in the years to come.

Once it was clear that the lab space would be on 2 main floor levels, and the offices confined to 2 tower levels, Jerne decided connecting the labs of the upper and lower levels with spiral staircases [QR1969_23]. With some hesitation the architects accepted Jerne's request. He explained that wherever he had worked, he had experienced what he termed a "floor syndrome". In Pittsburgh he had worked on the sixth floor and realized that he rarely met people from the fifth or seventh floors. With spiral staircases he wanted to encourage openness and mutual interaction between the members of staff. He wanted the "upper" and the "lower" labs to share instruments and equipment (e.g. ultracentrifuges, incubators). He wanted people to bump into each other!

Finally, Jerne wanted the staff to be lured into an attractive, very central place within the institute. "This place", he said, "shall be the cafeteria in the center of the main floor. Nobody should have to walk more than 30 seconds from lab to cafeteria (or from office to cafeteria). The cafeteria will guard against self-interest and claustrophobia. Directly above the cafeteria we shall position the main seminar room." The offices in the tower were meant for scientists writing manuscripts and for a couple of members who did not intend to do experimental work. But even they would be

QR1969_23 BII

in the immediate vicinity of the cafeteria. Jerne's idea of creating a floor with offices was based on the model of the Institute of Advanced Studies in Princeton, USA.

The architects and the subcontractors required specific and detailed information on everything. How many heavy instruments (e.g. ultracentrifuges) will be in a particular lab? How much heat will they produce? Will work be done standing or sitting at the benches, how many of each was needed in each lab? How high should the benches be? How many electric sockets should there be? How many for 380 V and how many for 220 V? Where should the sinks be located? What about the supply of warm and cold water? Will deionized water be needed?

At each meeting with the architects a new set of floor plans (and later plans of individual laboratories) were handed over to Lefkovits, showing innumerable technical details (in different color coding for electricity, water, air conditioning). Lefkovits had to approve and sign each plan. In several instances he signed without being quite sure of the full implications of the decisions. Areas for sterile tissue culture work and for molecular biology, as well as areas safe for the use of elevated amounts of radioactive isotopes had to be marked – again with additional color coding.

Jerne did not interfere with any of the technical issues. His only categorical decisions were: all walls, benches and cupboards were to be white. The offices should look like laboratories: no teak, no extravagancies, just plain and frugal in appearance. The floors should be made of gray linoleum. And the doors should have the color and texture on which one could write with chalk.

The Rheinfelden Meetings

Eventually Niels Jerne stepped down from his position at the Paul Ehrlich Institute, and Prof. Günther Heymann took over the directorship in Frankfurt. Assuming that the construction arrangements in Basel were "in good hands", Jerne finalized his plans for the round-the-world journey to meet potential candidates for positions at the BII. Mrs. Pfenninger (secretary to Prof. Pletscher) prepared the travel itinerary, as she handled the administrative work until a permanent secretary was hired. But before leaving, Jerne still wanted to meet the mini-nucleus of the BII. Since the last meeting (March 4th, 1969), 3 months had passed, a period during which the construction had greatly advanced. The meeting was set for May 28th to 29th, and it was to be held in Rheinfelden (some 20 km from Basel, upstream the river Rhine). The participants

As Socrates pointed out, the essential difficulty of scientific research is that you are searching for the unknown or, in other words, that you do not know what you are searching for.

were: Brigitte (Ita) Askonas, Ruggero Ceppellini, Louis Du Pasquier, Hans Halbach, Niels Jerne, Andrew Kelus, Ivan Lefkovits, Fritz Melchers, Ben Pernis and Klaus Rajewsky.

The venue of the Rheinfelden meeting was the Hotel Schiff [QR1969_24]. Jerne set an agenda consisting of 3 issues: concept of the institute, construction of the building and scientific projects. Jerne welcomed the participants, some of them present for the first time (Brigitte Askonas from London, Fritz Melchers from Berlin and the USA, Louis Du Pasquier from Bordeaux and, as a non-scientific staff participant, Hans Halbach from Geneva). Jerne wanted to convey the idea that the problem of "specificity" was the most important issue in immunology, and that it was an issue that could be approached and solved. Of the numerous important themes, *antibody specificity and its origin* would be the best unifying leitmotif for the institute. If a scientist wished to study the biology of macrophages, monocytes or the biology of the complement system, the question should be asked if acquiring this particular knowledge would advance the understanding of the specificity of the immune system.

Of the numerous important themes, *antibody specificity and its origin* would be the best unifying leitmotif for the institute.

Jerne proposed that the research at the BII should include several animal models: mice, rats, rabbits, chickens, frogs and perhaps sheep. He did not mention guinea pigs, and he was very reserved about human models. The argument for choosing these animal species became a recurring one. Andrew Kelus explained how animal breeding stations for rabbits are established, and reported on the facilities for mice at Roche and those planned for the new institute. Lefkovits reported on his interactions with the ar-

QR1969_24 BII

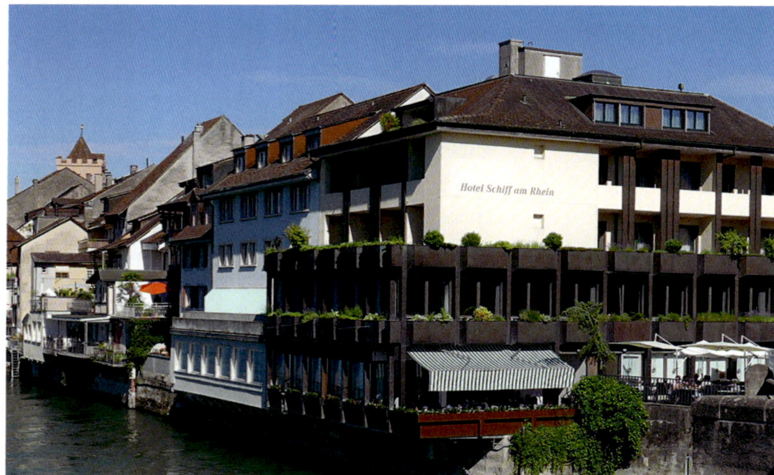

Hotel Schiff, Rheinfelden: venue of a BII planning meeting

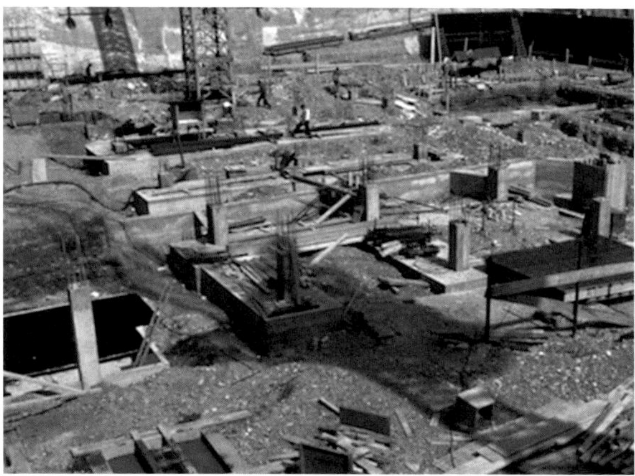

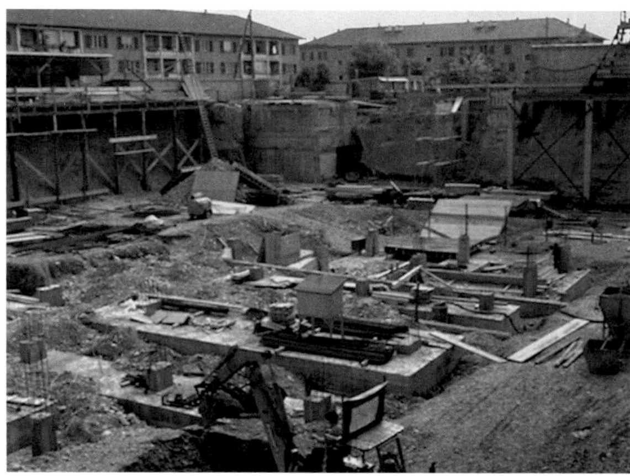

Views of the early stages of construction

chitects, emphasizing that the schedule for completing construction by October 1st, 1970, would be upheld. He distributed questionnaires related to the building and equipment (to be collected the next day) and explained "what is where" in the building under construction.

The meeting was well in progress when the last participant, Ruggero Ceppellini, arrived. He had come from Italy by train and was perplexed that the train had passed through Rheinfelden without stopping. From the main railway station in Basel he returned to Rheinfelden on a slow train. There he asked the first person he met how to get to the Hotel Schiff. The man, identifying Ceppellini's Italian accent, asked him, "lei cerca lavoro?" (Are you looking for a job?). Ceppellini truthfully admitted that this was the case. To which the Italian said, "Albergo Schiff cerca un capo cuoco" (Hotel Schiff is looking for a chef).

The participants briefly described their interests, especially in view of what Jerne had outlined at the onset of the meeting. Of course emphasis was placed on what research they wanted to do in the institute. The meeting was suspended for a few hours in order to visit the construction site, after which it continued back in Rheinfelden.

The following day, when the meeting was over and the participants had left, Jerne asked Lefkovits and Kelus how they perceived the meeting. It was not only a rhetorical question, as Niels indicated that there was something bothering him. He was puzzled that most of the participants mentioned whom they were going to include in their group instead of talking about their own experiments. And Jerne continued: "My original idea of 12 groups with 12 group leaders is wrong; if I go along this path, my influ-

First-class scientists attract first-class scientists; second-class scientists attract third-class scientists.

Jerne's creed

ence in running the institute will be limited to the choices of the 12 group leaders." And he continued: "Everyone at the meeting stressed how good are those young colleagues whom they want to bring to the institute; then it dawned on me that we would rather need more of those young people than their bosses." This statement turned out to be the birth of the idea to establish a horizontal structure.

Jerne carried on: "The institute will consist of 50 scientists, all having equal status as 'members'. Of course we shall have a handful of permanent members, but this will be to ensure continuity. And as we will have a large majority of members staying for a period of 2–3 years, the turnover will ensure the adaptability of the entire institute to keep the momentum." And as a postscript: "Technical assistance will be limited to 1 technician per scientist, and this constraint will force members to collaborate with each other within a horizontal structure."

As an aftermath of the Rheinfelden meeting, Jerne phoned – one by one – Ben Pernis, Ruggero Ceppellini and Göran Möller, and explained his objection to the original plan of 12 groups and his inclination to create a horizontal structure based on "members". Pernis replied that he had already sensed Jerne's "shift" and embraced the new idea. Ceppellini did not like the idea, and Möller said that calling all members equal smelt of an Orwellian kind of equality, but eloquently suggested "intermediate" models, such as reserving some lab units for a special type of turnover, e.g. having a Swedish laboratory as an outstation of Karolinska Institutet. Jerne left this particular issue open (to be elaborated on later).

Recruitment from Round the World

Late in August 1969 Jerne started his round-the-world journey – spending time in Australia, afterwards in the USA [QR1969_25]. The trip was highly successful, and his reports back to Basel from places he visited described the recruitment progress. Names such as Theo Staehelin, Ethel Jacobson, Zoltan Tökes and Helmut Pohlit arose and were included in the list of people who should receive a contract.

QR1969_25 BII

On October 9th Niels had a dinner with Max Delbrück. On the following day Delbrück received "the" phone call from Stockholm with the news that he, Salvador Luria and Alfred Hershey were awarded the Nobel Prize for Medicine. Jerne referred to this dinner with Max Delbrück as "The Last Supper". Jerne returned to Europe in mid October 1969. His home was no longer in Frankfurt but in Provence, where earlier he had purchased a castle, the renovation of which had required major input and energy from his wife, Alexandra [QR1969_26]. She welcomed Niels to a beautiful, representative castle with a huge refurbished fireplace, and space for everything they had accumulated over the years. After a few weeks in Provence, Jerne came back to Basel. Although he had been kept up-to-date with the pace of construction during his absence, he was pleasantly surprised to see how far the building had progressed. Jerne was preoccupied with a complication that concerned his good friend and colleague Eduard Kellenberger, and he intended to settle it immediately.

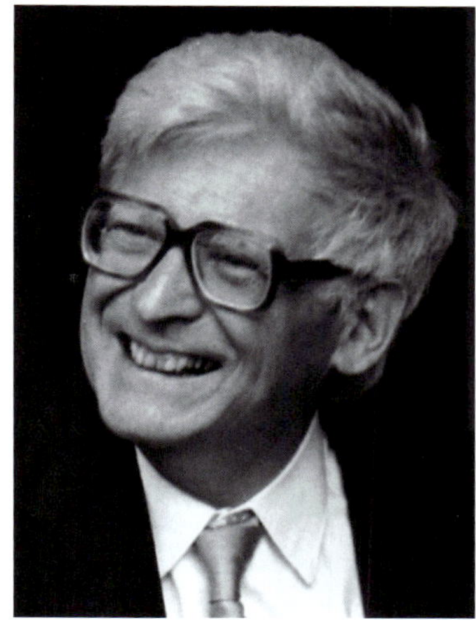
Eduard Kellenberger, Director of the Biozentrum, Basel

This needs a digression. Besides the planned BII, there was another nascent institute in Basel. It was the Biozentrum [QR1969_27], to be built by the state, financed from various sources (the canton of Basel-Stadt, the Swiss Confederation and some pharmaceutical companies) and have Eduard Kellenberger as its director.

In the arena of science, academia and private industry at that time there were 5 people who played a decisive role in planning the future of science in Switzerland and particularly in Basel, the metropolis of pharmaceutical research. Documents from the Biozentrum list them as follows:

The most important promotors from science, academia, and private industry were:

- Eduard Kellenberger (scientific researcher in Geneva at the time; professor at the Biozentrum from 1970)
- Alfred Pletscher (head of research at Hoffmann La Roche at the time)
- Hubert Bloch (head of pharmaceutical research at Ciba at the time)
- Christoph Tamm (professor of Organic Chemistry at the time, and later Rector)
- Arnold Schneider (head of the Department of Education at the time)

These 5 – and others – gave the Biozentrum the highest priority. Although the Biozentrum had been planned and the foundation stone laid considerably before the BII project was conceived, its construction was proceeding at a much slower pace than that of the BII building. Kellenberger's department in Geneva was expected to close in autumn 1970, and he would not have a workplace until the Biozentrum was ready. Therefore, Jerne came up with a solution.

QR1969_26 BII

QR1969_27 BII

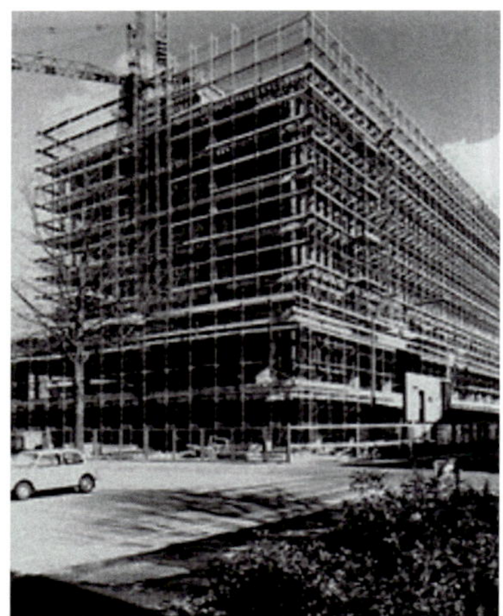

The Biozentrum under construction on the Schällenmätteli site, Basel

Freely paraphrased Jerne said: "I shall accept you and your group in my institute for a period of 1–2 years. I shall include you in our budget (except salaries), and you will be our guest until the Biozentrum is ready. We shall profit from you twofold: you will help us to 'warm up the engine', and by temporarily filling the available lab space, I can recruit members without the pressure of time."

Roche agreed with this arrangement, and a handshake between Jerne and Kellenberger made the problem disappear. This solved another issue that Jerne, Kellenberger and Lefkovits discussed over a glass of wine soon after the aforementioned agreement. Kellenberger had suggested on several occasions that Lefkovits might profit by contacting Kellenberger's coworker, Mr. Jacques Bron, who was involved in the construction of the Biozentrum. Now that Kellenberger and his group were BII guests, Jacques Bron could help Lefkovits to organize the future BII infrastructure.

On October 1st Ingrid Schnurr was appointed head of the temporary secretariat of the BII that was located in Building 52 of Roche [QR1969_28]. She took over all the administrative duties from Mrs. Pfenninger, and all the work preparing contracts previously handled by Lefkovits. Later, when additional secretarial help was acquired, Miss Schnurr worked for Niels Jerne until his retirement a decade later. She will be mentioned frequently as the BII story develops. At the time Miss Schnurr was hired, the first 2 technicians, Yolanda Magnenat and Rosemarie Liske, started work in the temporary lab in Building 7.

Rheinfelden Two

Now that Niels Jerne had settled the situation regarding Eduard Kellenberger, he decided that it was time to call a meeting of people who had either accepted the positions he had offered them or were seriously considering doing so. Similar to "Rheinfelden one" (May 1969), he now proposed holding a "Rheinfelden two" meeting, which would again take place in the Hotel Schiff, this one from December 10th to 13th, 1969. Ingrid Schnurr was entrusted with the organization of this meeting. Many questions from the architects (and from individual subcontractors) were awaiting answers. Lefkovits sent all prospective participants a list of questions. In particular he hoped to receive answers on specific points regarding equipment needed. Only a few of the participants complied with this request, while most of them said that they did not mind

whatever "gadgets and utensils" were chosen. Twelve persons participated in the meeting, most of those who were at "Rheinfelden one".

The Rheinfelden meeting was conceived as a scientific meeting. Jerne presented his new theory about the generation of antibody diversity. The manuscript had been ready for a few months, but at that time only 3 scientists outside of Basel had the details: Max Delbrück, Klaus Rajewsky and Morten Simonsen. At several places in this book, the tenets of Jerne's hypothesis of generation of antibody diversity will be discussed in detail. Here, suffice it to say that the hypothesis assumed that only a miniscule portion of specificities is inherited (transmitted from generation to generation), and the enormous repertoire of specificities arises somatically during ontogeny. Jerne did not intend to convince the participants of this, but wanted the principal dichotomy, "somatic vs. germ line", to receive attention. The meeting was of course accompanied by discussions, questions and clarifications, and its main aim was fulfilled: to establish the question of "specificities" as central to future research directions.

Part of the meeting was concerned with the construction of the institute, emphasizing the urgency of providing answers requested by the architects and subcontractors. Kellenberger also announced that in January Lefkovits could depend on the support and competence of Jacques Bron in setting up the BII infrastructure. The meeting was over, people wished each other a Merry Christmas.

It surprised Lefkovits that shortly afterwards Mr. Altenbach called for a meeting on December 23rd, so close to Christmas. Jacques Bron was summoned to Basel to participate in that meeting, and in all following ones. Kellenberger's generous gesture that the BII could "borrow" Jacques Bron and co-opt him onto the construction committee was of decisive importance. From that moment onwards, the floor plans had to be signed by Bron, and he rapidly became indispensable. Only after this meeting could they toast to a "Happy New Year 1970", a decisive one for the BII.

Treasure Trove 1968–1969
The database contains documents related to the BII in a broader context (lists, series of photographs, etc.).

The Year 1970

First contracts were signed. Jerne called a foundation meeting, later referred to as "the first Krafft meeting". An advisory board and a board of consultants were established. On October 1st, 1970, the institute opened. In 7 laboratories 25 scientists started to work (A. Kelus, I. Lefkovits, T. Staehelin, S. Fazekas, E. Jacobson, T.-W. Tao-Wiedmann, C. Steinberg, L. Du Pasquier, F. Loor, D. Braun, J.-C. Jaton, H. Pohlit, G. Roelants, B. Askonas, D. Dresser, J. Andersson, O. Sjöberg, J. Hay, J. Obel, V. Miggiano, D. Bernoco, S. Shin, A. Falvey, W. McKeehan, M. Schreier).

First Contracts Signed

By spring 1970, the not yet existing BII was the "gossip topic number one" in the world of immunology.

The year 1970 started with contracts being issued to 6 prospective members of the BII [QR1970_01]: Theophil Staehelin from Basel, then Ann Arbor, Stephen Fazekas from Canberra, Ethel Jacobson from New York, Seung-il Shin from Seoul, then USA and Bruges, Fritz Melchers from Berlin and the USA, and Tien-Wen Tao-Wiedmann from Boston.

Jacques Bron took up his assignment and relieved Lefkovits of certain duties. As time went by, a problem concerning Jacques arose. He was loyal to Eduard Kellenberger with whom he had worked for many years and he was conscientious regarding his work at the Biozentrum, but he started to "fall in love" with his assignment at the BII. More than once he pointed out this quandary to Lefkovits, who, having finally got the message, arranged with Jerne and Kellenberger that Bron should be released from the Biozentrum and join the BII on a permanent basis.

By spring 1970, the not yet existing BII was the "gossip topic number one" in the world of immunology. Visitors (future members or just those curious about it) dropped in, and this started to be a logistics problem. Because of the visitors, Lefkovits was more often brewing espresso on his Pavoni machine than doing experiments. But more problematic was the fact that visitors felt the urge to visit the building site on their own initiative. According to the strict safety rules this was forbidden without prior arrangement.

QR1970_01 BII

The problem was solved by Alfred Pletscher's generous offer of a villa at Schwarzwaldallee 47 (located roughly halfway between the BII and Roche) to be used until the construction work on the BII was finished. It was very spacious and the rooms could

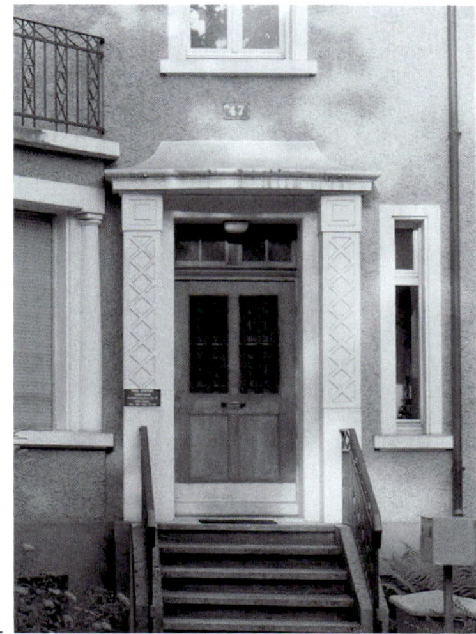

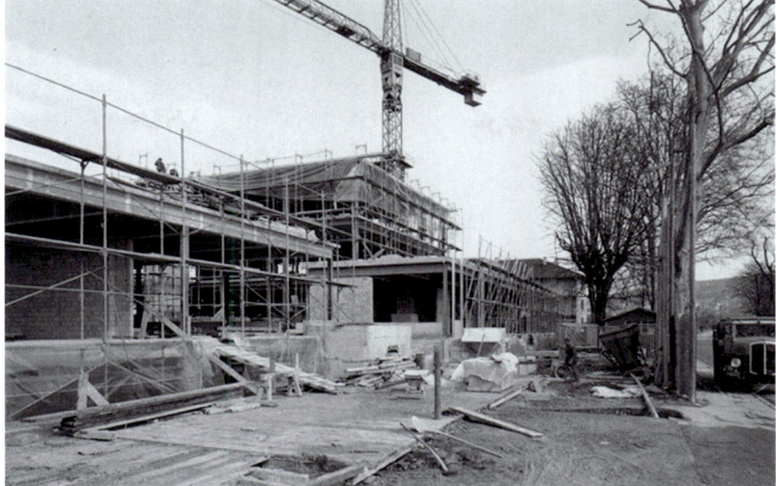

1 Villa at Schwarzwaldallee 47

2 View of construction site from Grenzacherstrasse

easily be converted into offices so everything could be concentrated at one place. Ingrid Schnurr moved there from Building 52, and Niels was given an office (but used it rarely). Importantly, visitors could be shepherded there, thus not being a nuisance at the building site. Floor plans could be spread out for visitors to look at. The visitors were coming and going, and were usually booked into the Hotel Krafft. It was a modestly priced hotel, and Jerne cultivated this kind of Protestant frugality. A reading room was designated in the villa – with copies of *Nature* and *Science* available – to keep at least some of the visitors quiet. It was agreed that about 12 journals would be available on the day the institute opened, and some back issues as well. To set up the library, Mrs. Zdena Joukl was hired; she was installed in a spacious office at Schwarzwaldallee and started ordering journals and books for the future library of the institute.

The 1st Krafft Meeting

The number of new members was already considerable, and Jerne summoned another meeting to be held in the Hotel Krafft [QR1970_02] from April 30th to May 3rd, 1970. The participants were: Dwight Anderson, Jan Andersson, Brigitte Askonas, Dietmar Braun, Ruggero Ceppellini, David Dresser, Louis Du Pasquier, E. Eikenberry, Richard Epstein, Stephen Fazekas de St. Groth, William Ford, Melvin Greaves, Hans Halbach, Ulrich Hämmerling, Jean-Claude Jaton, Niels K. Jerne, Eduard Kellenberger, Andrew Kelus, Heinz Köhler, Ivan Lefkovits, Francis Loor, Fritz Melchers,

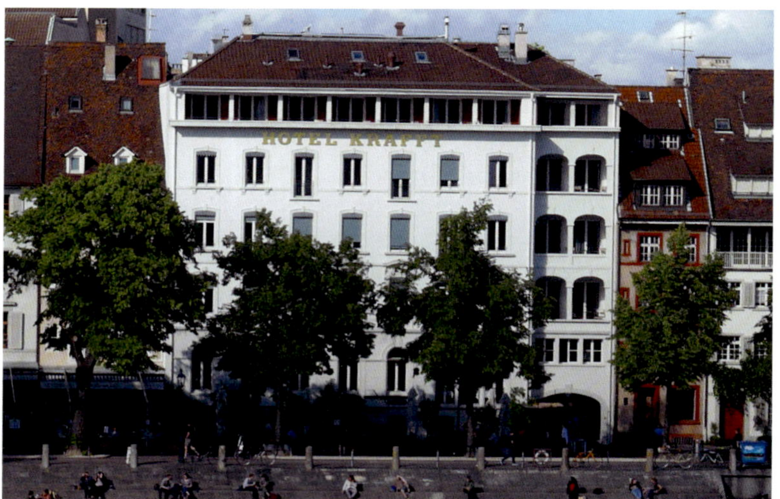

Hotel Krafft, Basel:
venue of a BII planning meeting

Vincenzo Miggiano, Göran Möller, Al Nordin, Benvenuto Pernis, Helmut Pohlit, Klaus Rajewsky, Hansruedi Ramseier, Eric Ruoslahti, S. Sarkar, Seung-il Shin, Olof Sjöberg, Theophil Staehelin, Charles Steinberg, Glauco Tocchini-Valentini, Zoltan Tökes, Zdenek Trnka and Tien-Wen Tao-Wiedmann.

The Krafft meeting was set up as a conference with an itemized agenda and times allotted to the speakers. There were several sessions, the purpose of which was to depart from a "one-man show" that Jerne was against (he definitely preferred to listen rather than to talk). Thus, Jerne only explained the "basics" about the institute, thereafter participants presented their research reports or proposals. While the talks were going on, small groups (always 5–6 people, in order not to interfere with the daily routine at the construction site) made site visits to the institute. In spite of the fact that all necessary information had been circulated to everyone, the Krafft meeting had a different status from just ordinary information gathering: it was more an opportunity for future colleagues to meet. It was not uncommon for participants to ask each other:

"Are you coming?" – "Well, if you come I shall come too."

The meeting finally gave Lefkovits a chance to ask people about equipment and instruments. Some people were very specific about their needs, while others nonchalantly said that they would be satisfied with whatever was supplied (later not remembering this attitude). Fritz Melchers greatly helped by suggesting the formation of an "instrument committee" [QR1970_03]. It was decided that Melchers, Bron and Lefkovits would visit (later that

QR1970_03 BII

year) the ACHEMA Fair in Frankfurt to inspect the latest laboratory equipment and discuss it with the suppliers.

As in Rheinfelden, at this meeting too the question of technicians was raised. The plan was to have 1 technician per scientist, thus one would need to hire 50 technicians. Were there enough Swiss technicians "on the market"? Jerne pointed out that the issue was not only whether there were enough qualified technicians around, but also that they should be "English-speaking". Not for the convenience of the scientists, but because an internationally functioning institute must have English as its working language. Göran Möller fully agreed with Niels, saying that "on this continent there are two countries where technicians speak good English – England and Sweden". Göran continued, "I am willing to advertise in the *Svenska Dagbladet* [QR1970_04], and I am sure that I will find any number of highly qualified technicians. And I am willing to interview them and make a kind of pre-selection". This was agreed upon, and it was a great success.

The Krafft meeting was over, and Jerne now had a list of scientists to whom contracts were to be issued. Soon afterwards, Mr. Altenbach asked Lefkovits for a private talk. He was very concerned, realizing that all these people at the meeting were indeed expecting the institute to be ready by October 1st. Altenbach paused, and said: "I will make sure that the institute opens on October 1st, but only about half of it will be 'bezugsbereit' (ready for occupation). The rest will be finished by April 1st, 1971. Between October and April any remaining WIVO furniture will be installed."

With a grim face Lefkovits reported back to Jerne and was surprised by his reaction: it was fine by him, as it would allow a less hectic start. Jerne then wrote to all newly hired scientists and adjusted their starting dates to the alternatives of October 1970 or April 1971.

Countdown to the Opening

At the next meeting with the architects, both Lefkovits and Bron were present; Mr. Altenbach – greatly relieved and in a good mood – distributed floor plans with color coding of the areas that would not be ready initially and showing that the garage would be inaccessible until April 1971.

After the Krafft meeting Jerne went to Provence for a few weeks, returning to Basel on June 1st, 1970, to take up permanent residence. He rented an apartment at Rümelinsplatz in the old town of Basel.

QR1970_04 BII

The progress of science consists partly of replacing preconceived ideas by better ones and partly of collecting experimental data related to these ideas. The latter exercise facilitates the former.

One of the new members of the institute was Zdenek Trnka [QR1970_05]. He came from Geneva, from the same office at the WHO where Jerne had worked a decade earlier. Zdenek's original affiliation was the Czechoslovak Academy of Sciences in Prague, from where he relocated to Geneva in 1965 for an assignment at the WHO. Upon the Soviet occupation of Czechoslovakia in August 1968 his position was (expectedly) not prolonged. He could complete his term, but then he either had to return to Czechoslovakia or become a refugee. Jerne valued Trnka's contribution to science, but had in mind to get him involved in administrative duties, especially those related to science. A small problem arose as Jerne had already promised the administrative position to Hans Halbach, another person from the WHO. This potential conflict vanished as Hans Halbach was asked by Roche to advise on interactions between the company and the WHO. Clearly Zdenek would have been happier to be offered scientific membership and a lab. However, it turned out to work very well for him, also in terms of true experimental work, which will be reported later. Lefkovits passed some of the administrative duties over to Trnka, but retained all those aspects related to ensuring that the deadline for the opening of the institute in a few months' time would be kept.

Göran Möller kept his promise and placed several ads in a Swedish daily newspaper. Even a single ad would have been enough, so great was the response. He interviewed each applicant, selected a short list and sent the dossier to Lefkovits. Göran was so conscientious that not only did he write about the qualifications of the technicians, but mentioned also other attributes, such as "long legs" and "beautiful dark eyes". Göran, at the age of 30, was already a famous immunologist and probably the youngest professor in Sweden. The "summary of the interviews" contained statements for which today he would be brought to court. At that time it did not, but his secretary photocopied the letter and pinned it on the notice board at the Karolinska. Explanations and apologies were in order. Here in Basel "the scandal" became common knowledge, but it is fair to say that the "attributes" mentioned in the dossier did not play any role in the hiring procedure. In all the years of the institute's existence, more than 30 Swedish technicians were employed. Their qualifications were superb and their loyalty to the institute exceptional [QR1970_06].

QR1970_05 BII

QR1970_06 BII

The first Swedish technicians recruited by Göran Möller (Anita Söderberg and Lena Skarvall) received their contracts and joined the temporary lab in Building 7. Although the institute's opening was still 4 months away, Ethel Jacobson, Theo Staehelin and Stephen Fazekas arrived and helped with preparations for the move into the new building. Especially important was Theo Staehelin's input: he had extensive knowledge of modern research facilities and was a native Swiss. There were many suitable Swiss in the vicinity, but he was a repatriated Swiss who understood the expectations and problems of the institute to be.

There are values valid for an individual or a population even when, from the subjective point of view of some opinion leaders, such values are not endorsed or accepted.

Modified from *Stanford Encyclopedia of Philosophy*, E.N. Zalta (2009 ed.)

Advisors and Consultants

Jerne had a sixth sense in bringing compatible people together. He decided to create an "Advisory Board" with the function of advising the director on issues that could arise during the running of the institute. For Jerne it was an easy task to select the most suitable board candidates, as he already knew from his recruitment journey who those were who had a keen interest in the institute. Jerne's choice of board members was made by approaching outstanding scientists of indisputable international reputation, obviously people whose personalities he trusted. It was his intention that the board members should come from many different countries, because this emphasized the board's "internationality" and "prominence".

He knew very well that Swiss scientists should also be on the board, but how was he to choose a few from the dozens or so from Basel, Zurich, Bern, Geneva, Davos or elsewhere, as no unpleas-

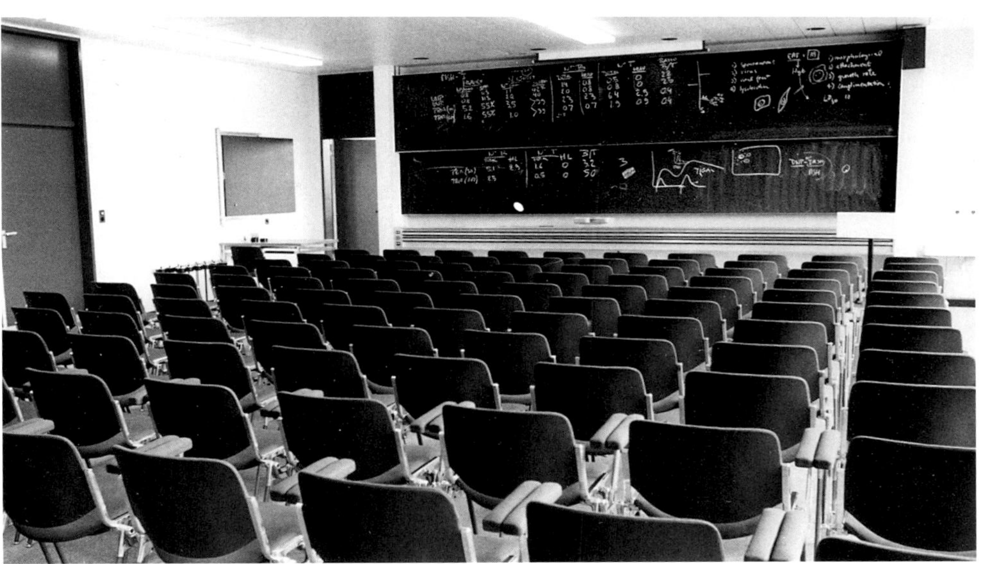

Large seminar room in the BII

ant feelings should be stirred up in those left out? After all, Switzerland is a small country where everyone knows everyone. The Jernean solution was to establish, besides the International Advisory Board, a second board, a Swiss one. It was implemented immediately in 1970 and was maintained throughout and beyond Jerne's directorship. Thus the BII had two independent boards: the International Advisory Board and the Swiss Board of Consultants.

The initial board members were to be appointed by Jerne. They were to rotate so that a complete renewal would be achieved in 3 years (except during the initial period when some of them would have to step down to make place for new members). The International Board had a slightly different function from that of the Swiss Board, which would focus on the relationship with the Swiss scientific community and on social matters. The Swiss Board would appoint 2 delegates to be co-opted onto the International Board. This was a very convenient procedure, as it elegantly solved the delicate problem of participation of Swiss scientists on the International Advisory Board.

At that time when neither fax nor e-mail existed, and sending letters was too slow, Jerne contacted potential Board members by phone – ticking off the names on his neatly written list. Within days he had established an International Advisory Board [QR1970_07], and with help from Henri Isliker he had set up a Swiss Board of Consultants. In the last month before the institute's opening 3 meetings were planned: the Board of Consultants, the International Advisory Board, and also a second Krafft meeting. The venue of both board meetings was to be the villa in Schwarzwaldallee 47.

The Board of Consultants [QR1970_08] assembled for its first meeting on August 28th, 1970, and the International Advisory Board on September 14th and 15th. The agendas for both board meetings revolved around the deadlines for the completion of the first and second stages of the BII (October 1970, April 1971).

QR1970_07 BII

The 2nd Krafft Meeting

Ingrid Schnurr and Ivan Lefkovits prepared a second Krafft meeting. There were two categories of participants: scientists, who were to move into the labs within weeks, and others, who watched the hectic interactions, but were to move to the BII half a year later, in April 1971. Everything revolved around the floor and lab plans, and about identifying items that must be available in the labs from day one. Great concern rose about the preparation of

QR1970_08 BII

media and establishing the animal facilities. Madame Gisèle Bron, the wife of Jacques, was to supervise the media kitchen, as she had been head of the media kitchen in Kellenberger's department in Geneva. Some people stayed on in the Hotel Krafft after the meeting was over, and discussions often continued long into the night in the nearby Rheinkeller restaurant.

The Opening, October 1970

On October 5th, 1970, the BII opened: laboratories 1–6 remained off zone, laboratories 7–13 were ready. The earlier arrivals – Stephen Fazekas, Ethel Jacobson, Theo Staehelin and Tien-Wen Tao-Wiedmann – were joined by 19 newcomers: Jan Andersson, Brigitte Askonas, Domenico Bernoco, Dietmar Braun, David Dresser, Louis Du Pasquier, Amy Falvey, Jack Hay, Jean-Claude Jaton, Francis Loor, Wally McKeehan, Vincenzo Miggiano, Jan Obel, Helmut Pohlit, Georges Roelants, Max Schreier, Seung-il Shin, Olof Sjöberg and Charles Steinberg; with Jerne, Kelus, Lefkovits and Trnka, that made a total of 27 scientists: on October 19th the first agar plates were prepared by Gisèle Bron.

The BII adventure had started.

Research Interests in Brief

It was an entirely heterogeneous group of scientists, and although it is not practicable to attach a "label" of interests to each person, a brief "who is who" in terms of their preferences follows:

Andrew Kelus	Anti-idiotypic responses in rabbits
Ivan Lefkovits	Microcultures of stimulated lymphocytes
Theo Staehelin	Regulation of protein synthesis
Stephen Fazekas	Antigenicity of mutants of influenza viruses
Ethel Jacobson	Antibody-induced suppression in mice
Tien-Wen Tao-Wiedmann	*In vitro* organ culture systems
Charles Steinberg	Genetics
Louis Du Pasquier	Amphibian tadpoles and their immune responses
Francis Loor	Immunofluorescence of cells of the immune system
Dietmar Braun	Streptococcal polysaccharide antigens (rabbits)
Jean-Claude Jaton	Amino acid sequencing of protein species
Helmut Pohlit	Antigenically cross-reacting carriers
Georges Roelants	Proliferation of cells during stimulation
Brigitte Askonas	General aspects of cell proliferation
David Dresser	Thymus-dependent and thymus-independent antigens

Jan Andersson	Microfluorometry and autoradiography on single cells
Olof Sjöberg	Concanavalin A responses and mitogenicity
Jack Hay	Draining lymph nodes of sheep and recirculation
Jan Obel	Antigen presentation
Vincenzo Miggiano	Mixed leukocyte cultures in humans and mice
Domenico Bernoco	Unidirectional MLC and blast transformation
Seung-il Shin	Cell fusion of lymphocytes
Amy Falvey	Initiation factors in protein synthesis
Wally McKeehan	Elongation factors in protein synthesis
Max Schreier	Translational control and mRNA

Niels Jerne "hand-picked" the majority of these scientists, though he readily acknowledged suggestions from already accepted members. Göran Möller, who hoped to establish a Karolinska subsidiary in Basel, suggested Olof Sjöberg and Jan Andersson, while Georges Roelants came from Ita Askonas' laboratory and teamed up with her and Jan Obel. Two Italian scientists, Vincenzo Miggiano and Domenico Bernoco, came from Ceppellini's group and were considered as "Ceppellini's people", although they soon gained considerable independence due to the horizontal structure of the institute. Theo Staehelin was a special case as he came to Basel with a vision to establish a molecular biology unit within an immunology environment. Jerne conceded that this group needed a certain size (somewhat larger than the horizontal structure would allow), and he expected Max Schreier (a postdoc of Hans Noll) to join it, along with Wally McKeehan and Amy Falvey. This occurred in November 1970. In that month Takeshi Matsunaga joined Andrew Kelus, Matthias Cramer joined Dietmar Braun, and Walter Gerhard teamed up with Stephen Fazekas.

By the end of 1970 the earlier mentioned number of 27 scientists had increased (with Matsunaga, Cramer and Gerhard) to a final count of 30.

The range of scientific interests of the founding group of members was broad, although the above-mentioned "label" was sufficient only for a basic orientation. The full scale of pursuits soon became obvious.

Preparing for Scientific Endeavors, 1970

Do Tadpoles Have an Immune System?

L. Du Pasquier

An amphibian tadpole has less than a million lymphocytes, but this "modest" number of cells is sufficient for mounting an immune response. Whether the specificity of the response is as good as in large animals was not known. Since the clonal selection dogma assumed that one cell makes one molecular species of antibody, and an organism was supposed to be ready to cope with a large spectrum of antigens, constraints of the response in terms of specificity and antibody quality (affinity) were expected to occur. Niels Jerne was keen to have this question clarified and put Louis on the job offer list that stemmed from the 1967 EMBO course in Frankfurt. In addition, the issue of metamorphosis (from a tadpole to a frog) occurring without compromising the immune system called for an explanation. Louis came to Basel with the idea to employ various antigens and several methodological approaches for measuring the quality (affinity) of antibody.

How Does the Immune Response Start?

I. Lefkovits

Although it was known that an immune response could be carried out by cells outside of the organism (under tissue culture conditions), the cells that participate in the actual response were only starting to be understood. An important test, the so-called plaque-forming assay developed in 1963 in Jerne's laboratory in Pittsburgh, enabled the identification of individual antibody-producing cells. This test revolutionized the quantitation of processes occurring during the immune response. It became possible to monitor the appearance of antibody-forming cells upon addition of antigen to spleen cells, and to perform various tests employing cells from mice that lacked a thymus (nude mice). Microcultures of mouse spleen cells were subjected to a fluctuation test, and all-or-none responses of small aliquots of cells were studied. Proportions of cultures that responded were expected to provide information on the number of cells capable of initiating an antigen-specific response. Nude mice were found to be a promising source of B cells for studying clones producing antibody of single molecular species.

Homogeneous or Monoclonal?

D.G. Braun, J.-C. Jaton, M. Cramer

For studying the structure of immunoglobulins, a source of well-defined antibody samples was required. Any natural sample of antibody – whether from blood or other body fluid – was always a complex mixture of molecules. In fact, the only truly homogeneous supply of antibodies was the myeloma protein samples obtained from patients with a cancer of antibody-forming (plasma) cells. These pathological immunoglobulins flood the blood stream and are readily retrieved for structural studies. However, immunization protocols existed that resulted in the induction of high levels of antibody of defined specificity and homogeneous molecular properties. This was the case through immunization of rabbits with streptococcal and pneumococcal polysaccharide antigens. Antibody obtained by such procedures was useful not only for elucidating amino acid sequences of these molecules, but also as a model for studying the properties of antibody-combining sites, as well as inheritance of idiotypes. The expressions "homogeneous" and "restricted heterogeneity" were often used to mean "monoclonal", which of course was not correct, as the era of the "monoclonal" antibody had not yet started.

Response or Tolerance?

H. Pohlit

Several well-defined antigens had been used for eliciting immune responses. The terms "epitope" and "paratope" (for antigenic determinants and for the combining site of the antibody) entered the vocabulary of immunologists, and "hapten carrier" models (epitopes attached to a larger structure – usually a protein entity) were scrutinized. Antigenically cross-reacting carriers allowed cross-stimulation under different ontogenic conditions to be studied. Tolerance to one of the carriers was used as a model for studying heterogeneity distribution.

What Does the Thymus Do?

D. Dresser

The broad spectrum of antigens falls conceptually into two categories. One is such that the immune response can be elicited only in animals with an intact thymus, while with antigens of the other category the response is also induced in animals lacking a functional thymus. Experimental protocols were worked out for studying not only stimulation, but also "reverse" processes, i.e. the induction of tolerance. Thymus-dependent and thymus-independent antigens allowed the study of the contribution of T and B cells to response and tolerance.

What Suppresses What?

E. Jacobson

Although the terms tolerance, suppression, paralysis and unresponsiveness were often used synonymously, there was always a certain contextual difference of the meanings. A special case was the antibody-induced suppression of the immune response. In vitro systems using immunoglobulin molecules with precisely defined molecular markers (allotype markers) allowed the study of the contribution of cell populations in the process of establishing antibody-induced suppression of the immune response. It was of importance that one kind of antibody was capable of interfering with another kind of antibody. This was the starting point of defining the idiotypic network, which for several groups became a major future research task.

How Do Mouse Strains Differ?

T. Matsunaga, A.S. Kelus

One of the reasons why mice became so popular for studying immunologically relevant problems was the notion that they are easily bred and maintained. But more importantly, there had been a large variety of different strains, some inbred or simply colony-maintained. Mixed antiglobulin tests and immunofluorescence were employed to detect allotypic determinants and histocompatibility antigens on mouse strains differing in their genetic makeup. Availability of specific antisera marked the beginning of proper genetic typing of lymphocytes.

Antigens or Mitogens?

O. Sjöberg, J. Andersson

Antigens and mitogens differ in their mode of interaction with cells of the immune system. A tiny portion of cells is involved in antigen-specific events, while entire populations are engaged in mitogen-induced activities. Concanavalin A and antithymocyte globulin were used to stimulate lymphocytes and to quantify the progress of RNA transcription on a single cell level (RNA transcription was meant to be an indicator in dissecting the stages of cell responses). Acridine orange microfluorometry and autoradiography of single cells were used for quantitation.

Is a Sheep Any Different from a Mouse?

J.B. Hay

Some conceptual enquiries of the immune system, like lymphocyte trafficking and recirculation, cannot be suitably handled in small animals like mice. Sheep became a useful model for studying the fate of cells during the immune response in large animals. Chronic lymphatic fistulae of the draining popliteal lymph nodes of sheep were used to study the characteristics of the cells (and antibodies) that leave a stimulated lymph node.

QRalpha_10 BII

What Makes a Lymphocyte Turn into an Antibody-Producing Cell?

G. Roelants, B. Askonas, J. Obel

Although it was known that B lymphocytes are predestined to become antibody-producing cells, the actual occurrences were yet to be determined. The starting point of the scrutiny was to study the proliferation of cells and their differentiation into antibody-forming cells. The immune stimulation model enabled the study of B cell memory formation.

QRalpha_11 BII

Cell Culture or Organ Culture?

T.-W. Tao-Wiedmann

Some researchers claimed that cell suspensions are easier to control than samples taken from organs. Cell suspensions form "fair samples", while slices of organs (e.g. spleen or lymph nodes) differ depending on the structure of the organ. Both organ cultures and cell suspension cultures became standard models for decades to come. An in vitro organ culture system using rabbit lymphoid tissues (spleen and lymph nodes) was used to study the initiation and maturation of the antibody response. The bacteriophage ΦX 174 became a standard antigen model for studying affinity of the formed antibody.

QRalpha_12 BII

How Do Cells from Newborns Behave?

V. Miggiano, R. Ceppellini

Lymphocytes can both "recognize" and "be recognized". Such recognition can be measured in an MLR assay (mixed lymphocyte reaction). A catalog of reactivity of lymphocytes from spleen, peripheral blood, thymus and bone marrow from mothers and newborns has been established in the human species. Lymphocytes of two sources that do not react to each other (MLR being negative) are said to be "compatible" which is an important status in the field of transplantation. The causes of the reciprocal hyporeactivity (of some of the populations) and the conditions under which this is achieved were worthy of deeper scrutiny.

QRalpha_13 BII

What Is Needed for Protein Synthesis?

T. Staehelin, M. Schreier, W. McKeehan, A. Falvey

Ingredients required for the synthesis of protein molecules were known, while factors that regulate the actual synthesis were only starting to be defined. Regulation of protein synthesis at the translational level in mammalian cells was used to investigate control mechanisms in the synthesis of antibodies. Studies using ribosome subunits, initiation factors, globin mRNA and other components allowed the definition of conditions for the initiation of protein synthesis.

QRalpha_14 BII

What Can One Detect by Immuno-Fluorescence?

F. Loor

Microscopes of ever-increasing resolution became excellent tools, with added value once fluorescence reagents became available. Molecules with fluorescence tags were used to detect the ability of lymphocytes to bind various structures. Ontogeny of Ig receptors on lymphocytes was studied by immunofluorescent spot techniques. It was found that thymus cells never express any detectable level of Ig receptors.

QRalpha_15 BII

How to Prevent Lymphocytes from Blasting?

D. Bernoco, R. Ceppellini

The vast majority of lymphocytes in the organism are idle, while a small portion that becomes involved in a response undergoes (as a first step in a chain of events) a "blast transformation". It was found that the presence of certain antibodies (alloantisera) in mixed lymphocyte cultures (MLC) greatly inhibits blast transformation. Studies were done to clarify whether the anti-HLA immunoglobulins are involved in the observed inhibition.

How Do Influenza Viruses Differ from Each Other?

S. Fazekas, W. Gerhard

Even minor alterations in the structure of antigens are recognized by the immune system. Closely related antigenic mutants within the group of influenza viruses revealed differences in the resulting immune responses, and the heterogeneity of serological responses was amenable for scrutiny by various analytical tools. Equilibrium measurements and thermodynamic measurements were used as a criterion to test antigens differing by known single-step mutations.

Can a Lymphocyte Fuse with Another Lymphocyte?

S. Shin

Techniques of cell fusion were adopted for long-term maintenance of lymphocytes from normal and immunized mice. Various mutants of myeloma cell lines were derived, with the aim of establishing procedures for "lymphocyte-lymphocyte" fusion.

First Internal Seminar:
Ruggero Ceppellini: Human Histocompatibility System

Everyone wanted to know about the skills and interests of other members, and of course they wanted also to keep good contacts to other institutions. The earliest ad hoc informal seminars were not documented. The very first recorded internal seminar was by Ruggero Ceppellini on October 27th, 1970, on the human histocompatibility system. It was part of a block of 4 seminars on 4 consecutive days: Tien-Wen Tao-Wiedmann (October 28th), Stephen Fazekas (October 29th) and Francis Loor (October 30th).

First Formal Seminar: *Klaus Rajewsky*

The first formally announced seminar recorded in BII documents was by Klaus Rajewsky from Cologne [QR1970_09]. He spoke on "Cell cooperation, antigen presentation versus information transfer". Klaus was a welcome guest at the BII and one of its strongest supporters.

In November and December a further 7 seminars were given (Ivan Lefkovits, Ethel Jacobson, Louis Du Pasquier, Helmut Pohlit, Andrew Kelus, Theo Staehelin and Max Schreier).

BASEL INSTITUTE FOR IMMUNOLOGY

Lecture by

Professor Klaus Rajewsky
Institute for Genetics
University of Köln
Germany

on

Cell Cooperation - Antigen Presentation
Versus Information Transfer

Monday, 16 November 1970 at 19.30 in the
Seminar Room.

QR1970_09 BII

Treasure Trove 1970

The database contains documents related to the BII in a broader context (lists, series of photographs, etc.).

QR1970_treasure BII

Next page: Antibody-forming cell in the center of a plaque

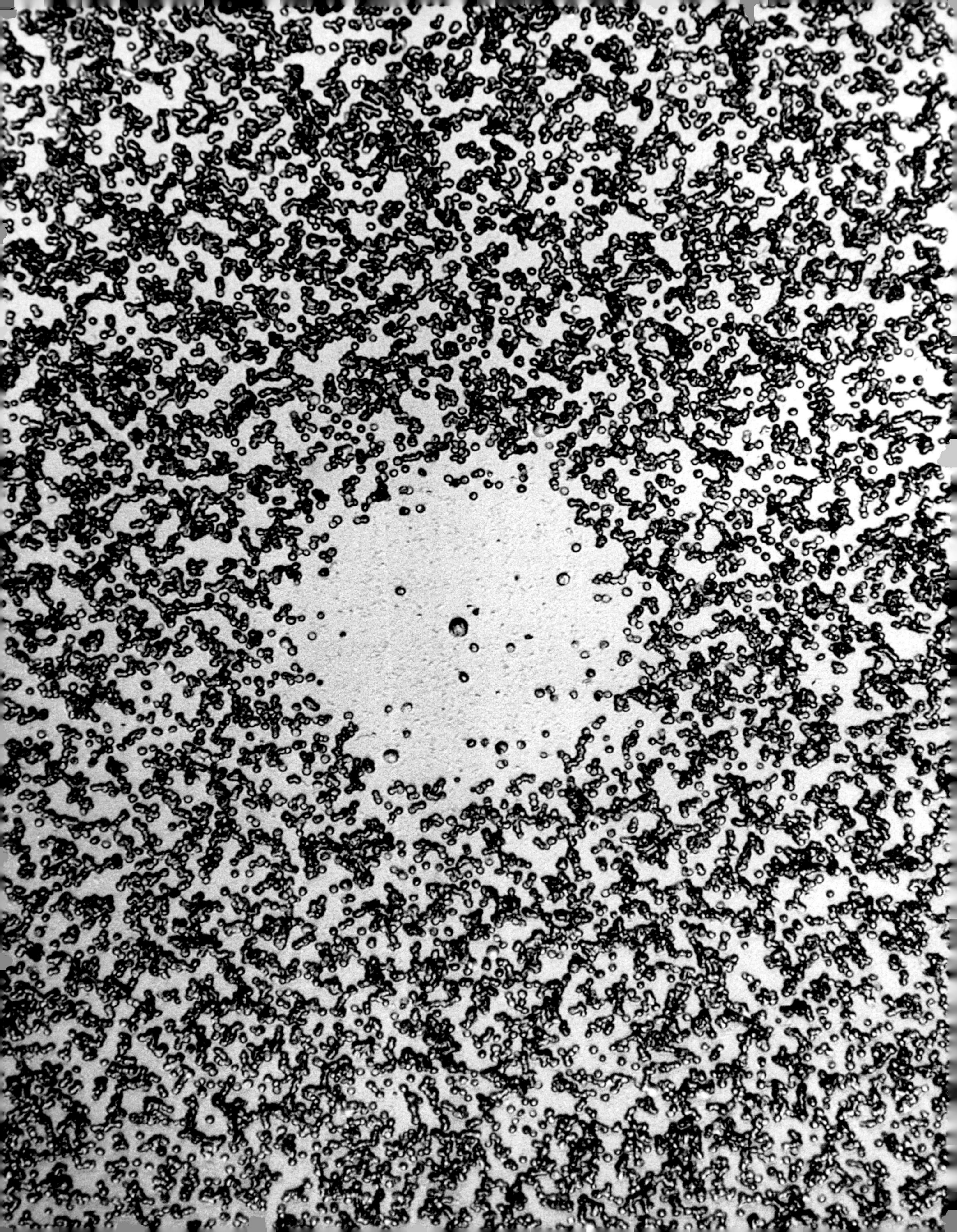

The Year 1971

Six months after the "partial" opening, the remaining areas were completed. On June 17th the official inauguration of the institute took place. Tinguely's Double Helix (a present from Maja and Paul Sacher) was installed. Niels Jerne delivered at the conference "The Challenge of Life", organized by Roche, a lecture entitled "Newer Knowledge of Immunobiology". Monday lunch seminars were initiated. Several courses were held including the EMBO course on homogeneous antibodies. Tonegawa started to work on the project of generation of antibody diversity. By the end of the year, 17 papers had been published. The Santa Lucia celebration completed the year.

In January 1971, Ruggero Ceppellini arrived into the fully equipped lab of Miggiano and Bernoco. Susumu Tonegawa arrived in mid January, and from the first day he received guidance and support from Charles Steinberg; now the number of scientists had increased to 32.

For scientific endeavor is a natural whole the parts of which mutually support one another in a way which, to be sure, no one can anticipate.

Albert Einstein, *Out of My Later Years*

The description of scientific interests and the synopsis of the work during the first 6 months of the BII showed that the working conditions were conducive to a "good start", and, furthermore, the research projects gave an indication as to future directions of work at the BII. There was an emphasis on studying heterogeneity and homogeneity of cells and molecules; already at this early stage a successful diversification of animal models (mouse, human, sheep, amphibian) was achieved, and, last but not least, team formation had begun. It will become clear throughout this narrative that scientists cooperated for a while to initiate joint projects and dissociated later in order to try something else, and that the great plasticity in the interactions was an integral part of the horizontal structure.

At some point Jerne was asked why he only rarely went down to the laboratories. He explained that he did not want to create a feeling that he was checking up on the scientists, and also he did not want to make distinctions by going to some laboratories and skipping others. But in his office he had discussions with scientists every day. Ingrid Schnurr fetched them and ensured that everyone had the opportunity to benefit from his knowledge.

The person not mentioned in any of the above projects is Charley Steinberg, a founding member of the BII. Charley was a theoretician, a geneticist by education, who stood behind many of the projects mentioned in this treatise, and most importantly he helped Susumu Tonegawa to get on the right track.

Niels Jerne took many decisions just by "saying what he wanted", but once his wishes in terms of "initial conditions" were implemented, he refrained from interfering with further developments. He discussed science with every newcomer, and did so individually and in groups. Discussions took place during the daytime and continued long into the night. It was a busy time both in setting up experimental work and discussing science in general.

There were not only discussions among the two dozen scientists, but due to a large "throughput" of visitors, many seminars were held. Some of them were duly announced, others occurred ad hoc, when visitors knocked on the door. The discussions, the spontaneity of dialog and the openness of argumentation became highly significant features of the institute, and a separate chapter will be devoted to this issue.

Six months after the "partial" opening of the BII, construction of the remaining areas of the institute was completed, and the entire institute became functional.

The Machine Is Switched On

Those first 6 months could have been tedious, but they were not. During the construction there was a spirit of mutual respect between the construction workers and the scientific staff. A minimal emission of noise was achieved, with work that caused noise or vibration being done at night. Not a single worker entered the "ready area" of the institute, and the work force had a separate entrance through the garage level. All this was negotiated with Mr. Altenbach, and interactions with the architects were excellent from the first to the last day. And the scientists did not look behind the partitions. There was an important exception to this, which will be mentioned later.

On March 31st, 1971, the partition between the construction zone and the functioning part was removed, the cleaning crew swept the floor and made the area ready for the next day.

On April 1st several scientists arrived: Ben Pernis was greeted by Niels Jerne and went to Francis Loor's lab to look at the fluorescence microscopy results; Fritz Melchers, already on the BII payroll since October 1970, also arrived on April 1st just to complete equipping his laboratory. Soon thereafter Fritz accepted Georges Köhler as his first PhD student in Basel.

Importantly, Eduard Kellenberger and his group (A.H. Doermann, J. Dubochet, B. and T. Hohn, F.A. Eiserling and L. Boehner) arrived and moved to the newly completed laboratories (Labs 4 and 5) [QR1971_01]. Also among the scientists who arrived was Hansruedi Ramseier from Zurich, who had been considered by Jerne in view of his earlier joint research project with Jean Lindenmann, although the latter could not join the institute.

In May 1971, Peter Lachmann joined the institute for a sabbatical year, and Alma Luzzati started to work with Ben Pernis. Later on another 21 scientists arrived from various countries: Irene Baldi, Ron Citronbaum, Susan Cullen, Arnold Feinstein, Yossi Haimovich, John Hamilton, Hansruedi Kiefer, Berenice Kindred, John Lightbody, Tom Mandel, Wolfgang Mayr, Tommy Meo, Markus Nabholz, Richard Pink, José Quintáns, Donald Shreffler, Zoltan Tökes, Giorgio Trinchieri, Jordi Vives, Niki Weiss, Siraik Zakarian [QR1971_02].

Simultaneously many technicians arrived and started their assignments. They were mostly of British or Swedish origin, although several were French, Italian and Belgian.

The newcomers had a contract in their hands, but "behind the scenes" various arrangements had to be done to enable their smooth transition from abroad to Switzerland. To work in Switzerland [QR1971_03] every foreigner required a residence permit, and in terms of quota regulation the Swiss Foreign Police handled this. The Foreign Police *(Ausländerpolizei)* of Canton Basel-Stadt gave an instruction to their office to reserve a certain number of permits for future BII employees. In spite of this, the permits were allotted on a one-by-one basis, and the Foreign Police meticulously checked each application. The Roche Personnel Department had filled in the forms, and in most instances the police approved the applications without question.

QR1971_01 BII

The Personnel Department made a collective statement to the Cantonal Employment Office *(Arbeitsamt)* that for positions to be filled by foreigners, nobody with equivalent qualifications could be found on the Swiss work market. Scientists arrived at the border with their passport and the necessary Assurance of Residence permit *(Zusicherung der Aufenthaltsbewilligung)*.

QR1971_02 BII

The proportion of foreigners in Switzerland was quite tightly regulated. From the point of view of the Foreign Police, the Basel Institute was a "good institute" as its scientists left Switzerland after completing their work contract. Every foreigner who "came and left" was, in the parlance of the statisticians, a good foreigner. Thus the institute was not refused (except on rare occasions) any

QR1971_03 BII

... and all Monday lunch seminars for the next 30 years started at 13.07.

requested residence permits. It was easier for the institute to hire foreigners than it was for the pharmaceutical companies.

Newcomers (scientists, their families, technicians – everybody) received adequate support with regard to finding accommodation and schools, opening a bank account and all other issues. In addition, Roche arranged the transfer of personal effects (except furniture). While positions of scientists and technicians were filled mostly from abroad, all the other positions, such as workshop and technical staff, animal caretakers, etc., were given to applicants from Switzerland or from the border regions in France and Germany.

The Monday Lunch Seminar 13.07

On Monday, April 5th, Ben Pernis gave a seminar describing the results of fluorescent staining of lymphocytes, and this event was held in the large seminar room (first floor). It was scheduled for 13.00, but the question had to be settled whether 13.00 meant 13.00 s.t. or 13.00 c.t. (sine tempore or cum tempore). Since the academic quarter was usually maintained at academic teaching institutions, and the BII was not a "true" teaching institution, a compromise was established to start at 13.07. This decision became set in stone, and all Monday lunch seminars for the next 30 years started at 13.07. Future Monday lunch seminars were habitually held in the small seminar room (on the top floor), and generally the room was full; crowded conditions were felt to be right. At Pernis' seminar, Francis Loor showed fluorescence microscope pictures already made at the BII.

Inauguration of the BII, June 1971

More than 3 years had passed since Jerne and Jann shook hands to agree on the establishment of an immunology institute. Jerne received a 10-year guarantee for the existence of the institute. But 10 years since when? When was the actual "day zero" of those 10 years? Although it was not essential to be precise about the date, it was convenient to count from the time when the institute became fully functioning – that gave a true "full" 10 years, with the likelihood of continuing beyond that.

QR1971_04 BII

"Zero day" was chosen by Jerne to be June 17, 1971, and this was then the day on which the inauguration of the BII was set [QR1971_04]. The date was selected to coincide with the meeting of the International Advisory Board.

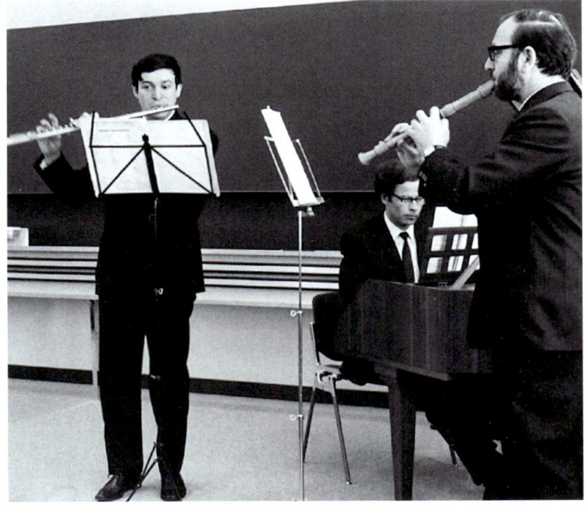

Louis Du Pasquier, Arnold Feinstein
(Helmut Pohlit at the harpsichord)

BASEL

INSTITUTE FOR IMMUNOLOGY

INAUGURATION

17th June, 1971

Gut zum Druck

Buchdruckerei zum Basler Berichthaus AG
Dufourstrasse 40, Telephon 061 23 10 77

Wir bitten Sie, diesen Probedruck nach erfolgter Prüfung möglichst bald zurückzusenden und ihn durch Ihre Unterschrift als «Gut zum Druck» zu bezeichnen. Da wir für stehengebliebene Fehler oder nachträgliche Änderungen am Satz jede Verantwortung ablehnen müssen, sind Korrekturen genau anzugeben. Das Original erbitten wir mit dem Probedruck zurück.

Auflage:

Datum: 14. 6. 71

Stempel und Unterschrift: Ivan Lefkovits

An die Buchdruckerei
zum Basler Berichthaus AG
Dufourstrasse 40
4000 BASEL

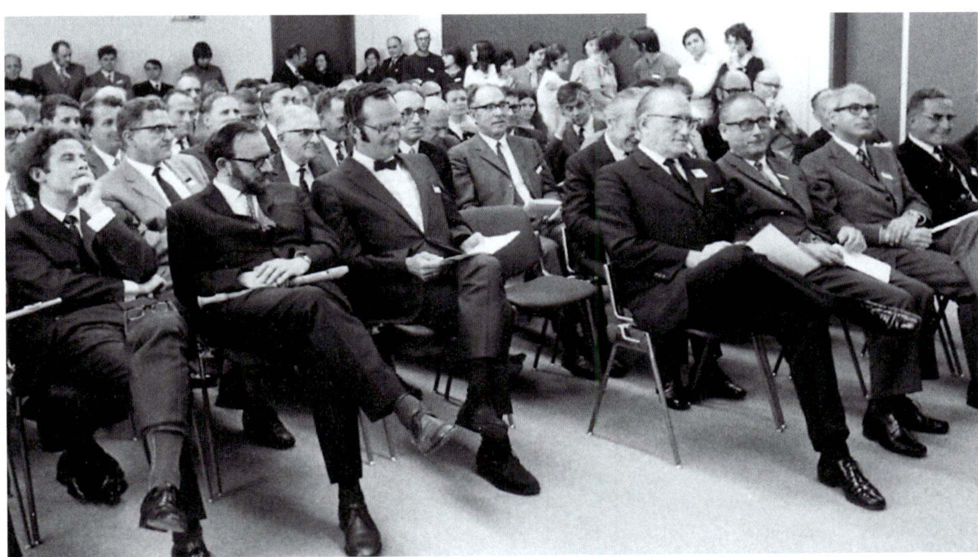

Lectures at the BII inauguration. Front row left to right: Helmut Pohlit, Arnold Feinstein, Howard Goodman, Adolf Jann, Alfred Pletscher and two representatives of the Roche Verwaltungsrat

The ceremony started with a musical prelude played on the treble recorder, flute and harpsichord by 3 members of the BII: Arnold Feinstein, Louis Du Pasquier and Helmut Pohlit, who interpreted pieces from Johann Sebastian Bach and Georg Friedrich Handel.

Adolf W. Jann, Alfred Pletscher, John H. Humphrey, Ernst Sorkin, Christoph Tamm, Hubert Bloch, Howard C. Goodman and Niels K. Jerne gave addresses. The speeches were followed with pieces by Henry Purcell, Carl Friedrich Abel and Claude Debussy, played by the above-mentioned members.

As our circle of knowledge expands, so does the circumference of darkness surrounding it.

Albert Einstein

The entire afternoon was reserved for science. Three lectures were given, all three on *diversity*. Niels Jerne and Stephen Fazekas each spoke about antibody diversity, and Ita Askonas about lymphocyte cell diversity. Board members moderated each lecture: the first lecture by Maaloe and Edelman, the second by Westphal and Sela, and the third by Dulbecco and Nossal.

The next day the Advisory Board convened with an agenda related to the experience of the past 8 months since the opening of the first section of the institute. Charley Steinberg and Ben Pernis assembled a synopsis of projects under way in the institute, and Niels Jerne reiterated the main research direction: diversity and heterogeneity of the components of the immune system (which was of course evident from the 3 lectures of the previous day). The board members prepared a report on the institute's activities, addressed to the Board of Trustees, and the Chairman of the Board, John Humphrey, and Vice-Chairman, Michael Sela, met Adolf Jann and handed over the Advisory Board statements. The meeting concluded with an invitation for dinner with Maja and Paul Sacher at their home in Frenkendorf [QR1971_05].

Tinguely's Double Helix

The institute was offered a present from the founding company Roche, and it was to be a sculpture signifying a cultural symbol related in some way to the new building. The artist designated to create the piece of art was Jean Tinguely [QR1971_06], a longstanding friend of the family of Maja and Paul Sacher. Obviously it was not a finished sculpture from the artist's warehouse, but rather a piece made to mark the institute and all it promised to become.

For Niels Jerne, a purist of science, this was a serious issue, and he and Tinguely met for many hours to discuss the project. Jerne explained the immune system and the basis of it, DNA, and Tinguely understood Jerne's point that without knowing the basic components of inheritance – the double helix of DNA – immunology could never become a solid scientific discipline.

QR1971_05 BII

When Jerne mentioned the spiral staircases connecting the labs between two floors, the idea to create a metallic counterpart of the biological double helix imprinted itself in Tinguely's mind. There was an extremely cordial relationship between Jerne and Tinguely. Jerne knew that it would be inappropriate to give Tinguely any further "instructions", nevertheless Jerne's last words were: "It could turn eternally, but it is not supposed to make any noise."

QR1971_06 BII

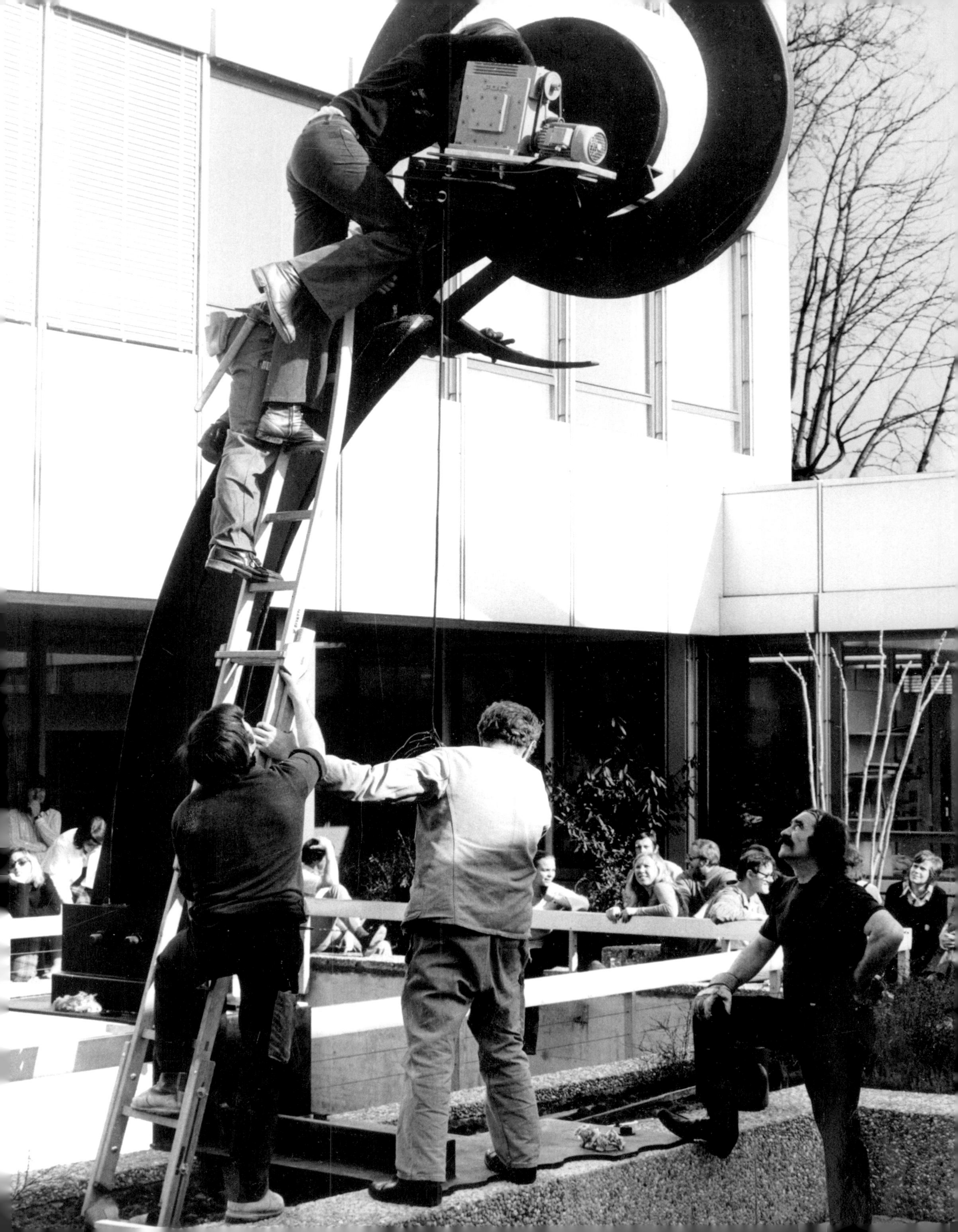

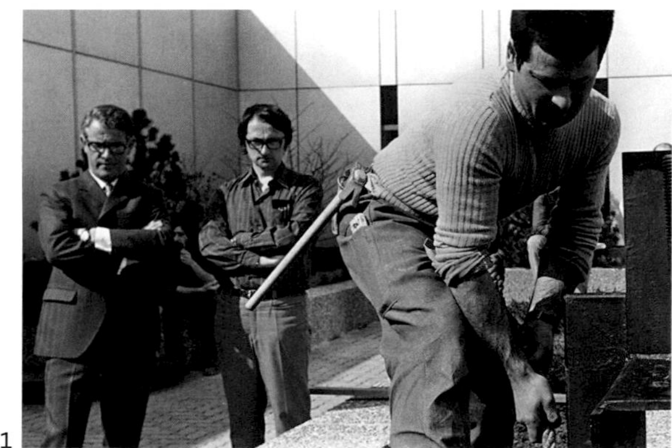
1

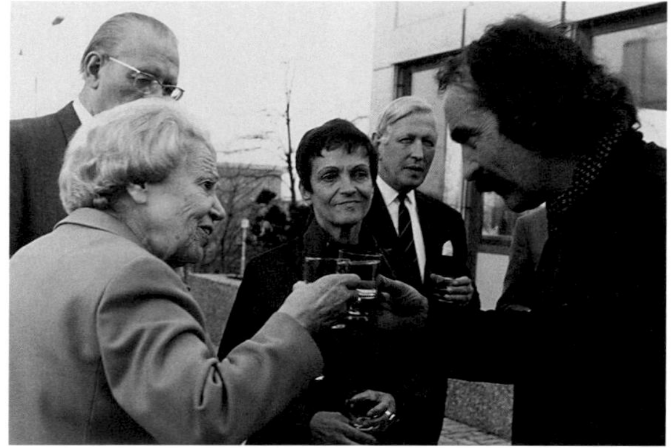
2

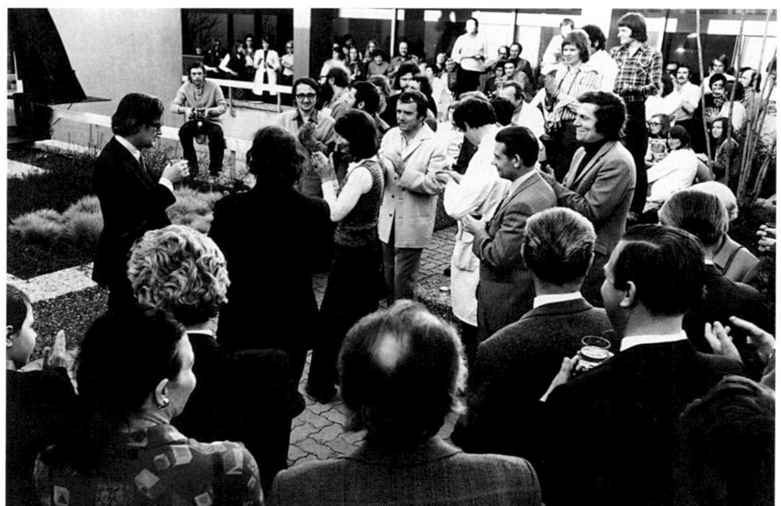
3

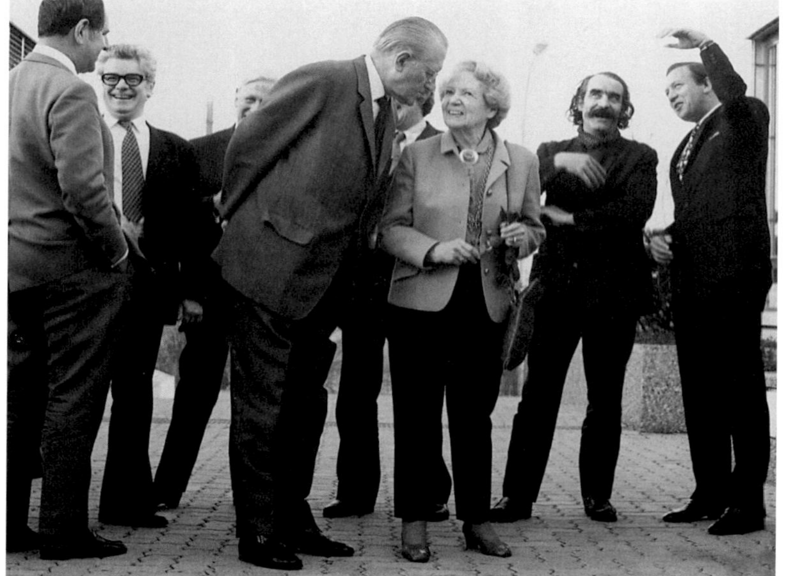
4

(Previous page) Tinguely supervises the Double Helix installation

1 Architect Mr. Wicki with Ivan Lefkovits

2 Maja Sacher and Jean Tinguely

3 Members of the BII at the inauguration

4 Adolf Jann listening to Maja Sacher

The Double Helix was installed at a festive occasion, and thereafter it turned day in, day out (except on rare occasions for maintenance) until the last day the BII existed. Now the Double Helix (to be mentioned in Book 2 of this treatise) is installed on the roof of the Tinguely Museum, and every visitor to Basel, arriving on the motorway from Zurich or Bern, sees the sculpture – not any more as an emblem of the BII, but of the city of Basel.

Gerry Edelman at the BII Lab Bench, 1971

Although Gerry Edelman came to Basel for the inauguration festivities of the BII and for the meeting of the Advisory Board, he spontaneously asked Niels Jerne whether he would be welcomed to stay for a few weeks at the BII, to make his hands wet with some experiments he had in mind but could not find time to get them done at home. Niels was very pleased, and Gerry got a lab bench (in Laboratory 12), technical help from a Swedish technician, and he made experiments on the attachment of lymphocytes to ConA-derivatized nylon fibers.

He promised to come back to Basel (to work), but the Nobel Prize that he received a year later kept him too busy. Nevertheless he came regularly for the Advisory Board meetings. He became a devoted friend of the BII, and in discussions with Adolf Jann, the President of Roche, he repatedly praised the wise and generous decision of creating the BII. From Basel he traveled directly to the First International Congress of Immunology in Washington.

The Challenge of Life

A few months after the inauguration of the BII, in September 1971, Hoffmann-La Roche organized a symposium called "The Challenge of Life" [QR1971_07] with the subtitle "Biomedical Progress and Human Values". It was a symposium to celebrate 75 years of Roche's existence, and it was a conference to show the deep commitment of the company to pursue biomedical science.

Roche invited eminent people from many branches of science and various cultural areas in order to start a dialog on the problems of biomedical progress. One of the speakers was Niels Jerne with a lecture entitled "Newer Knowledge of Immunobiology and Its Applications".

QR1971_07 BII

Among the speakers were Salvador Luria (MIT Cambridge, USA), Joshua Lederberg (Stanford University), Seymour Kety (Harvard Medical School) and also Margaret Mead (American

Museum of Natural History), Lord Zuckerman (Adviser to HM Government, London) and Jacques Monod (Collège de France, Paris). All the speakers and several participants visited the BII after the symposium. A book with the same title as the symposium's name was published a year later.

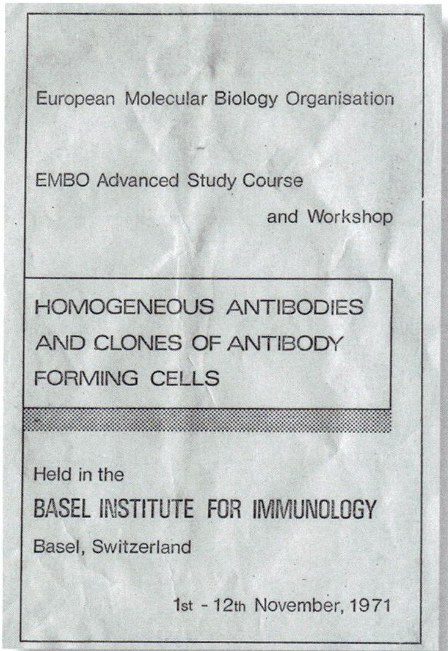
European Molecular Biology Organisation

EMBO Advanced Study Course
and Workshop

HOMOGENEOUS ANTIBODIES
AND CLONES OF ANTIBODY
FORMING CELLS

Held in the
BASEL INSTITUTE FOR IMMUNOLOGY
Basel, Switzerland

1st - 12th November, 1971

EMBO Advanced Study Course 1971

On November 1st, 1971, the first EMBO experimental course at the BII with the title "Homogeneous Antibodies and Clones of Antibody-Forming Cells" was organized [QR1971_08]. It was remarkable that a research institution – at such an early stage – was able to provide adequate facilities to carry out a course that required considerable resources and good logistics. It tested the functioning of the new institute to the limit.

The main emphasis was on producing antibody with restricted heterogeneity, as pioneered by Dietmar Braun and Jean-Claude Jaton. Besides that, the course dealt with induction of antibody-forming clones both in conventional cultures and in microcultures. The teaching staff, alongside Dietmar Braun and Jean-Claude Jaton, included Ivan Lefkovits, José Quintáns and Tien-Wen Tao-Wiedmann. There were 14 external participants and 8 BII members.

The course fulfilled its aim to disseminate information on emerging methodology.

Balance Sheet of 1971

For some members 1971 already marked a "complete" year of activities, while for many others it was just a period of instatement. Whether the institute was on a successful path was too early to judge, but at least it could be said that it was evidently not a flop. Three aspects of 1971 are worth emphasizing: (a) the institute became attractive for the entire world scientific community – scientists traveled to Basel to give seminars (and to watch the "marvel" of the BII coming into being); besides that, the First International Congress of Immunology took place in Washington, and the BII was a hot subject for corridor talks; (b) scientists became productive with an ease as if there were no gap between past and present; members who took up their appointments just months earlier became productive almost immediately; (c) publications, abstracts and reports from the institute started to surface in good journals, and 1971 was also the year in which the *European Journal of*

Immunology was founded, becoming an important platform for the publication of scientific papers from the BII.

Continuous Colloquium throughout the Year

As mentioned earlier, immediately after half the institute had opened in October 1970, scientists from all over the world came to give seminars. They presented results from their past and ongoing research, but they also wanted to check out the place they had heard about on the grapevine or from scientists already working there. In several instances the result of their visit was that they subsequently applied for a position. From the list of seminar speakers it was apparent that the spectrum of their research was considerably broader than the range of projects at the BII. Nevertheless the overall depth of presentations also served as a stimulus for Jerne to broaden his priorities and to include some additional aspects of immunology missing from his original choice.

There were 68 seminars given during 1971, and each one contributed to building a network of lasting interactions, resulting in collaborations and joint projects. These contacts were also utilized in the recruitment of instructors for the future international courses given at the BII.

Science in the Seminar Room

Visitors gave 53 seminars in 1971 [QR1971_09]:

K. Rajewsky, G. Pontecorvo, A. Bussard, G. Rossi, Y. Yagi, G.I. Holt, A.J. Munro, L.G. Caro, L. Cooper, M. Raff, P.J. McCullouch, T. Brunner, A.B. Edmundsen, C. Jenlin, I. McConnell, G.F. Mitchell, J. Cairns, J. Sterzl, W. Braun, V. Bockisch, G. Marin, K. Eichmann, A. de Weck, P.R. Carnegie, E. Möller, G.N. Edelman, D. Naor, W. Byrd, C.F. Fox, J. Dwyer, F. Modabber, F.W. Stahl, H.L. Spiegelberg, D. Metcalf, I. Pecht, G. Tridente, E. Vinuela, C. Brack, P. Valembois, S.W. Glover, C.W. Tedd, H. Frank, H. Strack, G. Cudkowicz, W. Ostortag, L. Suter, A. Durham, U. Schwarz, G. Bahr, M. Feldman, E. Kownatzki, C. Baglioni, S. Dray.

BII members gave 15 seminars [QR1971_10]:

Vincenzo Miggiano, Louis Du Pasquier, Dwight Anderson, Thomas Hohn, John Hay, Dietmar G. Braun, Eduard Kellenberger, Hansruedi Ramseier, Peter Lachmann, Jean-Claude Jaton, Arnold Feinstein, Susumu Tonegawa, Charles Steinberg, Ivan Lefkovits, Tien-Wen Tao-Wiedmann.

Science at the Bench

By the end of 1971 all the laboratories were functional and fully occupied by scientific staff as follows:

Laboratory 01	J.R.L. Pink, J.-C. Jaton
Laboratory 1	D.G. Braun, M. Cramer
Laboratory 2A	L. Du Pasquier, J. Haimovich, N. Weiss
Laboratory 2B	A.S. Kelus, T. Matsunaga
Laboratory 3A	J.B. Hay
Laboratory 3B	H.R. Ramseier, S. Zakarian
Laboratory 04	F. Melchers, R. Citronbaum, G. Köhler
Laboratory 4	H.R. Kiefer
Laboratory 5	R. Ceppellini, D. Bernoco, W. Mayr, S. Cullen, J. Lightbody, G. Trinchieri (shared with the group of E. Kellenberger)
Laboratory 6A	Z. Tökes
Laboratory 6B	S. Shin
Laboratory 7	J.A. Hamilton
Laboratory 8A	E.B. Jacobson
Laboratory 8B	F. Loor, B. Pernis, A. Luzzati
Laboratory 09	J. Andersson, O. Sjöberg, G. Möller, J. Obel
Laboratory 9	T. Meo, G. Vives, D. Shreffler, V.C. Miggiano I. Baldi, M. Nabholz
Laboratory 011	B. Kindred
Laboratory 11	S. Fazekas de St. Groth, W. Gerhard
Laboratory 012A	T.-W. Tao-Wiedmann, D. Dresser, J. Obel
Laboratory 012B	S. Tonegawa
Laboratory 12	I. Lefkovits, J. Quintáns
Laboratory 013	T. Staehelin, M. Schreier, W. McKeehan, I. Sundkvist, A. Falvey
Laboratory 13	G. Roelants, B.A. Askonas
Laboratory EM	T. Mandel
Laboratory ISO	H.M. Pohlit

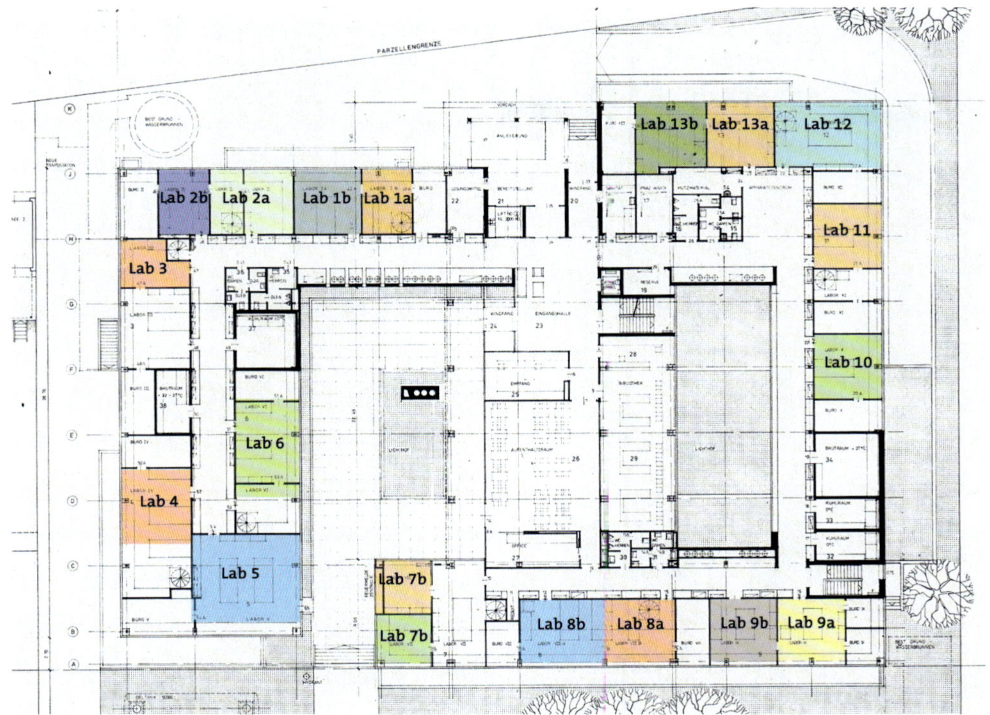

BII main floor (laboratories 1–12)

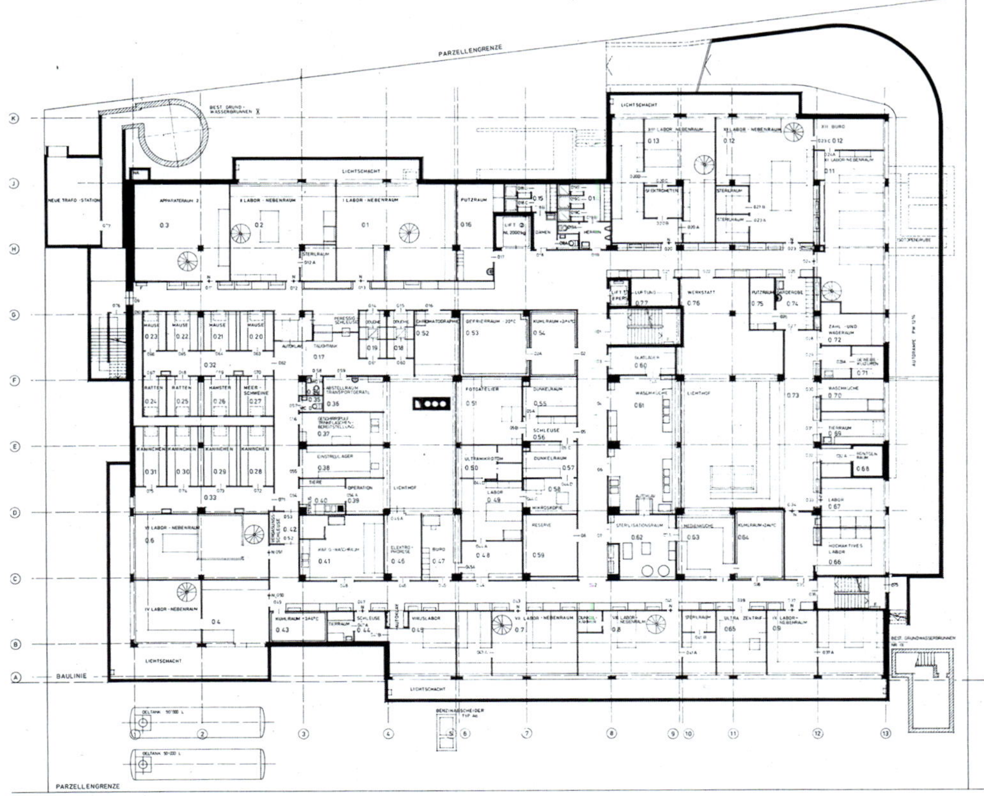

BII level 1 UG (laboratories 01–012)

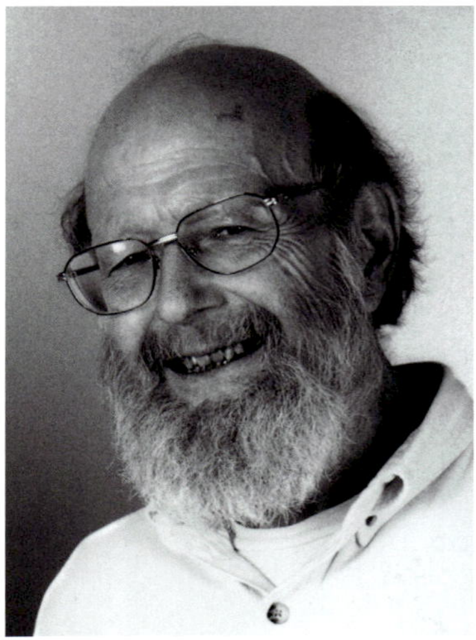

Charley Steinberg

The production of formal Annual Reports started only a year later. Therefore, information on science during 1971 was available only from a compilation of reports assembled by Charley Steinberg and Ben Pernis, prepared for Niels Jerne on the occasion of the Advisory Board meeting. The document was known as "Pernis-Steinberg Working Document 1971" [QR1971_11].

Niels Jerne reported at this Board meeting on the events of the year. He identified 16 research directions (lumping several projects together) which he presented as a synopsis. His list was as follows:

- Protein synthesis, initiation and elongation factors
- Intracellular and extracellular immunoglobulin in plasma cells and B cells
- Number of DNA copies for κ Ig light chains
- Antibodies of restricted heterogeneity
- Origin of antibody diversity
- Clones of cells producing antibody against phage
- Antigen-antibody reactions
- Lymphocyte membrane and receptors
- Lymphocyte triggering
- Regulatory factors released by lymphocytes
- Cell cooperation
- Allelic exclusion
- Somatic cell genetics
- Major histocompatibility complex
- Chimerism in mouse and man
- Genetic control of the immune response

These 16 areas of research did not imply 16 collaborative efforts, since the associations were loose ones. Nevertheless, the predilections of scientists led to future interactions. It is easy to decrypt that the topics were listed "from molecules to cells, to organism, to species". Within each topic, research projects were "lumped together" that Jerne considered as belonging together. For example, the entry "Origin of antibody diversity" carries the names of 6 scientists: Richard Pink, Louis Du Pasquier, Yossi Haimovich, Andrew Kelus, Georges Köhler, Stephen Fazekas. Each of these scientists had his own project, using his system and model, but nevertheless there was a common denominator, and Jerne provided a gentle hint: get together. And indeed interactions across all fields occurred.

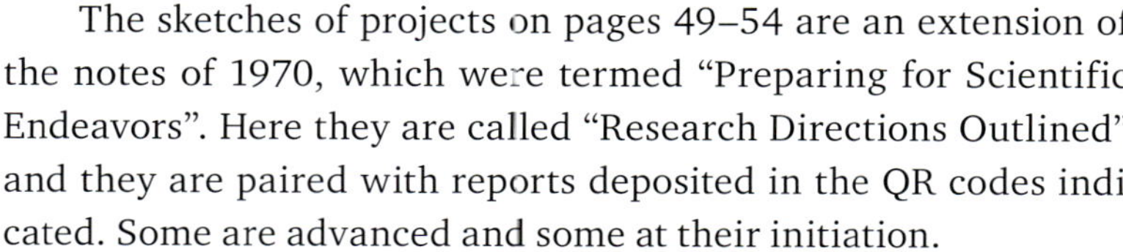

The sketches of projects on pages 49–54 are an extension of the notes of 1970, which were termed "Preparing for Scientific Endeavors". Here they are called "Research Directions Outlined", and they are paired with reports deposited in the QR codes indicated. Some are advanced and some at their initiation.

QR1971_11 BII

Research Directions Outlined, 1971

Protein Synthesis, Initiation and Elongation Factors

T. Staehelin, M. Schreier, W. McKeehan, I. Sundkvist

Although the protein synthesis in its general principles had been clarified, there were many important issues that had to be resolved before further advances on antibody synthesis could be accomplished. Using the model of synthesis of globin polypeptides it was found that the initiation of the synthesis of the two globin chains (α and β) occurs at different rates. But since both chains are required to be present in the cell at an equimolar ratio, the disbalance of the synthesis had to be compensated "somehow", and it was found that this is achieved by a higher copy number of mRNA for that chain that is synthesized at a slower rate, i.e. mRNA for α-chain. Minute alterations of Mg^{2+} ion concentration (in the translation system) greatly affect the ratio of α- to β-chain synthesis. Importantly, it was found that factors that are essential for the initiation of protein synthesis bind to the smaller subunit of ribosomes and can be removed by high salt. These factors are forming an initiation complex with Met-tRNA(F) and ribosomes, which was found to be true for both mammalian and bacterial mRNA translational systems.

With the above knowledge on the initiation of protein synthesis, experiments became feasible to study the events related to the "growing polypeptide", i.e. the elongation of the nascent protein molecule.

Intracellular and Extracellular Immunoglobulin in Plasma Cells and B Cells

F. Melchers, J. Andersson, R. Citronbaum

B cells were known to be the precursors of the actual antibody-forming cells. Upon antigenic stimulation, small B cells clonally expand into a population of blast cells, and these turn into plasma cells that are capable of synthesizing and secreting large amounts of antibody molecules. When zooming into subcellular components of such cells, it was found that different subcellular fractions of plasma cells differ in carbohydrate content, such that rough membranes contained N-acetylglucosamine and mannose residues, while smooth membranes contained also galactose and N-glycolylneuraminic acid. Through pulse-chase experiments the actual assembly line for immunoglobulin molecules that are ready to be secreted from the cells has been identified.

In parallel, immunoglobulin synthesis and secretion in small B lymphocytes were studied upon nonspecific stimulation of cells by locally concentrated concanavalin A. The time course of intracellular synthesis of IgM early after stimulation was established, and the conditions for the secretion of IgM were identified. It was found that the intracellular precursor IgM exists as a 7S structure, while the secreted IgM exists in 19S form. The two forms had different carbohydrate residues. The number of glucosamine, mannose, galactose and fucose residues present in free and membrane-bound immunoglobulins was found to be characteristic of the state of synthesis and secretion.

Number of DNA Copies for κ Ig Light Chains

S. Tonegawa

First steps towards determining the number of DNA copies for immunoglobulin light chains were done by concentrating on a special variant of the myeloma cells (70E). This variant has the distinct property that instead of secreting entire immunoglobulin molecules, it synthesizes and secretes light chain molecules only. RNA preparation isolated by Staehelin's method through sucrose gradient centrifugation, separating messenger RNA from ribosomal RNA, was subjected to polyacrylamide gel electrophoresis. Out of 25 detected autoradiographic bands, the band of 180,000 Da molecular mass was assigned for the Ig light chain mRNA, as verified by in vitro translation by Schreier and Staehelin.

Antibodies of Restricted Heterogeneity

Y. Haimovich, J.-C. Jaton, J.R.L. Pink, D.G. Braun, M. Cramer, A.S. Kelus

Although immunization in general does not aim at creating "degenerate" conditions in which the resulting antibody has a very narrow spectrum of specificities, there is at least one special case where such antibody is needed. Studies of structural properties of antibody, especially the amino acid sequence, relied on the availability of "homogeneous samples". For various species different immunization schemes were developed through which antibody production of restricted heterogeneity was achieved. Guinea pigs, rabbits and mice were used as experimental animals, and DNP-protein conjugates, pneumococcal and streptococcal polysaccharides, were applied as antigens. These experiments were done years before the advent of monoclonal antibody. Therefore, antibody populations of restricted heterogeneity had to play "temporarily" the role of homogeneous antibody. The methodology of amino acid sequencing was still in its infancy; nevertheless, these experiments paved the way for new experimental approaches. Tryptic peptides were analyzed, idiotypic and allotypic markers identified, genetic background scrutinized, and selective breeding established; the dose of antigen and route of injection were optimized. The wide range of animal species available in the institute (mouse, guinea pig, rabbit, sheep and to some extent human) enabled the comparison of segments of immunoglobulin chains of one species that were similar to the homologous segments in other species with other segments that appear to be highly variable.

Origin of Antibody Diversity

J.R.L. Pink, L. Du Pasquier, Y. Haimovich, A.S. Kelus, G. Köhler, S. Fazekas de St. Groth

The functional requirements of the immune system do not allow the dominance of homogeneity, but quite to the contrary, they are based on heterogeneity. Several research groups contributed to elucidating the repertoire of antibody production and to the regulation of the immune responses that promote the heterogeneity of the resulting antibody. Chickens, mice, rabbits, frogs (tadpoles) and also marsupials were used to follow antibody responses to DNP and TNP, to bacteriophage ΦX, to β-galactosidase and to Proteus vaccines. Readout of the heterogeneity was performed by analyzing isoelectric focusing patterns, antibody titer in the sera, and by measuring the affinity of the antibodies.

An assortment of findings was attained: the chicken served as a suitable model for studying cellular events occurring in the bursa, spleen and in other immunologically relevant organs; antibody was found to be heterogeneous not only when immunizing the adult but also young chicken, though the avidity of the antibodies was lower in the young than in adult chicken; maturation of the immune machinery in the chicken was well documented; tadpoles containing less than a million lymphocytes were able to mount an antibody response although with resulting antibody of low affinity; inactive mutant enzymes (β-galactosidase) were activated by distinct populations of antibodies within the serum of a rabbit; a bacteriophage neutralization assay offered itself for studying the kinetics of primary and secondary antibody response to bacteriophage ΦX; location of idiotypic determinants on immunoglobulins both in mice and rabbits served as a measure of the heterogeneity of the resulting antibodies.

Clones of Cells Producing Antibody against Phage

J. Obel, T.-W. Tao-Wiedmann, H. Pohlit

Bacteriophage was not only the most powerful tool of molecular biologists, but it found also its way into the field of immunology. This was the case both because of its antigenic properties and as a highly sensitive target for studying the fine specificity and homogeneity of antibodies. With bacteriophage ΦX it was possible to detect antibody-specific inactivation levels of phage mutants that were far superior to the sensitivity of classical hemolytic or hemagglutination titrations.

Antigen-Antibody Reactions

S. Fazekas de St. Groth, W. Gerhard, T.-W. Tao-Wiedmann, D. Dresser, H. Pohlit, F. Melchers

Various models were established to study the interaction of antibody with its immunizing and boosting antigens. Offering the newly introduced definition of epitopes and paratopes it became possible to define the property of these complementary entities with great precision. Antibody populations specific for influenza viruses were scrutinized to discover the effect of sequential vaccination with cross-reactive influenza viruses. The quality of antibody was established by measuring equilibrium constants against immunizing and boosting antigens. It was found that single-step antigenic mutants yielded antibody of increased affinity, though the prevalent antibody that is produced is the kind which was produced on the first encounter (doctrine of the original antigenic sin). Another approach of the antigen-antibody reactions was based on rigorous mathematical analysis of affinity distributions obtained for the hapten/monovalent antibody system. Further a cellular assay for enumerating cells producing antibodies against bacteriophage (ΦX as a model) by "reverse plaquing" was used to define the property of antigen-antibody interactions. Activation of β-galactosidase mutants by antibody that is directed to a special epitope of the enzyme enabled the activity of single molecules of the enzyme to be measured. Besides the others, it was possible to establish that the Michaelis-Menten constant of antibody-activated enzyme is lower than that of the wild-type enzyme.

Lymphocyte Membrane and Receptors

N. Weiss, L. Du Pasquier, H.-R. Kiefer, S. Cullen, D. Bernoco, V.C. Miggiano, R. Ceppellini, J.A. Hamilton, B. Pernis, F. Loor

The basics of B cells and T cells had been established through work of many laboratories worldwide. In Basel the scrutiny was extended to inspecting the cells of the immune system in several additional species. It was a surprise that a subpopulation of amphibian thymocytes express (at least transitionally) immunoglobulin molecules on their surface, revealed by staining with an Ig-specific antiserum. Some controversial observations appeared in respect of the nature of T cell receptors. Nevertheless, one solid finding prevailed, i.e. anti-θ serum selectively destroyed T cells.

Numerous approaches were tried out to selectively bind lymphocytes to various antigen-derivatized solid supports, such as hapten-derivatized nylon meshes, or antigen coupled to the surface of Petri dishes or to various sorts of beads. This was done either for counting the proportion of cells with demonstrable binding properties or for actual fractionation of (native or hapten-primed) lymphocytes. This led to first estimates of frequencies of antigen-binding cells (1 in 20,000 nonprimed cells recovered from the derivatized fibers, in contrast to close to 1 in 100 cells from the primed population).

A major study revealed a profound mobility of components of the lymphocyte membrane. It was found that the distribution of Ig receptors on the membrane of untreated cells is truly homogeneous. Admixture of anti-Ig causes binding to Ig receptors, which induces cross-linking, followed by patch formation and finally "cap" formation. After a time period the cap disappeared by endocytosis, and new Ig receptors reappeared in increased numbers.

The work on "patch" and "cap" formation prompted experimentation on the clearance of anti-HLA antibodies from the membrane of human lymphocytes. The topography of HLA molecules on the membrane was scrutinized. It was found that human lymphocytes are susceptible to complement-dependent lysis only if they were tested "immediately" after allowing HLA antiserum to be absorbed to human lymphocytes. When cells that scored positive for several HLA antigens were sensitized with a monospecific serum and then tested for their ability to endocytose the complex of the HLA antigens, only those HLA molecules that were not reacting with the monospecific serum were endocytosed.

Lymphocyte Triggering

J. Andersson, O. Sjöberg, J. Obel, I. Lefkovits, B. Askonas, G. Roelants

It was well known that the immune response is based on clonal proliferation of lymphocytes. The actual processes, however, like the nature of signals needed for triggering the lymphocytes to enter cell division, and to steer the progeny towards antibody production, were not yet elucidated.

Induction of the primary antibody response by isolated mouse lymphocytes in vitro offered a powerful tool for studying the triggering events at the initiation of the immune response. The methodology existed also in a scaled-down system (a microculture system) that was used to estimate the number of precursor cells involved in the response and also to estimate the size of the resulting antibody-forming clones.

Extensive work has been done on antigen-specific and non-antigen-specific B cell regulation, on signals affecting cell division, and on the role of syngeneic and allogeneic T cells and their products. Both antigens (sheep red cells and various hapten carrier models) as well as mitogens (especially LPS) were applied. Primary and secondary responses were studied with the important finding that B memory cells transferred to irradiated hosts (mice) became functional in the new environment, such that a dose of one million primed cells yielded 1–4 anti-DNP clones in the recipient mouse. This work was refined using hapten carrier permutations, e.g. primary response induced by a certain antigen and followed by challenge with a cross-reacting or non-cross-reacting antigen.

Conditions for participation of B cells and T cells in the antigen-driven response were established, and also conditions under which a response could be prevented or suppressed.

Regulatory Factors Released by Lymphocytes

J. Hay, I. Lefkovits, M. Schreier, T. Staehelin

For a long time there were reports on various soluble factors that affect the cells of the immune system. It was not clear whether they had anything to do with the specificity of the immune response or maybe with some other side aspects of the immune system. In the years when T and B cell interaction was scrutinized, it was not even clear whether T cell-B cell interaction occurs via cell-to-cell contact or through soluble mediators. Therefore attention was given to factors released by lymphocytes and other cells of the immune system.

One of the most prominently studied soluble factors was macrophage migration inhibitory factor (MIF). MIF was originally discovered as a soluble factor involved in delayed hypersensitivity and in various macrophage functions, including phagocytosis, and tumoricidal activity. Several protocols were developed to produce MIF, and several neat systems were used to test the activity – mainly the "migration inhibitory" activity of macrophages (as the name of the factor indicates). Experiments in those days were of importance, but later the structure (and function) became fully clarified, and MIF importance has been seen in fields other than immunology.

Several laboratories shared the interest in the production, isolation and characterization of the T-cell-replacing factor. Collaborative efforts were made such that some groups produced the factor (most effectively by allogeneic interaction of T cell populations of different histocompatibility background), while others attempted fractionation, purification and characterization of the obtained preparations. These efforts were of importance then and helped to advance the field; nevertheless, only decades later (due to molecular cloning) did the structural definitions become available. T-cell-replacing activity fell into several groups: T-cell-replacing factors 1, 2, 3, etc. Tentative names were given to different interleukins. One of the T-cell-replacing factors was found to be identical to "B cell growth factor II". Two main interleukin activities targeting B cells were: products involved in B cell proliferation (BCGF) and products involved in B cell differentiation (BCDF), mostly responsible for maturation of activated B cells into immunoglobulin-secreting cells. Even this classification is being reexamined and unified.

Cell Cooperation

B. Kindred, T.-W. Tao-Wiedmann, D. Dresser

T cell-B cell cooperation was successfully studied in systems in which cell populations could be admixed at will to create functional responding systems. Useful models were established using athymic nude mice, but also thymectomized or irradiated mice. Nude mice were especially suitable as they not only lacked a functional thymus but also displayed a very low level of immunoglobulin in the serum. Nude mice available at the BII were obtained by (partial) backcrossing to C57BL/6 background, thus possessing H-2b alleles. It was found that long-lasting cooperation (in terms of mounting a full immune response) was achieved only if the cells (B and T) had the same H-2 alleles.

Parallel to the question of requirement of matching histocompatibility alleles there was a question whether or not immunological memory can be induced in the absence of T cells. In most attempts establishing of memory under such conditions (in nude mice) failed. Both problems were addressed using an in vivo situation, since reconstitution of responses in vitro was always achievable due to the allogeneic effect. Helper function involved in the in vitro reconstitution experiments was not antigen-specific. The finding that the necessity for using the same hapten-carrier conjugate, both in primary and secondary response, is overcome in a GvH situation. This was a strong indication that the allogeneic effect supports cell-cell cooperation in an antigen nonspecific manner in terms of T cell carrier specificity.

Cell cooperation in the responses to bacteriophage ΦX was studied both in the mouse (nude, thymectomized, normal) and also in organ cultures of rabbit lymphoid tissue. It was found that initiation of primary and memory responses in terms of IgM and IgG responses to ΦX epitopes was successful using organ culture of rabbit lymphoid tissues. The absence of the thymus (thymectomy, irradiation) diminished the response to ΦX.

T cell help was shown to be required both for clonal proliferation and differentiation into antibody-secreting cells, though for proliferation help it is required to a lesser extent than for differentiation.

Allelic Exclusion

B. Pernis, A. Luzzati, A.S. Kelus, J.A. Hamilton, I. Lefkovits

Several years before the BII was created, Pernis (founding member of the BII) discovered that from the two alleles that the lymphocyte possesses in terms of immunoglobulin expression, only one is expressed. This expression profile that is clonally inherited was called allelic exclusion. Allelic exclusion became an important subject for scrutiny both in mice and rabbits. Genetic markers for allotypes were established, and antiallotypic antisera were produced. It was shown that allotypic suppression both in rabbit and mouse species could be induced. Attempts were made to break allotype suppression by cell transfer into irradiated recipient animals.

The expression of allotypes enabled analysis at the clonal level in cell cultures with a limiting number of rabbit peripheral blood cells. Studies related to the switch from IgM to IgG were done; the results showed that the allotype is maintained after the switch and that the allelic exclusion is a stable feature of the resulting clones.

Several other experiments, of some importance at that time, were performed: implantation of normal cells into the peritoneal cavity of suppressed mice; resolving whether B cells may be primed in the absence of thymus, and histological survey of the inability of nude mice to switch from IgM to IgG, studied with particular emphasis on the formation of germinal centers.

Somatic Cell Genetics

S. Shin, I. Baldi, V. Miggiano, M. Nabholz, D. Shreffler

The institute brought together people experienced in somatic cell hybridization. Hybrids between cells of mouse and human origin were obtained by Sendai virus-mediated fusion, followed by HAT selection. The main emphasis of the studies was on the enzymology and immunochemistry of the HGPRT (hypoxanthine-guanine phosphoribosyl transferase). The aim was to study the nature of somatic mutations. Since these experiments have foreshadowed the era of monoclonal antibody, a relevant quote from the report of Seung-il Shin is reproduced here: "We set out to produce hybrids from lymphocytes and lymphocyte-derived cells in order to analyze the control mechanisms governing antibody synthesis..." Other attempts were towards establishing man-mouse hybrids for studying cell surface structures (HLA, immunoglobulins, viral receptors) and following their chromosomal content. Serologically the expression of man and mouse histocompatibility markers was analyzed.

Major Histocompatibility Complex

A.S. Kelus, L. Du Pasquier, J. Theodor, S. Zakarian, D. Bernoco, W. Mayr, R. Ceppellini, J. Lightbody, V.C. Miggiano, G. Trinchieri, T. Meo, G. Vives

Histocompatibility antigens were to play a major role in most immunologically relevant research endeavors. This was the case for histocompatibility models of the human (HLA) and mouse (H-2), and it has been recognized that there is a (not yet elucidated) common principle of histocompatibility organization in man and the mouse. Many methodological approaches were developed, the aim of which was to measure reactions of cell compatibilities (mixed-lymphocyte reactions, cell-mediated lympholysis, and in vitro equivalents of graft-versus-host reactions). The main emphasis (that of clinical relevance) was on the survey of the distribution of HLA antigens in the population of the world. Issues that were far beyond the basic research, like establishing blood donor panels, were prominently discussed. The fact that antigenic structure of corals was also studied was only logical in the context of conservation or divergence in evolutionary context of the histocompatibility.

There was strong emphasis at the BII to study the histocompatibility system. The structure of the institute prevented strong expansion of some projects at the cost of other equally important projects. The HLA research developed into a strong collaborative effort that included many other laboratories, and in a later portion of this book there will be a special chapter just on this issue.

Chimerism in Mouse and Man

T. Matsunaga, A.S. Kelus, D. Bernoco, V. Miggiano, R. Ceppellini

Chimeric mice became a usable tool in immunological research, as they allow investigation of special conditions in animals that have two distinct genetic pools. Since in mouse chimeras the inner cell mass of implanted blastocysts contributed to all cell lineages, studies on immune competence and mutual tolerance became feasible, and lymphocyte mosaicism and immunoglobulin gene expression has been investigated, and mutual tolerance was confirmed. Tolerance and pathology in tetragametic (allophenic) human chimera was studied.

Genetic Control of the Immune Response

R. Ceppellini, S. Fazekas de St. Groth, B. Kindred

Besides an experimental approach in studies of histocompatibility antigens, an attempt was made to combine classical genetics with the findings on immune responsiveness to specific antigens. Convergence of the results with those from other groups led to the discovery of immune response (Ir) genes (Ir genes were defined as being closely linked to major histocompatibility loci of the species).

In the mouse species, studies of responsiveness to various mutants of influenza virus were undertaken. A unifying mechanism for the genetic control of the immune response to influenza virus was proposed, based on the asymmetric nature of the antigenic cross-reactions observed between parent viruses and their mutants selected in the presence of neutralizing antibodies.

Published Papers and Submitted Manuscripts of 1971

By the end of 1971, a total of 17 papers had been published [QR1971_12] and 46 manuscripts submitted for publication. Most importantly, there was Niels Jerne's paper on somatic generation of immune recognition. It was "paper number one" of the newly founded periodical *European Journal of Immunology* (it was the first article in issue 1, volume 1, 1971).

For this year and for all those to follow, the publications were the only measurable output of the institute's activity, and in turn this was also the criterion for measuring the contribution of individual members to the "rich cornucopia" of scientific knowledge. Other scientometric criteria, such as "impact factors" or "H-indices" were not yet widely used. During the institute's 30 years of existence, over 3,000 papers were published, as will be described in later sections of this book.

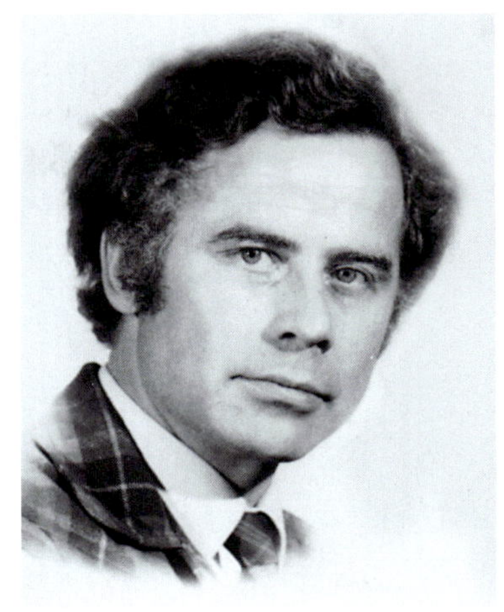

Helmut Pohlit

Papers published in 1971

Jerne NK, Eur J Immunol 1971;1:1–9
Kelus AS, Pernis B, Eur J Immunol 1971;1:123–132
Dubochet J, in Principles and Techniques of Electron Microscopy, ed Hayat MA, New York, Van Nostrand Reinhold Publishing, 1971
Wolf B, Janeway CA Jr, Coombs RRA, Catty D, Gell PGH, Kelus AS, Immunology 1971;20:931–944
Coombs RRA, Kelus AS, in Human Anti-Human Gammaglobulins, ed Grubb R, Samuelsson G, Oxford, Pergamon Press, 1971
Ceppellini R, in Progress in Immunology, ed Amos B, Academic Press, 1971, p 973
Loor F, Immunology 1971;21:557–564
Ramseier H, Lindenmann J, Eur J Immunol 1971;2:348–351
Lightbody J, Bernoco D, Miggiano VC, Ceppellini R, Virol Immunol 1971;64:243–254
Bernoco D, Mattiuz PL, Miggiano VC, Ceppellini R, Virol Inmunol 1971;64:272–284
Rajewsky K, Pohlit H, in Progress in Immunology, Academic Press, 1971, pp 337–354
von Borstel RC, Cain KT, Steinberg CM, Genetics 1971;69:17–27
Tao TW, Proc IVth Int Congr Radiation Res, 1971, p 100
Ramseier H, Lindenmann J, J Exp Med 1971;134:1083–1094
Ramseier H, Eur J Immunol 1971;1:433–441
Ramseier H, Lindenmann J, Eur J Immunol 1971;1:441–446
Jerne N, in Ontogeny of Acquired Immunity, Ciba Foundation Symposium, Elsevier, 1971, pp 1–15

QR1971_12 BII

First International Congress of Immunology, 1971

The Immunology Congress in Washington, D.C., in August 1971 [QR1971_13] was an event of prime importance, and the congresses that followed (in 3-year intervals) became even more prominent.

QR1971_13 BII

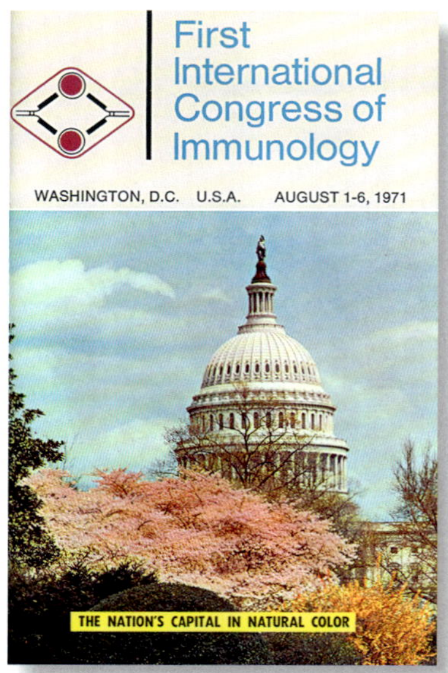

In Washington, the foundation of the BII had been a hot topic of conversation; Gerry Edelman just completed a visit at the BII and told the world about the wonder in Basel.

The President of the Congress was Maurice Landy, who soon after the congress settled permanently in Switzerland (Davos) and remained a good friend of the BII.

Two papers authored (and co-authored) by BII members were presented at the congress and published in the congress proceedings (Progress in Immunology, Academic Press, 1971).

BII List of Scientists in 1971

The list below gives the names of scientists who were members of the BII in 1971 [QR1971_14]. All these scientists and the projects they were involved in have been portrayed in the previous chapters:

Jan Andersson, Brigitte Askonas, Irene Baldi, Domenico Bernoco, Dietmar G. Braun, Ruggero Ceppellini, Ronald Citronbaum, Matthias Cramer, Susan E. Cullen, David W. Dresser, Louis Du Pasquier, Stephen Fazekas de St. Groth, Joseph Haimovich, J.A. Hamilton, John B. Hay, Ethel B. Jacobson, Jean-Claude Jaton, Andrew S. Kelus, Hansruedi Kiefer, Berenice Kindred, Georges Köhler, J. Lightbody, Ivan Lefkovits, Francis Loor, Alma L. Luzzati, Tom Mandel, Takeshi Matsunaga, Wolfgang R. Mayr, Wallace L. McKeehan, Fritz Melchers, Tommaso Meo, Vincenzo C. Miggiano, Göran Möller, Markus Nabholz, Jan Obel, Benvenuto Pernis, John R.L. Pink, Helmut Pohlit, José Quintáns, Hansruedi Ramseier, Georges E. Roelants, Max H. Schreier, Seung-il Shin, Donald C. Shreffler, Olof Sjöberg, Theophil Staehelin, Charles M. Steinberg, Ingegerd Sundkvist, Tien-Wen Tao-Wiedmann, Zoltan A. Tökés, Susumu Tonegawa, Giorgio Trinchieri, Zdenek Trnka, Jorge Vives, Niklaus Weiss, Siraik Zakarian.

This makes a total of 56 scientists. Members of the Kellenberger group (Dwight Anderson, Gus Doerman, Jacques Dubochet, Frederick A. Eiserling, Thomas and Barbara Hohn, Eduard Kellenberger) are not included in the list as they were guests with the distinct status of "Biozentrum group", as explained elsewhere.

Three scientists who left the BII before the end of 1971 do not appear on the list: Peter Lachmann, Arnold Feinstein and Klaus Rajewsky (these three scientists kept coming repeatedly to the BII in later years – for shorter or longer visits). John Griffith was on the members' list but sadly died during 1971, and was known only to the starting nucleus of BII members.

QR1971_14 BII

BII List of Technicians in 1971

Selecting good scientists did not mean selecting for the ability to perform adequate research and run good experiments. To do that, good technicians had to be hired [QR1971_15]. It was mentioned earlier that Göran Möller from Stockholm and Ita Askonas from London offered to head-hunt for good technicians. This worked out very well, and from 1970 to 1971 there were 57 technicians (49 female, 8 male):

Kerstin Andersson, Theo Baltz, Marietta Bernoco, Inga Birgen, Roberto Boccardo, Karin Burvall, S.M. Chambers, Michel Couture, Kerstin Dahlberg, Allan D'Arcy, Susan Davies, I.K. Dale, Nancy M. Erhardt, Panfilo Federico, Luciana Forni, Ingeborg Gerstner, Monica Gidlund, Pamela Grant, Chantal Guiet, Lena-Britt Hägg, Birgitta Hagström, John Hatton, Moira Henderson, Kerstin Hild, Elisabeth Hillebrand, Hansjörg Hoch, Laurence Hoch, June Hornby, Walter Hunkeler, Wendy J. Hunter, Janet Irwin, Reto Jaeggi, Dorothee Jablonski, B. Johansson, I. Kinell, Birgitte Elisé Kugelberg, Ann Langeveld, Pierre Lix, Jennifer Lowe, Dorothy D. Mauce, Dorothea Mayr, Mary Patricia McNally, Ingrid Möllegard, Pauline Moorhouse, Mary B. Oliver, Doris Plüss, Anne-Marie Rijnbeek, Aina Rydén, Monica Schöld, Marianne Schweizer, Helena Skarvall, Melvin Slaughter, Anita Söderberg, Ruth Stewart, Irene Sträuli, Ingegard Sundquist, Reet Tees.

Technicians should be under the supervision of the scientist in whose work they participate and in no way be under the control of the administration with respect to such matters as weekly working hours.

The strength and also the weakness of the institute was that the academic freedom was only intended for scientists. Technicians with considerable formal qualifications (technicians trained at specialized schools and also some with a BSc degree) were included in research projects, but with the explicit goal of helping scientists to perform experimental work.

In many instances technicians were co-authors of publications, and there was an unwritten rule for including or not including them as co-authors. The prerequisite for co-authorship was that the technician understood the project, and was able to give a seminar or to explain the procedures to a third party (e.g. by presenting a poster).

The horizontal structure of the institute had foreseen that each scientist received help from 1 technician. Mini-groups of 2 scientists + 2 technicians worked out well. There were, however, special experimental techniques that required additional pairs of hands (e.g. protein chemistry and amino acid sequencing).

The work contracts for scientists and technicians were different. Scientific staff (except for permanent members) had time-limited contracts, while the technicians were hired as regular employees. In spite of the fact that scientists had their "academic freedom" and technicians were "regular employees", there was rarely a problem with this incongruence. Scientists expected that the technicians worked extra hours and on weekends. The technicians fulfilled this expectation and received compensating free time (e.g. a long weekend) without additional payment for extra hours.

QR1971_15 BII

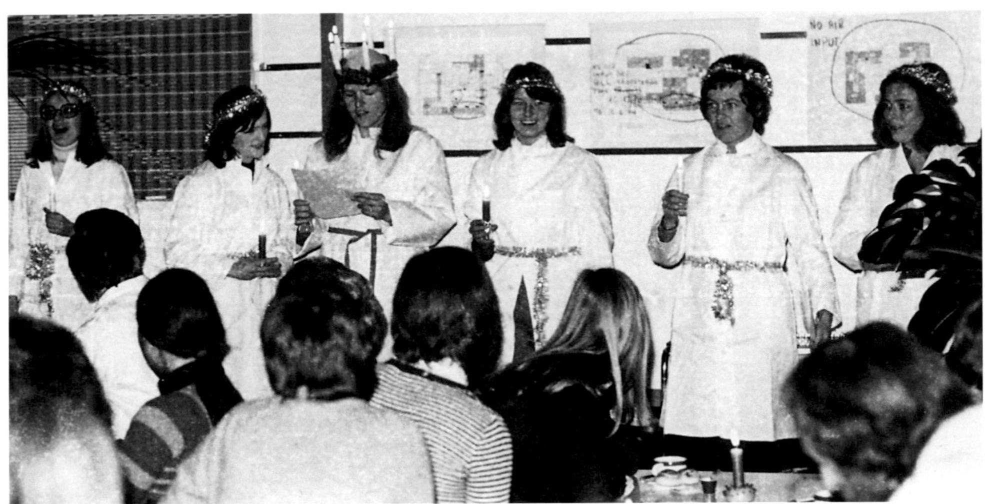

Santa Lucia with Swedish lyrics and Neapolitan songs

The technicians recruited in the starting years of 1970 and 1971 worked for scientists who were only insignificantly older than they were. As time went by, a "demographic shift" took place, and the technicians became senior in age to newly arriving scientists. Thus, in the decades of their work at the BII, due to the turnover of scientists, they had 6, 7 or more bosses who were getting younger and younger than they were.

Furthermore, technicians were the driving force behind many social activities: parties, outings, etc. One event – initiated in December 1971 – became a beautiful tradition of the institute, and it was the celebration of Santa Lucia on December 13th.

The BII Facilities

Although the inauguration of the institute was in June 1971, two months earlier, i.e. by April 1st, 1971, all the laboratories were completed and started functioning. The institute comprising 1,800 m^2 laboratory space (including the radioisotope unit, X-ray facilities and electron microscopy unit), 100 m^2 library, 150 m^2 cold rooms and incubator rooms, 200 m^2 cafeteria and reception area, 500 m^2 animal facilities, 200 m^2 media kitchen and workshop, and 600 m^2 space in the tower (a seminar room, guest rooms, offices for scientists and administrative staff) changed from the architects' hands to institute management. Lefkovits signed the last floor plan to ratify the completion of the institute's construction.

It was intended that the BII accommodate some 150 employees: 50 scientists, 50 technicians and 50 maintenance staff (administration, workshop, animal care, cafeteria, library, etc.). Niels Jerne was convinced that all successful research institutes were crowded, not only because good institutions attract more people than they have room for, but also because crowding promotes interaction among scientists.

The administrative infrastructure comprised secretarial services, art work office, photographic lab, library, telephone operator and receptionist, animal care, mechanical and electronic workshop, media preparation and wash kitchen, cleaning personnel, drivers and some highly specialized services such as the cell sorting facilities and the radioisotope lab. Surprisingly, 50 people (later 60) were able to take care of everything. It all worked well, people smiled and were happy…

The head of infrastructure from the early planning phase until the devastating fire at the institute (1985) was the unforgettable Jacques Bron [QR1971_16]. He was considered by everyone to be very kind, very efficient and somebody who was able to please everyone, and do everything needed for the smooth running of the institute.

Although the main emphasis in this volume is placed on science and on the people doing the science, all the other activities and the facilities that made the institute so attractive to scientists are described as well.

QR1971_16 BII

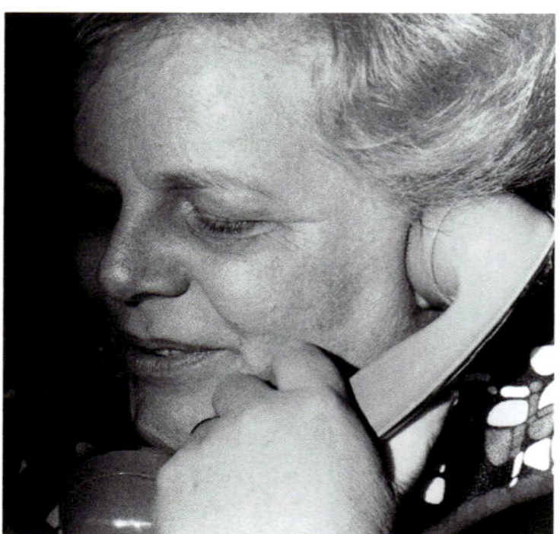

Elsi Degen

Reception

The reception area [QR1971_17] was considered to be the "friendly face" of the institute. There was no formal registration of visitors but they usually stopped at the desk. During the entire era of the BII the key person at reception was Elsi Degen. Elsi had both profound visual recognition ability and an infallible memory for numbers, names, addresses and data. She knew everybody, remembered every phone number and was kind to everybody. Scientists who left the institute would call and ask Elsi to find a telephone number or address of colleagues or institutions from years back. She was the closest to what Google provides today. For her a special term could be coined: "audiopedia"; she recognized the voice of everyone, she anticipated with whom the person wanted to talk, she took messages. She would remember voices for years after people had left the institute. During holidays and on those rare instances of illness, others – whoever was free – helped out and sat at the reception desk.

Elsi Degen died a year after the BII was closed down.

Workshop

Otto Kamber was head of the workshop for many years [QR1971_18]. The main emphasis of the workshop was on:

- Maintenance of instruments
- Construction of prototypes of equipment
- Daily checking of all instruments
- Arranging guarantee maintenance and contracts for outsourcing
- Interaction with companies producing plexiglass components and electronic equipment

The workshop team was always enthusiastic and willing to spend extra hours on related jobs, e.g. recording the proceedings of symposia and meetings, restructuring and refurbishing laboratories for new scientists, and last but not least, dealing with emergencies. The contact to scientists was direct and immediate, without hierarchy.

Some members of the workshop who found team work too demanding chose niches, and there were several, e.g. maintaining microscopes and other optical devices, or constructing small instruments from plastic materials, etc.

In addition to the workshop staff, Branko Badovinac, Johannes Büchler, Denes Szabo and Camille Weber were responsible for the maintenance of the heating and air conditioning.

QR1971_17 BII

QR1971_18 BII

Radioisotopes

For several years the radioisotope unit [QR1971_19] was run under the supervision of Helmut Pohlit, and when he left the BII, the unit continued functioning under the management of Ruedi Frech and Juerg Widmer.

The main function of the radioisotope unit was irradiating mice and cells with the ^{59}Cs source, and monitoring the purchase and use of radioactive isotopes, mainly ^{35}S-methionine, ^{14}C amino acids, ^{32}P and ^{33}P isotopes, and in some instances ^{131}I. There was a specially equipped lab for work with higher radioactive doses, the so-called C-lab. Brigitte Schaumburg and Rolf Merkle were part of the team. Brigitte was responsible for checking radioactive cleanliness in all the laboratories.

Cell Sorter Facility

Lee and Len Herzenberg were the first scientists to bring up the question of acquiring cell sorter facilities, and some years later a cell sorter was purchased. It was probably the first cell sorter in Europe and was initially run by Tim Knaak [QR1971_20].

Animal Facilities

The institute with its wide range of projects had to have a large number of animal species for use in experimental research: mice, rats, rabbits, chickens, frogs, sheep and, rarely, guinea pigs. The animal facilities [QR1971_21] were localized on two floors in the BII building, and in addition there were farms in Rodersdorf and Münchenstein.

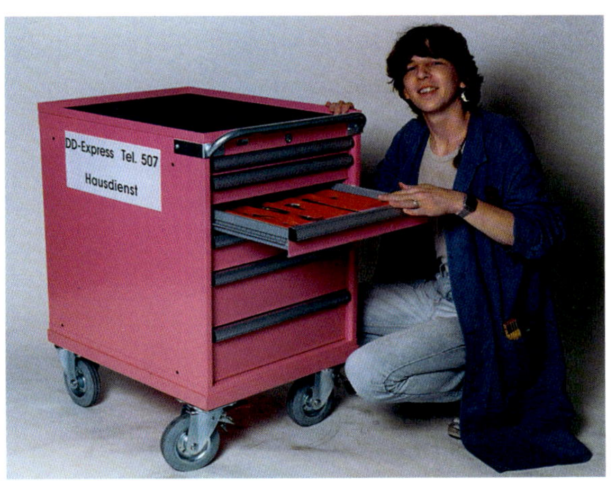

Maintenance service of the workshop

In the early days, the logistics of interactions between scientists and the staff at the breeding sites (including those at the animal facilities of Roche) were complex and often tedious, as the large numbers of different strains of mice, and the breeding requirements, were exceptionally demanding. Experiments on lymphocyte recirculation were performed on the sheep model. The responsibility for keeping the sheep model over the years was in the hands of Zdenek Trnka, who furthered this research alongside his function as administrator.

The first animal caretaker was John Hatton, whose main work was to supervise the maintenance of the rabbit colony of Andrew Kelus.

A vivarium for the frogs was specially constructed for Louis Du Pasquier. Later it was used by Jim Kaufman for his axolotls and John Hansen for his trout.

Media Kitchen

Gisèle Bron was head of the media kitchen [QR1971_22] and the glassware washing facilities for many years. This unit was one of the best of its kind: the most efficient, not only in Basel, but also in the entire region. The preparation of distilled water and ultrapure quartz-distilled water was a true art, and guaranteed the excellent quality of the media.

Programmable autoclaves for sterilizing glassware and media were adopted long before the computer era (on punched cards). There was a standard selection of media, and in addition each scientist could deposit his media protocol (or protocols for various buffers) and that was prepared and placed in the adjacent cold room. Scientists who had "standing orders" did not even have to contact the media kitchen for replenishment; the shelves were checked, and stocked up when necessary.

The technicians brought dirty glassware to the washing facilities, and it was washed in such a manner that glassware from different laboratories was not mixed up. The following morning the technicians retrieved the containers with the washed glassware.

Thirty-eight books of "recipes" from laboratories at the BII were stored in the media kitchen so that any of the media or buffers could be prepared when needed. It was not rare that scientists who had left the institute later contacted the media kitchen to obtain a photocopy of a particular recipe.

QR1971_22 BII

Laboratory and Institute Cleaning

The institute was a pleasantly clean place. It was cleaned before work started in the morning and thoroughly cleaned in the evening. For many years the head of the cleaning team was Mrs. Adelina Mosimann [QR1971_23].

Purchasing/Budgets/Travel

Purchasing was arranged as an independent facility, i.e. it was not part of the Roche purchasing system. The pride of the purchasing department was that any order form handed in by 11 a.m. was processed the same day. Ordering was done by phone or fax, and speedy delivery was ensured. In the lean structure of this department Isabelle Altounian became a well-remembered person, helpful to everybody although sometimes critical and outspoken. Dorothy Poms, with great enthusiasm, arranged the travel itinerary for the scientists. From the bills submitted, she knew exactly who liked what kind of food, and she also knew who liked Bordeaux wine and who preferred Australian Shiraz [QR1971_24].

Secretarial Facilities

From the start Ingrid Schnurr was employed as Niels Jerne's secretary, and Lesley Gut worked for Zdenek Trnka. The next priority was typing the manuscripts, for which a secretarial pool was established. The secretaries first used IBM magnetic card machines, which were followed by Wang word processors and finally by Macintosh computers. Only much later were "editorial assistants" employed with the aim to prepare proceedings of the workshops and symposia held at the institute. This is elaborated in Book 2.

QR1971_23 BII

Library

The first librarian of the BII was Zdenka Joukl. In the early days, keeping the library functional was an easy task. The number of books on the shelves and the number of journals were easy to oversee. There was just one single photocopier in the institute.

QR1971_24 BII

Over the years the library became too small, the book shelves had to be placed in the corridors, and an additional reading area was set up near the seminar room.

One of the duties of the librarian was to maintain the collection of reprints of published articles. Later the reprints were bound and made available to the members of the institute [QR1971_25].

QR1971_25 BII

Artwork and Photography

Hans-Peter Stahlberger [QR1971_26] was responsible for the artwork from the very beginning until his retirement. His artwork features in most of the publications of the BII, and he was instrumental in designing the Annual Report covers.

Mirek Pazdera was head of the photography unit for about two decades. Scientific photography and the technical photography of electrophoresis gels were his main domain.

Computer Infrastructure

In the early seventies, prior to the computer era, the first Hewlett-Packard programmable calculators (HP 65) with magnetic strips became available. The institute purchased 12 of them, which was all that were available "locally". Everything else had to be performed on the Roche IBM mainframe computer. Charley Steinberg was a frequent visitor to the Roche facilities, writing and running programs there. The possibility to introduce word processing typewriters was recognized when IBM put typewriters with magnetic cards on the market (IBM Mag Card Executive). Bert Temminck strongly believed in Apple Macintosh computers, so all the computers (except those which were part of instruments – such as cell sorters) were Macs from the very beginning. A local network, with document transfer through a "go-between", was established. Randy Baron and Jerome Aarden joined the IT department at a later stage of the institute [QR1971_27].

The very first Mac computer at the institute was an Apple IIe purchased for the fluorescence activated cell sorter (FACS) I machine to help with Don Gerson's studies of the early phases of mitogenic stimulation of lymphocytes. The Roche Physics group designed and made a real-time linear-to-log converter to compress the range of the FACS data, enabling digitized plots and quantitative analysis of FACS data to be obtained, rather than the previous Polaroid screenshots (details of this innovative approach are given in the QR code).

QR1971_26 BII

QR1971_27 BII

Transport

As with all the other services, transportation was a highly efficient and reliable facility. Transporting experimental animals, blood, mail, parcels and all other necessary items (instruments for repair, material for the mechanical workshop, etc.) was part of the duties of the transportation group. Peter Menini and Rolf Bieri worked as

CAFETERIA PRICE LIST	
Coffee	Fr. 1.–
Tea	Fr. 1.–
Extra cream	Fr. -.15
Extra sugar	Fr. -.10
Ovomaltine, chocolate, warm or cold	Fr. 1.25
Milk, warm or cold	Fr. -.90
Orange juice, small glass	Fr. 1.–
Orange juice, large glass	Fr. 1.10
Croissant, Schwöbli (two-halved bread roll)	Fr. -.65
Wholemeal roll, Schlumbi (round bread roll)	Fr. -.60
Open sandwiches	Fr. 1.55
Butter (portion), Jam (portion)	Fr. -.40
Cheese spread	Fr. -.85
Cold Plate	Fr. 3.80
Cheese: Appenzeller or Gruyère	Fr. 1.90
Fresh fruit	Fr. -.90
Yoghurt	Fr. 1.10
Small pastry	Fr. 1.10
Season's fruit tart	Fr. 1.20

drivers, and Jean-Paul Rudloff and Mihaly Dekany were amongst those responsible for the distribution of material to the laboratories, media kitchen and other facilities [QR1971_28].

Cafeteria

Besides providing food, the cafeteria [QR1971_29] was a very important meeting place for scientists. People came to the cafeteria to have a cup of coffee between two centrifugation runs, and they also sat there when planning their experiments. It almost became a tradition to refer to the cafeteria when new ideas came up. The paper napkins played an important role.

The food was good and became more varied over the years. In the beginning, open sandwiches, *Birchermuesli* and *Gipfeli* were part of the standard range of available food. Then soup was added and, at a still later stage, hot and cold plates could be ordered. The food was delivered fresh every day at noon from the main Roche canteen.

QR1971_28 BII

Electron Microscopy

The electron microscopy laboratory was designed according to Eduard Kellenberger's ideas, although on a modest scale, as Kellenberger and his group were only staying at the BII for a limited period (until the Biozentrum was completed). It was not intended to become a "service laboratory", and indeed a succession of scien-

QR1971_29 BII

tists carried out high-end research projects relevant to basic immunology. After Kellenberger had left, Tom Mandel (from the Walter and Eliza Hall Institute in Melbourne) took over, followed by Stefanello de Petris (from Milan), and later Christine Brack headed the laboratory. Christine (as mentioned in a later section) stayed in the Basel area.

On his return to Australia, Tom Mandel encouraged Rhodri Ceredig to apply to the BII. Due to a mix-up (delayed mail delivery) Rhodri ended up in Lausanne. Years later, however, his wish to join the BII was fulfilled when he spent a sabbatical there, joining Jan Andersson, Ton Rolink and Fritz Melchers to work on the analysis of various aspects of B cell development.

Other Facilities

Several other facilities, such as peptide synthesis, oligonucleotide synthesis or transgenic animal preparations, were added later and will be mentioned elsewhere.

Political Issue: Women in Switzerland, 1971

Historical note: In 1971 women in Switzerland were given – by popular vote – the right to vote at the federal level [QR1971_30]. This was long overdue, Switzerland being one of the last countries to give women the vote. At the cantonal level, Vaud and Neuchâtel were the first cantons to give women the vote, in 1959. In the years to come, the trend to introduce equal rights for women materialized throughout the political spectrum. In several parliamentary periods, they even had the majority in the government. Subsequently, 3 presidents of the confederation were female, and the issue of gender became a "non-issue".

QR1971_30 BII

Treasure Trove 1971

The database contains documents related to the BII in a broader context (lists, series of photographs, etc.).

QR1971_treasure BII

Next page: Niels Jerne's experimental protocol for the adoptive transfer of cells into various strains of mice

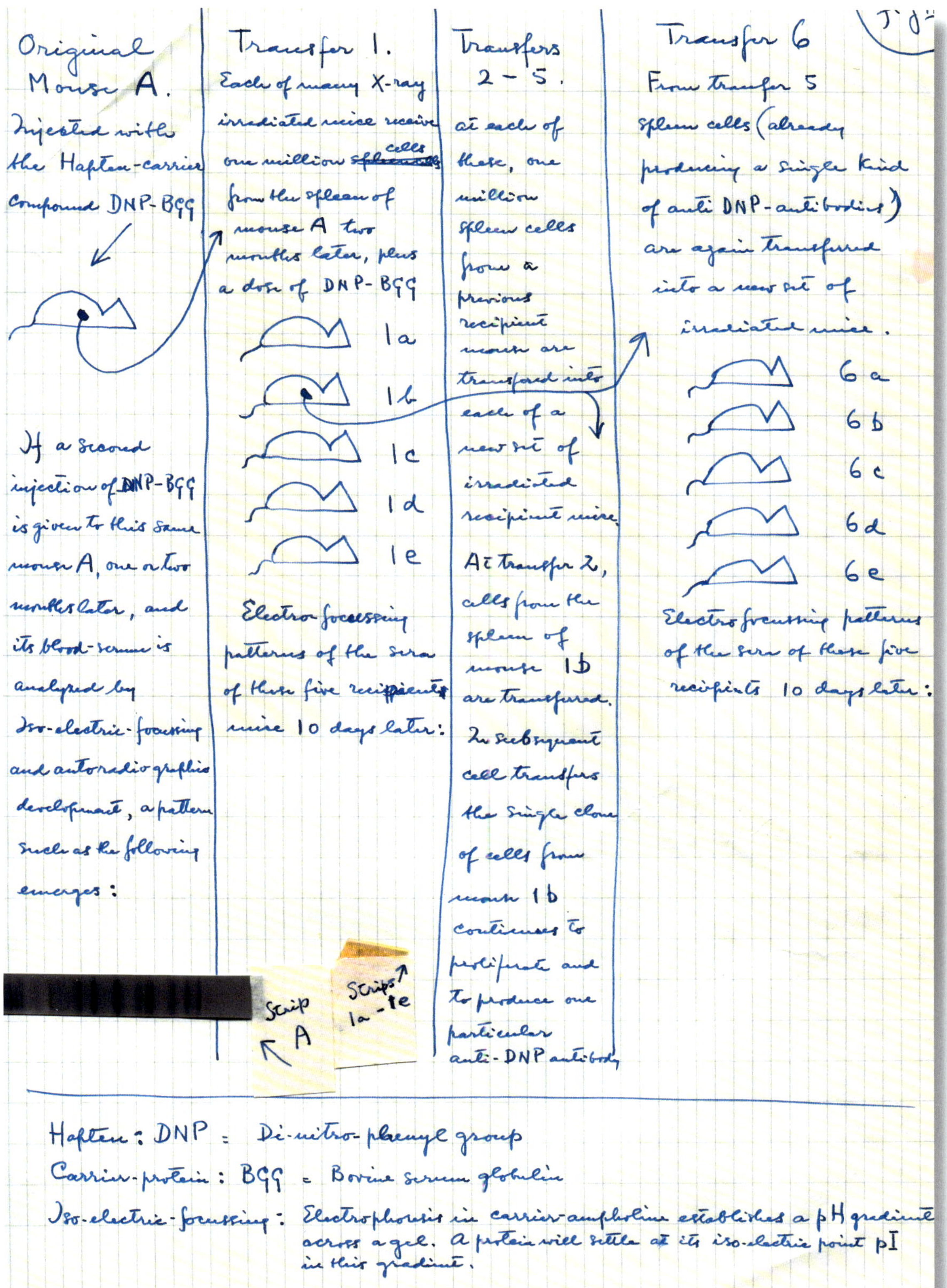

Original Mouse A.
Injected with the Hapten-carrier compound DNP-BGG

If a second injection of DNP-BGG is given to this same mouse A, one or two months later, and its blood-serum is analysed by Iso-electric-focussing and autoradiographic development, a pattern such as the following emerges:

Transfer 1.
Each of many X-ray irradiated mice receive one million cells from the spleen of mouse A two months later, plus a dose of DNP-BGG

1a
1b
1c
1d
1e

Electro-focussing patterns of the sera of these five recipients mice 10 days later:

Transfers 2 – 5.
at each of these, one million spleen cells from a previous recipient mouse are transferred into each of a new set of irradiated recipient mice.

At transfer 2, cells from the spleen of mouse 1b are transferred.

In subsequent cell transfers the single clone of cells from mouse 1b continues to proliferate and to produce one particular anti-DNP antibody

Transfer 6
From transfer 5 spleen cells (already producing a single kind of anti DNP-antibodies) are again transferred into a new set of irradiated mice.

6a
6b
6c
6d
6e

Electro-focussing patterns of the sera of these five recipients 10 days later:

Strip A
Strips 1a – 1e

Hapten: DNP = Di-nitro-phenyl group
Carrier-protein: BGG = Bovine serum globulin
Iso-electric-focussing: Electrophoresis in carrier-ampholine establishes a pH gradient across a gel. A protein will settle at its iso-electric point pI in this gradient.

The Year 1972

The BII became fully functional. The scientific activities were matched by contributions at meetings, symposia and workshops. Several members took up teaching responsibilities at various universities in Switzerland and abroad. The institute established several boards to ensure that the high standards of the institute were achieved and then maintained. These boards were: the International Advisory Board, the Swiss Board of Consultants and the Board of Trustees.

Arrivals 1972 (15)
In January 1972 several new members joined the institute and filled places in the laboratories. The 15 scientists who joined the BII in 1972 are listed below:
Wesley W. Bullock, R.N.P. Cahill, Mario De Marchi, Amy K. Falvey, Walter Gerhard, Joel W. Goodman, John R. Kettman, Louis Lafleur, John Russell Little, Jacques F.A.P. Miller, Graham F. Mitchell, Stanley E. Read, Jonathan Sprent, Felix O. Wettstein, David Stott.

Came and Left in the Same Year (2)
Giovanna Luciani, Jennifer Phillips.

Leavers 1972 (11)
Brigitte Askonas, Maria Irene Baldi, Susan Cullen, David Dresser, Amy Falvey, Walter Gerhard, Berenice Kindred, Tom Mandel, Seung-il Shin, Donald Shreffler, Olof Sjöberg.

QR1972_01 BII

Visiting Research Workers

Throughout the year, a large number of visiting research workers came and went; there were 33 of them. They joined various laboratories for performing collaborative work. Some of these visitors became co-authors of papers published by BII members:

Stephan Arrenbrecht, Zuhayr Awdeh, Antony Basten, Manfred Braun, Angelo O. Carbonara, Lois Carrasco, Marco Castagneto, Erwin Diener, William L. Ford, Eugen Gander, Ingrid Gedutin, Philip G.H. Gell, Raymond Gesteland, Dominique Granato, Eckhart Hahn, Felix Harder, Nurit Hollander, John Horton, Gabrielle Jobin, D. Kolakowski, Judy Lewis, Walter Messer, Mia Pacher, R. Piazza, Philippe Roch, Sergio Romagnani, Jörgen Rygaard, Sören Freisleben Sörensen, P.F. Spahr, Werner Stolp, Andrew Stuart, A.S. Süssman, Jacques Théodor.

For the BII, 1972 started optimistically. The New Year's Eve celebrations were similar to everywhere else in Europe, but perhaps even more exuberant. The "scent" of the *Santa Lucia* celebration (a new event introduced by Olof Sjöberg and Jan Andersson) was felt in the air over the remaining days of 1971. In some labs, the Christmas lights were also left on during the holidays, but once the New Year started, the research projects again became the scientists' main concern.

Some of the projects were extensions of projects initiated and carried out in 1971, while others were newly conceived. The ongoing ones were related to

- "purification of mRNA, translation of exogenous mRNA, initiation factors, intracellular transport of Ig, allotypic markers of chicken Ig" (Tonegawa, Baldi, Schreier, Pink, Askonas, Haimovich, Jaton) [QR1972_01],

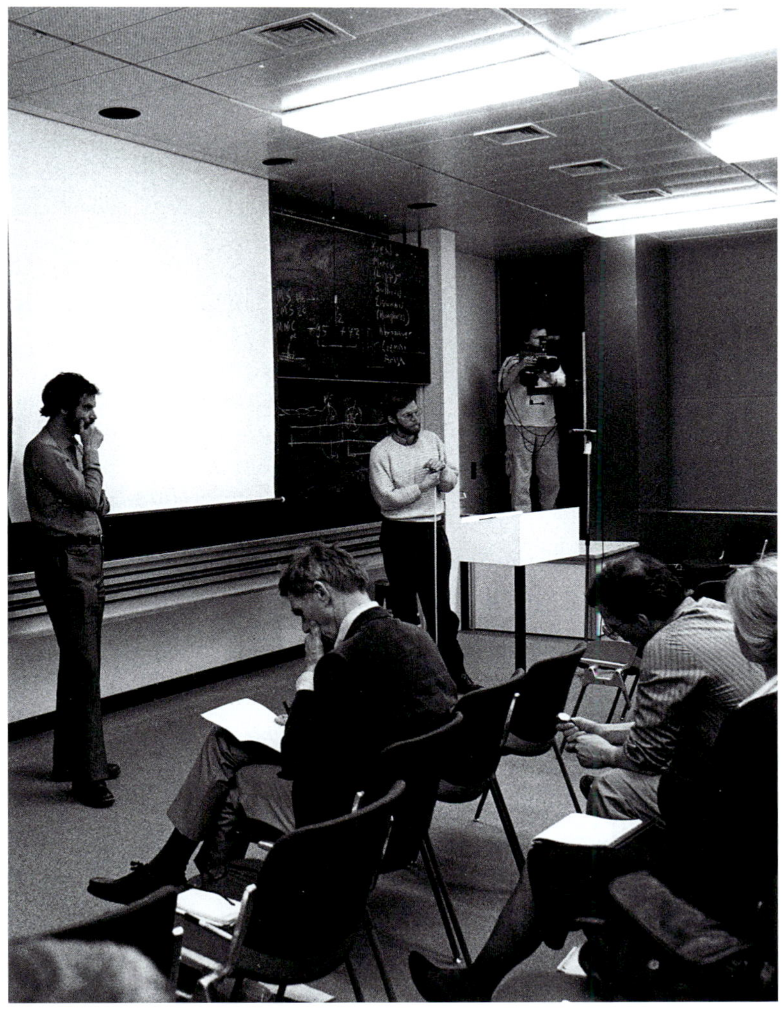

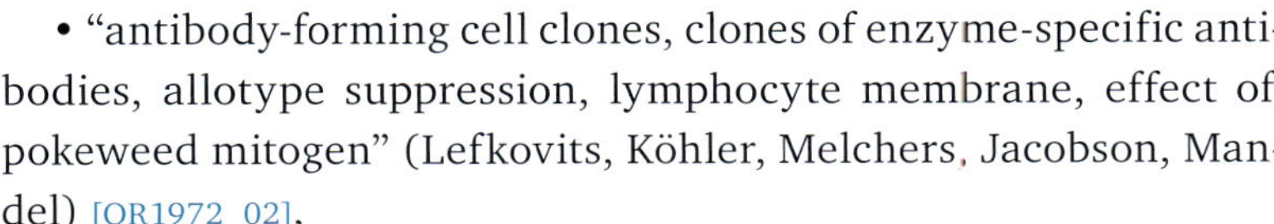

• “antibody-forming cell clones, clones of enzyme-specific antibodies, allotype suppression, lymphocyte membrane, effect of pokeweed mitogen” (Lefkovits, Köhler, Melchers, Jacobson, Mandel) [QR1972_02],

• “HLA system, MLR in *Xenopus laevis*, inhibition of GvH, antigen-carrying macrophages, MIF from sheep” (Bernoco, Ceppellini, Du Pasquier, Miggiano, Weiss, Zakarian, Askonas, Lachmann) [QR1972_03],

• “complementation of responses in nude mice, memory in the absence of T cells, allophenic mice, original antigenic sin, antibody against β-galactosidase” (Kindred, Matsunaga, Meo) [QR1972_04], and are linked to the four QR codes.

Research Directions 1972

Outlines of the projects initiated during 1972 are given below. They are only an "indication" rather than a representative description of the work.

Rosette-Forming Cells for Studying Precursor Cells

Graham Mitchell, Louis Lafleur

Graham Mitchell arrived from Australia and Louis Lafleur from Canada. It was known that one and the same variable portion of immunoglobulin can be joined to two different kinds of constant parts of immunoglobulin, forming either IgM or IgG molecules. Graham and Louis felt that they could address the question whether the cells expressing either one or the other type (IgM/IgG) had a common intermediate precursor, or alternatively belonged to two separate lineages. They applied the methodology of rosette-forming cells, knowing that "more compact" rosettes can be separated from the "looser" ones. Rosettes were formed by incubating sheep red cells with mouse spleen cells, and those with low binding capacity for antigen were dissociated by vigorous agitation. Portions of rosettes were transferred to irradiated mice (together with T cells), and the ability of mice to give rise to antibody-forming cells was measured. Results suggested that IgM and IgG precursors can be separated on the basis of antigen-binding capacity. This opened the possibility to determine whether the higher binding capacity of IgG precursors is due to a higher density of receptors or higher binding affinity.

Cap Formation with TL Antigens

John Russell Little, Francis Loor

John R. Little joined the already functional lab of Francis Loor who was an expert on studying differential expression of protein molecules on membranes, applying the methodology of "cap formation". In the joint project these two members studied the molecule named "thymus leukemia" cell membrane antigen (TL). The expression, disappearance and re-expression of this molecule on the membrane of lymphocytes were intimately related to the function of the cell. John Russell Little brought with him to Basel anti-TL serum, and Francis offered antisera conjugated to fluorescein and to rhodamine. Since the two dyes fluoresce with different colors, it was possible to distinguish (using protocols that allowed or prevented cap formation) the "original" TL determinants from "newly expressed" TL determinants. With TL+ leukemia cells, newly expressed TL antigen could be detected even before capping was completed. This protocol became widely applied in various studies of sequential appearance of cell surface molecules. Francis Loor developed the so-called lipid raft hypothesis in membrane microdomains.

T-Cell-Independent Response

John Hamilton, Graham Mitchell, Louis Lafleur

Although the main effort of cellular immunology was geared towards establishing the rules of cell-to-cell interaction, it was known that there exist well-defined responses of B cells that take place in the absence of T cell influence. John Hamilton, Graham Mitchell and Louis Lafleur decided to study one such type of response. Pneumococcal polysaccharide (SIII) is such a persisting antigen that leads in vivo to T-cell-independent antibody responses. It was also known that DNP-lysine is a hapten that can be readily conjugated to the pneumococccal polysaccharide (SIII). Graham, John and Louis were able to demonstrate that anti-DNP responses were elicited in this system, but the injection of the free hapten readily inhibits IgM responses, while it does not affect IgG responses.

Inhibition of the Antihapten Responses with Hapten Coupled to Erythrocytes

Jacques F.A.P. Miller

Graham Mitchell's and John Hamilton's interest in models that dissociate IgM and IgG responses (as demonstrated in the joint project with Louis Lafleur using persisting antigens) was extended in experiments with Jacques Miller using another experimental setup in which inhibition of the antihapten responses with hapten attached to syngeneic and allogeneic mouse erythrocytes was scrutinized. When a mouse was injected with hapten NIP coupled to an immunogenic carrier, a vigorous IgM and IgG response was achieved. A single injection of syngeneic erythrocytes coupled to a hapten NIP caused a complete inhibition of IgG anti-NIP response and a partial reduction of IgM anti-NIP response. The unresponsive state can be transferred into irradiated recipients by injecting spleen cells, provided that multiple injections of the hapten-coated erythrocytes are given prior to transfer. NIP-coated mouse erythrocytes persist for long periods in mice.

Sindbis Virus

Felix Wettstein, Theophil Staehelin

Felix Wettstein was a former coworker of Theo Staehelin and co-author of famous papers on "ergosomes", a name that became better known as "polysomes". Felix joined the BII for a sabbatical, and his main interest in Basel was to study the synthesis and integration of proteins into cell membranes. As a model he used Sindbis virus coat protein. His experiments and some proposals about utilizing stearoyl derivative of the carbohydrate for studying the switch of IgM to IgG were later integrated in the experiments of other research groups in Basel.

Activation of Lymphocytes through B Cell and T Cell Mitogens

Wesley Bullock, Jan Andersson and the "Swedish lab"

Wesley Bullock joined Jan Andersson to participate in Jan's ongoing projects, but he also continued projects initiated at the Karolinska Institute in collaboration with Antonio Coutinho (who later joined the BII). The laboratory was nicknamed the "Swedish lab", and indeed Olof Sjöberg, and Göran and Erna Möller were involved in many projects. The starting point of Wes' work was the finding that mouse spleen cells cultured without antigen frequently undergo large increases in numbers of cells secreting immunoglobulins reactive against sheep red cells and also against various haptenic determinants. Spontaneous activation seemed to be due (at least in part) to a direct stimulatory effect of fetal calf serum on the cultured cells. Syngeneic normal mouse serum added at the start of culture suppressed the appearance of such antibody-forming cells. Primary antibody response to SRC was not inducible in the absence of fetal calf serum. If, however, the serum-free cultures were supplemented with optimal concentrations of mitogens (concanavalin A or lipopolysaccharide), a primary specific antibody response to SRC could be induced. Experiments utilizing a combination of suboptimal and optimal doses of mitogens, and blending with mixed lymphocyte reactions, were devised to define the rules governing the in vitro responses. Other experiments performed in collaboration with Jan Andersson concerned the findings that concanavalin A activates DNA synthesis with a dose response curve that shifted when compared to serum-containing and serum-free medium. Concanavalin A had no activating effect on spleen cells from nude mice, indicating involvement of T cells. Similar studies were performed using other mitogens, some of them acting on B cells, like lipopolysaccharides and purified protein derivatives. Wes and Jan found also that mitogens such as lipopolysaccharides were capable of bypassing the requirement for binding antigenic determinants to specific Ig receptors, and as a result they promoted "nonspecific" activation of B cells.

Lymphocyte Recruitment by Single Lymph Nodes

Ross Cahill, Jack Hay, Zdenek Trnka

The sheep model was introduced to the BII by Ross Cahill and Jack Hay, but the true promotor of the sheep project was actually Zdenek Trnka. Zdenek, a decade-long friend of Bede Morris of Canberra, was inspired by the sheep model that seemed ideally suited to study the recirculation of cells involved in the immune system. The experimental model of Morris had been used to monitor the cellular events in the lymphatic system of sheep, following establishment of chronic drainage fistulae from single lymph nodes. Increased traffic of lymphocytes from blood to lymph had been found to be a characteristic early event in any immune response of a single lymph node. Antigen-reactive cells have been assayed throughout the immune response to allogeneic lymphocytes. It was found that although a large nonspecific element was associated with lymphocyte recruitment, there was a disappearance of specific, antigen-reactive cells in the local efferent lymph. Not only did this occur in the lymph from the regional node, but also in the systemic pool, as assayed in the efferent lymph from a contralateral node. These findings opened up experimental approaches for monitoring the circulating pool during an ongoing immune response.

Allogeneic Antilymphocyte Antibodies in Recipients of Repeated Transfusions

Mario De Marchi, Angelo Carbonara, Maurizio Savi, Wolfgang Mayr

Mario De Marchi joined the BII to work on a project, with Angelo Carbonara (Torino) and Maurizio Savi (Parma), related to allogeneic antilymphocyte antibodies in recipients of planned transfusions. Together with Wolfgang Mayr the response against antigens of the lymphocyte surface was evaluated in the context of individuals who have received, over the years, repeated blood transfusions from known donors. Techniques employed included standard complement-dependent lymphocytotoxicity tests, blocking of lymphocyte reactivity and the methodology of "co-capping" and immunofluorescence. No evidence of antibodies against antigens controlled by genes outside the HLA linkage group was obtained.

Analysis of Influenza Virus-Specific Antibody Populations

Walter Gerhard, Stephen Fazekas de St. Groth

Walter Gerhard joined Stephen Fazekas to work on influenza viruses. Using the notion of senior and junior antigens antisera to junior antigens were tested in terms of quality and quantity against senior ones. The measurements were performed on hyperimmune rabbit sera, using the homologous and cross-reactive influenza antigens. It was found that when an animal immune to a junior virus is boosted with a senior antigen, the cross-reactive species of antibody are selectively enriched. The results of testing the equilibrium constants were in good agreement with the hypothesis of original antigenic sin postulated by Stephen Fazekas.

Immune Response to Small Mono- and Bifunctional Determinants

Joel W. Goodman, Georges Roelants

Joel W. Goodman joined Georges Roelants for a sabbatical in order to explore the immune response of guinea pigs to L-tyrosine-*p*-azobenzene arsonate (RAT), which was known to induce a cellular immune response by itself and which can serve as a carrier for conjugated haptens. The anti-DNP responses to bifunctional antigens, such as DNP-RAT, are frequently more homogeneous than those made in response to DNP-protein conjugates. The complementary charge effects between antigens and antibodies were investigated by isoelectric focusing patterns of the resulting antibody, and the correlation to anti-RAT cellular responses was established.

Modulation of the in vitro Immune Response by Pokeweed Mitogen

Jack Kettman, Ivan Lefkovits, José Quintáns

Jack Kettman came from Dick Dutton's lab with many ideas that he hoped to address with colleagues at the BII. He ran his own laboratory and only later (and then regularly almost every year) returned to join Ivan Lefkovits' lab. The work he started in Basel was related to the effect of pokeweed mitogen (PWM) that was known to be a B cell mitogen. In vitro immune response in the presence of PWM yields either a profound stimulation or a depression in the number of antibody-forming cells, depending on the number and specificity of T cells present in the culture.

Another project that Jack initiated in Basel was the involvement of T cell factors modulating the immune response in vitro, especially in the context of other "nonspecific agents" like mercaptoethanol and/or B cell mitogens. This was also the starting stage of joint projects with Ivan Lefkovits and José Quintáns on precursor cells specific to SRC in nude mice. A dilution scheme for B cells has been applied to estimate the frequency of precursor cells specific to SRC present in the spleens of nude mice. Jack added another "dimension" to the ongoing limiting dilution experiments by scrutinizing the contribution of macrophages to the number of precursor cells engaged in the response, and on clone sizes achieved.

Studies on Immune Response Enhancement by Adjuvants

Jennifer Phillips, David Dresser

Jennifer Phillips joined David Dresser to study a special aspect of adjuvanicity. Jennifer had chosen several substances that were known for having an "adjuvant effect" in the immune response and asked the question whether the achieved enhancement is directed towards B cells or T cells. Dresser and Phillips coined the expression "orientation of adjuvants", and upon comparing 3 adjuvants (pertussis, lentinan and lipopolysaccharide) they found that LPS was a B-cell-oriented adjuvant, lentinan a T-cell-oriented substance, and pertussis was correlated with both B and T cell responses.

Human T Lymphocyte Rosettes

Stanley Read, Alma Luzzati, Ben Pernis

Stanley Read joined Alma Luzzati and Ben Pernis in order to elucidate a strange phenomenon that a large proportion of human T lymphocytes has the ability to bind sheep erythrocytes (SRC). This binding property can be observed under the microscope by so-called rosette formation. Stanley examined this phenomenon to determine whether or not it had any relationship to the immunological function of the T cell. Stanley found that rosette formation is blocked by pretreatment of lymphocytes with sodium azide, indicating that membrane activity is essential. He concluded that the ability of T cells to bind SRC does not depend on T lymphocyte receptors specific for SRC but rather upon the membrane mobility of the cells. Which membrane moieties have the affinity for the SRC was not detrimental. Rosette formation remained a useful "diagnostic" tool for identifying human T lymphocytes.

Migration of Activated T Lymphocytes

Jonathan Sprent, Jacques F.A.P. Miller

Jacques Miller and Jon Sprent arrived from Australia; Jacques came for a sabbatical, while Jon stayed in Basel for several years. The starting point of their investigation was the finding that parental strain thymus cells when transferred to heavily irradiated F1 mice proliferate extensively in the spleen and lymph nodes, and then appear as blast cells in thoracic duct lymph. These thymus-derived thoracic duct lymphocytes (T.TDL) were shown to consist of a nearly pure population of T cells activated only to the antigens which provoked their formation. A proportion of T.TDL do migrate to the intestines, while other cell populations, e.g. bone marrow cells, migrate to other organs, e.g. the liver. There they release DNA (or its breakdown products), perhaps as a result of cell death.

Another project that Jon Sprent and Jacques Miller tackled was the specific unresponsiveness of adoptively transferred lymphoid cells. They found that the failure of cells from recently primed donors to respond to the priming antigen on adoptive transfer could be overcome by supplementing with normal spleen cells, but not with thymus cells alone or bone marrow cells alone. This implied that unresponsiveness involved both T and B lymphocytes and was not due to a suppressive influence exerted by T cells.

Extramural Lecturing

BII members gave seminars in 38 different cities. The geographic spread indicates the network of interactions. The places are listed in the time order of the scheduled event: Geneva, Bern, Vienna, Giessen, Lausanne, Paris, Göttingen, Havana, Cologne, London, Turin, Berlin, Frankfurt, Copenhagen, Toronto, Canberra, Rochester, Lyon, Zurich, Hamburg, Melbourne, Zagreb, La Jolla, Carry-le-Rouet, Madison, Moscow, Philadelphia, Boston, New York, Rome, Rehovot, Tsakhadzor, Naples, Freiburg, Innsbruck, Chicago, Evanston, Heidelberg. At some places, several members gave seminars on different occasions, 82 altogether. Incidentally, Tsakhadzor is in Armenia.

Several QR codes refer to the extramural activities [QR1972_05] [QR1972_06] [QR1972_07] [QR1972_08].

QR1972_05 BII

Contributions at Meetings, Symposia and Workshops

BII members lectured at numerous symposia and workshops, but these activities will be mentioned separately (events from several years will all be listed together in a later section). In March 1972, a major conference on "Leukocyte cultures" was organized by Gerd Riethmüller in Tübingen [QR1972_09]. Two members of the BII (Georges Roelants and Ivan Lefkovits) presented their experimental systems there.

QR1972_06 BII

QR1972_07 BII

QR1972_08 BII

QR1972_09 BII

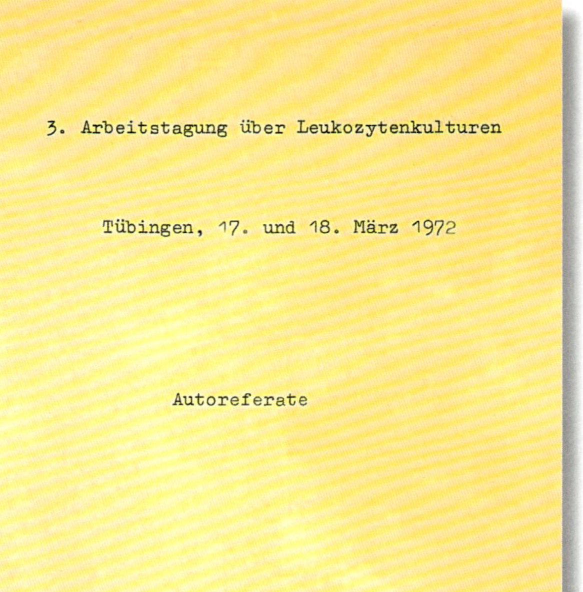
3. Arbeitstagung über Leukozytenkulturen

Tübingen, 17. und 18. März 1972

Autoreferate

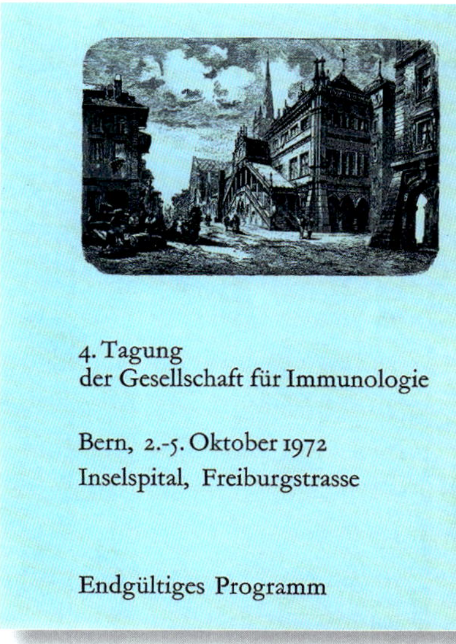

4. Tagung
der Gesellschaft für Immunologie

Bern, 2.–5. Oktober 1972
Inselspital, Freiburgstrasse

Endgültiges Programm

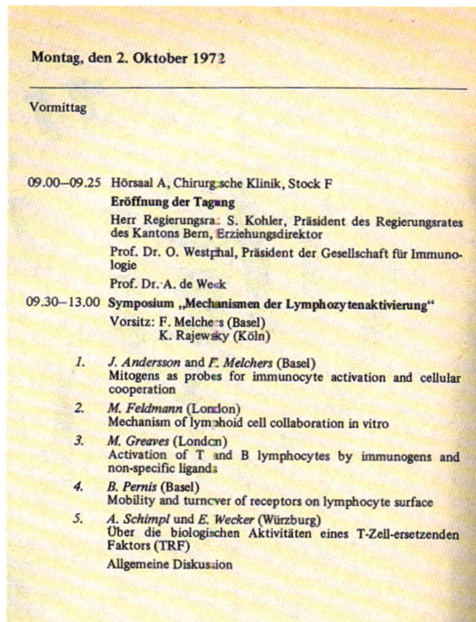

Montag, den 2. Oktober 1972

Vormittag

09.00–09.25 Hörsaal A, Chirurgische Klinik, Stock F
Eröffnung der Tagung
Herr Regierungsrat S. Kohler, Präsident des Regierungsrates des Kantons Bern, Erziehungsdirektor
Prof. Dr. O. Westphal, Präsident der Gesellschaft für Immunologie
Prof. Dr. A. de Weck

09.30–13.00 **Symposium „Mechanismen der Lymphozytenaktivierung"**
Vorsitz: F. Melchers (Basel)
K. Rajewsky (Köln)

1. *J. Andersson* and *F. Melchers* (Basel)
Mitogens as probes for immunocyte activation and cellular cooperation
2. *M. Feldmann* (London)
Mechanism of lymphoid cell collaboration in vitro
3. *M. Greaves* (London)
Activation of T and B lymphocytes by immunogens and non-specific ligands
4. *B. Pernis* (Basel)
Mobility and turnover of receptors on lymphocyte surface
5. *A. Schimpl* und *E. Wecker* (Würzburg)
Über die biologischen Aktivitäten eines T-Zell-ersetzenden Faktors (TRF)

Allgemeine Diskussion

Dienstag, den 3. Oktober 1972

Vormittag

Sektion I Hörsaal A, Chirurgische Klinik, Stock F
Zellkooperation (09.00–10.45)
Vorsitz: K.U. Hartmann (Tübingen)
P.G. Munder (Freiburg)

09.00 *27.* *H. Warnatz, F. Scheiffarth, U. Staerk (Erlangen)*
Untersuchungen über die Hapten-Carrier-Spezifizität antigenbindender Zellen.

09.15 *28.* *P. G. Munder, W. Raetz, G.A. Luckenbach. M. Modolell (Freiburg)*
Ein neues System zur Antikörperbildung in vitro

09.30 *29.* *M. Modolell, W. Raetz. P.G. Munder (Freiburg)*
Untersuchungen zum Wirkungsmechanismus von Adjuvantien in der Gewebekultur.

09.45 *30.* *J. Quintans, I. Lefkovits (Basel)*
Antibody production by spleen cells from nude mice in microculture.

10.00 *31.* *K.U. Hartmann (Tübingen)*
Vergleich der Aktivität von B-Zell-Mitogenen mit aktivierten T-Zellen.

10.15 *32.* *B. Perren, G. Schumann, P. Dukor (Basel)*
Disoziation von Cytotoxizität und Helferaktivität bestrahlter Thymuszellen.

10.30 *33.* *W. Droege (München)*
On the nature of the suppressive effect of thymus cells.

10.45 Pause

In October 1972, Alain de Weck of the Inselspital Bern organized a conference of the "Gesellschaft für Immunologie", which was a joint meeting of German and Swiss immunologists [QR1972_10]. It was the first time that scientists from the BII could introduce themselves and their work on the Swiss scientific stage. A large number of projects was presented and received widespread attention.

Venia Legendi

Most of the institute's members came from places where they had had both teaching and research responsibilities. The newcomers enjoyed the work arrangements at the BII, having neither administrative duties nor the "burden" of teaching. Nevertheless, several scientists did take up extramural teaching activities, and some of them did so from the early days. Fritz Melchers and Dietmar Braun were involved in teaching in Freiburg. Soon they were offered a "Habilitation" (Venia legendi, Privatdozent) [QR1972_11]. Louis du Pasquier's teaching affiliation at the Pasteur Institute was called "Chargé de cours". Theo Staehelin and Charles Steinberg were "Titular professors" at Basel University. Besides that, Ruggero Ceppellini and Ben Pernis kept their professorships in Turin and Milan. Years later Ivan Lefkovits habilitated at the Philipp's University in Marburg. Teaching in Lausanne, Marseille and at other

QR1972_10 BII

QR1972_11 BII

Ultimately, man is looking forward to the elimination of disease, for sounder minds and bodies, abundant and nutritious food supplies, the highest standards of personal care and hygiene and a longer lifespan for all people everywhere on earth.

W. Mattia, Roche, Nutley

places became regular activities for those who felt that contact with students is of mutual benefit. Later in this book, the teaching activities at the University of Basel will be mentioned.

Roche Nutley Creates the V.D. Mattia Award, 1972

When the BII was busy establishing its own identity, Roche Nutley was too far distant from everyday considerations; nevertheless the BII noticed with satisfaction that Roche Nutley established an award named after V.D. Mattia, its former president and one of the strongest supporters of basic research [QR1972_12]. As already mentioned, it was Mattia who ignited in Alfred Pletscher a fascination for modern approaches to biological research.

Thus it was of no surprise that Roche Basel considered creating an award of its own, albeit in a somewhat different form. So it established the Roche Research Foundation for Scientific Exchange and Biomedical Collaboration, with an endowment of 10 million Swiss Francs.

Adolf Jann and the English-Language Kindergarten

It became clear that for newcomers' families one institution was missing: an English-language kindergarten. This issue became even more urgent when the Biozentrum opened and more English-speaking families with pre-school-age children were coming to work in Basel. Fritz Melchers, with a network of friends at the Biozentrum, was the driving force for attempting to establish an English-language kindergarten. A quick solution could only be achieved by "negotiating" at the highest level, and the president of Roche, Adolf Jann, made it happen [QR1972_13]. The kindergarten was established at the lower end of the Grenzacherstrasse (maybe Grenzacherstrasse 22), equipped with adequate furniture and run by volunteer teachers recruited from newcomers' families.

QR1972_12 BII

Whenever Niels Jerne visited Adolf Jann at the Roche headquarters (Building 21) Jann always enquired about the kindergarten. For several years, the well-being of the kindergarten was a topic which warmed up their conversation. Among the kindergarten teachers was Judie Mitchell, the wife of Graham Mitchell.

QR1972_13 BII

The kindergarten existed for many years and was open also for children from other institutions, such as the Biozentrum and the Friedrich Miescher Institute.

Yellow Submarine

Jörgen Rygaard (University of Copenhagen) and Ivan Lefkovits started a collaboration on athymic mice with so-called *nu/nu* mutation. These mice had to be bred and maintained under specific pathogen-free conditions, preferentially kept apart from other strains of mice. A special cubicle with positive pressure and a lockable double-door entrance was built to maintain some 300 nude mice with a backcross program to obtain a congenic strain, *nu/nu* C57BL/6. The shape of the cubicle invoked a submarine, so the staff dubbed it "the yellow submarine" (Beatles song 1966: *In the town where I was born, Lived a man who sailed to sea, And he told us of his life, In the land of submarines)*. Soon after the installation of the submarine, enough nude mice were available for running several projects [QR1972_14].

Self-Service in Affluent Settings

The corridor in the 1UG (lower main floor) had 26 spacious cupboards in which everything that was needed for standard lab work was stored and could be accessed by the laboratory staff. There were no formalities, no ordering forms, and no slips to be filled in. Glassware of every kind, beakers, flasks, cylinders, Petri dishes, Pasteur pipettes and everything else were available 24 hours a day. Sterilized and non-sterilized items were on store. A person was responsible for checking and replenishing the cupboards.

The self-service of culture media was organized on a similar basis. A cold room was accessible from the corridor, and sterile media could be taken at any time. The staff of the media kitchen entered the same cold room through the inner door of the media preparation facility and checked the cold room shelves, knowing that media on demand had to be supplied at certain intervals. Media that expired were removed. If a lab planned a large experiment, it arranged for a special supply.

The self-service was soon extended to other items beyond lab supplies. Paper, envelopes, writing blocks, stationery, pencils, ballpoint pens and sellotape: all items were available and replenished every day.

It was noticed that items which were "reliably available" in self-service cupboards were not hoarded in the labs. It was much less wasteful than material purchased through a standard ordering procedure.

QR1972_14 BII

The Advisory Structures

Although the institute's inception was reliant on a handshake between Adolf Jann and Niels Jerne, several structures were put into place to ensure that the high standard of the institute was achieved and then maintained. Two of them, as explained earlier, were brought to life by Jerne, and one was established by Roche.

The purpose of these three bodies was set out as follows:

- The International Advisory Board (IAB) scrutinized the scientific progress and programs of the institute, as well as all matters relevant thereto
- The Swiss Board of Consultants (SBC) consisted of immunologists working in other laboratories in Switzerland. Its terms of reference were similar to the Board of Advisors, and, in addition, it encouraged cooperation among immunologists in Switzerland
- The Board of Trustees BII (BT-BII) was responsible for supervising the operation of the institute and for ensuring its independence

Members of the IAB and SBC in later years changed due to rotation, and the alterations throughout the years are recorded in the corresponding QR codes [QR1972_15], [QR1972_16] and [QR1972_17].

For the starting period the members of all three boards are given below.

QR1972_15 BII

QR1972_16 BII

QR1972_17 BII

Members of the International Advisory Board (IAB)

Renato Dulbecco	Salk Institute for Biological Studies, San Diego
Gerald Edelman	Rockefeller University, New York
John Humphrey	Chairman of the National Institute for Medical Research, London
Ole Maaloe	University of Copenhagen, Copenhagen
Gustav Nossal	Walter and Eliza Hall Institute, Melbourne
Michael Sela	Vice-Chairman of the Weizmann Institute of Science, Rehovot
Otto Westphal	Max-Planck-Institut für Immunbiologie, Freiburg

Members of the Swiss Board of Consultants (SBC)

Johann-Rudolf Frey	Research Department of F. Hoffmann-La Roche, Basel
Alfred Hässig	Chairman of the Blood Transfusion Service, Swiss Red Cross, Bern
Henri Isliker	University of Lausanne
Eduard Kellenberger	Biozentrum, Basel
Jean Lindenmann	University of Zurich
Peter Miescher	University of Geneva

Ernst Sorkin	Schweizerisches Forschungsinstitut, Davos
Pierre Vassalli	University of Geneva
Alain de Weck	Inselspital, Bern

Members of the Board of Trustees (BT-BII)

Adolf Walter Jann	Chairman of the Board of Directors, Roche
Alfred Pletscher	General Director of Research, Roche
René von Graffenried	General Director for Legal Affairs, Roche
Niels Kaj Jerne	Director of the Basel Institute for Immunology

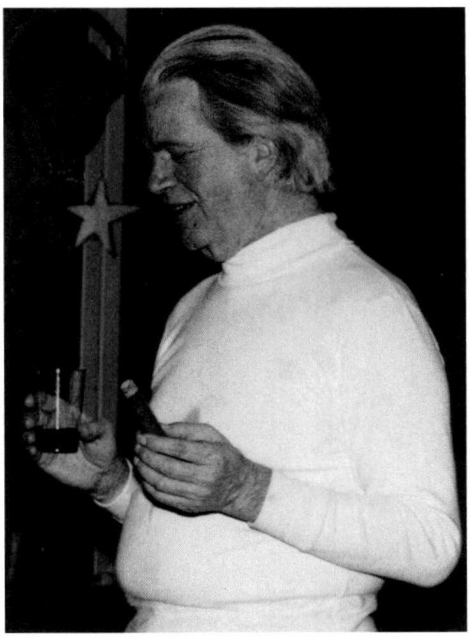

Ole Maaloe, supervisor of Niels Jerne's PhD thesis

Renato Dulbecco was a long-standing friend of Niels Jerne, and it was him who proposed hiring the young scientist Susumu Tonegawa who then played an important role in the fame of the institute. Besides inventing a culture medium named after him (Dulbecco's modified Eagle's medium), his main scientific contribution was to establish a link between genetic mutations and cancer. He was awarded the Nobel Prize in Physiology or Medicine in 1975. Dulbecco had been a member of the Italian resistance during World War II.

Gerald Edelman was keenly interested in the BII and spent 2 months there soon after it opened. Edelman was the first to establish the amino acid sequence of the immunoglobulin light chain. In Basel he initiated studies on binding cells to concanavalin A-coated nylon strings.

John Humphrey had been, for Jerne, a profound source of knowledge on cells involved in the immune system.

Ole Maaloe was Jerne's friend and colleague from old times in Copenhagen. Although Maaloe was 3 years younger than Jerne, he had been the supervisor of Jerne's PhD thesis.

Gustav Nossal was a "recent" friend of Jerne – their friendship had been established during the first part of Jerne's round-the-world journey. Niels Jerne and Sir Macfarlane Burnet were the key figures in natural selection theories (Jerne 1955, Burnet 1957), and Nossal was a worthy successor of Burnet in the Walter and Eliza Hall Institute. Not only was Nossal a member of the Advisory Board, but he was also a frequent visitor to the BII.

Michael Sela was acquainted with Jerne from the time of Jerne's directorship of the Paul Ehrlich Institute. Jerne was highly interested in the synthetic antigens that were developed and used in Sela's laboratory in Rehovot. The reason for this specific interest was Jerne's wish to define the "minimal size" of an antigenic determinant (epitope), and Sela's synthetic antigens were the closest to these definitions. Sela, of Polish origin, was stationed in Czechoslovakia after World War II to help Czech and Slovak Jews leave the country for the future state of Israel.

Otto Westphal was helpful to the BII from the first days of its existence. There were excellent interactions between Basel and Freiburg due to their proximity, and also due to Westphal's involvement in the German Immunology Society.

Within the Board of Consultants, Johann-Rudolf Frey played a prominent role (mentioned elsewhere in this volume), as he was the one who suggested that the research direction of the institute should be the study of the immune system. Alfred Hässig already knew Jerne from his time in Copenhagen, and they had interacted again during Jerne's WHO appointment in Geneva. Hässig founded the Swiss blood donation system and was one of the first scientists to take out products from the blood in order to make plasma for the treatment of chronic diseases. Henri Isliker's role has been mentioned earlier; he remained a strong supporter of the BII throughout its existence. Eduard Kellenberger was connected to Jerne not only due to personal friendship, but also through many colleagues working on bacteriophages, which had also been of interest to Jerne. Both Kellenberger and Jerne considered themselves disciples of Max Delbrück.

Although Jean Lindenmann is best known for his discovery of interferon, his acquaintance with Jerne occurred outside this field. They interacted during the short period when Lindenmann worked as a bacteriologist at the Bundesamt für Gesundheit in Bern and Jerne worked in Geneva. Later, when working in Zurich, Lindenmann sent Jerne the manuscript of a paper (Lindenmann and Ramseier) on the "product of antigenic recognition (PAR)". Jerne wanted Lindenmann to join the BII – at least for a sabbatical – to work on PAR, and although this did not come about, he was highly influential as a member of the SBC.

Peter Miescher is best known for his work on circulating immune complexes. He was introduced to Jerne in Geneva by Eduard Kellenberger. Ernst Sorkin, who had been working in a remote place in Switzerland (Davos), warmly welcomed Jerne's arrival to Switzerland – he knew Niels from Copenhagen. Sorkin was an immunologist, interested in completely different aspects of science than Jerne (chemotaxis, neuroimmunology), but he remained a great friend of the institute and was a valuable source of contacts in the Swiss network. Pierre Vassalli played an important role in establishing contacts to immunologists in the Suisse Romande. Alain de Weck had been a long-standing friend and colleague of Johann-Rudolf Frey, and through him he had contacts to Roche. Alain de Weck was a highly influential scientist in Switzerland, both in basic and in clinical immunology.

In practical terms the reports of the two scientific boards (IAB and SBC) were addressed to the Board of Trustees, with the Chairman of the IAB personally handing over the report to the Chairman of the Board of Trustees.

The first meetings of the SBC and of the IAB convened in August 1970, at the villa in Schwarzwaldallee. The second board meetings were to be held in the BII itself, to take place within a few months upon completion of the final stages of construction.

From Niels Jerne's Notes

The description of the projects of scientists who arrived during 1972 was intended to provide a platform to illustrate their contributions. With the following excerpt from Jerne's "Introduction to the Annual Report 1972", an overall picture of the research landscape becomes apparent [QR1972_18]. The selection is modified to such an extent that it should be considered only as "Jerne-derived" thoughts. It is in line with Jerne's philosophy that either one provides all names or none; the text that follows, taken from Niels Jerne's notes, avoids giving names.

The extreme heterogeneity of antibody molecules makes it difficult to study their properties. Use has been made of particular situations in which animals produce large quantities of homogeneous antibodies, either because of neoplastic lymphocyte proliferation, or as a result of immunization with certain antigens such as bacterial polysaccharides or of the transfer of single antibody-producing cell clones into irradiated animals. The properties investigated included amino acid sequences, idiotypic determinants and isoelectric points of these antibody molecules. The use of these properties as genetic markers has given some insight into the extent to which they are determined by the genome of the zygote.

Following synthesis of antibody, the secretion of the molecules by a cell requires that they penetrate reticular membranes and the outer cell membrane. Successive attachments of carbohydrates to the molecules appeared to guide this process. Apart from idiotypes, antibody molecules display other antigenic markers, allotypes, which are determined within a species by allelic genes. In heterozygous animals a given antibody-forming cell, as well as its clone of progeny cells, expresses only one allotypic allele. This allelic exclusion was used for characterizing clones of cells. A search for further allotypic markers in rabbits, mice, guinea pigs and chickens was undertaken to increase the range of applications of these genetic tools. Allotype

QR1972_18 BII

suppression showed that B lymphocytes expressing a given allele on their receptors can be suppressed by antibodies directed against these allotypic determinants, and that specific T cells can maintain the suppression of B cells. For bursa cells and B lymphocytes it was relatively easy to demonstrate that receptors are antibody-like molecules which enable the cell to recognize antigens. Membrane fluidity permits the receptors to move over the cell surface and, under certain conditions, to aggregate and to form a cap over one pole of a lymphocyte. Although it has been shown that a lymphocyte may simultaneously display receptors of more than one antibody class, all receptor molecules on one cell have identical combining sites and light chains. T lymphocytes appeared to be as discriminating as B lymphocytes in specific antigen binding. This was shown by incubating T cells with radioactive antigens, and also by demonstrating that T cells specifically adhere to antigen-coated nylon fibers. It has been more difficult to demonstrate unequivocally that T cell receptors are antibody-like molecules. An attempt to obtain a better general understanding of membranes has been made by electron microscopic and other techniques. Apart from the antibody-like receptors, many other proteins occur in the membranes of lymphocytes and other immunologically relevant cells. Special attention was paid to those proteins that express structural genes present on the chromosome that carries the histocompatibility locus, named H2 in the mouse and HL-A in man. The rejection of transplanted organs and tumours is a consequence of differences in these histocompatibility loci of donor and recipient. Rejection processes can be mimicked in vitro by mixing lymphocytes from two human donors, or from two mice. Such a mixed lymphocyte culture results in lymphocyte stimulation that can be assayed by demonstrating DNA synthesis, and is followed by a second step, which is a cytotoxic action of the lymphocytes against target cells. The antigens that are recognized by the aggressor lymphocytes are HL-A or H2 related. The first step of stimulation has been shown, however, not to be a consequence of recognition of serologically determined HL-A differences, but to depend on genes that are adjacent to HL-A or H2 and code for as yet unknown surface structures. These are perhaps related to the structures encoded by certain Ir-genes. Successful transfer of myelomas from one mouse to another mouse can be prevented by immunizing the recipient mouse with the myeloma protein, which can be interpreted as idiotypic determinants functioning as transplantation antigens. Lymphocytes can respond when their receptors recognize the presence of antigens; they can also respond when the antigens they display are recognized by the receptors of other lymphocytes, or by antibody molecules. Apart from these

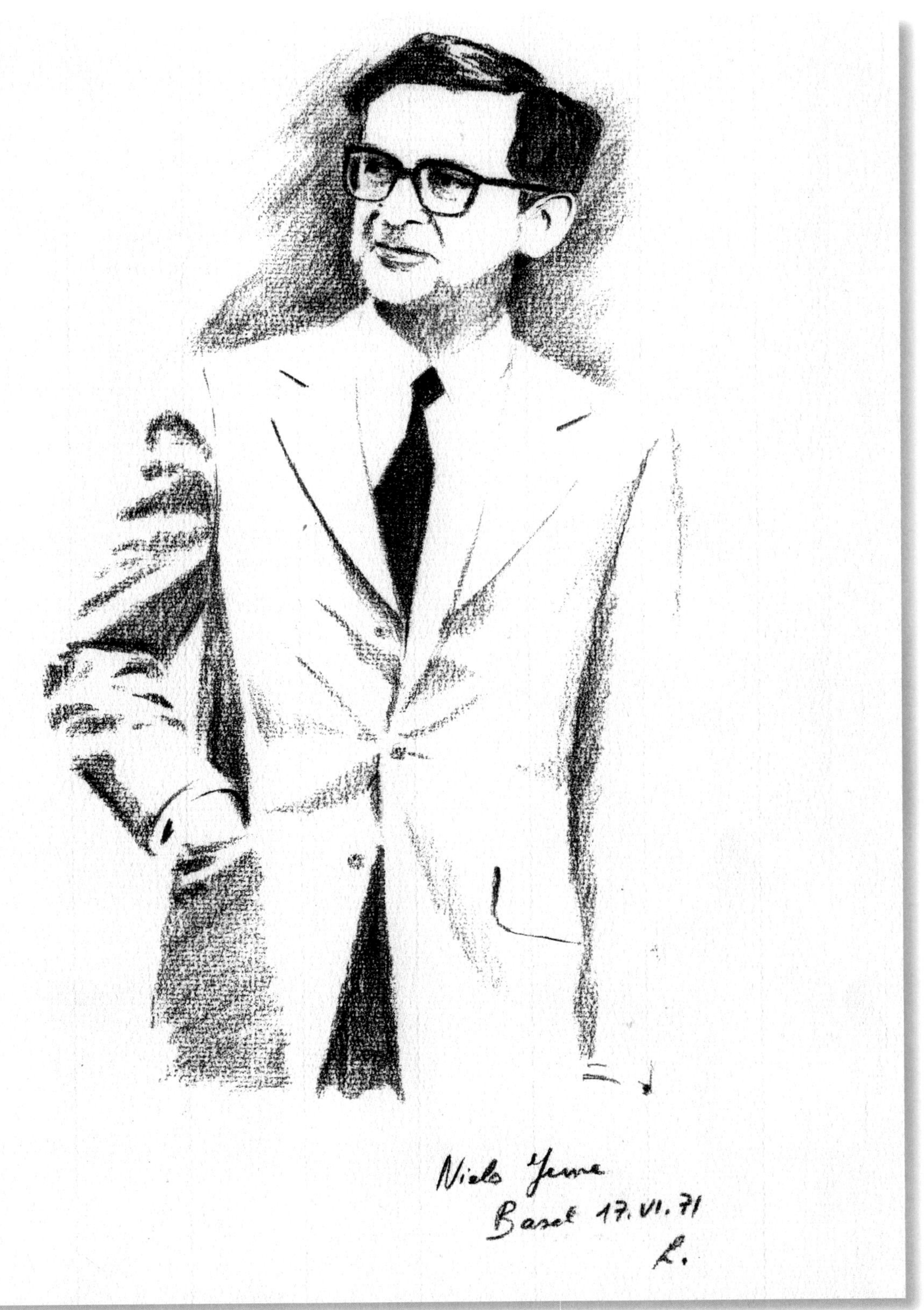
Niels Jerne
Basel 17.VI.71
L.

"specific" situations, lymphocytes can respond "nonspecifically" to a variety of substances such as lymphocyte mitogens, which bind to lymphocyte membranes. Responding B cells will produce antibodies to which these lymphocytes are committed and which are not directed against antigenic determinants of the mitogens. This has proven to be a powerful research tool, not least because T cells and B cells respond differently to different mitogens. Whereas antibody synthesis and secretion is a B cell function, T cells are responsible for the various manifestations of cell-mediated immunity such as delayed hypersensitivity. It has been shown, however, that interaction between T and B cells is a frequent requirement for the full expression of an immune response. Studies of the "helper" function in promoting B cell activity became feasible. These include the characterization of active substances secreted by T cells, and studies of the differences in action of syngeneic and allogeneic T cells. Nude mice (lacking thymus) were useful for studying conditions in which T cells restore immune responsiveness. This has been done by thymus grafting or by T cell injections in vivo as well as by culturing the lymphocytes of nude mice in vitro in the presence of antigens and of T cells from donor mice. The latter technique has permitted an approach to determining the frequency of precursor B cells that can respond to a given antigen. In microcultures antibody-producing cells can be induced which appear to belong to a single clone derived from one precursor cell. Single clones derived by this technique from cultures of lymphocytes of heterozygous rabbits present one allotype only. Clones of antibody-forming cells arising in immunized animals can be enumerated by analysis of the banding pattern of serum antibodies in isoelectric focusing. In view of the enormous diversity of antibody molecules produced by a single animal, it is difficult to imagine the presence in the zygote of all structural genes required. Various theories, therefore, propose an ontogenic generation of antibody gene diversity. The tolerance of the immune system to "self" antigens is known to be acquired in ontogeny. This has been confirmed in studies of the responsiveness of lymphocytes from allophenic mice in mixed lymphocyte cultures. Other ontogenic studies made use of bursectomy in developing chickens. The parameters describing antibody heterogeneity with respect to affinity towards the antigen are important because a main feature of antibody diversity is the fact that a given antibody-combining site can fit a variety of antigenic determinants with different degrees of precision, and vice versa. It remains astonishing that the immune system of a small tadpole, possessing only about two million lymphocytes, appears to be able to discriminate between related antigens, just as well as a large animal, such as a goat, does.

One should bear in mind that Jerne's text was written in 1972, and it carries the stamp of that time. Nevertheless, it shows his skepticism towards certain interpretations, e.g. on the nature of the TCR (T cell receptor), which, in the strict sense, turned out to be of a very different kind, although in more general terms the TCR is still a member of the immunoglobulin superfamily that is generated by somatic rearrangement, as will be shown later.

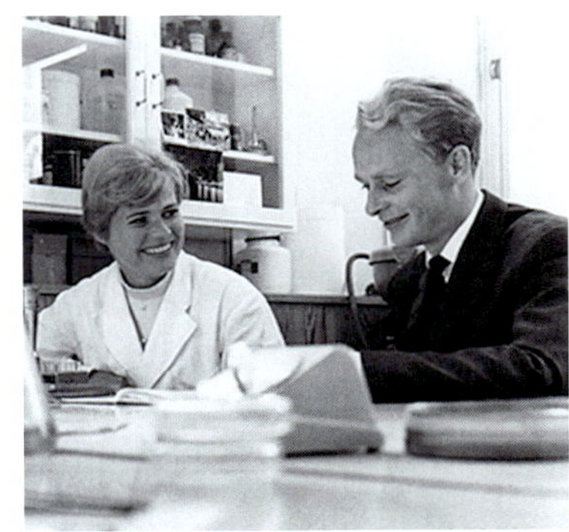

Erna and Göran Möller from the Karolinska Institute

Gerald M. Edelman, Member of the BII Advisory Board, Nobel Prize Winner 1972

Gerry Edelman, a member of the Advisory Board of the BII, won the Nobel Prize for Medicine and Physiology 1972 (shared with Rodney Porter) [QR1972_19]. The announcement of the Nobel Prize committee was: "*Immunebodies or antibodies is the designation of a group of proteins in the blood that play an important part in the defense against infections and in the development of many different diseases. Their perhaps most characteristic property is the capacity to react and combine with substances, foreign to the organism, so-called antigens and to do so in a highly specific manner. There probably exist more than 50,000 different antibodies in the blood, each of them reactive against one particular antigen. Their main features are similar but they show individual characteristics and constitute, therefore, an extremely heterogeneous group. Since, in addition, they appear as very large molecules of a complex structure, it is understandable that the study of their chemistry for a long time offered great difficulties.*"

QR1972_19 BII

Erna Möller and Göran Möller Visiting the BII at the Early Stage

During the planning of the institute, both Erna and Göran provided Niels with exceptional support and helped to establish a Swedish nucleus (scientists and technicians) in Basel.

Treasure Trove 1972

The database contains documents related to the BII in a broader context (lists, series of photographs, etc.).

QR1972_treasure BII

The Year 1973

Most of the new scientists joined existing groups. Jerne's office became the place for discussing the state of knowledge and future projects. Besides publications in prestigious journals, institute members participated in a number of workshops and conferences (London, Innsbruck, Brighton, Stockholm, New Delhi and other places). Roche became involved in conflicts regarding the pricing policy of their drugs in the UK. The BII Annual Reports became an invaluable source of information – distributed to every major immunology laboratory worldwide – with 123 reports for 1973.

Arrivals 1973 (18)
Eighteen scientists joined the institute in 1973, some of them arriving straight after the New Year, while others started at various times throughout the year: *Peter Baumann, Armando Bernardini, Melvin Cohn, Robert Cone, Wulf Droege, Stanislaw Dubiski, Hansjörg Forster, Heiner Frost, Haim Ginsburg, Leslie Hudson, Hans Huser, Peter Krammer, Angelika Kunz, Gabriel Michael, Stefanello de Petris, Harald von Boehmer, Matthias Wabl, Andreas Ziegler.* Some of them joined existing groups, others established their own laboratories. The institute achieved its optimal (planned) size, and from this year on there was a well-tuned balance between arrivals and departures.

Came and Left in the Same Year (1)
Gabriel Michael.

Leavers 1973 (22)
Jan Andersson, Wesley Bullock, Mario De Marchi, Stephen Fazekas de St. Groth, Joel Goodman, Joseph Haimovich, John Hamilton, Jack Hay, Ethel Jacobson, ▶

The Director in His Office

The New Year, 1973, started unusually early for Niels Jerne. For several reasons, he did not take the traditional Xmas time off to go down to Castillon. One was that he had just moved to the "zum Trillen" apartment in the old town of Basel (Rümelinsplatz). Besides that, a meeting about the Biozentrum was scheduled to be held with Eduard Kellenberger. Thus, Niels could be visited in his office right at the beginning of 1973. And people did visit.

It has already been mentioned that Niels did not go to the laboratories too often. He did not feel comfortable doing so. He felt that visits were always loaded with expectation and with thoughts about "why that lab and not ours". But his office was open to everybody any time.

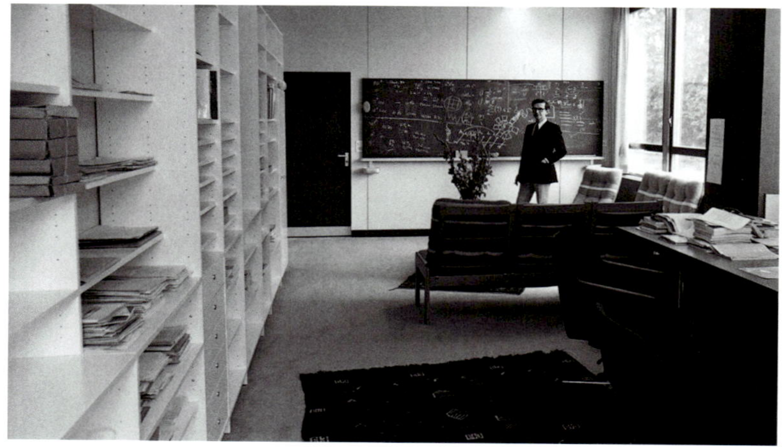

Niels Jerne at his famous blackboard in his office at the BII

Jerne's office was spectacular. The room had two important features: an extraordinarily large blackboard (blackboards at the BII will be mentioned elsewhere) and a huge desk along the entire length of the office. The desk was covered with items arranged in an orderly manner: journals, manuscripts, letters, and books – all neatly placed.

On first glance it became evident that he worked on several things simultaneously. However, he did concentrate on one issue, and when he was finished with it, or when he felt that "it was enough", he started on another pile.

Ingrid Schnurr (later Westen) was Niels' personal secretary throughout his entire directorship. Ingrid was not involved in handling the administrative matters of the institute, as Jerne delegated the entire administration to "others", and this will be described later. Ingrid made sure that Jerne had all his manuscripts typed, itineraries of journeys arranged, but importantly, she made sure that the stream of visitors was adequately controlled. Ingrid's office was accessible from the corridor, and the door was always open. Door signs, "do not disturb", were unknown to her. Ingrid not only spoke several languages, but she could type them perfectly. It was the "pre-computer age"; if a major "typo" occurred, she retyped the page. Even if she was busy, it was not hectic in her office. She was perfectly willing to type other people's manuscripts as well.

A small conference room was next to the secretary's office, and that of Zdenek Trnka, the administrator, was two doors away.

Jerne's bureau could be entered via the office of his secretary, and also through a door leading to the large seminar room. That door was rarely used, certainly not by visitors. It meant that Niels could enter the seminar room directly from his office, but he felt that this was not right as it attracted too much attention. He usually entered the seminar room via the main door, as did everybody else.

▶ *John Kettman, J. Russell Little, Takeshi Matsunaga, Wolfgang Mayr, Wallace McKeehan, Jacques F.A.P. Miller, Graham Mitchell, Hansruedi Ramseier, Stanley Read, Tien-Wen Tao-Wiedmann, Jorge Vives, Niklaus Weiss, Felix Wettstein.*

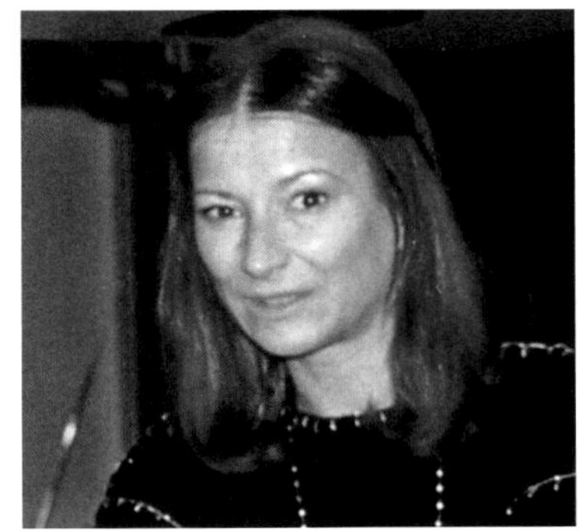

Ingrid Schnurr

Conferences and Symposia, 1973

1973 was a year with many commitments at international conferences, symposia and workshops. The first one was in February, the last in November. At each of them several members participated. The conferences are listed below:

- Workshop and Conference on Cellular Immunity in Mice, London Hospital Medical College
- 4. Arbeitstagung über Leukozytenkulturen: "Lymphozytenfunktion *in vitro*", Innsbruck

- International Conference on "The Spleen, Its Pathophysiology", Cluj, Romania
- International Symposium on Immunogenetics of Laboratory Animals, Prague
- British Society for Immunology, Brighton
- Hoffmann-La Roche Research Department, Basel, research projects of clinical importance (see next page)
- Demonstrations at the BII for the 6th Postgraduate Course in Experimental Medicine, University of Zurich (see below)
- Ninth International Congress of Biochemistry, Stockholm
- Joint Meeting of European Societies of Immunology, Strasbourg
- Society of General Physiologists, Symposium on "Cellular Secretion and Regulation in the Immune Response", Woods Hole
- IUIS-WHO Symposium on "Differentiation and Function of Lymphoid Cells", Sinaia, Romania
- British Society for Immunology, London, Annual Meeting
- First International Workshop on Nude Mice, Aarhus
- WHO course on "Biosynthesis of Immunoglobulins", New Delhi

Demonstrations at the BII for the 6th Postgraduate Course in Experimental Medicine, University of Zurich

One of the courses, in July 1973, was special, as it was organized for the participants at a postgraduate course of the University of Zurich. Seventeen BII labs were involved in organizing lectures and demonstrations for the 22 students attending the course:

D.G. Braun	"Specificity of antigen-antibody reactions"
I. Lefkovits and	
J. Quintáns	"Antibody-forming cells"
A.S. Kelus	"Allotypy and idiotypy"
J.R.L. Pink	"Isoelectric focusing"
M. Cramer	"Protein structure of immunoglobulins"
F. Loor	"Immunofluorescence"
L. Du Pasquier	"Antibody formation in lower animals"
H. Kiefer	"Fractionation of lymphocytes"
Z. Trnka and	
R.N.P. Cahill	"Traffic of lymphocytes and mediators"
J. Sprent	"Thoracic duct cannulation"
V.C. Miggiano	"MLC"
R. Ceppellini and	
D. Bernoco	"HLA typing, CML"
G.F. Mitchell	"Thymectomy"
W.W. Bullock	"Antibody formation *in vitro*"

B. Kindred	"Inbreeding and nude mice"
H. Ginsburg	"Target cell destruction"
T. Staehelin, M. Schreier and F. Wettstein	"Protein synthesis and immunology"

Lectures at Hoffmann-La Roche Research Department, Basel

There was also a certain (though not an overwhelming) interest from the Research Department of Roche in interacting with the "new" institute. Prof. Alfred Pletscher strongly encouraged such interactions. On 2 occasions (April and May 1973) 2 days of lectures were organized for the Research Department of Roche. The lectures took place in the Roche main building.

J. Haimovich	"The antibody-combining site"
J.F.A.P. Miller	"Lymphocytes – the immunologically competent cells"
F. Melchers	"Synthesis and secretion of antibodies"
G. Roelants	"Lymphocyte receptors"
S. Fazekas	"Viruses and antibodies: interaction of antigens and antibodies"
R. Ceppellini	"Histocompatibility antigens"
B. Pernis	"Problems in clinical immunology": I. The impact of immunology on medicine II. Tumor immunology
J. Andersson	"Mitogens as probes for immunocyte activation"

Roche Conflicts, 1973

A serious conflict between Roche and the British government came about when the British Parliamentary Undersecretary of State ordered the price of Valium and Librium to be reduced [QR1973_01]. The debate in the British Parliament started as follows: *This Order 1973 (Regulation of Prices of Tranquillising Drugs) relates to drugs sold by the Roche Group, comprising Roche Products Limited, SAPAC Corporation Limited and F. Hoffmann-La Roche and other associated companies, mainly as Librium and Valium. The purpose of the Order is to give effect to the Report of the Monopolies Commission, which recommended substantial reductions in Roche's prices for these drugs.*

This conflict seemingly had nothing to do with the BII, but it surprised Niels Jerne to receive a call from the head of a British parliamentary delegation requesting "a site inspection at the BII". Whether this violated some rules or laws was not the issue; a group of people appeared at the institute, and instead of talking to the director, they went directly and randomly into various laboratories with a set of questions: (a) What kind of drugs are you

QR1973_01 BII

It surrounded you with the best scientists on the planet, in an environment where all things were possible if you were good enough to get them. There was no excuse for failure other than you were not good enough.
Don Bellgrau

developing? (b) What happens with the results? (c) To whom at Roche are you reporting? With incredulity they noticed that scientists and technicians had not a clue what the questions meant, and the delegation concluded that the institute did not work on developing drugs – neither directly nor indirectly.

This deposition turned out to be of importance for Roche as, according to British law, a company was not allowed to add costs for developing new drugs to the price of existing drugs, but indeed it was acceptable to add costs for basic research. The price of Valium and Librium had to be reduced, but to a substantially lesser extent than if the institute's costs were taken into consideration in the Roche price calculations.

Jerne's Quote on the 1973 Research Projects

The gestation of a single research project extends over several years. More than a year usually goes by in designing and executing the work and in interpreting and publishing the results obtained. Additional time is needed for the scientific community to absorb and evaluate these results in comparison with the existing body of knowledge and with sometimes apparently conflicting results obtained in other laboratories. It is therefore difficult to assess current advances in immunology at yearly intervals.

New Projects Added, 1973

The projects outlined below are described in more detail in the Annual Report for 1973. All in all, there were 123 research reports comprising 80 pages, and they were the joint efforts of all the members and technicians. The technicians are not listed as "contributors" although in many instances they were more than helping hands. Jerne addressed this aspect in a separate document [QR1973_02].

QR1973_02 BII

Treasure Trove 1973
The database contains documents related to the BII in a broader context (lists, series of photographs, etc.).

QR1973_treasure BII

New Projects Added, 1973

The description of scientific achievements at the BII is based on the first-hand information given in the research reports, and thereafter in publications. But it would be beyond the scope of this book to detail projects that are explained in the Annual Reports; the sheer volume of material precludes such an undertaking. Nevertheless, it is important – at least when describing the "pioneering years" – to give space to the projects of the newly arriving scientists. This was done for 1972, and below it is done for 1973.

From the 18 newcomers, 4 did not submit a report (Mel Cohn, Peter Krammer, Angelika Kunz, Matthias Wabl) to be presented in the Annual Report 1973, while others, among them David Stott, though having arrived in 1972, completed their first project report in 1973. Mel Cohn enjoyed special member status and interacted by giving seminars, which bore his name (the Mel Cohn seminar series).

Reiteration Frequency of Antibody Genes

Armando Bernardini

The aim was to estimate the number of genes coding for the variable region of immunoglobulin polypeptide chains. The work was based on hybridization of mRNA and DNA preparation. A preparation of light chain mRNA was labeled with ^{125}I and hybridized to mouse liver DNA. Analysis of the results of such experiments indicated that nucleotide sequences coding for the entire C-region and most of the V-region are unique (this is defined by the so-called reiteration frequency that states how many copies of a certain gene sequence are present in the genome). The results suggested that in the mouse there is a very limited number of genes coding for the variable regions of immunoglobulin chains. This was of some importance, since others thought (and argued without experimental findings) that there were many.

N-Terminal Amino Acid Sequences of Immunoglobulin Light Chains

Susumu Tonegawa, Jean-Claude Jaton, Richard Pink, Max Schreier, Brigitte Askonas

When purified mRNA coding for immunoglobulin light chains is submitted to a cell-free translation system, the resulting polypeptide is about 20 amino acid residues longer than the secreted light chain. The "extra" portion (dubbed "leader sequence") consists of mostly hydrophobic amino acid residues and this part of the molecule is absent from the secreted light chain.

Structure and Function of Mammalian Ribosomes

Ingegerd Sundkvist

The main aim of Ingegerd's work was to characterize the functional activity of ribosomal subunits obtained through different procedures. In one method, polyribosomes were converted into single ribosomes upon completion of polypeptide chain synthesis (natural process); in another method, polyribosomes were incubated at high ionic strength with puromycin to cause premature polypeptide chain release (puromycin method). Three initiation factors were identified and partially purified.

The Role of J Chain in the Synthesis and Assembly of IgM

David I. Stott

A new component of IgM and IgA molecules, called J chain, had recently been discovered. It was a polypeptide chain with 6–7 cysteine residues found in polymeric IgA and IgM at a ratio of one J chain per molecule. It was absent from the monomeric forms. Mouse myeloma Y5781 was used to study the role of J chain in the assembly of IgM in the cell. It was found that anti-IgM serum specifically precipitated the J chain, together with the IgM molecule. Since upon reduction the J chain is released from the complex, it was concluded that the two components are attached through disulfide bonds.

Allotypes of Rabbit and Mouse Immunoglobulin

Stanislaw Dubiski

The institute's rabbits were bred for the purpose of maintaining a colony with defined genotypes for immunoglobulin markers (allotypes). The work on rabbit IgM allotypes revealed that one of the allotypic systems (Ms3 system) is absolutely specific for IgM, while two new IgM allotypes (Ms7 and Ms8) behave like alleles of Ms3. Antisera with defined specificity against the discovered allotypes were made available for further genetic typing and biochemical studies.

Selective Breeding for Specific Antibody Clones in Rabbits

Dietmar G. Braun, Hans Huser, Jean-Claude Jaton, Andrew S. Kelus

Rabbits were bred selectively for restricted responses to the streptococcal group A variant polysaccharides. It was investigated whether rabbits, when injected with the same antigen as their parents were immunized, produce antibodies similar to those of the parents in terms of their heavy and light chain allotypes, amino acid sequences, idiotypic specificities and isoelectric focusing properties. Breeding from 1 high responder male and 2 restricted high responder (to Av-CHO) female rabbits resulted in segregation of high and low responder progeny after 2 generations. Homologous anti-idiotypic antisera were raised against 6 restricted streptococcal group-specific antibodies. Two of these idiotypic systems have been analyzed in detail for idiotypic cross-reactions.

IgM Producing Tumors as a Model for B Cell Maturation

Jan Andersson, Ronald Citronbaum, Fritz Melchers, Benvenito Pernis, David I. Stott

Several adjuvant-induced Balb/c tumors producing IgM were characterized by analysis of the cellular distribution of IgM and by biochemical study of immunoglobulin synthesis, turnover and secretion. The cells of different tumors appear to represent different stages in B cell maturation when compared to normal, LPS-stimulated B cells. These tumors therefore represent a useful model for studying IgM synthesis and for other processes which change during B cell maturation.

Interaction of Surface Ig and Concanavalin A and Mechanism of Capping

Stefanello de Petris

The interaction of Con A and surface Ig was studied by electron microscopy. Fluorescein-conjugated Con A was capable of inducing cap formation at 37°C in a major portion of spleen cells and to a lesser extent in thymus cells. By using vinblastine (microtubule disruptive drug), colchicine (inhibitor of microtubule polymerization by binding to tubulin) and cytochalasin B (inhibitor of actin filament polymerization), conditions were found in which reversible inhibition of cap formation was obtained. The results indicate that microfilaments play an important role in cap formation. Freeze-etching of cells prefixed with glutaraldehyde revealed that components of the membrane that do not become constituents of the cap (intramembranous particles) remain randomly distributed over the cell membrane.

Surface Immunoglobulin of Sheep Peripheral Lymphocytes

Heiner Frost, Francis Loor, Ross Cahill, Zdenek Trnka

Rabbits were immunized with several preparations of sheep immunoglobulin, and the resulting antisera were characterized by immunoelectrophoresis and by the Ouchterlony technique. Specific antibodies were detected against IgG1, IgG2 and Fab. All antibodies with the exception of anti-IgG2 were present in high titers. Antibodies against non-Ig proteins were removed by adsorption with fetal lamb serum, and the Ig from the adsorbed antisera was conjugated with fluorescein isothiocyanate. These conjugated anti-sheep Ig antisera showed various degrees of binding to the surface of a proportion of sheep peripheral lymphocytes.

Origin of Immunoglobulin Bound to Activated T Lymphocytes

Leslie Hudson, Jonathan Sprent, Jacques F.A.P. Miller

Synthesis of immunoglobulin (Ig) by T lymphocytes was a controversial issue. Previous work has shown that Ig is readily detected by indirect immunofluorescence on the surface of activated T cells obtained from thoracic duct lymph of irradiated F1 mice injected with parental strain thymus cells. In order to establish the identity of this Ig, thoracic duct lymphocytes (TDL) were passed through anti-Ig columns with the aim of removing "residual" B cells. Using this protocol a strong reduction of the detected surface Ig was obtained. This was considered as evidence that the IgM on TDL is predominantly antihost alloantibody derived from B cells in the thymus cell inoculum from which the TDL were prepared.

T Cell Tumors

Peter Krammer, Benvenuto Pernis

In some strains of mice, e.g. AKR/J, there is a high incidence of spontaneous development of thymomas (at the age of about 12 months the tumor incidence reaches about 90%). The etiological agent responsible for tumor development is the Gross leukemia virus, which is vertically transmitted in these animals. We have found that all thymomas maintained in our laboratory stain positively with an anti-MSLA antiserum (an antiserum raised in rabbits, specific for mouse T cells) and thus show another independent T marker. Receptors for complement were studied by rosette formation with ox red blood cells sensitized with rabbit IgM antibodies plus mouse complement. The thymoma model offers a tool for studying the nature of the T cell receptor.

Exploration of Cell Surface Topography by Specific Antisera

Robert Cone, Domenico Bernoco, Giorgio Trinchieri

Antibody-mediated aggregation of molecules at the outer membrane layer of lymphocytes enabled the topography of the cell surface to be explored. The rearrangement of molecules (upon application of antibody followed by labeled anti-Ig) was followed visually by immunofluorescence. The formation of complexes at the cell surface makes the cell specifically resistant to complement-dependent lysis for all determinants carried by the molecular population that was aggregated. The 6 HLA antigens on the surface of cells from a donor heterozygous at all 3 "serum determinant" (SD) loci aggregate independently. This suggests that each SD locus is a cistron whose HLA product is expressed at the cell surface on a distinct molecular species.

Formal Genetics of the HLA System

Peter Baumann

A panel of more than 700 unrelated individuals (volunteers working at Roche) were typed for all known factors of the HLA system and for many other genetic polymorphisms (red cell antigens, salivary secretions, enzymes, serum proteins). Studies with this panel have proven the existence of a third SD (serologically defined) locus, SD-3, within the HLA region. SD-3 antigens were found expressed on all lymphocytes of the peripheral blood and on platelets. The panel was also used for analyzing the evolution of allogeneic antibodies during planned transfusions. Attempts were made to serotype the MLC determinants with allogeneic antisera by indirect immunofluorescence using fluorescent antirabbit complement from guinea pigs. This test became a usable alternative to the complement-dependent lysis techniques.

Function of Lymphocyte Subpopulations in the Mixed Lymphocyte Reaction

Harald von Boehmer, Jonathan Sprent

The mixed lymphocyte reaction (MLR) is thought to result from recognition between lymphocytes of different genetic origin. Genes coding for some of these determinants are located in the major histocompatibility complex, others segregate independently of MHC. T lymphocytes of certain mouse strains will recognize syngeneic B lymphocytes and respond with proliferation. Responsiveness to syngeneic lymphocytes declines as the animals mature. These observations prompted a closer study of the cells which interact in MLR. Evidence was obtained that T cells, even though mitomycin C-treated or X-irradiated, can recognize MLR determinants on the untreated cells. This recognition results in the formation of a factor which stimulates the untreated cells to synthesize DNA. It is well possible that somatic interaction of lymphocytes early in ontogeny generates immune response patterns that are later observed in adult mice.

Changes in MLC-Reactive Cells during the Allogeneic Response by Single Lymph Nodes

Ross Cahill, Heiner Frost, Jack Hay

The immune response of a single sheep lymph node to allogeneic lymphocytes has been examined. It did not differ from responses to a wide variety of other antigens studied in this system. MLC-reactive cells specific for the donor allogeneic lymphocytes were followed in one-way MLC reactions, where the donor lymphocytes were prevented from responding by prior irradiation with 4,500 R. A kinetics study of the proliferative response revealed profound changes in ^{3}H-thymidine incorporation throughout the MLC, thus providing a precise characteristic of the responsiveness of the cell population.

Induction of Primary Cell-Mediated Immune Response to Mycoplasma in Cell Culture

Haim Ginsburg

Mycoplasma is the smallest microorganism that can grow outside of cells. Pathogenic mycoplasma organisms multiply extensively in the respiratory tract, while in cultures of rat lymphocytes they grow as small clusters on the cell membrane. Treatment of rat lymphocyte cultures with chlortetracycline successfully eliminates infectious mycoplasma particles with a net result of explosive multiplication of the blast cells. If these "new lymphocytes" are re-exposed to *M. pulmonis*, all lymphocytes are retransformed to blast cells within 16 h. Essential components of cellular immunity (blast cells and the hypersensitive lymphocytes) are obtained by interaction of rat lymphocytes with intact mycoplasma.

Fractionation of Sheep Lymph Containing Biologically Active Factors

Ross Cahill, Max Schreier, Heiner Frost

The lymph draining from stimulated lymph nodes of the sheep contains 2 biologically active substances. By salt fractionation of lymph plasma, which is strongly inhibitory for macrophage migration, 2 inhibitory components (fraction I and II) were separated. Fraction I is a powerful inhibitor of macrophage migration, but it is probably not a lymphokine but rather a component of the clotting system. The active component of fraction II (MW 25–40,000) seems to be the lymphokine MIF.

Thymus Dependence of Reaginic Antibody Formation in Mice

Gabriel Michael

Reaginic antibodies to several protein antigens will not be formed in nude mice unless these mice are first given normal thymus grafts or are injected with normal thymus cells. Injection of a high dose of Balb/c cells (5×10^7) allowed a moderate level of reaginic antibodies to be formed. More importantly, it was shown that a higher level of reaginic antibody (and a longer-lasting one) is achieved when a smaller number of thymocytes, i.e. 5×10^5 per *nu/nu* mouse, is administered. It is suggested that IgG is immunoregulatory in suppressing reaginic antibody formation, since under conditions of maximal IgG formation IgE formation is suppressed.

Induction of B Cell Tolerance to Sheep Erythrocytes in vivo

Graham F. Mitchell, Louis Lafleur

Experiments have been performed to test the hypothesis that some precursors of antibody-forming cells (B cells) are susceptible to tolerance induction when confronted with antigen in the absence of T cells. Evidence for the hypothesis came from studies in mice using haptenated pneumococcal polysaccharide (DNP-SIII), D-amino acid synthetic polymers (DNP-D-GL) and self-structures (e.g. NIP mouse red cells). Hapten-specific tolerance follows from the injection of such conjugates. B cells of high antigen-binding capacity are inhibited by contact with antigen unless T cells are present. B cells of low antigen-binding capacity encounter less antigen and are not susceptible to "T cell-independent" tolerance induction. Low doses of SRBC ($<10^7$ SRBC) did not lead to tolerance in this nude mouse system.

Isolation of the Protein Antigens Present on the Surface of Influenza Virus

Andreas Ziegler,
Stephen Fazekas de St. Groth

Two different protein species are present on the surface of influenza virus: hemagglutinin and neuraminidase. It has been established that serological mutants of influenza virus, selected under antibody pressure, show changes in the hemagglutinin molecule. Antihemagglutinin antibodies raised against mutants (senior antigens) show strong binding to the antecedents of these mutants (junior antigens), whereas weak binding can be observed in the reaction of senior antigens to antijunior antibodies. Antisera raised against whole virus contain antibodies against the neuraminidase. These methods for the isolation and purification of the surface proteins involve enzymatic cleavage of the proteins of purified virus by bromelain, followed by the purification by column chromatography.

The Year 1974

A new category of "visiting scientists" was established (in order to comply with the strict cantonal quota for foreigners). A major innovation in the building was the conversion of laboratory 011 into a teaching laboratory. Two courses were given there: Advanced Course on Protein Biosynthesis and Advanced Study Course on Lymphocytes. In Brighton, at the Second International Congress of Immununology, 14 members delivered lectures. Tonegawa and colleagues published 4 papers on the generation of antibody diversity. Georges Köhler completed his doctoral thesis.

Arrivals 1974 (19)
Nineteen scientists joined the BII in 1974. Gordon Sato was a senior member both by age and reputation, pairing with Sir Macfarlane Burnet (Nobel Prize for Medicine 1961), who is listed in the category of scientists arriving and leaving in the same year.
Andrei Augustin, Humberto Cosenza, Tommy Douglas, Bruce Elliott, Bernhard Erni, Werner Haas, Geoffrey Hoffmann, Berenice Kindred (for a second time), Heinz Köhler, Gaston Matthyssens, Zoltan Nagy, Walter Riesen, Luciana Rovis, Gordon Sato, Jörg Schmidt, Rita Schuller, Bela Takacs, Bernd Weimann, Siegfried Weiss.

Came and Left in the Same Year (5)
Giovanna Azzini, Armin Boschetti, Sir Macfarlane Burnet, Ingrid Harbitz, Robert Phillips.

Leavers 1974 (17)
Peter Baumann, Armando Bernardini, Ronald Citronbaum, Melvin Cohn, Robert Cone, Matthias Cramer, Stanislaw Dubiski, Haim Ginsburg, Georges Köhler, Angelika Kunz, Louis Lafleur, Tommy Meo, Jonathan Sprent, David Stott, Ingegerd Sundkvist, Zoltán Tökés, Siraik Zakarian. ▶

In the chapters for the 4 preceding years, new BII members are introduced cursorily, in order to show the steady "build-up" of the research activities. These chapters conclude with descriptions of the new scientists' projects. Thus, the opening scene (1970) represented the "primeval soup" of talents of the founding group of scientists, then the projects became focused (1971), and later (1972, 1973) emphasis was placed on demonstrating "the integration of new members into the fully functioning research enterprise". It was a central issue to show the process of "being and becoming".

In the chapter for 1974 and those following, the emphasis will be on describing how the achievements of the BII unfolded, outlining the multifaceted aspects (science, courses, lectures, extramural activities, anniversaries, theater performances and others); nonetheless, innumerable projects will be referred to, both in the narrative and as QR notes.

The Teaching Laboratory and the Blackboard

BII was conceived as a basic research institute without a direct link to the university education system. Teaching on a postgraduate level was considered, but it did not have a high priority during the initial period. The decision was based on Jerne's belief that the institute consisting of a relatively modest number of scientists had not only to minimize the time spent on administrative duties, but also not be distracted from the main goal by taking up teaching activities. This decision was carefully tuned in such a manner that teaching was not completely excluded, but it was abridged to training at an "expert level".

The laboratory 011A was converted into a teaching laboratory in spring 1974, and the course to inaugurate it was the "Advanced Course on Protein Biosynthesis" held in August 1974. The layout of the teaching laboratory was such that it was suitable for holding experimental courses for 16–24 participants. It was a large laboratory having 4 large benches, each providing space for 4–6 participants. It had a blackboard along one of the walls.

The laboratory was used as a research facility when no courses were given. Usually courses were planned to be held at times when, due to staff turnover, the lab was empty in order to be prepared for a new group. When this was not possible timewise, the members moved out and were temporarily hosted by other research groups. Some members considered this arrangement a nuisance, while others enjoyed the hospitality of recipient labs, which in turn allowed for new contacts and often the initiation of joint projects.

Two courses were held in 1974 (July and October), one on protein biosynthesis, the other on lymphocytes.

Course I: Advanced Course on Protein Biosynthesis

The "Advanced Course on Protein Biosynthesis" was sponsored by the Schweizerische Kommission für Molekularbiologie, which was part of the Swiss National Science Foundation [QR1974_02]. The instructors were Theo Staehelin and Armin Boschetti of the BII and Tom Bickle from the Biozentrum, Basel.

The course covered some of the basic experiments employed in the elucidation of the genetic code, as well as in the reconstitution, and functional and structural characterization of bacterial ribosomes. In the mammalian field, the students prepared and tested ribosome subunits and initiation factors according to procedures developed mainly at the BII. They also performed some new modifications of experiments, such as combining a mammalian translation system with a bacterial transcription system.

The students were:

Steven Alasdair, Dominique Belin, Silvain Berner, Walter Bossart, Olivier Civelli, Albert Egg, Wendy Gibbs, Martin Glor, Robert Hetzel, Hans Hosbach, Ulrich Kaufmann, Douglas Marvil, Jean-Jacques Mermod, G. Miozzari, Ernst Peterhans, Hermann Polger, Ross Smith, Christine Steinheil, Richard Voellmy (all from Zurich, Basel, Geneva and Paris).

▶ Visiting Scientists 1974 (29)
A new category of "visiting scientists" was introduced in 1974. To have such a group was somewhat against the "all-members-are-equal" principle, but this arrangement grew out of necessity, as Switzerland had a strict quota for providing residence permits for foreigners (see the QR note [QR1974_01] on the Überfremdungsinitiative 1974). Scientists staying for 6 months or less were not included in the quota.
Jan Andersson, La Jolla; Kamala Balakrishnari, New Delhi; Florence Bovey, Basel; Franco Celada, Rome; Xavier Chardonnens, Geneva; Cees Cornelisse, Leiden; Alastair Cunningham, Canberra; Mario De Marchi, Turin; Antonio Fantoni, Rome; S. Fazekas de St. Groth, Sydney; Josef Haimovich, Rehovot; Raymond Hamers, Brussels; Günther Hämmerling, Cologne; John Hay, Toronto; Claudia Henry, Berkeley; Herman Kalckar, Boston; Edwin S. Lennox, La Jolla; Dorothea Mayr, Vienna; Wolfgang Mayr, Vienna; Indira Nath, New Delhi; Alberto Piazza, Turin; Edgar Pick, Tel Aviv; Johan Ploem, Leiden; Philippe Roch, Bordeaux; Roland Scollay, Sutton; Herman Waldmann, Cambridge; Robert Walen, Paris; Peter Wernet, New York; Jadwiga Wojtulewicz, Warsaw.

QR1974_01 BII

QR1974_02 BII

Course II: Advanced Study Course on Lymphocytes

The "Advanced Study Course on Lymphocytes" was sponsored jointly by the WHO, ICRO and UNESCO, and organized by Vincenzo Miggiano and Georges Roelants, with a large staff of instructors from the BII, and guest instructors from Lausanne, Turin, Florence, Berkeley and Ann Arbor [QR1974_03].

The program included a general introduction to lymphocyte separation, characterization and reactivity in vitro, and instruction in techniques related to automation and miniaturization, and various other methods as indicated in the QR note.

The students were selected from many countries, including from the Soviet Union, Hungary and Czechoslovakia:

Vagn Andersen (Denmark), Ignaz Auer (Germany), Roland Ball (England), Patricia M. Chisholm (Scotland), Marc De Bruyre (Belgium), Jean-Pierre Dessaint (France), Ilaria Dishkant (USSR), Ralf S. Geha (Lebanon), Shan Soh Ha (Singapore), Turgut Imir (Turkey), Anil N. Jayawardena (Ceylon), Jens Jensenius (Denmark), Roger Kennett (USA), Filip Lulo (Yugoslavia), Marcella Pediconi (Italy), Philippe Roch (France), Nazario Rubio (Spain), V.M. Rumjanek (Brasil), Gabriella Sarmay (Hungary), Alexander Sarokin (USSR), Jacob Shoham (Israel), Carol H. Sibley (USA), Peter Sima (Czechoslovakia).

From Basel to Brighton, 1974

The Second International Congress of Immunology, Brighton, UK [QR1974_04], was undeniably the most important scientific event of 1974. The preceding conference – 3 years earlier – had taken place in Washington, D.C. There the foundation of the BII had been a hot topic of conversation in "corridor talks", while in 1974 the participation of BII members was a high-profile opportunity for 14 of them to participate and present their work, with 6 of them being workshop chairmen.

R.E. Cone	"Biochemistry of lymphocyte receptors" and "Dynamics of lymphocyte membranes"
R. Pink	Co-chairman of the workshop on "Genetic coding for immunoglobulins"
L. Hudson	Co-chairman of the workshop on "Enrichment of lymphocyte populations by affinity chromatography"
S. de Petris	Chairman of the workshop on "Techniques of immune-electron microscopy"
B. Pernis	"Behavior of cell surface components in immunological phenomena"
F. Melchers	Co-chairman of the symposium on "Synthesis and secretion of Ig"
D.I. Stott	"J chains" and "Assembly of the immunoglobulin molecule"

QR1974_03 BII

QR1974_04 BII

I. Lefkovits	"The nature of the clonal response to antigen"
D.G. Braun	"Idiotypic antibody" and "Antibody synthesis *in vitro*"
M. Cramer and D.G. Braun	"Antibody responses of restricted clonability"
H. von Boehmer	Co-chairman of the workshop on "Analytical cell electrophoresis"
L. Du Pasquier	Chairman of the workshop on "Primitive vertebrate immunology"
H.-R. Kiefer	"Specific cell separation"
J.-C. Jaton	"Rabbit allotypes", "Variable region structure" and "The structure of the antigen-binding site"

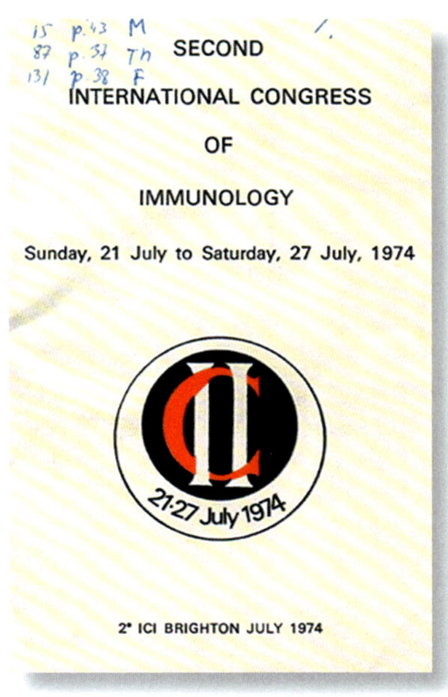

Georges Köhler's Doctoral Thesis, 1974

Fritz Melchers' scientific interest prior to his arrival at the BII was related to 2 subjects: secretion of immunoglobulins and β-galactosidase. On the activation of mutant β-galactosidase by specific antibodies, Fritz had a fruitful collaboration with Walter Messer. The work on the β-galactosidase project continued when Fritz' first doctoral student, Georges Köhler, made it the subject of his thesis. In 1974 Georges defended his thesis entitled *Eine Analyse der Heterogenität von Antikörpern gegen das Enzym Beta-Galactosidase aus E. coli* at the University of Freiburg [QR1974_05].

Upon obtaining his doctorate, Georges looked for a position where he could continue to investigate the heterogeneity of antibody. He took up a postdoctoral fellowship at the Laboratory of Molecular Biology in Cambridge, UK, where he began working with César Milstein to investigate the mechanism that underlies the diversity of antibodies. During this work, Köhler and Milstein devised their hybridoma technique for the production of antibodies. In the chapter for 1976, Georges' return to the BII is described.

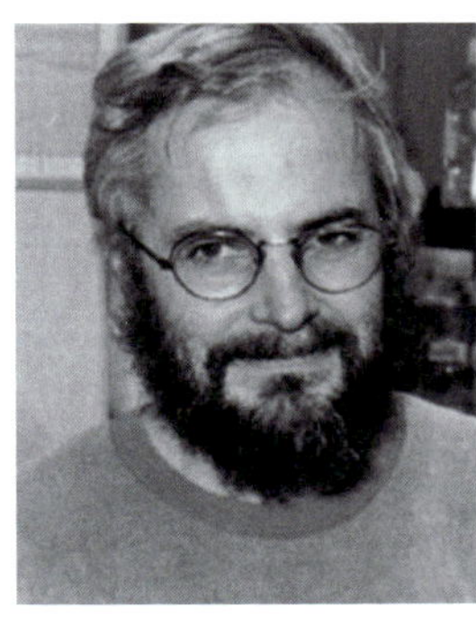

Georges Köhler

Werner Haas Joins the BII

Werner Haas came from Gus Nossal's laboratory (Walter and Eliza Hall Institute, Melbourne, Australia). He joined Harald von Boehmer and soon became not only a valuable coworker, but also one of the most critical and outspoken members of the BII.

Werner had studied medicine in Freiburg in Germany. His thesis in the laboratory of pathologist Harald Noltenius dealt with Burnet's clonal selection theory, new at that time. After his final exams, Werner worked in various hospitals in Berlin (1971/1972) and then decided to go back to research. His fascination with Burnet's clonal selection theory led him to apply to the Walter and

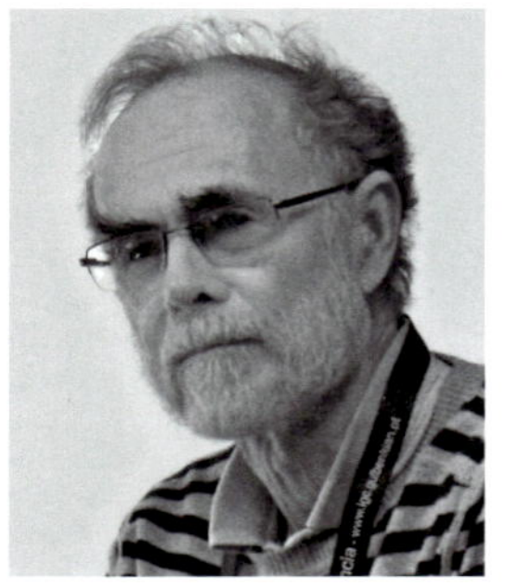

Jonathan Sprent

Eliza Hall Institute. He was accepted and became Gus Nossal's PhD student, working in the lab of Alex Szenberg on the overall theme of isolation of antigen-specific lymphocytes. From Harald von Boehmer he learned about Niels Jerne's paper on "The somatic generation of immune recognition", which was the first paper published in the newly established *European Journal of Immunology*. Harald completed his PhD work on the separation of B and T cells by cell electrophoresis in the laboratory of Ken Shortman, and then Harald and his wife Monica moved to Basel. Soon afterwards, on Harald's suggestion, Werner applied for a position at the BII, he was accepted, and in the autumn of 1974 started his career there [QR1974_06].

Tommy Meo to Ann Arbor, Then to St. Louis and Back to Basel

Tommy Meo was born in Forino (near Avellino, Italy), studied medicine in Turin, and in 1970 he was introduced to research in the Genetics Department, headed by Ruggero Ceppellini. Tommy was accepted at the BII in 1971 and became involved in genetic and serological studies on MLR determinants in the H-2 lr region. From Basel he moved to Donald Shreffler's laboratory in Ann Arbor and in St. Louis (1974–1976), where he explored the central portion of the MHC providing important clues to the evolutionary relationships of the HLA and the H-2 complexes. Tommy Meo returned to Europe for his second term at the BII (1976–1978). His next steps will be described in the later sections of this book.

Jon Sprent to London

After 3 years in Basel Jon accepted an offer from University College London, and later he moved to the Scripps Clinics in San Diego. His research interests concerned the life span of B and T cells circulating in the mouse, thymus function, T cell differentiation and homeostasis, and immunological tolerance. More about Jon, especially his development to become one of the most prominent immunologists, is given in the chapter for 1977.

QR1974_06 BII

QR1974_07 BII

Graham Mitchell and Melbourne Zoo

After 2 years at the BII, Graham Mitchell returned to Australia [QR1974_07]. Graham obtained a PhD at the Walter and Eliza Hall Institute in 1969. A large number of papers of "Mitchell & Miller" and "Miller & Mitchell" with discoveries in cellular immunology had populated the *Journal of Experimental Medicine* and other prominent journals since 1970. Besides Basel, he worked in the USA and UK, and finally settled in Australia to establish a new program in immunoparasitology at the Walter and Eliza Hall Institute. Graham has been a director of the Royal Melbourne Zoological Gardens.

Graham was a Gold Medallist of the University of Sydney and was awarded the honor of the "Officer of the Order of Australia for Services to Medical Science".

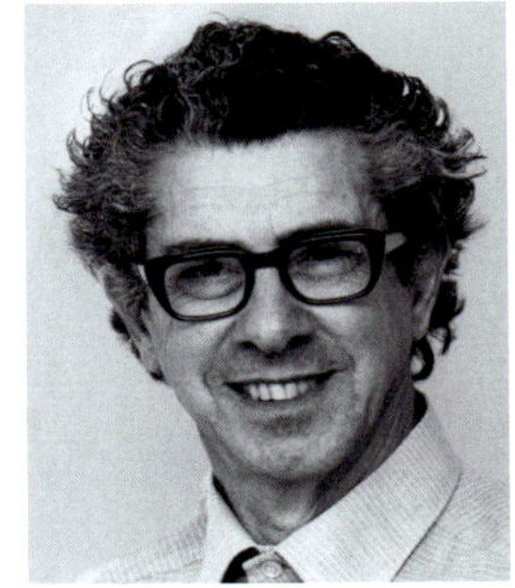

Jacques F.A.P. Miller

Roche Successes, 1974

Although this narrative concerns the Basel institute, certain Roche developments were of importance. New drugs such as 5-fluorouracil, Lexotanil and Rohypnol were launched and new institutes created. Roche Japan set up a new research center with Prof. Yashuo Yagi as head, and a Marine Pharmacology Institute in Dee Why, Australia, was established under the leadership of Joseph Baker.

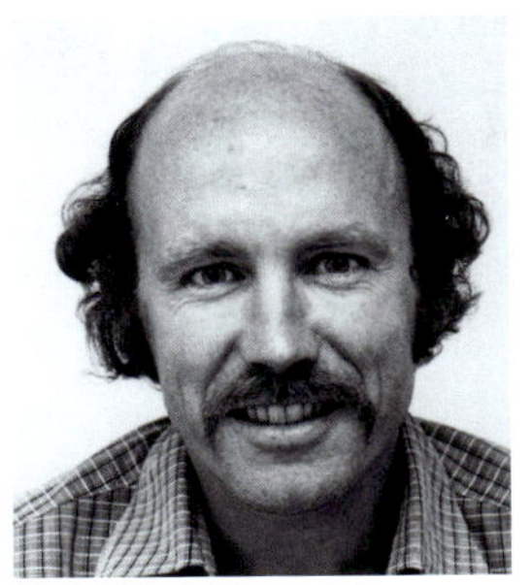

Graham Mitchell

Nobel Prize for Christian de Duve, a Long-Standing Friend of the BII

Members of the staff were happy to learn that a long-standing friend of the institute and prospective member of the Advisory Board, Christian de Duve [QR1974_08], was awarded the Nobel Prize for Medicine 1974. He shared this prize with Albert Claude and George Palade *"for their discoveries concerning the structural and functional organization of the cell"*.

QR1974_08 BII

Treasure Trove 1974

The database contains documents related to the BII in a broader context (lists, series of photographs, etc.).

QR1974_treasure BII

Next page: DNA strands (C. Brack) as detailed on p. 190

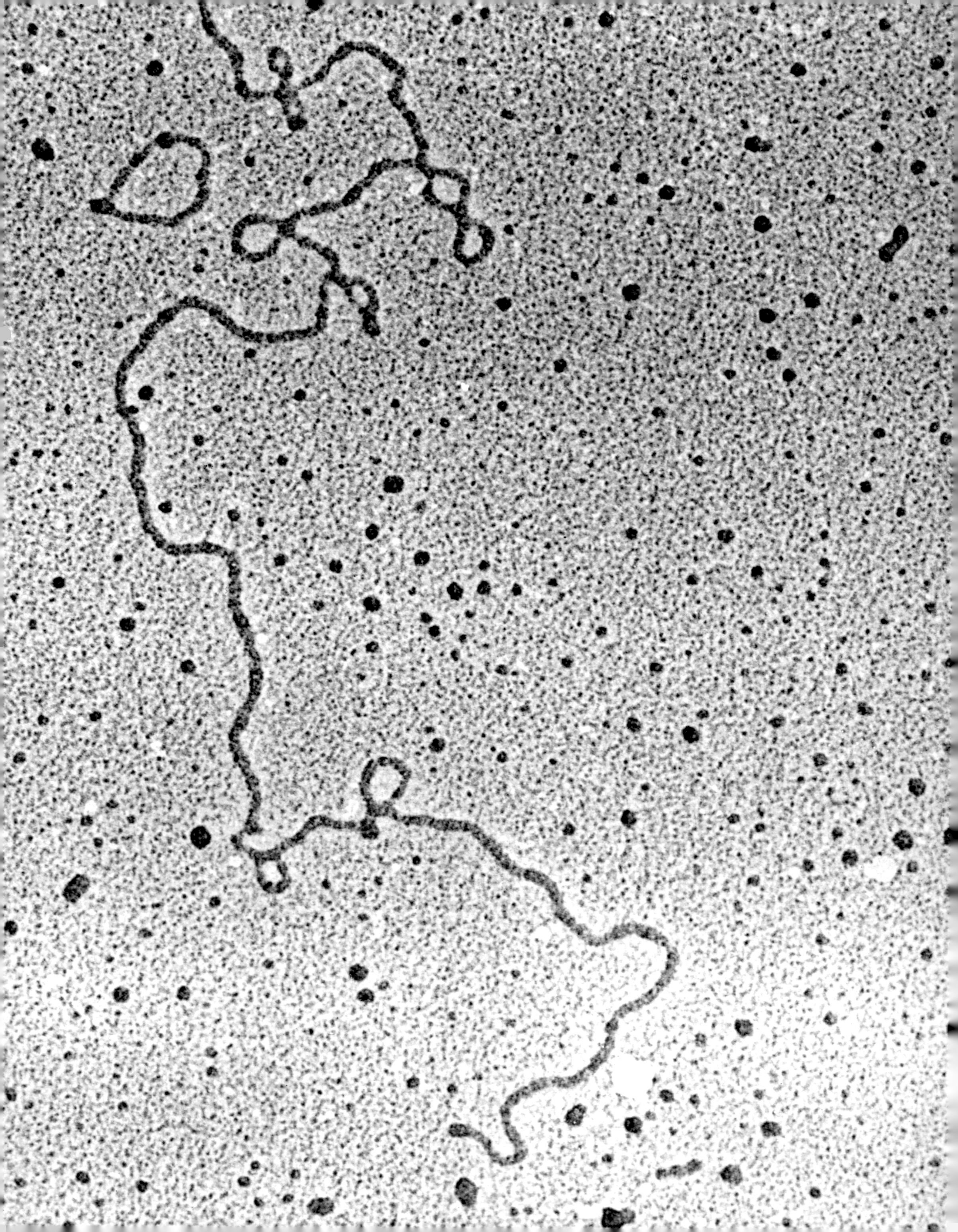

Reporting and Disseminating Results, 1974

The number of published papers kept increasing steadily. Again quoting Jerne: *More than a year usually goes by in designing and executing the work and in interpreting and publishing the results obtained.* By 1974 – since the conception of the institute – 313 publications had appeared in various peer-reviewed journals and proceedings.

Scientists who had spent 2 or more years at the BII were successful in having their research published. During the 2 years reported, the most prolific 23 authors published 210 papers (this grand total is not entirely correct, as some papers were counted twice due to multi-authorships). The number of papers authored or co-authored in 1973 and 1974 are given in parenthesis: *D.G. Braun (11), R. Ceppellini (7), R.E. Cone (4), M. Cramer (5), W. Droege (5), L. Du Pasquier (10), J.-C. Jaton (11), N.K. Jerne (7), B. Kindred (9), I. Lefkovits (15), F. Loor (17), F. Melchers (16), T. Meo (8), V.C. Miggiano (10), M. Nabholz (9), B. Pernis (7), J.R.L. Pink (4), J. Quintáns (10), G.E. Roelants (13), J. Sprent (15), S. Tonegawa (4), G. Trinchieri (9), H. von Boehmer (4).*

Although quantity is not always correlated with quality, the above list allows the identification of scientists who were fully productive in the new environment and were obtaining results worth reporting.

The research projects highlighted below meant to indicate the emerging picture of the immune system. The wealth of knowledge is of course incomparably larger than what is shown here.

Clonal Selection, Network Theory

Niels K. Jerne combined his vision, wisdom and intuition, and emphasized his view on the immune system, clonal selection, network theory and last but not least on the methodology of quantitating the numbers of antibody-forming cells.

Generation of Antibody Diversity

Susumu Tonegawa, in a combined effort with **Charley Steinberg**, reached the "home straight" towards solving the problem of the generation of antibody diversity. Evidence for the somatic nature of the generation of diversity was overwhelming.

Genetically Identical Toads

Louis Du Pasquier and **Matthias Wabl**, in collaboration with **Hans-Ruedi Kobel**, obtained genetically identical toads by activating diploid eggs by irradiated sperms. They studied in these *Xenopus* toads the antibody heterogeneity upon response to some defined antigens. This was the start of several research projects on nuclear transfer in the coming years.

Turnover of Immunoglobulin Molecules

Fritz Melchers continued studying B lymphocyte populations. In collaboration with various groups he investigated the turnover of immunoglobulin molecules; he did so by radiolabeling small and large splenic lymphocytes, and he established the rate of synthesis and the half-life of secretion of IgM molecules. This work enabled the classification of B lymphocytes from various lymphoid organs (lymph nodes, thoracic duct, spleen and bone marrow). At this stage **Harald von Boehmer** had set up a free-flow electrophoretic system for cell separation; thus Melchers had access to separated cell fractions.

Immunoglobulin Synthesis in Fetal Liver

Bob Phillips pursued the work on immunoglobulin synthesis in fetal liver, and he did it with **Fritz Melchers** and **Francis Loor**. They pulsed a fetal liver cell suspension with a radioactive amino acid and measured the radioactivity in precipitates with anti-Ig serum. They found significant Ig synthesis in samples of 13 and 19 days of gestation. Parallel to this, fetal liver cells were stained with fluorochrome-labeled antisera. Presence of Ig in the cytoplasm was shown on day 14 of gestation.

Chicken Model of the Immune System

Richard Pink scrutinized human myeloma proteins, subjecting them to isoelectric focusing in polyacrylamide gels. None of the samples studied gave identical focusing patterns. These results were the benchmark for further studies on clones of anti-streptococcal group A antibody from the chicken model he established at the BII.

Specificity of Anti-Idiotypic Determinants

Humberto Cosenza and **Heinz Köhler** succeeded in identifying idiotypic reactive cells in Balb/c mice upon immunization with phosphorylcholine. They measured plaque-forming cells displaying specificity to the immunizing antigen and to the anti-idiotypic determinants. Cosenza concluded that the antibody synthesized during the immune response combines with the respective antigen, which in turn serves as a carrier for the idiotypic determinants.

Network Hypothesis

Geoff Hoffmann was a theoretician, and his primary interest was in substantiating Jerne's network hypothesis. His main concern at the early stage of his work was the definition of the complementary sets of the responding sets and anti-idiotypic sets of cells.

Maternal Effect in Antibody Response

Berenice Kindred and **Georges Roelants** established in the mouse that immunization of a mother with DNP causes restriction of the anti-DNP antibodies produced by her offspring. This work was a starting point in studying the so-called maternal effect in antibody response.

Initiation of Clonal Responses

Ivan Lefkovits and **José Quintáns** collaborated with **Humberto Cosenza** on the assortment of clones producing antibody against phosphorylcholine and anti-idiotypic antibody. T cell involvement in the response was studied. They concluded that T cells are not needed for initiating clonal responses, though they are needed for clonal expansion.

The Year 1975

The turnover of scientists balanced out: 7 scientists left, and 18 scientists replaced them. The terrarium was converted into a vivarium to accommodate additional species of amphibians. Eighteen BII members participated at workshops and conferences in Basel, Aarhus, Amsterdam and Mainz.

1975 was an important year for research in the institute, as 5 years' existence would unmercifully show whether the high expectations were matched by true achievements. *Vorschusslorbeeren* only last for a short while. The "indicators" were positive: the number of publications in high-impact journals was satisfactory, the number and the quality of applicants were very good, and the BII remained as attractive as it had been at the onset.

In this section the procedure for selecting new members is described. Furthermore, additional animal species (especially cold-blooded animals), in which the immune system and its evolutionary aspects could be studied, were introduced into the BII. Courses held at the institute are listed, and last but not least the projects of scientists newly joining the institute are described. These features are interlaced with several quotes from Jerne's Annual Report introductions.

Arrivals 1975 (18)
Clinton Ballou, Nicholas Cohen, Ronald Corley, Antonio Coutinho, Pierre Dolivo, Garrison Fathman, Hans Hengartner, Nobumichi Hozumi, Judith Johnson, Michael Julius, Katherine Knight, Michael Pawlita, David Poskitt, Irmtraut Schmid, Edwin Seegmiller, Michael Taussig, Hans Trachsel, Takeshi Watanabe.

Came and Left in the Same Year (1)
Albert Nordin.

Leavers 1975 (7)
Leslie Hudson, Heinz Köhler, Peter Krammer, Jan Obel, Georges Roelants, Gordon Sato, Giorgio Trinchieri.

Procedure for Selecting New Members

Years previously Niels Jerne had said: "I want to recruit the best people available." He did not say "best people", but rather "best people available". And by 1974 he had achieved a full house, and it was a full house according to his choice. A new era started when a balance had been reached, and further new staff had to be recruited from candidates who formally applied for a position.

It became widely known that the institute offered time-limited contracts, and that the applicants had to present a proposal for a project. Thus, except for students (to be explained elsewhere) the positions were meant as a "second postdoc" position. Applicants knew that they had to explain in a letter what they had done previously (maybe at their first postdoc position), and what research they wanted to do at the BII, if accepted. Often it was the case that they had already participated at a BII course – as students

Moving to the Basel Institute was to come to the center of the world.

Antonio Coutinho

or lecturers – and had a clear idea of what the BII expected from its staff. Another group of candidates were those who read the Annual Report of the BII, which within the first 3 or 4 years (see QR note on Annual Reports) had become a major source of information in the world of immunology and could be found on the shelves of every major immunology lab.

Jerne appointed a Scientific Staff Selection Committee, which read the applications and had ad hoc meetings when needed. Charley Steinberg was one of the key members of the committee. If an applicant said that he had heard about this famous institute, would like to work there and was willing to undertake whatever project was offered him, his application had little chance of being considered. A candidate with a well-defined project (if it fitted into the general framework of BII activities) had a good likelihood of being accepted.

Interestingly, a new member was not obliged to stick to his "promise" to work on the project he had described in his application. He could change his mind and work on something else. Nevertheless, there could be a conflict between his promise and his actual work. When the contract neared its end, a confrontation might arise when the scientist approached Jerne to negotiate a prolongation.

If, in a hypothetical case, the applicant had abandoned the originally envisaged project and worked on something else, Jerne could have expressed his appreciation and prolonged the contract, or he might have said "sorry, your contract will not be prolonged, as you did not do what you intended to do, and were not successful in the alternative project you chose".

In 1974 (and for years thereafter) the turnover was such that "arrivals" and "departures" of scientists balanced out. Overall the number of applications was 70–100 per year. This "indicator" of attractiveness of the BII was one of the "inner criteria" to measure the success of the institute.

The Terrarium Becomes a Vivarium for Cold-Blooded Species

1975 started in a stable manner with one minor reconstruction to be completed: the conversion of the terrarium into a vivarium – plainly said, space was needed for work on amphibians. Years previously, when the institute only existed in form of floor plans, Louis Du Pasquier explained to Jerne that he would need a different type of animal facility for his research than that used for rodents.

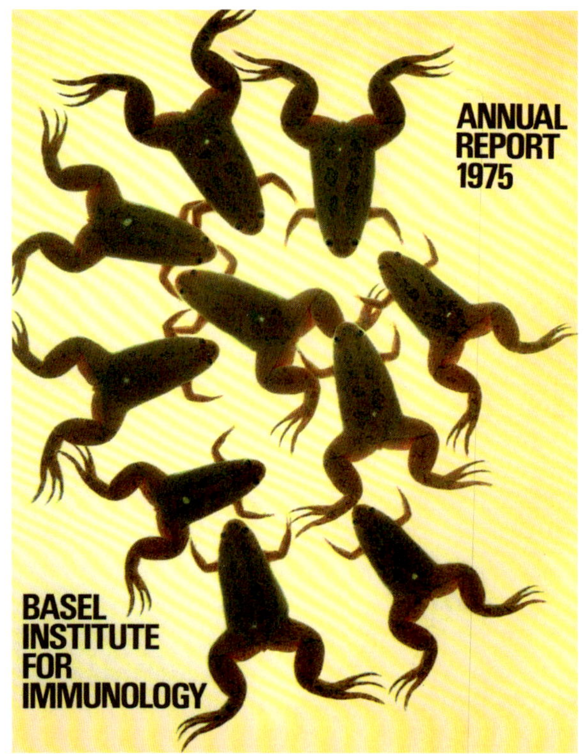

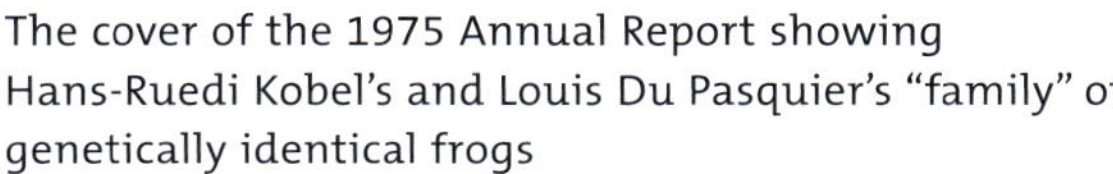
The cover of the 1975 Annual Report showing Hans-Ruedi Kobel's and Louis Du Pasquier's "family" of genetically identical frogs

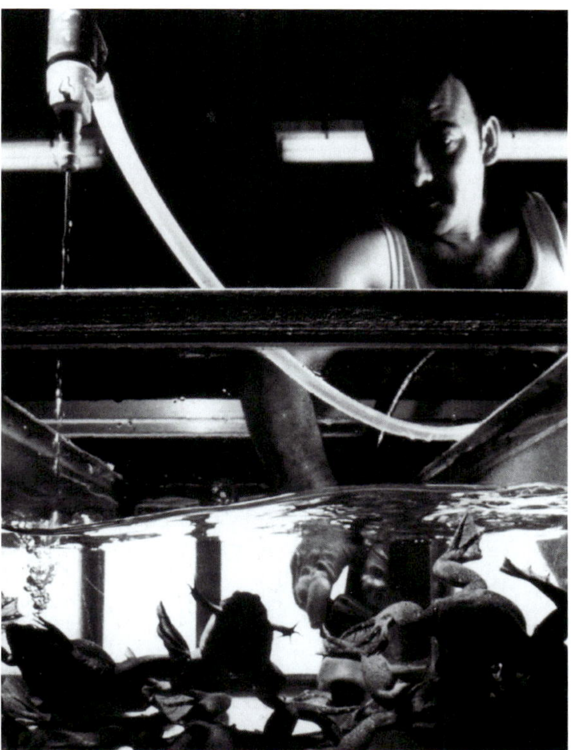
Vivarium

The main animal facility of the BII was mouse oriented, besides that there was a farm for rabbits at Rodersdorf, and a chicken farm at Frick. When Louis saw the floor plans (back in 1970), he realized that an atrium-like space existed which would be suitable for housing frogs and other cold-blooded animals.

On the first set of floor maps that area was conceived as an "open" space, but soon it was agreed that it would be covered by a glass roof. In the plans it was referred to as a "terrarium". With ground heating and watering systems it was an ideal place to keep the semi-terrestrial amphibian species. As the space was adjacent to the workshop, the maintenance of the facilities was delegated to the workshop employees.

Over the years, it became clear that bullfrog tadpoles and adults would remain a model for long-range projects, but another species of amphibian, *Xenopus*, being fully aquatic and easier to breed, would prove to be the model of choice. Thus, the terrarium had to be transformed into a set of hundreds of glass aquaria able to

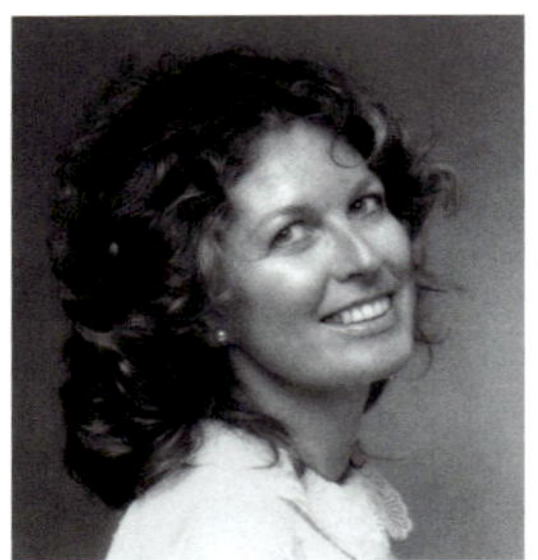

Irma Schmid

host about 3,000 specimens, especially the new species collected during an expedition to Africa. The "vivarium" with filtered and heated water, and equipped with various safety features, was copied from the blueprint of Prof. Fischberg's facility in Geneva University, and improved on by the BII workshop [QR1975_01]. Years later the vivarium facility was adapted to keep axolotls and trout as well.

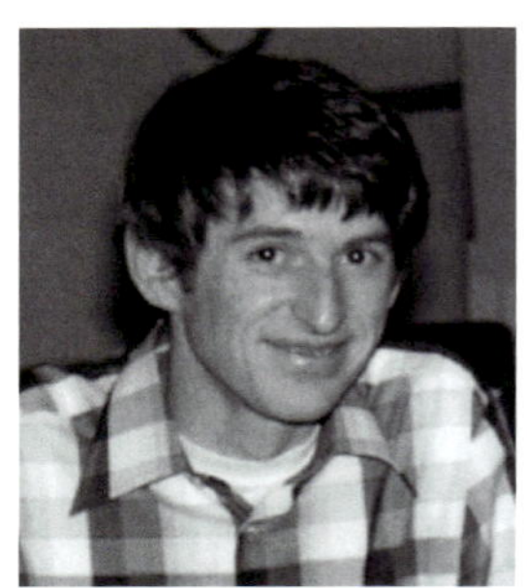

Max Schreier

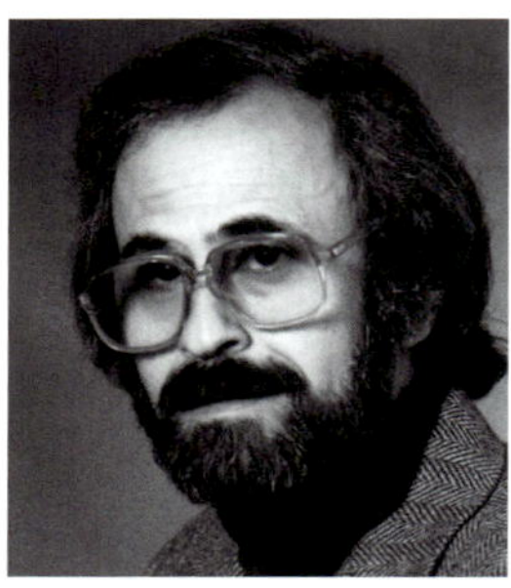

Nick Cohen

Who Joined Who, 1975

All the new scientists joined fully functioning research laboratories, but nevertheless some of them initiated their own projects. Those who made prior arrangements to integrate into existing groups were Nick Cohen, who joined Louis Du Pasquier to embark on a project of immunoregulation during metamorphosis, and Ed Seegmiller, who joined Max Schreier to study immunodeficiency related to blocks in purine metabolism.

Irma Schmid first joined Max Schreier's lab, where she contributed to the project to analyze colony formation of lymphocytes in soft agar; later she moved to Dietmar Braun's research group. Michael Julius was awaited with great expectation, as he came from Lee and Len Herzenberg's laboratory and intended to evaluate whether a fluorescence-activating cell sorter (FACS) would be a suitable tool to be introduced to the institute – at that time only prototypes of the FACS existed. Michael's immediate project was with Andrew Kelus and Ben Pernis to identify events in IgM to IgG switch. This was satisfactorily done in rabbit species, and it was especially fitting that Andrew Kelus had a strain in his rabbit colony with an allotype marker restricted to the IgM b4 allotype. Michael also started a project on T cell dependence on the development of B cell memory.

Antonio Coutinho came from Göran Möller's laboratory and continued work on projects which had been initiated by the Swedish group (including Jan Andersson who had returned to Uppsala from Basel; listed as a visitor in 1974) with the main emphasis on maturation of B lymphocytes after mitogenic stimulation. After improving culture conditions, Coutinho and Melchers achieved extensive cell proliferation in up to 8 days.

Pierre Dolivo's main interest was the formal genetics of HLA, studying samples from patients suffering from ankylosing spondylitis. Ronald Corley's first projects involved the study of lymphocyte responses resulting from priming to alloantigens.

Judith Johnson embarked on studies of precursor cells in mosaic mice. She developed a model of stable immune system chimer-

QR1975_01 BII

ism by injecting fetal liver cells from 2 strains of mice into irradiated F1 mice.

Michael Taussig had chosen the difficult and treacherous research direction of studying T cells sharing idiotypic determinants with antibody (and with B cells). He wanted to detect V-region antigenic determinants on T cell factors. Since several of these findings turned out to be faulty, it is relevant to mention that Taussig in his reports noticed that in a "number of experiments poor or negative results were obtained".

Reports on the projects of the remaining 6 newcomers – Clinton Ballou, Katherine Knight, Al Nordin, David Poskitt, Hans Trachsel and Takeshi Watanabe – are given in the QR notes [QR1975_02], [QR1975_03], [QR1975_04] and [QR1975_05].

QR1975_02 BII

QR1975_03 BII

QR1975_04 BII

QR1975_05 BII

Twenty Categories

The previous paragraphs provided a glimpse of the activities of new members. But of course these are only a fraction of all the work carried out in the institute. The research was not formally categorized; nevertheless, when assembling the research reports for the Annual Report this became necessary. In the 1975 Annual Report the research is divided into 20 categories:

- The origin of antibody diversity
- Protein synthesis
- Growth and maturation of lymphocytes in culture
- Structure of immunoglobulin genes
- Structure of immunoglobulins
- Allotypes and idiotypes
- Regulation of the immune response
- Genetics of immune responsiveness
- Clones of antibody-forming cells
- Differentiation of lymphocytes
- The lymphocyte surface
- Chemical studies of membrane components
- Histocompatibility antigens
- Mixed lymphocyte reactions
- Cell cooperation

- Specific unresponsiveness
- Lymphocyte recirculation
- Lymphocyte subpopulations
- Viruses and tumors
- Laboratory methods

The 1975 Annual Report comprises 136 research reports. Assuming that publications in *Nature* and *Science* indicate more general interest, it should be noted that 3 papers appeared in *Nature* and 1 paper in *Science*.

Workshops and Conferences, 1975

Four major workshops and conferences with a strong participation of BII members were held in Basel, Aarhus, Amsterdam and Mainz:

- 6th Workshop on Leukocyte Cultures, Basel
- 6th International Histocompatibility Workshop Conference, Aarhus, Denmark
- 10th Leukocyte Culture Conference, Amsterdam, The Netherlands
- Annual Conference of the "Gesellschaft für Immunologie", Mainz, Germany

Details of these four conferences are given in the QR notes [QR1975_06], [QR1975_07], [QR1975_08] and [QR1975_09].

Jerne on the Endocrine System and on the Nervous System

In his "Introduction to the AR 1975" Jerne writes: *The analysis of the immune system into its elements must be followed by the integration of these elements into a functional system. This task can be compared to the assembly of a jigsaw puzzle from an incomplete set of pieces. Studies of regulatory phenomena in the immune system represent partial integration attempts, since all regulation involves interactions between cells. Interaction either requires direct cellular contact (as in the nervous system), or it can be mediated by secreted molecules (as in the endocrine system). As lymphocytes circulate throughout the body, both these types of interactions occur. Both involve molecular components of lymphocyte surface membranes ("re-*

ceptors"), which can interact with components of other cells ("stimulators") or with molecules released by other lymphocytes (factors, antibodies) [QR1975_10].

Coutinho on Protein A Plaque Assay at Christmas, 1975

The protein A plaque assay, a technique which allows for the class-specific detection of all cells secreting immunoglobulin irrespective of antigen specificity (and later adapted to detect all cells secreting any protein), was finalized around Christmas day 1975. Soon published by Gronowicz, Coutinho and Melchers in the *European Journal of Immunology* (1976, vol. 6, p. 588), the paper's echo reached over 1,000 citations within 20 years of publication. This was an important addition to Jerne's plaque methodology invented a decade earlier.

QR1975_10 BII

Nobel Prize 1975 for Renato Dulbecco, Advisory Board Member

On October 10th, Niels Jerne, with great pleasure, telephoned Renato Dulbecco to congratulate him on winning the Nobel Prize for Medicine, 1975 [QR1975_11]. It was Dulbecco who had suggested to Jerne that he offer Susumu Tonegawa a position in the BII. Dulbecco shared the Nobel Prize with David Baltimore and Howard Temin. A few years later Baltimore became a member of the BII Advisory Board.

QR1975_11 BII

Treasure Trove 1975

The database contains documents related to the BII in a broader context (lists, series of photographs, etc.).

QR1975_treasure BII

The Year 1976

Ben Pernis, a founding member of the BII, accepted a call to Columbia University, New York. An EMBO course on lymphocyte physiology was held at the BII. Niels Jerne called for an extramural conference on idiotypes (Baumanière, France). At the 41st Cold Spring Harbor Symposium, 8 members presented their results, among them Susumu Tonegawa with work that led to his Nobel Prize. Georges Köhler returned to Basel to establish a hybridoma technology research group. In a factory belonging to Roche, Italy, an explosion occurred, releasing dioxin into the air.

Arrivals 1976 (9)
Eleven members joined the institute, 2 of them only staying for part of the year: *Sefik Alkan, Jack Cowan, Christoph Heusser, Norman Iscove, Georges Köhler, Tommaso Meo, Wolfgang Schalch, Marc Shulman, John Stocker.*

Came and Left in the Same Year (2)
Susumu Ohno, Iver Heron.

Leavers 1976 (17)
Clinton Ballou, Domenico Bernoco, Nicholas Cohen, Pierre Dolivo, Tommy Douglas, Wulf Droege, Heiner Frost, Jean-Claude Jaton, Katherine Knight, Markus Nabholz, Zoltán Nagy, Benvenuto Pernis, José Quintáns, Walter Riesen, Luciana Rovis, Rita Schuller, Edwin Seegmiller.

A certain shift in the focus of scientists, especially in respect of their interests on T cells and regarding the role of these cell types in the immune system, became apparent. Nevertheless, attention in the clarification of the origin of antibody diversity remained unabated.

The Annual Reports, compiled and edited by Charley Steinberg, were distributed to all major university departments and institutes around the world. In some countries the demand was such that their research institutions reprinted (with permission of the BII) a considerable number of copies for "local" distribution (e.g. in South Korea). Niels Jerne's introductions became "cult" chapters read by scientists and laymen. The introduction to the 1976 Annual Report is an especially striking example of a summary of the work accomplished by BII scientists that year.

In the chapter for 1975 it was shown that the BII had fulfilled, by all criteria, the high expectations that had been raised by the world scientific community in the preceding years. In the process of writing about the initial stages of the institute, it was of central importance to introduce, year for year (1970 onwards), the new members and their projects. During that period, many scientists left the BII on completion of their contracts.

Turnover of Scientists at the BII Creates an Alumni Network

Sixty-four scientists left the BII from the time when it opened until the end of 1975. In the first part of this chapter, the "procedure of leaving" and the new positions of those departing are described.

The "goodbye" parties were the enjoyable aspect of someone leaving. It was an exception if a scientist left without throwing a party (see the section on parties); here, it suffices to say that a goodbye always included a promise to return, and indeed people kept coming back.

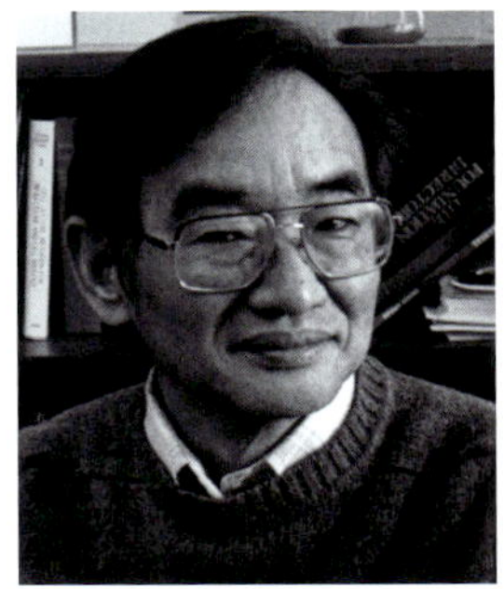

Gordon Sato

The 64 Scientists Who Left the BII up until the End of 1975

Jan Andersson, Brigitte Askonas, Irene Baldi, Peter Baumann, Armando Bernardini, Armin Boschetti, Wesley W. Bullock, Ron Citronbaum, Melvin Cohn, Robert Cone, Matthias Cramer, Susan Cullen, Mario De Marchi, David Dresser, Stanislaw Dubiski, Amy Falvey, Walter Gerhard, Haim Ginsburg, Joel W. Goodman, Yossi Haimovich, John Hamilton, Ingrid Harbitz, Jack Hay, Leslie Hudson, Ethel Jacobson, John R. Kettman, Heinz Köhler, Peter Krammer, Angelika Kunz, Peter Lachmann, Louis Lafleur, John Lightbody, J. Russell Little, Giovanna Luciani, Sir Macfarlane Burnet, Tom Mandel, Takeshi Matsunaga, Wolfgang Mayr, Wally McKeehan, Gabriel Michael, J.F.A.P. Miller, Graham F. Mitchell, Göran Möller, Albert Nordin, Jan Obel, Jennifer Phillips, Robert Phillips, Hansruedi Ramseier, Stanley E. Read, Georges Roelants, Gordon Sato, Seung-il Shin, Donald Shreffler, Olof Sjöberg, Jonathan Sprent, David Stott, Ingegerd Sundkvist, Tien-Wen Tao-Wiedmann, Zoltan Tökes, Giorgio Trinchieri, Jorge Vives, Niki Weiss, Felix O. Wettstein, Siraik Zakarian.

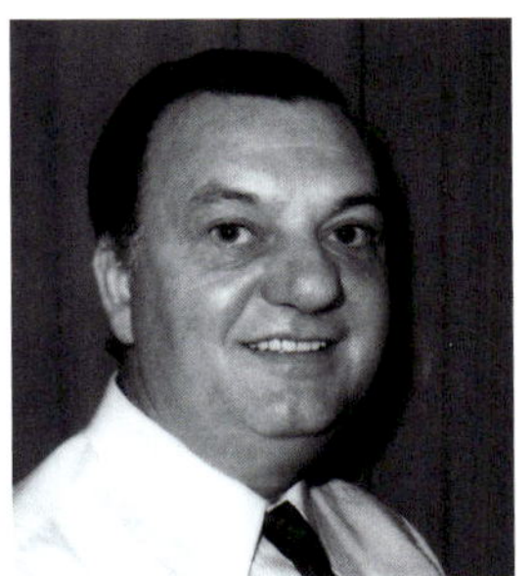

Domenico Bernoco

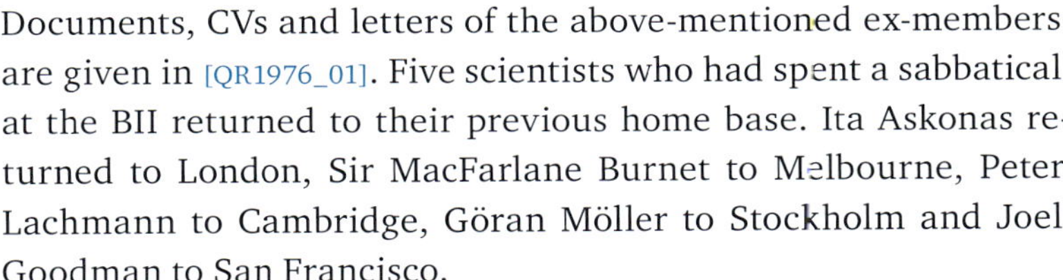

Documents, CVs and letters of the above-mentioned ex-members are given in [QR1976_01]. Five scientists who had spent a sabbatical at the BII returned to their previous home base. Ita Askonas returned to London, Sir MacFarlane Burnet to Melbourne, Peter Lachmann to Cambridge, Göran Möller to Stockholm and Joel Goodman to San Francisco.

The numbers are not entirely correct: some scientists left but later returned again as members, some returned as "visiting scientists", within the said period (e.g. Stephen Fazekas, Berry Kindred, Tommy Meo – so they are not mentioned in the turnover list).

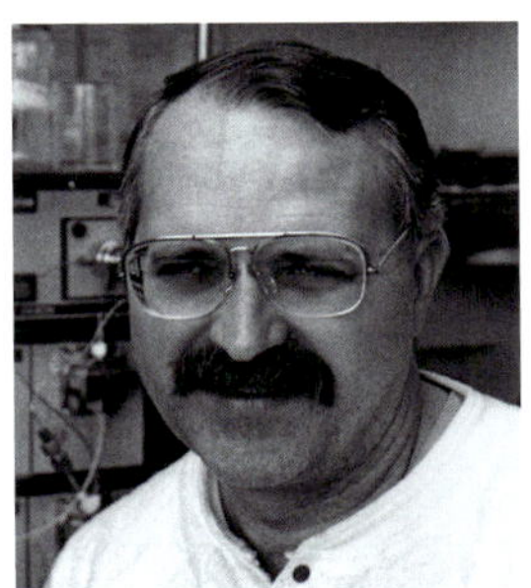

Wally McKeehan

Returns to the institute were arranged either because some collaborative experiments had to be completed or manuscripts written; in some instances former members became regular visitors with ongoing collaborations with BII staff.

Those scientists who came for a sabbatical had an easy task when leaving – they gave up their furnished apartment and returned to their home environment. In many instances, however, a young family had pre-school-age children and/or children at school. What the family experienced was decisive as to whether or not the scientist applied for a prolongation. Usually families adjusted well to the Swiss way of life. Some were critical, often overcritical. The criticism was sometimes superficial, e.g. shops closing

QR1976_01 BII

at 6.30 p.m. did not meet with approval by American families. Other criticisms were made about the inapproachability and often intolerance of Swiss people, who like to keep their distance, and about the many rules and regulations.

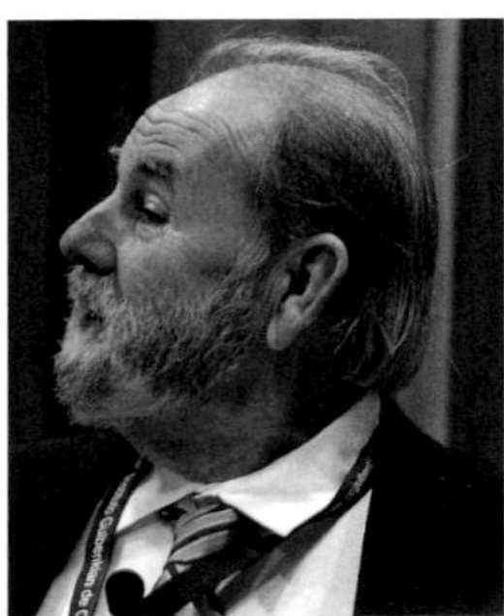

Jack Kettman

Although this chapter is included under the year 1976, it was characteristic for the preceding period and for the years to come that scientists and their families adjusted to Switzerland so well that they often were not ready to leave when their contracts expired. Many scientists and their families remained in Switzerland forever, moving to other research institutions, universities or pharmaceutical companies, and, in some instances, by simply retiring in their comfortable Swiss surroundings. There is a section in this book on those scientists who remained in Switzerland.

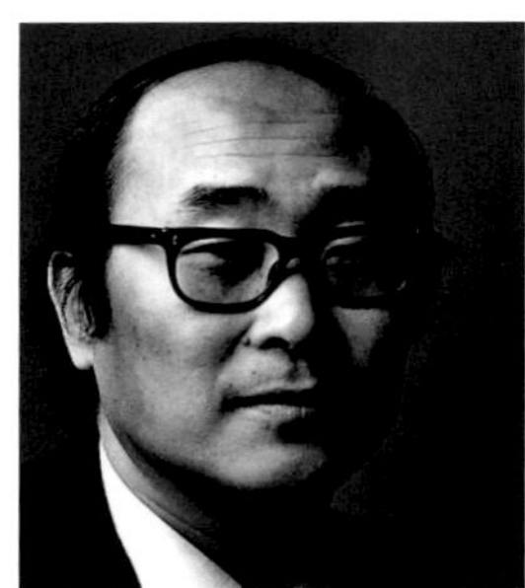

Seung-il Shin

Although Jack Kettman left Basel to settle in Dallas, he soon found that both research at the BII and Europe's cultural life were worth him becoming a regular commuter between the two continents. At the time when Ron Citronbaum and Seung-il Shin left the institute, it was by no means clear that Ron would become a successful doctor, or that Seung-il would become an important scientific administrator in his country of origin – South Korea. Now, decades later, Seung-il lives in California.

At the time of reviewing these data (spring 2016) 14 members mentioned earlier are no longer alive: Brigitte Askonas, Ron Citronbaum, Ethel Jacobson, Georges Roelants, Göran Möller, Jan Obel, Joel W. Goodman, Sir Macfarlane Burnet, Ben Pernis, Wulf Droege, Tommy Meo, Zdenek Trnka, Ruggero Ceppellini.

I am leaving Basel for some time and therefore I am having a party on Tuesday the 31st at 1930. You are very wellcome to "Zum Letzen Batsen" , Schlossgasse 11 in Binningen. Take the elevator to the ground floor.

Göran Möller

Ben Pernis Leaves for Columbia University, New York, 1976

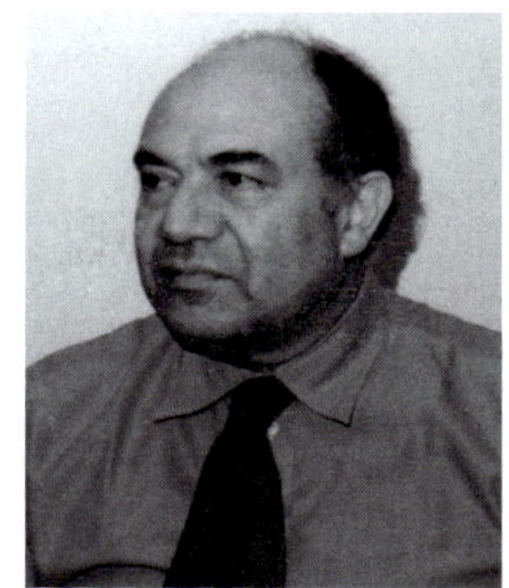

Ben Pernis

Ben Pernis was the first permanent member to give up this position; in 1976 he was recruited by Columbia University, New York, to become a Professor of Microbiology and Medicine [QR1976_02]. Ben was highly esteemed by all his colleagues in Basel and also in his home country Italy (Milan). Niels Jerne and Ben Pernis were not only friends and colleagues, but Niels expressed the hope that Ben might return to Basel as his successor. At that time, it was assumed that the next director of the institute would be chosen from "outside" candidates. This did not come about and Pernis remained at the Columbia University until his retirement.

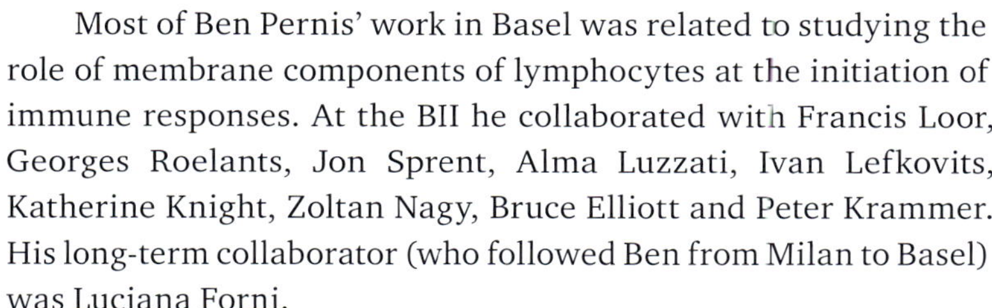

Most of Ben Pernis' work in Basel was related to studying the role of membrane components of lymphocytes at the initiation of immune responses. At the BII he collaborated with Francis Loor, Georges Roelants, Jon Sprent, Alma Luzzati, Ivan Lefkovits, Katherine Knight, Zoltan Nagy, Bruce Elliott and Peter Krammer. His long-term collaborator (who followed Ben from Milan to Basel) was Luciana Forni.

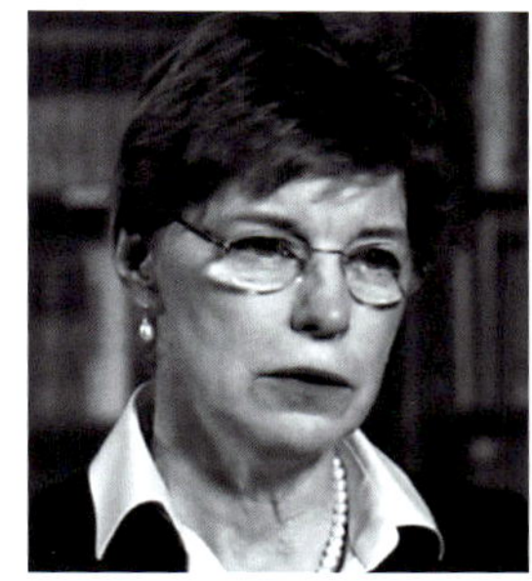

Katherine Knight

The keywords of his projects were "membrane IgD", "patch formation", "capping" and "allelic exclusion". He and his abovementioned colleagues were the first to establish the meaning and consequences of the redistribution of molecules on the fluid two-dimensional membrane of lymphocytes.

Katherine Knight to Chicago, 1976

Katherine Knight worked at the BII with Ben Pernis and Andrew Kelus on B lymphocyte development and on the generation of the antibody repertoire, and this theme she followed up at her new position at the Loyola University in Chicago.

For her investigations she used normal and transgenic rabbits as well as rabbits genetically modified by nuclear transfer techniques. For the purpose of studying B cell development she developed or adopted molecular genetic, immunochemical and cell culture techniques, including DNA cloning and sequencing and in vitro gene expression.

Katherine served on the American Association of Immunologists Council from 1991 to 1996 and was president of the AAI from 1996 to 1997. In 2013 Katherine was awarded the AAI Lifetime Achievement Award.

Zoltan Nagy to Hungary 1976, Then (with a Delay) to Canada

Zoltan A. Nagy came to the BII in September 1974, with a fellowship awarded to him by the Hungarian Academy of Sciences. At the institute he worked together with Benvenuto Pernis, Markus Nabholz, Peter Krammer and Bruce Elliott on the mechanism by which activated T cells acquire surface immunoglobulin passively. This work helped to eliminate the wide-spread belief that surface Ig might represent the antigen receptor of T cells. Already "converted" from an immunohistologist into a cellular immunologist Zoltan came in 1976 for a short second stay at the BII, and then he accepted an invitation from Bruce Elliott to spend a year in his laboratory in Canada, which materialized upon a "back and forth to Hungary" in 1978. Thereafter he received a job offer from Jan Klein in the Immunogenetics Department at the Max Planck Institute for Biology in Tübingen, Germany. There he made significant contributions to the biology and genetics of the murine MHC [QR1976_03]. Subsequently, he held various positions in the pharmacological and biotech industries, working on T cell recognition and autoimmunity. Recently he has summarized his thoughts on the field and memories of the participants in a history book (*A History of Modern Immunology: The Path toward Understanding*, Academic Press, 2014).

EMBO Course on Lymphocyte Physiology, 1976

EMBO courses had already become a tradition – this year the course was on lymphocyte physiology (March 15th–27th, 1976) [QR1976_04].

The program included demonstrations, experiments and workshops on the origin, differentiation, physiology and circulation of lymphocytes. Lymphocyte subpopulations were characterized with respect to cell size, surface charge and the presence of surface membrane markers. The rate of turnover of immunoglobulins, migration patterns and tissue distribution served further to distinguish subpopulations.

A series of lectures dealt with the conceptual framework of current research in lymphocyte physiology.

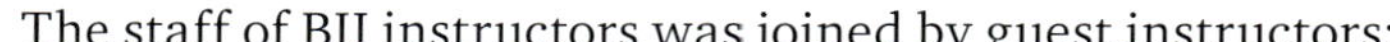

The staff of BII instructors was joined by guest instructors:

H. Cantor (Boston), N. Le Douarin (Nantes), W.L. Ford (Manchester), R.L. Gardner (Oxford), J.D. Horton (Durham), J.C. Howard (Cambridge), P.W. Kincade (New York), A. Matter (Basel), H.S. Micklem (Edinburgh), G. Möller (Stockholm), R. Nezlin (Moscow), D.G. Osmond (Montreal), R.A. Phillips (Toronto), J. Sprent (London), S. Strober (Stanford), P. Vassalli (Geneva).

The students came from many countries:

K. Bighouse (England), B. van Camp (Belgium), A.A. de Freitas (Scotland), B. Reguiro Garcia (Spain), E. Gerassi (Israel), L. Hammarström (Sweden), A.H. Handyside (England), V. Hooghe (Belgium), R. Joho (Switzerland), F. Jotereau (France), K. Karjalainen (Finland), H. Lemke (Sweden), M.H.J. van Oers (The Netherlands), C. Penit (France), G. Rannie (England), J.J. Rimmer (England), J.G. Saal (Germany), K. Sege (Sweden), M. Shinitzky (Israel), M. Wioland (France).

Science is not a deductive exercise of moving from one logical conclusion to the next experiment, but it is imagination in action, patching scraps of knowledge into something rich and new.

N.K. Jerne

Conference on Idiotypes in Les-Baux-de-Provence, April 1976

Niels Jerne usually delegated the organization of conferences to colleagues. The conference on idiotypes was in a certain sense his "private conference", as he wished to clear his mind about the role of idiotypes in the regulation of the immune system. He wished to have the conference in a quiet place somewhere near his home in Provence, and so the beautiful Hotel Baumanière in Les Baux-de-Provence was chosen as the venue. The single theme of the conference was "Antigens on the Antibody Molecules" [QR1976_05].

"Are idiotypes important in the regulation of the immune system?"

Jerne's opening statement was: "All vertebrates produce antibody. Millions of specific antibody molecules. These millions of different antibody molecules are good antigens themselves."

The participants were asked to talk about their experiments, and why they did them. What was it that they wanted to find out? The participants were not encouraged to present *lectures* but rather to speak freely without manuscript about their concepts and experimental findings.

The participants could be critical of themselves and of others. Some ideas were dismissed as phantasy, some experiments discounted as unsound, some reagents were challenged as unreliable, some generalizations were considered inadmissible. The debates during the days and nights of the conference were pervaded by a general feeling that it was all important and worth listening to, in the hope of acquiring ideas that are needed for making progress. Jerne repeatedly stated that science is not a deductive exercise of moving from one logical conclusion to the next experiment, but it is imagination in action, patching scraps of knowledge into something rich and new.

Jerne's question "Are idiotypes important in the regulation of the immune system?" was not really answered. But he insisted: "Even if this turns out not to be the case, idiotypes may still have some importance as tools in experiments, where the shape of the epitope has to be defined by different means."

QR1976_05 BII

Mirrors would be well advised to think twice before reflecting images.

Jean Cocteau

IDIOTYPES

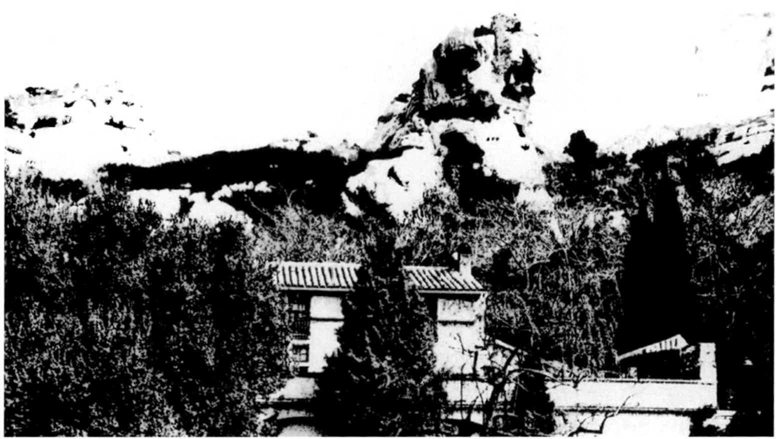

Four "take home" questions were put to the participants:

1. Where does the collection of idiotypic determinants (or idiotopes) occur on the variable domain?
2. How many different variable domains are there in the immune system of one animal?
3. Do two mice of an inbred strain have the same set of combining sites?
4. Are some idiotypes absent in some mice, say in low responders, or in animals with some predetermined responsiveness?

The conference was recorded on tape and transcribed (all this was before the computer era).

The transcripts were sent to the participants to rectify misunderstood words and sentences, but not to change what they had actually said. Afterwards Ingrid Schnurr compiled the conference proceedings book.

Hilary Koprowski from the Wistar Institute in Philadelphia praised not only the culinary aspects of the conference "the best cuisine within 5,000 miles of Philadelphia", but he also stated in his summary of the conference "that it has shown how biologists, confronted with poorly defined concepts and baffling findings, try to grope their way towards clarification".

To a journalist Koprowski said: "Non-immunologists might have expected a dozen serious immunologists to discuss problems of curing infectious diseases, cancer, allergy and other disorders, no, they discussed science."

An Excerpt from Jerne's Introduction to the Annual Report 1976

The term idiotype stands for the set of antigenic patterns (idiotopes) present on the variable domain of an antibody molecule. Idiotopes can be located at or near the combining site, and anti-idiotypic antibodies are readily prepared by injecting homogeneous antibodies into animals of other species. It has been shown that anti-idiotypic antibodies can also be made by animals of the same species or the same inbred strain and that an animal even produces antibodies against its own antibodies. Because of the enormous diversity of antibodies, we must conclude that every antibody molecule produced by the immune system is an anti-idiotypic antibody against some other antibody molecule produced by the same immune system. It has been found that the injection of minute amounts of anti-idiotypic antibody into a normal mouse profoundly influences the ability of this mouse to produce antibodies of the corresponding idiotype. All this points towards the existence of a functional idiotype/anti-idiotype network among B cells and their products.

41st Cold Spring Harbor Symposium, 1976

Eight members of the BII presented their work at the symposium "Origins of Lymphocyte Diversity". Susumu Tonegawa's presentation received special attention and was significant in his groundbreaking research which led to his Nobel Prize.

N.K. Jerne	Opening Address, "The Common Sense of Immunology"
S. Tonegawa	"Immunoglobulin Genes"
M.H. Julius, A.A. Augustin and H. Cosenza	"Idiotypes and Anti-Idiotypes as Probes in Analysis of Immunoregulation"
B. Weimann	"Induction of Immunoglobulin Synthesis in Abelson Murine Leukemia Virus Transformed Mouse Lymphoma Cells in Culture"
H. von Boehmer	"The Influence of H-2 Gene Products on Cell-Mediated and Humoral Immune Responses"
L. Du Pasquier	"The Ontogenesis of Lymphocyte Diversity in Anuran Amphibians"
F. Melchers	"Immunoglobulin Synthesis and Turnover and Mitogen Reactivity of Murine B-Lymphocytes during Ontogeny"
B. Pernis	"Synthesis of Multiple Immunoglobulin Classes by Single Lymphocytes"

It has already been mentioned that Susumu Tonegawa received great support and coaching from Charley Steinberg. At the CSH Symposium this was palpable. Steinberg traveled to the symposi-

The most important presentation of this symposium was the Steinberg-Tonegawa talk.

um with the sole purpose of assisting Susumu [QR1976_06]. The presentation was very successful, and Charley participated in the corridor talks which strengthened Susumu's standing. At that time, Steinberg and Tonegawa were joint authors of several papers, and the research was generally referred to as the "Tonegawa-Steinberg" project. Jim Watson told Niels Jerne at the conference: "The most important presentation of this symposium was the Steinberg-Tonegawa talk." On 3 papers out of 4, Charley Steinberg was co-author. The CSH paper included Hozumi, Matthyssens and Schuller. Steinberg's name was not on it and did not appear on any further papers. Mention will be made later on of the work of Christine Brack, André Traunecker, Nobuchi Hozumi, Ora Bernard, Hitoshi Sakano, Bonnie Blomberg and several others. They all contributed to Tonegawa's later fame. Susumu's achievements were indeed astonishing, since he arrived at the BII as a "not-yet immunologist", repeatedly stating that all the immunology he needed, he learned from Ita Askonas.

It was (and perhaps still is) a fine tradition of the CSH Symposia that the introduction and the summing-up are made by an eminent representative of the field. In 1967 Jerne had already played this role when he presented a highly acclaimed lecture "Waiting for the End". At the symposium 9 years later, Jerne gave the opening address entitled "The Common Sense of Immunology".

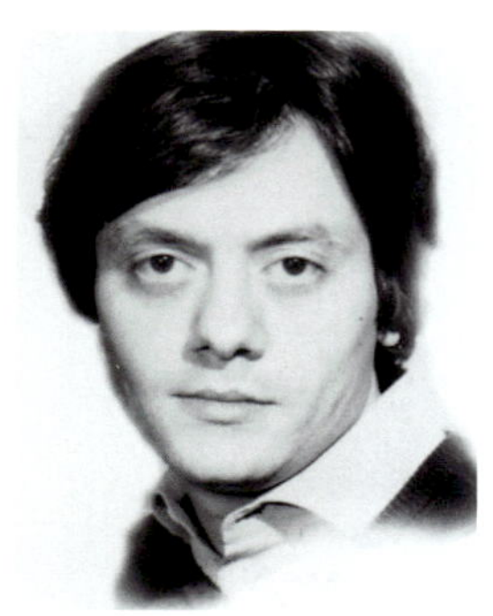

Tommy Meo

Tommy Meo's Move to Munich and the Final One to Paris

Tommy Meo demonstrated during his second term in Basel (1976–1978) the MHC association of a "hitchhiker gene", indicating evolutionary conservation of these complexes over long distances. During this second term in Basel he also identified the first chromosomal localization, showing that the same homolog of mouse chromosome 12 determines the simultaneous expression of IgM and IgD [QR1976_07].

QR1976_06 BII

Tommy obtained an attractive offer to join Gert Riethmüller's new Immunology Department in Munich in 1978, where he worked on the cloning of mouse complement C4 gene. He then moved to Paris, to set up in 1982 the Immunogenetics Unit of the Pasteur Institute. Having characterized the genes encoding C4, he undertook a systematic search for new genes in the H-2-S region and discovered the RD gene and the cytochrome P-450 21-hydroxylase genes. Tommy died in Paris in 1997.

QR1976_07 BII

Georges Köhler Returns to the BII, 1976

Georges Köhler completed his term at the Laboratory of Molecular Biology in Cambridge, UK, where he and César Milstein devised the hybridoma technique for the production of antibodies. Georges returned to the BII in 1976 where he remained for another 9 years. He became a permanent member, and with his new group he continued investigating antibody diversity. At the time of Georges' transfer from Cambridge to Basel, Klaus Rajewsky's laboratory gave him great support in order to ensure that adequate experimental conditions existed for the newly established hybridoma technology. Georges started to develop and use transgenic mice as a tool to understand the mechanism that underlies self-tolerance [QR1976_08].

The Seveso Disaster and Its Implications, 1976

In a manufacturing plant of a subsidiary of Hoffmann-La Roche in Seveso, Italy, an explosion occurred on July 10th, 1976. It resulted in the exposure of several areas to the substance dioxin. The industrial plant, located in Meda, was owned by the company ICMESA *(Industrie Chimiche Meda Società Azionaria)*, a subsidiary of Givaudan, which in turn was a subsidiary of Hoffmann-La Roche [QR1976_09].

QR1976_08 BII

QR1976_09 BII

Although the accident caused no fatalities, it created a very strong reaction in public perception in Italy (apart from a number of cases of people suffering with chloracne, there were no casualties). In the 1983 chapter, other aspects of this case will be mentioned, especially the consequences of the "disappearance" of barrels containing waste from the cleanup.

The Seveso case is mentioned here because it had damaging consequences on certain decision-making at the BII. Roche was and still is insured by Zurich Insurance, the president of which was, at that time, Fritz Gerber. Zurich Insurance handled the Seveso problem to the full satisfaction of Roche, but it is probable that the management of Roche was displeased with the lengthy bureaucratic negotiations with the Italian authorities. The other side of the coin was that the event caused frustration amongst Italian scientists, including those working at the BII. For instance, Ruggero Ceppellini showed distrust towards Roche by turning down the position, to which he had earlier committed himself, to become a head (with Theo Staehelin) of the Applied Research Project for Monoclonal Antibody.

More on this topic will be mentioned in the chapter for 1983.

Treasure Trove 1976

The database contains documents related to the BII in a broader context (lists, series of photographs, etc.).

QR1976_treasure BII

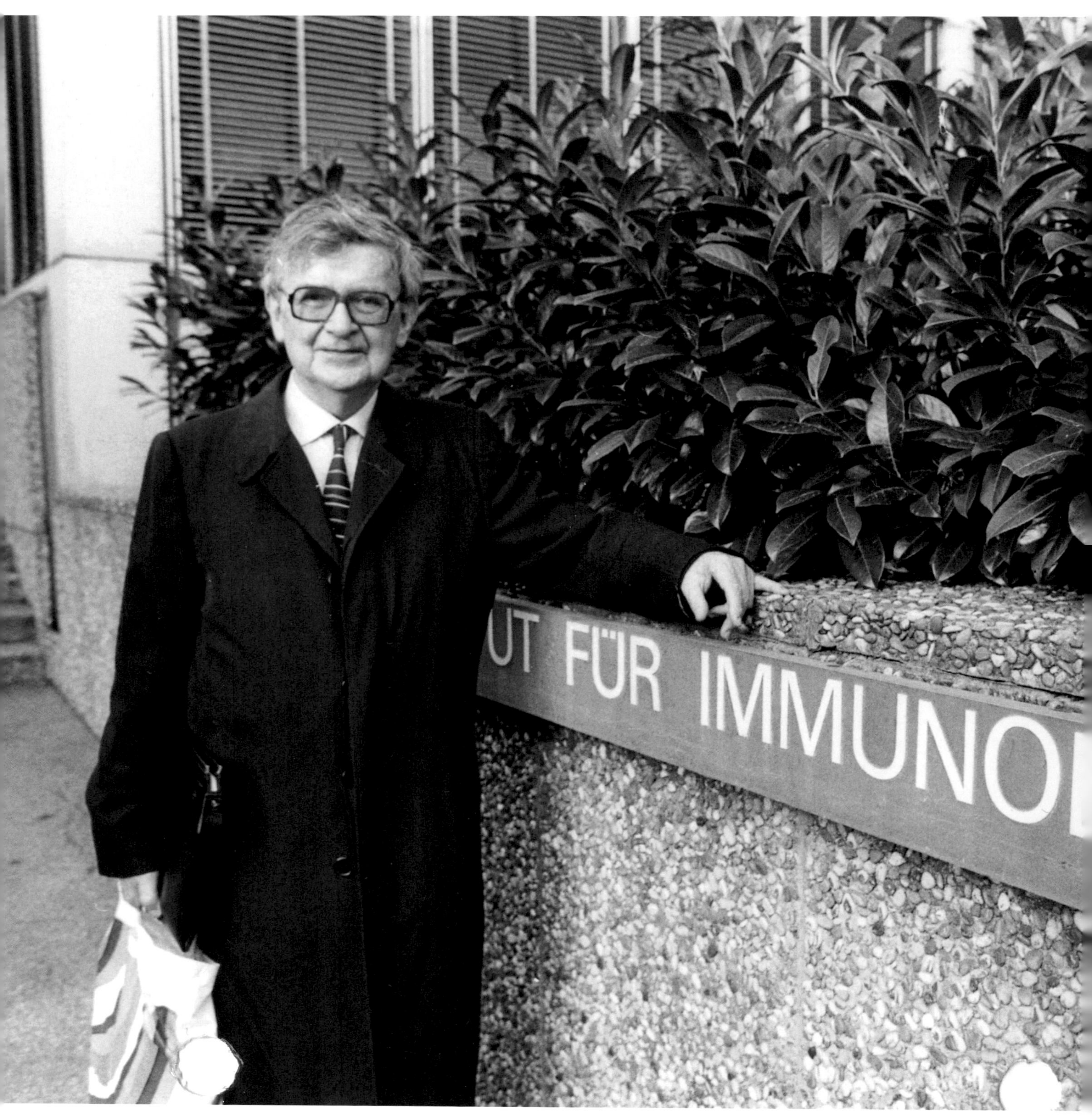
UT FÜR IMMUNO

The Year 1977

Theo Staehelin, a permanent member of the BII, accepted the position of head of the "Applied Immunology Project" at Roche. Berenice Kindred and Wulf Droege left for Heidelberg and Jonathan Sprent for London. The Roche Institute of Molecular Biology in Nutley celebrated its 10th anniversary. Several BII members participated as speakers or chairpersons at the 3rd International Congress of Immunology in Melbourne. Niels Jerne hinted that he had health problems and started discussing his succession.

Scientific Concepts by Niels Jerne, 1977

During the first part of the 20th century, until 1960, immunology had developed in isolation from the mainstream biology. Immunology was nothing but a catalog of phenomena for which immunologists invented a special terminology, e.g. *humoral immunity, cellular immunity, hypersensitivity, tolerance, allergy, anaphylaxis, haptens*, etc. These terms had no parallels in other fields of biology, and the phenomena observed were not attached to the function of any known organ in the body. Immunology therefore remained an isolated area of biology, although it was compensated for this isolation by having a special relationship to medicine, to which it contributed vaccination, serological diagnosis and other important procedures.

Although antibody molecules, present in blood serum, had been discovered in 1890, it was still not known in 1960 which cells synthesize them. One of the reasons for this prolonged ignorance was the dominance of an erroneous concept, looking at antibody formation the wrong way, which blocked the path to further advances. This concept was the *antigen template theory*, which postulated that antibody molecules must acquire their complementary structure in direct contact with antigen. This idea was based on apparently sound reasoning, which essentially went as follows. The number of different antigens to which an animal can make specific antibodies is very large, if not infinite. These antigens include synthetic substances, which have never existed naturally. Therefore, the structure of specific antibodies cannot be genetically programmed, but must be determined by the antigens. It is therefore necessary that antigens enter into a cell to enable it to

Arrivals 1977 (12)
Twelve scientists, from Holland, Australia, Japan, Italy, the USA and also from Switzerland, joined the institute: *Lucien Aarden, Claude Bernard, Ora Bernard, Bonnie Blomberg, Christine Brack, Melvin Cohn, Stephen Fazekas de St. Groth, Minoru Hirama, Stanley Leibo, Roberto Poljak, Scott Rodkey, Massimo Trucco.*

Leavers 1977 (18)
Ronald Corley, Jack Cowan, Bruce Elliott, Bernhard Erni, C. Garrison Fathman, Hansjörg Forster, Hubert Jacot-Guillarmod, Berenice Kindred, Gaston Matthyssens, Vincenzo Miggiano, J. Richard Pink, Jörg Schmidt, Theophil Staehelin, Bela Takács, Michael Taussig, Hans Trachsel, Takeshi Watanabe, Andreas Ziegler.

produce a fitting antibody molecule. The lymphocyte is not a candidate for such a cell because it is not phagocytic. Every couple of years since 1915, reports were published showing the presence of antibody in the cytoplasm of lymphocytes. These reports were disregarded. How can antigens direct antibody formation by action at a distance, from the outside of a cell? Even scientists who found high antibody concentrations inside lymphocytes suggested that these cells were perhaps antibody storage cells.

In the 1940s, when plasma cells were demonstrated to secrete antibody, the conclusion was immediately drawn that plasma cells must be cells that descend from macrophages that had initiated antibody formation. It was only in the 1950s that ideas emerged that were not predicated on the need for phagocytosis of antigen to initiate antibody formation. The insight was simply that a cell can respond to a given antigen only if that cell possesses antigen-recognizing receptors. The molecules par excellence that can recognize antigens are antibody molecules. It therefore seemed evident that antibody molecules must be present before a foreign antigen arrives, otherwise that antigen could not be recognized as such. This is emphasized here because it may well be that some of the present seemingly self-evident concepts are also totally erroneous and delay further clarification of the immune system.

When the new notion that antibody molecules are made in the absence of antigen gradually became accepted in the early 1960s, many things suddenly fell into place, such as the fact that lymphocytes were important cells and that the clonal selection theory was probably correct. Happily, this insight coincided with important analytical work, which revealed the structural basis for the diverse specificities of antibody molecules. It was shown, moreover, that lymphocytes can be cultured in vitro, and that lymphocytes in culture, upon addition of antigen, will produce specific antibodies. It looked, and it still looks, as if lymphocytes that grow as disperse cells are ideal for the study of cell differentiation in vertebrate animals (abridged from the Introduction to the 1977 Annual Report [QR1977_01]).

QR1977_01 BII

Clonal Selection in Jerne's Words

QR1977_02 BII

I now come to a basic law of immunology, that is most probably correct: the law of the unispecificity of lymphocytes [QR1977_02]. *This law says that all antibody molecules produced by one lymphocyte have identical variable domains, and that all cells of a clone that descend from this lymphocyte likewise express only this same variable do-*

main in all antibody molecules they produce. This law is supported by innumerable experimental results. Accordingly, a B cell presents on its surface receptor antibody molecules of identical specificity, and this cell, when stimulated, will secrete antibody molecules of that same specificity. This leads to the simple picture of clonal selection as was understood in the 1960s, before T cells had been discovered. The population of B-cells consists of a large number of clones of cells. All cells of one clone produce antibodies of only one specificity. The term clone is here used to denote a set of cells synthesizing antibodies of identical specificity. It may therefore consist of the sum of several actual clones that happen to be identical in this respect. Entering antigen molecules encounter cells of several different clones that display variable domains fitting sufficiently well to bind this antigen. In some way, antigen attachment is followed by signals that cause these cells to proliferate, to differentiate, and to secrete antibody.

Joghem van Loghem, Lucien Aarden and the CLB

As Niels Jerne's name is mostly associated with cellular assays (plaque assay), it is often forgotten that not cells (lymphocytes) but their products (antibodies) were his main concern. Thus, he was an immunochemist rather than a cellular immunologist. Antibody in the blood and in the body fluids was the point of departure for all his studies. The Statens Serum Institut in Copenhagen had been his home base, and from there contacts to various "serum institutes" worldwide were initiated. One of his most important contacts was Joghem van Loghem in the Central Laboratory of the Netherlands Red Cross Blood Transfusion Service (CLB) in Amsterdam [QR1977_03].

Dr. van Loghem was the scientific director of the CLB from 1950 to 1978. He was the first person to detect the human platelet antigen 1a. A young scientist, Lucien Aarden, who studied anti-DNA antibody (diagnostic and prognostic tools for systemic lupus erythematosus) worked at the CLB. Lucien joined the BII in 1978 and worked there for several years.

Lucien remained attached to the BII throughout the decades, participating in joint projects, and teaching courses and summer schools. In Amsterdam he organized regular WHO courses for Central American students. A large number of BII members traveled to Amsterdam to teach at these courses. This was the start of several important CLB-BII collaborative projects.

QR1977_03 BII

Charley Steinberg and Manuscripts

Scientists who were not worried about getting overly strong criticism, or sarcastic comments, were happy to submit their manuscripts to Charley for correction. In the pre-computer age the corrected pages were covered in red ink; one such page is reproduced below, and other pages are shown in the QR note [QR1977_04]. Some former members treasure these pages, even now, three decades later.

QR1977_04 BII

One of the comments reads as follows: "The integers are by definition 'numerable', even though they are infinite. The number of lymphocyte sets is even finite, so they are definitely not 'innumerable'."

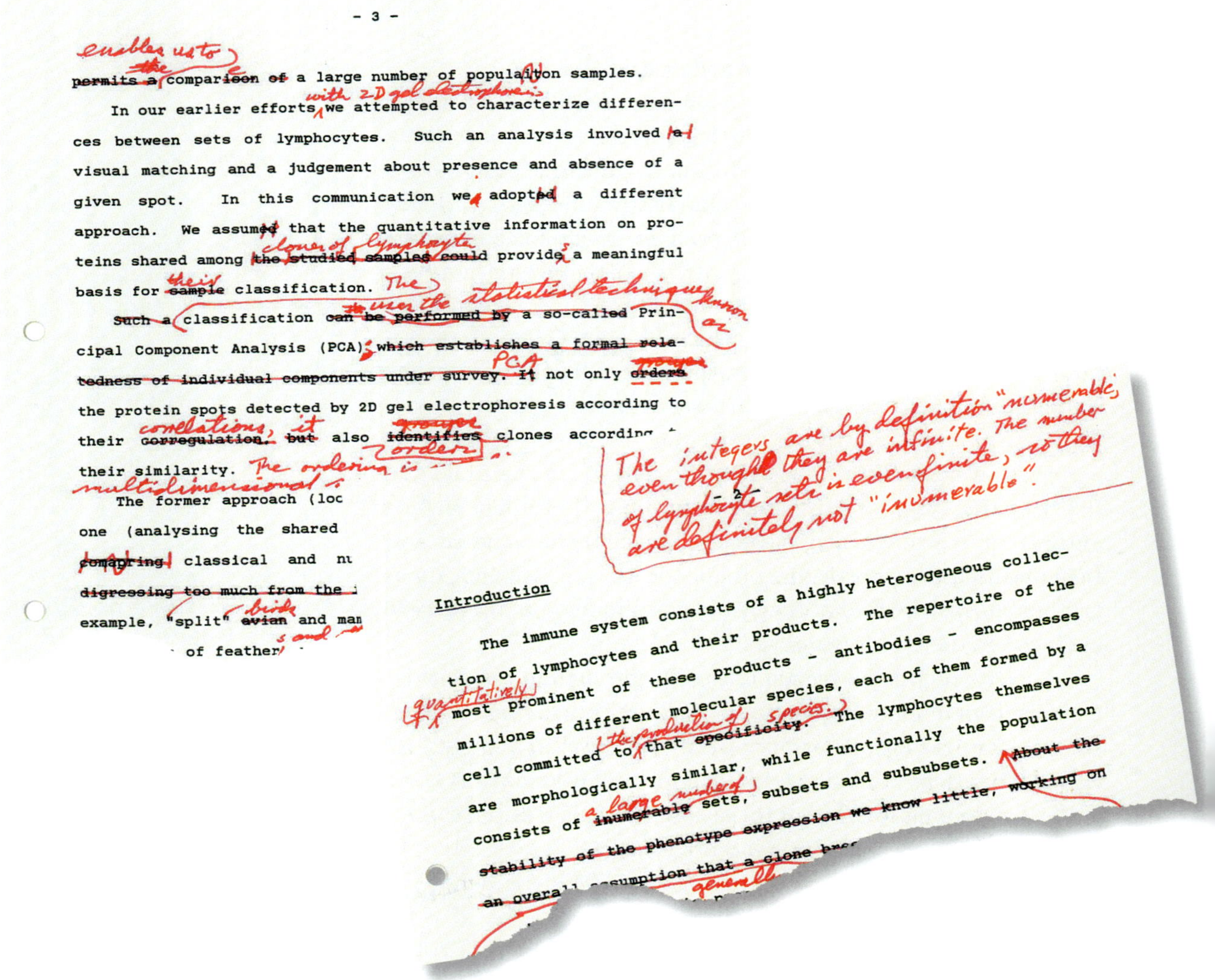

- 3 -

permits a comparison of a large number of population samples.

In our earlier efforts we attempted to characterize differences between sets of lymphocytes. Such an analysis involved a visual matching and a judgement about presence and absence of a given spot. In this communication we adopted a different approach. We assumed that the quantitative information on proteins shared among the studied samples could provide a meaningful basis for sample classification.

Such a classification can be performed by a so-called Principal Component Analysis (PCA) which establishes a formal relatedness of individual components under survey. It not only orders the protein spots detected by 2D gel electrophoresis according to their coregulation but also identifies clones according to their similarity.

The former approach (loc... one (analysing the shared ... comparing classical and n... digressing too much from the ... example, "split" avian and ma... of feather...

The integers are by definition "numerable", even though they are infinite. The number of lymphocyte sets is even finite, so they are definitely not "innumerable".

Introduction

The immune system consists of a highly heterogeneous collection of lymphocytes and their products. The repertoire of the most prominent of these products - antibodies - encompasses millions of different molecular species, each of them formed by a cell committed to that specificity. The lymphocytes themselves are morphologically similar, while functionally the population consists of innumerable sets, subsets and subsubsets. About the stability of the phenotype expression we know little, working on an overall assumption that a clone ...

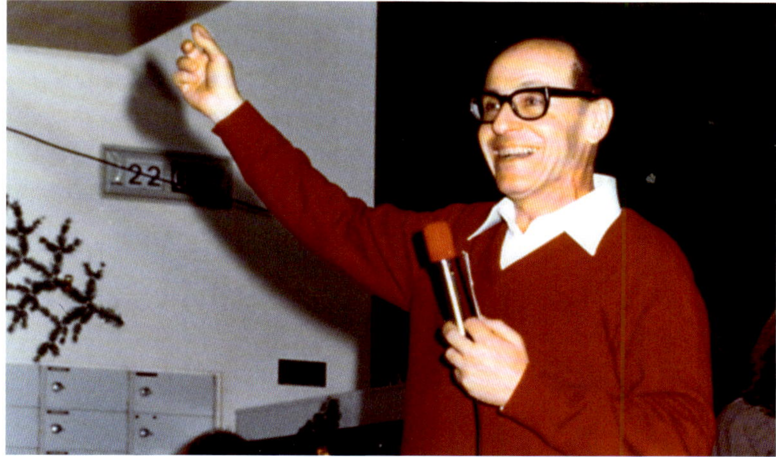

Mel Cohn

Mel Cohn's Seminar Series

"It is so boring, let's talk about things we do not agree upon."
Mel Cohn

It is difficult to assess what had driven Mel Cohn to leave his comfortable home in California and come year after year to Basel, to spend weeks or often months at the BII. Mel Cohn was and still is a highly extrovert scientist, ready to talk to everybody on all aspects of all theories of the immune system. Mel did not even wait to overcome his jet lag, and immediately started a seminar series, in which he "dictated" the theme, but was ready to digress when answering questions raised by people attending the seminars [QR1977_05].

The seminars were always about the model of B and T cell interaction, about "two-signal theory". The seminar room was packed, and the discussions were lively, continuing for long hours. Mel's personality was very different from Niels', but they got along very well.

Jerne never pushed to convince people, but people were convinced; Cohn pushed hard, but there was always resistance. And Mel liked that resistance. When it happened – rarely – that people were of the same opinion, Mel said: "It is so boring, let's talk about things we do not agree upon."

Mel argued with everybody, among others with Antonio Coutinho, who told Mel that a certain statement was messy. Mel said: "You might call it messy, but it is right", and Antonio replied, "It is better to be clear than to be right".

This statement of Antonio was remembered by many colleagues, and years later he was asked why he had said that; he replied, "because what was clear remained clear, but what was thought to be right was often (later) shown as wrong".

QR1977_05 BII

Alcohol and Spirit

It was customary to keep the laboratory doors open, and when late on Friday afternoons one walked along the BII corridors, parties were noticed. When someone had a major paper accepted for publication, corks flew on other weekdays as well. On the notice board in the entrance, it was often announced: *TGIF in the lab of D.G.* When Niels Jerne noticed the TGIF acronym, he was displeased that "Friday" among scientists received the "low-class" connotation of *Thank God It's Friday.* He felt that only non-scientific staff should celebrate the weekend "refuge".

Niels Jerne ignored TGIF parties, but a regular glass of wine in a pub – alone or with colleagues – was his custom. Mostly it was a glass or two, but there were special occasions when drinking became excessive. Google claims that the expression "he drinks like a Dane" is of Czech origin, but that notwithstanding, Jerne defined himself as a moderate social drinker. In some instances, when he felt the occasion merited it, he would "outdrink" everybody and make aggressive statements which he otherwise would not make. There were 2 or 3 scientists among Jerne's friends who enjoyed such confrontations.

Theo Staehelin Leaves for Roche, 1977

... and so the "Applied Immunology Project", with 22 positions, was established.

Theo Staehelin was the second permanent member to leave the BII. As mentioned, the first one who left was Ben Pernis, accepting a Professorship at Columbia University, New York. Under very different circumstances and with vastly dissimilar perspectives, Theo Staehelin decided to accept the position of head of the newly formed "Applied Immunology Project" at Roche Basel [QR1977_06]. He was offered this position by Prof. Alfred Pletscher, head of Roche Research.

Theo Staehelin (whom Jerne knew and valued from Pittsburgh) had been highly successful at the BII, and certainly his expertise in molecular biology was of extraordinary importance. But so it would be for Roche – at least judged from Alfred Pletscher's perspective. The circumstances of Staehelin's move were of exceptional significance, not only for him, but also for Roche, and had consequences for the BII too.

QR1977_06 BII

Some months earlier, Jerne and the permanent members held a small meeting to discuss Georges Köhler and César Milstein's paper (still in manuscript form) about the new method of hybridoma production. Jerne called Pletscher to convey his view of the potential importance of this new technology for Roche. The round table with Pletscher, Steinberg, Staehelin, Lefkovits, Ceppellini and Miggiano emphasized the urgency of the matter. Pletscher's immediate reaction was "great, go ahead". Once Jerne explained that the development would have to take place on Roche premises rather than at the BII – with strong help from the BII – Roche took measures to embark on this project.

Pletscher convinced Roche Management, and so the "Applied Immunology Project", with 22 positions, was established. For several weeks it looked as if it would be under the joint leadership of Ceppellini and Staehelin, but for reasons that are explained elsewhere, Ceppellini backed out of the project and Staehelin moved to Roche. His formal position was Vice-Director of Roche.

It is beyond the scope of this book to analyze the results of the project [QR1977_07], but suffice it to say that in spite of its convincing successes, Staehelin felt that he was not receiving adequate support for this undertaking. Part of the problem was that the main support had come from Alfred Pletscher, who had taken an opportunity to retire and devote his time to organizing the *Zentrum für Lehre und Forschung* (see the 1987 chapter in Bock 2 of this history). It is very probable that in the middle echelons of Roche there was animosity towards the BII (perhaps it was thought that the BII "now" intended to expand to Roche), and Theo felt the consequences. To reiterate, the presumed animosity was not coming from the "top" but from the "middle", with the final consequence that this would disadvantage the company. It is undeniable that Staehelin, with his team that included Miggiano, Jacot and several former BII members, had prepared the ground for the development of Roche's products which would bring the company revenues in billions of Swiss francs, i.e. the production of monoclonal antibody for diagnostics, and by providing essential support for the Interferon Project of Roche/Genentech, and also for the certification of "Roferon A" years later.

Eight years after the Roche adventure commenced, Georges Köhler asked Theo to join him in the Max Planck Institute in Freiburg, and Theo gladly accepted.

As a result, the translation of a new discovery into a marketable drug through research and development is now so costly in time and money, and so risky, that few but the very largest firms can even contemplate it.

Lord Todd, former President of the Royal Society and Nobel Laureate in Chemistry

Roche Recruits Scientists from the BII

Although the chapters for each year provide the basis for portraying the events as they occurred, this paragraph describes the transfer of scientists from the BII to Roche for the period from 1975 till the institute closed. The first move was in 1977, but then only Theo Staehelin, Hubert Jacot and Vincenzo Miggiano relocated to Roche

QR1977_07 BII

[QR1977_08]. When considering the entire time span of this history, the following list emerges:

Bela Takacs, Vincenzo Miggiano, Theo Staehelin, Hubert Jacot, Michael Steinmetz, Manfred Brockhaus, Richard Pink, Howard Etlinger, Johann-Rudolf Frey, Werner Haas, Hajime Karasuyama, Zlatko Dembic, John Stocker, Gianni Garotta.

Some of the scientists will be mentioned again at the appropriate time, so here it suffices to say that on the list are 2 permanent members (Staehelin and Steinmetz), while all others were scientists with limited contracts. Roche offered these scientists very good working conditions, and in most instances higher salaries than they had at the BII. But it was a fact that scientists with non-permanent contracts (often after several prolongations) were expected to find positions elsewhere in the world arena of science. Some scientists chose Roche because they clearly considered the offer adequate and attractive.

It was a *yin and yang* situation. People moving from the BII to Roche did not lose any time for adjustment (yin), and they were immediately useful and functional for Roche in their new position (yang). Admittedly, for some of the scientists, the work turned out to be disappointing, and they moved on to other places.

Elsewhere in this volume, the transfer of scientists to other institutions within Switzerland is summed up [QR1977_09]. A former member of the BII, Howard Etlinger, quoted another colleague, Don Bellgrau, who judged the BII to have the best research environment. The paraphrased quote is as follows: "Howard, did you notice that when you are on the pavement outside the institute, you can see scratch marks from the fingernails of scientists as they are dragged away when desperately trying to stay in this, the best place in the world to do research?" (Quoted with permission.)

QR1977_08 BII

Roberto Poljak and the 3D Structure of Proteins, 1977

QR1977_09 BII

Roberto Poljak was on Jerne's early list of potential BII members. The appointment did not materialize as Roberto's operation was far too large to fit into the BII's horizontal structure. Instead, Roberto was welcome to join the institute for a sabbatical, and that he did in 1977. His work attracted fame and recognition, and his stay there greatly enriched several research groups. Roberto has written a small document – especially for this book – which is reproduced in full [QR1977_10].

QR1977_10 BII

Here is an excerpt from the document: *"I arrived in Basel in September 1977 and joined the laboratory of Susumu Tonegawa as a visiting scientist. There I met a number of very active and bright researchers with whom I had daily interactions. These include Ora Bernard, Christine Brack, Nobu Hozumi, Minoru Hirama, Hitoshi Sakano, and several others. Staff members of other laboratories I saw frequently and whose company I enjoyed include Claude Bernard, Patricia Riegert, Ivan Lefkovits, Humberto Cosenza, Marc Shulman, Hans Hengartner, and many others.*

Charlie Steinberg had been one of my instructors at Cold Spring Harbor when I took the Phage Genetics course in 1964. I was somewhat surprised to learn that he had joined the BII, since I did not think immunology was his field of interest. However, I felt reassured by his presence because I knew he was a very fine person and a very intelligent scientist, capable of deep insights, as his record at the BII has shown. I had frequent discussions with him and always learned from his insights and advice.

I should add here that I very much enjoyed meeting and talking to Louis Du Pasquier. Our talks had to do with the generation of antibody diversity since his work on the generation of diversity in Xenopus *had become a classic in the field.*

I also enjoyed very much talking to Hans Hengartner, who had returned from the MRC in Cambridge. Recently I did some research in the maturation of antibody responses to protein antigens, a field in which Hans preceded me with a very important paper on the antibody response to the vesicular stomatitis virus."

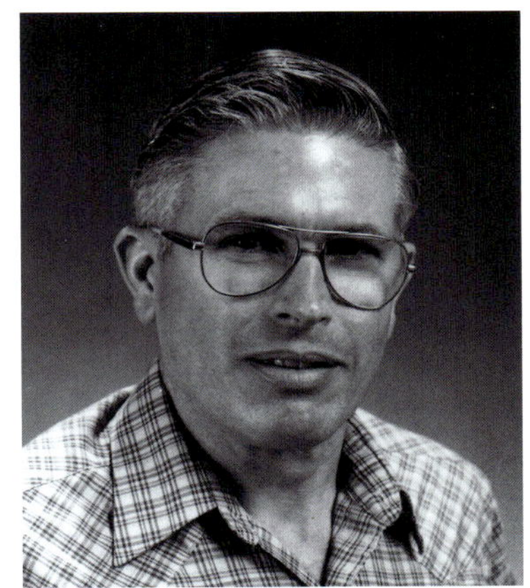

Scott Rodkey

Scott Rodkey Joins Dietmar Braun

Scott Rodkey's memories of the BII are given in the QR code [QR1977_11] – here are the introductory lines of his letter: "*My time at BII had a significant impact on my professional life. I was privileged to interact with a group of very talented and innovative people at BII. My lab home was in Lab 2, directed by Dietmar Braun. Dietmar was an enthusiastic and energetic colleague with whom I forged a lifelong friendship that flourishes still today. In addition to Dietmar, Wolfgang Schalch was in the lab then and provided excellent chemistry insight to many discussions in the lab and in the lunchroom. Others at the institute including Ivan Lefkovits, Charley Steinberg, Louis Du Pasquier, Harald von Boehmer, Michael Julius, Geoff Hoffmann, Andrew Kelus, Stan Leibo, Roberto Poljak, and of course Mel Cohn (a talented theoretician and truly gifted Starboy) were BII members who were valuable colleagues throughout many years following my time at BII. Professor Niels Jerne profoundly impacted my later career by sharing his philosophy of science and his keen insights into how science works.*"

QR1977_11 BII

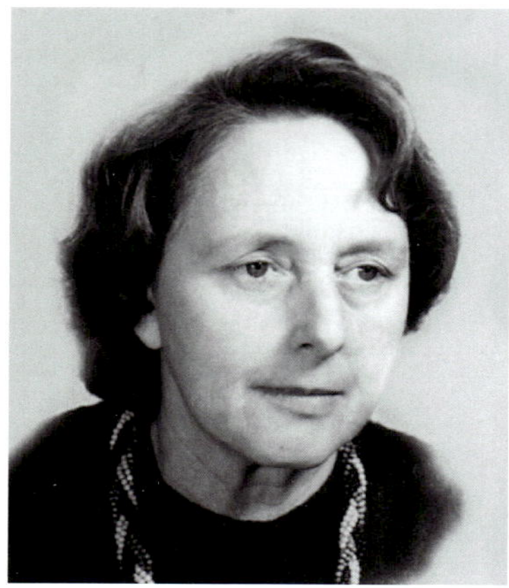

Berenice Kindred

Berenice Kindred Leaves for Heidelberg and Tübingen, 1977

Berenice Kindred was a member of the BII in two separate periods [QR1977_12]. She came in 1972 for 1 year from the University of Konstanz (department headed by Eberhardt Weiler). From 1974 to 1977 Berry's main work at the BII was on the genetics of immune responses in nude mice. She compared reconstitutions with allogeneic or syngeneic thymus cell suspensions, with grafts of neonatal thymuses, and with MLR-primed lymphocytes. She collaborated with Dietmar Braun, Ethel Jacobson, Francis Loor, Ivan Lefkovits and Ron Corley. She left for the German Cancer Research Centre, Heidelberg, and later she moved to the Max Planck Institute in Tübingen.

Wulf Droege Leaves for Heidelberg, 1977

Wulf Droege joined the institute in 1973 upon completing a postdoc position at Harvard University. His work on the suppressive effect of thymus-derived cells, and his collaborative work with Richard Pink, Vincenzo Miggiano and Andreas Ziegler, opened a door for him to obtain a prestigious position at the German Cancer Research Centre in Heidelberg in 1977. No research he carried out in Basel foreshadowed the key discovery he made in Heidelberg of the stimulatory effect of superoxide radicals and hydrogen peroxide on lymphocyte functions. This led to a series of studies on the role of reactive oxygen species, glutathione (and its precursor cysteine) in physiological and pathological processes. Wulf died in 2010 [QR1977_13].

Jonathan Sprent Leaves for London, 1977

After 3 years at the BII (1972–1975) Jon Sprent left for University College London, then went on to the Wistar Institute, Philadelphia, and later (1984) to the Scripps Research Institute, San Diego. Jon was already very well known when he arrived at the BII.

QR1977_12 BII

QR1977_13 BII

He graduated from the University of Queensland, and carried out his PhD studies with Jacques F.A.P. Miller at the Walter and Eliza Hall Institute in Melbourne. Jon's papers with his mentor Jacques were respected by the entire scientific community. Upon his arrival to Basel he immediately continued publishing prolifically. His papers on the lifespan of cells circulating in a mouse, and on the effect of priming with antigen caught the immediate interest of institute members. Collaborations with Harald von Boehmer,

Werner Haas, Georges Roelants, Francis Loor, Ben Pernis, Peter Krammer, Ivan Lefkovits, Leslie Hudson and others yielded a large number of frequently cited papers. Further aspects of Jon Sprent's career are given in [QR1977_14]; here, suffice it to say that he is considered as one of the most eminent immunologists of his generation. At the time of writing, Jon is Professor of Cellular Immunity at the Garvan Institute of Medical Research in Sydney, Australia.

Andreas Ziegler to Charité, Berlin

Andreas Ziegler carried out the work for his doctoral thesis at the BII on the major histocompatibility complex of the chicken and received his PhD degree at the University of Heidelberg in 1977. Following postdoctoral work at the MRC Laboratory of Molecular Biology in Cambridge, UK, on monoclonal antibodies against human and rodent cell surface antigens at César Milstein's laboratory, he became a staff scientist at the Universität Tübingen, where he continued working on human leukocyte differentiation antigens. After an intermediate appointment at the Universität Marburg, Andreas was chosen as a Director of the *Institut für Immungenetik*, Charité, Berlin. His research interests focus on structural and functional research of the MHC genomic region and its gene products. He was involved in the Human Genome Project for the analysis of chromosome 6. His translational interest is strongly related to antibody-mediated immunotherapy, both in oncology and transplantation medicine. He continued working on genes and antigens belonging to the extended major histocompatibility complex (xMHC) and their association with disease, but he was also interested in the molecular basis of mate choice, concentrating on xMHC-encoded odorant receptors and their involvement in reproduction. Since his retirement from the Charité in 2013, he works as CEO of Ziegler Biosolutions in Waldshut-Tiengen. His current research interests include the analysis of structure/function and dynamic relationships of membrane molecules. He is also involved in the problem of association of HLA-B*27 class I molecules with the rheumatic disease ankylosing spondylitis.

Sister Institute in Nutley, 10th Anniversary, 1977

QR1977_14 BII

Throughout this book it is maintained that the Roche Institute of Molecular Biology (RIMB) in Nutley and the Basel Institute were sister institutes, "the Nutley girl" being about 4 years older than "her Baloise sister". Although the charter of both institutes was very

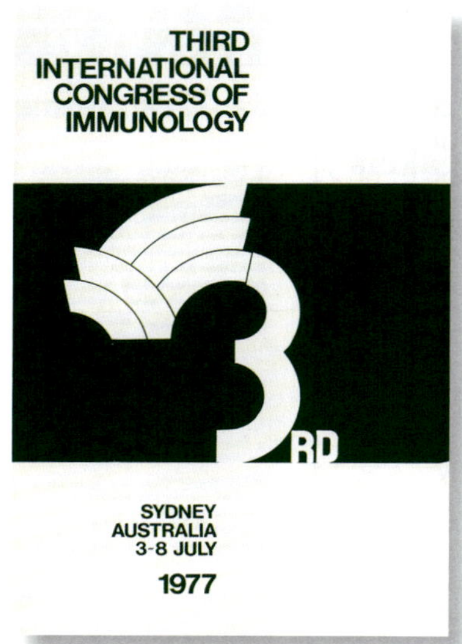

similar, one major difference was that the Basel institute kept emphasizing (with the benevolent understanding of Roche management) its *basic* research path. Nutley, instead, willingly maintained close ties to the Roche Research Laboratories. The RIMB established itself as a recognized center of excellence, and the achievements of its scientists were highly regarded worldwide. These achievements during its first 10 years are well documented in their Annual Reports [QR1977_15].

From Basel to Sydney, 3rd International Congress of Immunology, 1977

As with the 1st and 2nd International Congresses of Immunology (Washington and Brighton) the 3rd International Congress of Immunology in Sydney, Australia, attracted several thousands of immunologists from all over the world. Several participants from the BII attended and presented their work there [QR1977_16].

Roche Research Institute of Marine Pharmacology, Dee Why, Australia

The BII developed friendly research cooperation with another institute created by Hoffmann-La Roche (in Dee Why, Australia). This institute was conceived as a platform for a multidisciplinary approach to the challenge of isolating biologically active substances from marine organisms. Research facilities became operational in 1974 under the directorship of Joseph T. Baker [QR1977_17]. Several encouraging visits with the aim of establishing the envisaged cooperation took place. The research objectives were to isolate and characterize new molecules (one of which was methylaplysinopsin), to investigate biological activities and, as the foreseen joint project, to test the mitogenicity and immunogenicity of the substances. This cooperation did not materialize as Roche decided to close the Roche Research Institute of Marine Pharmacology in 1982.

QR1977_15 BII

QR1977_16 BII

QR1977_17 BII

Jerne on Retiring – Health Problems, Not Serious, but...

In the second half of 1977, Niels started to have some health problems, probably not serious, but he often felt tired and had to cancel his participation in several conferences. He talked individually to permanent members and colleagues from the previous era (mainly Gunther Stent and Klaus Rajewsky) and started to ask people whom they would consider as a successor. Jerne was aware that academic freedom is for the "here and now", while a large organization like Roche would not settle the question of a successor in an academic fashion. Companies are used to making decisions which are usually irrevocable. But still Jerne wanted to know.

Then in November 1977 Jerne explicitly asked some colleagues to put down on paper their thoughts and suggestions [QR1977_18]. Below are a few examples of replies:

QR1977_18 BII

INTERNE MITTEILUNG an: N.K. Jerne

Kopier an:

von : C.M. Steinberg Bau:

Datum : February 17, 1977 Tel.:

Betrifft: THE NEXT DIRECTOR

(1) Perhaps the Selection Committee or Roche wishes to start a new Institute under the present name and patronage. If that is the case, they are obviously not interested in the opinion of the present staff, including me. Therefore, in order to continue these comments, I must assume that this is not the case.

(2) There are no scientific institutes of comparable size which are run upon the same principles as the B.I.I. Hence, it is unreasonable to expect that the director of another institute would provide the necessary continuity.

(3) To select one of the present members would be one way of assuring continuity. In my opinion, none of the present permanent members possesses the scientific breadth and depth necessary to run the Institute and the scientific reputation in immunology necessary to attract first rate young people from all over the world. In addition, the choice of any of the present permanent members would be extremely divisive just at the time when unity is needed.

(4) The obvious solution is a former member – Ben Pernis.

(dictated to Sigrid over the phone)

After this preliminary consideration, while it would be too long to write about merits and drawbacks of the many excellent candidates that have been mentioned as your successors, I want to express my preference for Ben Pernis because :

In giving my suggestion for your successor, I restricted my choice to the people that I know personally. There are qualities (dignity, firmness together with humanity) which I wish the new Director to own, and can not be recognized through the value of scientific production. Walter Bodmer (Oxford) and Ben Pernis (New York) are the persons who, according to me, better approach you in this respect.

	Nossal	Lennox	Cohn	Pernis	Melchers
Breadth of vision	++	+++	+++	+++	++
Authority in immunology	++	++	+++	+++	++
Political acumen	+++	—	++	+++	++
Relations with staff	+++	+++	++	+++	+
Relations with employer					
1. getting on	+++	+	+	+++	+
2. standing up to	—	—	+++	+++	+++
Sum:	14	9	14	18	11

From the replies, preference for Ben Pernis became obvious. Interestingly, Niels would even have been ready to consider a generational handover (after all, in Australia the 35-year-old Gus Nossal was Burnet's successor), and Antonio Coutinho (then aged 32) would have been on his list. This point came up in Niels' conversation with Sydney Brenner.

BTA 1: Jerne and 65 + 1

A number of Niels Jerne's former colleagues and friends were invited to celebrate Niels' birthday in December 1977. It was a "1 year delayed" celebration of his 65th birthday, just dubbed as "65 + 1". The idea was not to let Niels know that besides BII members, friends from the old days would be present [QR1977_19]. They were to be the core of the birthday present: an oversized cardboard box was prepared as a "live parcel", with a ribbon round it that Niels had to cut.

It was followed by a play: it was a precursor of what evolved into the "Basel Theater for the Arts" (BTA). Michael Julius, as narrator, asked Niels Jerne to come up to the stage and open the box. A group of people disguised in black robes and masks sprang out and the individuals took a seat. Michael Julius directed a fictitious dialogue combined with pantomime. Jerne's task was to guess who those "individuals" were hidden behind their masks.

QR1977_19 BII

Among the actors were Claudia Henry, Gunther Stent, Eberhard Weiler, Werner Reichardt and Klaus Rajewsky. Jerne only recognized Klaus Rajewsky. These friends traveled incognito, but Claudia Henry caused a major turmoil when her purse with pass-

1 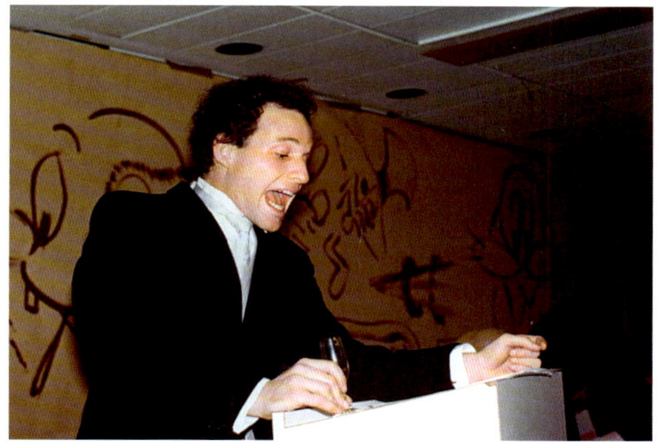

2 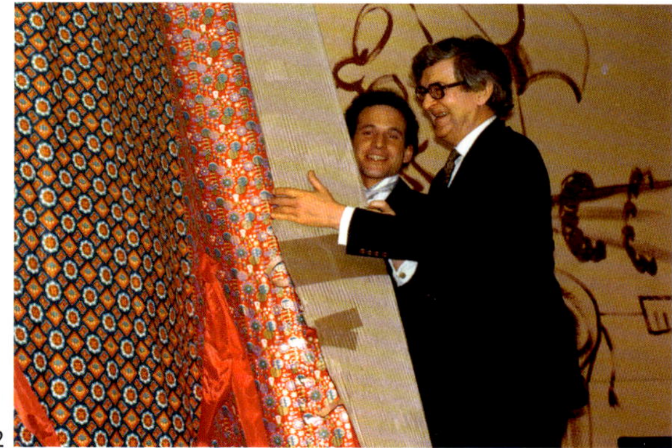

3 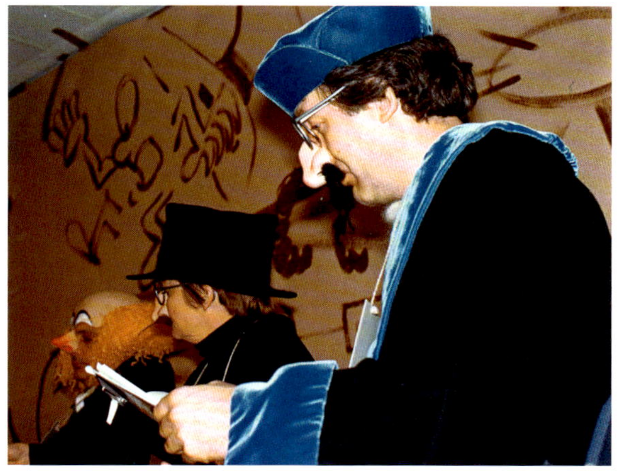

4 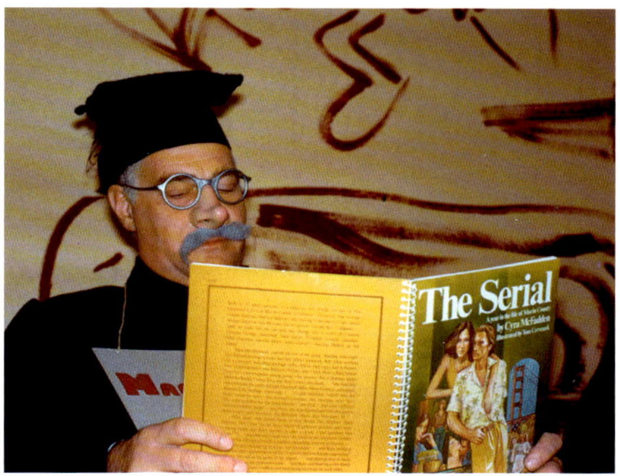

1 Michael Julius, narrator
2 Opening the giant present box
3 Klaus Rajewsky
4 Gunther Stent

port and address book was stolen – found by the police, who diligently phoned all the numbers noted in the agenda. The police intervention became a continuation of the "absurd theater".

In the collection of Niels' letters, there is a note to Gunther Stent which reads: "Gunther, it was wonderful of you to take the trouble to come all the way from California to surprise me on my so-called 65 birthday."

BTA 2: "Snow-White", the Second Performance of the Basel Theater for the Arts

The BTA's performance of Snow-White was a major event at the end of 1977. The script had been written and rewritten as a joint effort of several members and technicians [QR1977_20]. The performance took place soon after that of the short sketch known as "Jerne 65 +1". The enthusiasm for "65 + 1" led to the idea of producing a "proper" theater play, not just a sketch. It is not known whose idea

QR1977_20 BII

TO ALL PARTICIPANTS IN "SNOW-WHITE"

On Thursday next, 15th December, all participants will meet in the seminar room at 8 p.m. for a first rehearsal. If necessary, we shall have a second rehearsal sometime on Sunday, 18th December.

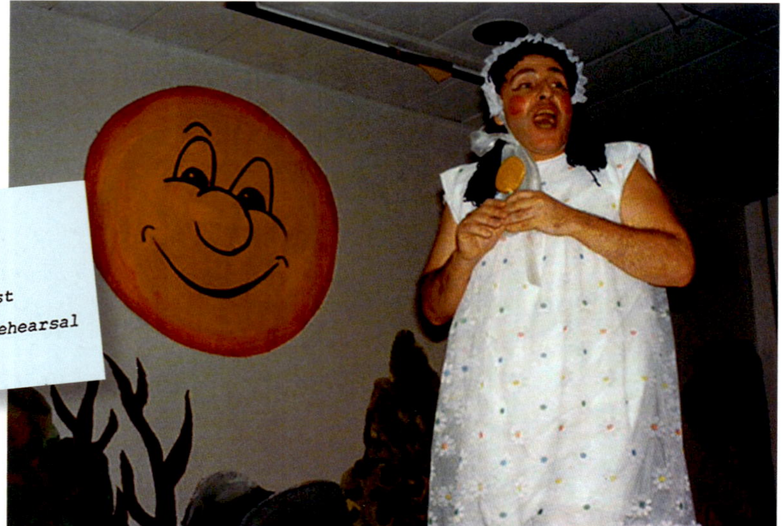

Mel Cohn

it was to perform the Snow-White fairytale, but certainly the facts that the characters of the 7 dwarfs could apply to several scientists and the mirrors could serve as a reflection of a scientist's ego were the decisive elements in embracing the idea of performing this play.

Ingrid Schnurr had a major role in the thinking, setup and practicing of the Snow-White play. Most of it was actually "invented" by her, Michael Julius and Antonio Coutinho, in the big house that Antonio shared for some time with Michael Julius and Bonnie Blomberg.

The basic script was written within days, but "egocentric modifications" continued up to the last minute, and some changes occurred during the performance itself. The play was put on stage on Monday, December 19th, 1977.

The 7 dwarfs were played by 14 people, and the mirror itself and its image alternated every so often (Ivan Lefkovits, Isabelle Altounian, André Traunecker, Jacques Bron and Klaus Rajewsky). There were several Snow-Whites and several Queens. Today, gender proponents would be very happy to see the mixing of the sexes. The Snow-Whites were Humberto Cosenza, Michel Delétraz, Ingrid Schnurr, Mel Cohn and Antonio Coutinho, whose appearance set the mood of the play: he mimed what the speaker read.

The first set of the 7 dwarfs was Alma Luzzati, Ora Bernard, Judith Johnson, Bonnie Blomberg, Max Schreier, Andrew Kelus and Christine Brack. The second set was Fritz Melchers, Harald von Boehmer, Bernd Weimann, Dietmar Braun, Susumu Tonegawa, Hansruedi Kiefer and Louis Du Pasquier.

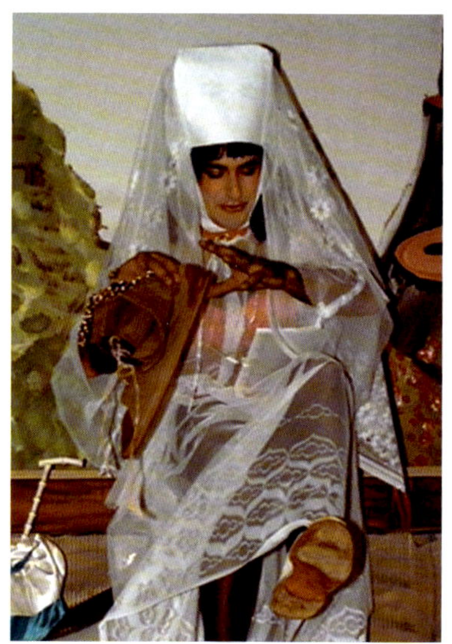
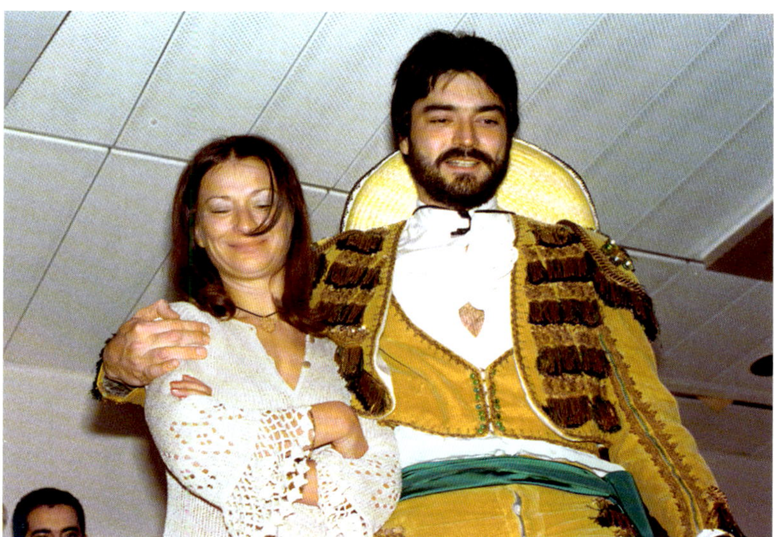

Scenes from Snow-White

What followed was pure Dadaism. The speaker continued to read the script, asking the fairytale questions, "who's been eating off my plate?", etc., while the dwarfs were immersed in another reality, "who has taken all my pipettes?", "who has been spitting in my water-bath?" Each dwarf spoke in his native language, and Ruggero Ceppellini, in his Italian bass voice, was the loudest. And when the Queen asked who was the prettiest lady, André Traunecker walked on stage in a T-shirt bearing the words "Scientific search committee".

The script mentioned the "Basel Theater for the Arts", and all future performances used this title.

Treasure Trove 1977

The database contains documents related to the BII in a broader context (lists, series of photographs, etc.).

WHILST THE SPEAKER ASKS ALL THESE QUESTIONS, EACH DWARF ASKS A DIFFERENT QUESTION, for example, Who has been spitting in my water-bath? and the like.They speak in their native languages.

The Year 1978

Georges Köhler organized the first workshop on hybridoma technology. The emphasis was on B lymphocyte fusions in the mouse system. Two permanent positions became vacant after Ben Pernis and Theo Staehelin had left the BII. They were filled by Georges Köhler and Harald von Boehmer. Susumu Tonegawa was awarded the Max Cloëtta Prize, the highest scientific recognition in Switzerland. Werner Arber, a valued member of the Advisory Board, was awarded the Nobel Prize for the codiscovery of restriction enzymes. Matthias Wabl (a close collaborator of Louis Du Pasquier and Charley Steinberg) left for the Max Planck Institute, Tübingen.

Arrivals 1978 (13)
Thirteen scientists from various places in Europe, the USA and Japan joined the institute: *Robbert Benner, Claudia Berek, Salvatore Cammisuli, Kirsten Fischer Lindahl, Johann-Rudolf Frey, Gianni Garotta, Ole Henriksen, Iver Heron, Sarah Howie, Claus Koch, Richard Maki, Hitoshi Sakano, Charles Sidman.*

Came and Left in the Same Year (2)
Robert Anderson, Christine Pellisard.

Leavers 1978 (20)
Dietmar Braun, Melvin Cohn, Humberto Cosenza, Minoru Hirama, Nobumichi Hozumi, Hans Huser, Judith Johnson, Stanley Leibo, Tommaso Meo, Michael Pawlita, Helmut Pohlit, ▶

T Cell Factors

Major research on soluble mediators that transmit cellular signals was initiated. A dozen projects were described in the 1978 Annual Report.

- Requirements for production of T cell growth factors
- Target cells of T cell growth factors
- T cell triggering is a two-step mechanism
- Characterization of T cell growth factors in humans and mice
- A part of the helper activity contained in Con A supernatants
- Analysis of the time course of helper factor formation
- Comparison of factors induced by Con A and PWM
- Molecular and quantitative analysis of helper T cell replacing factor
- The specificity of concanavalin A-induced helper T cell factor
- Cell-free mediators in the immune response
- Characterization of cell-free mediators in the immune response

The Antibody Repertoire

Continuing research on antibody heterogeneity was emphasized by Jerne in his introduction to the 1978 Annual Report [QR1978_01], as follows: *"The enormous diversity or repertoire of variable do-*

mains that one animal produces has always been the most fascinating aspect of immunology. Most immunologists would believe the size of this repertoire in mice and men to exceed one million, perhaps even by one or more orders of magnitude. One way of approaching the repertoire problem is to determine, among a population of lymphocytes stimulated in vitro, the frequency of cells that respond to a given antigen and produce specific antibodies. This has often been done in recent years, and for various antigens frequencies of about one in 10^5 B cells were often observed. These findings do not yield a good repertoire estimate: most antigens present several antigenic determinants (epitopes), and even against a single epitope many different antibody combining sites may show a detectable fit in the assays used. On the other hand, the in vitro conditions may not permit an optimal expression of all potentially capable B cells."

▶ *Roberto Poljak, David Poskitt, Scott Rodkey, Wolfgang Schalch, Irmtraut Schmid, John Stocker, Matthias Wabl, Bernd Weimann, Siegfried Weiss.*

The BII Workshop

The workshop was well equipped to design and construct any prototype of instrument required by the scientists. All prototypes were developed within the premises; when additional instruments

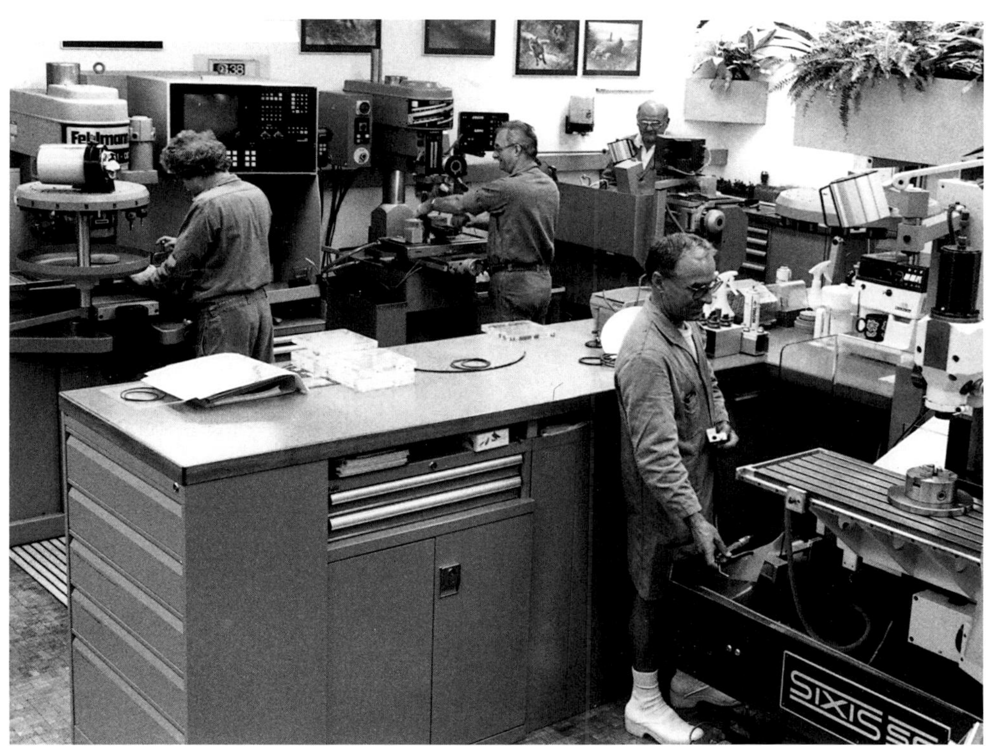

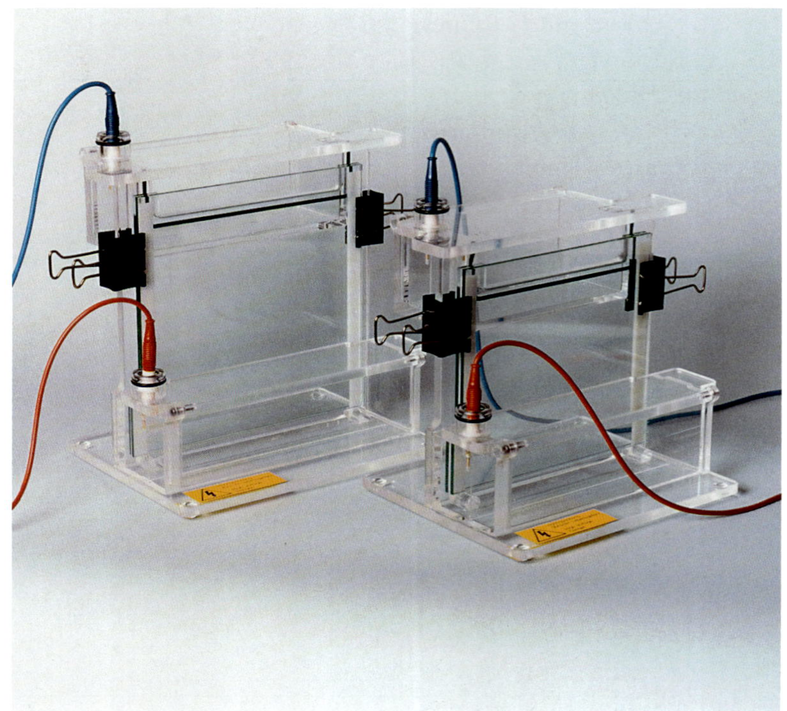

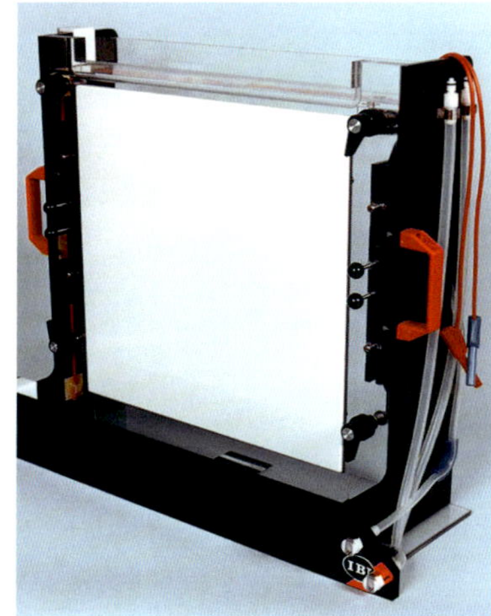

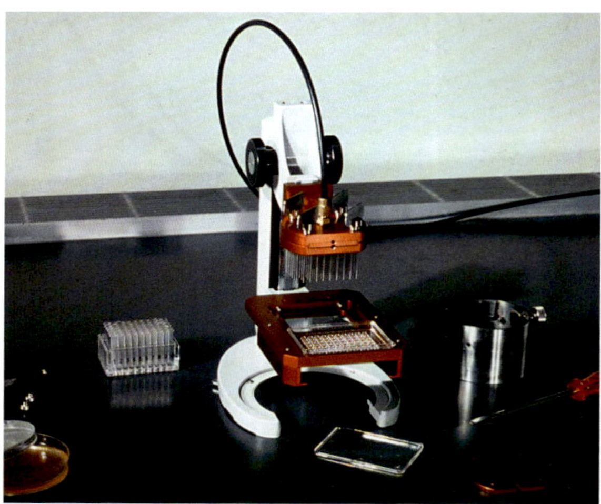

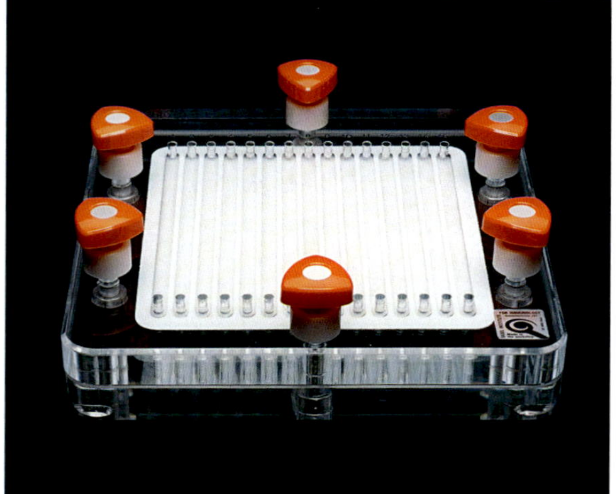

Examples of instruments made in the workshop

of the same kind were needed, small companies in Basel produced them, in order to keep the workshop staff free to construct new instruments. The BII workshop was among the first to have computerized a lathe *(Drechselbank)* that recorded the individual steps taken to design and construct each prototype, and which could automatically make identical copies of the same mechanical parts.

The ever-increasing prestige of the workshop and its importance in making competitive new laboratory instruments were exemplified by the decision to place one of the workshop products on the cover of the 1978 Annual Report. The equipment was dubbed "gynobatrachotron" (explained in the QR code [QR1978_02]).

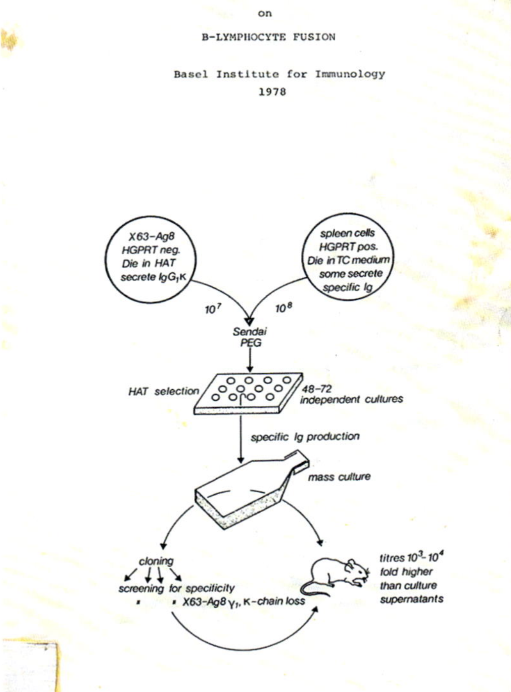

EMBO Laboratory Course on B Lymphocyte Fusion, 1978

Hybridoma technology was still in its infancy in 1978 but the scientific community's interest in it was great. At the EMBO course [QR1978_03], the main organizer of which was Georges Köhler, the participants were given first-hand information.

Matthias Wabl Leaves for the Max Planck Institute, Tübingen, 1978

Matthias Wabl completed his term at the BII in 1978 after fruitful collaboration with a number of scientists, especially with Louis Du Pasquier and Charley Steinberg. Matthias' first and second papers while at the BII (1975 and 1976) were published in *Science* and *Nature*. In the *Science* paper, Matthias and Louis had shown that "Lymphocytes of *Xenopus laevis* have the gene set for promoting tadpole development". This paper could have won a Nobel Prize but did not – instead, years later, John Gurdon received one.

Wabl made seminal contributions on the ontogenesis of lymphocyte diversity in amphibians and performed experiments (with Judith Johnson and Tommy Meo) showing that the genetic information for IgM and IgD expressed by a single cell lies on the same chromosome (chromosome 12).

QR1978_02 BII

Interestingly, after leaving Basel Matthias kept returning to the BII – for collaboration and for keeping up scientific and social contacts. Matthias has since developed transgenic mice with genetically optimized antibody-encoding loci, Heavy, Kappa and Lambda, and the V-D-J loci have been replaced by human coding regions that use mouse regulatory regions to produce antibodies that have entirely human variable regions in mice with fully functional immune systems. Antibodies from these mice can be fully humanized in a second step and produced in CHO cells to manufacture therapeutic monoclonal antibodies as pharmaceutical products. Many of his later publications were with his former colleagues at the BII [QR1978_04].

QR1978_03 BII

QR1978_04 BII

Dietmar Braun to Ciba-Geigy, 1978

Dietmar Braun

Dietmar Braun was one of the few BII members who was hired on a 5-year contract. Niels Jerne recognized that the buildup of a protein laboratory with highly specialized equipment and its maintenance required a somewhat different time scale. Dietmar became highly productive and published 67 papers during his years at the BII. His contract was prolonged several times, but then (1978) he left to join Ciba-Geigy, Basel [QR1978_05].

Dietmar came to Basel from Richard Krause's laboratory (NIAID Washington) with first-rate papers published in *PNAS*, and the *Journal of Experimental Medicine*. His main interest was in "homogeneous antibody" specific to streptococcal group A carbohydrate. With Jean-Claude Jaton he obtained the amino acid sequence of 69 N-terminal residues of heavy chain derived from a homogeneous rabbit antibody.

Dietmar joined the Pharmaceutical Division of Ciba-Geigy, Basel. He has risen there into the position of vice-director. His later scientific activities involved work in Vienna, Austria, and at several places in the USA.

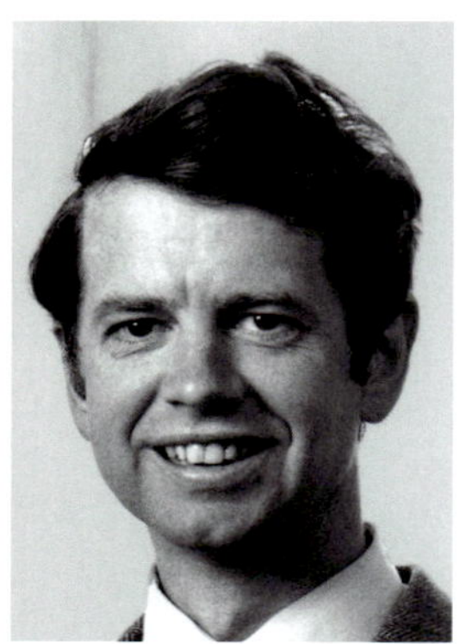

John W. Stocker

John W. Stocker to Roche, 1978

After 2 years at the BII, John took in 1978 a position with Hoffmann-La Roche, Basel. His first role at the Central Research Unit Roche involved the study of monoclonal antibodies and leading a task force investigating opportunities for scientific and commercial development of biotechnologically engineered vaccines. Later he served as Director of Pharmaceutical Research, Roche. In 1987, John returned to Australia as the founding Managing Director of the commercial biomedical company AMRAD Corporation Ltd., which was a bold attempt to establish an indigenous pharmaceutical industry in Victoria to capitalize on first-class medical research and to commercialize Australian biomedical discoveries.

Stocker was appointed the Chief Executive Officer of the Commonwealth Scientific and Industrial Research Organization (CSIRO) in 1990, with the aim of forming collaborative research and development efforts with private enterprises, which included clean and green food production, new biotechnology to revolutionize the production of drugs using gene shears (RNA self-cutting principle discovered by Wayne Gerlach and Jim Haseloff) as well as establishing disease-resistant crops.

QR1978_05 BII

In 1995 he was appointed as a member of the Prime Minister's Science, Engineering and Innovation Council, and Chairman of the Australian Science Technology and Engineering Council. In 1996, he was appointed as Chairman of the Australian Scientific, Technological and Engineering Council, with the aim of promoting public awareness of science, with the focus on the importance of Australian marine resources. He is Chairman of Sigma Company Ltd. of the Grape and Wine Research and Development Corporation. He is a Director of Telstra Corporation Ltd., Cambridge Antibody Technology Group plc and Circadian Technologies Ltd. More about the exciting career of John Stocker can be found in the QR note [QR1978_06].

Again Ten Permanent Members

Ben Pernis (in 1976) and Theo Staehelin (in 1978) resigned their permanent member positions. As there was no hierarchy among scientists, and no possibility of promotion to a "better" position, competition among scientists solely concerned scientific achievement. As long as the permanent positions were filled – there were only 10 – there was no rivalry regarding permanent status. Jerne (upon consultation with the Scientific Staff Selection Committee) made sure that the vacant positions were filled swiftly: chosen were Georges Köhler and Harald von Boehmer.

There was no formal procedure for selection, and as the institute was considered to have been "devised and designed" for Niels Jerne, it was basically his choice. The final decision was preceded by phone calls to members of the Advisory Board and the Board of Consultants, and probably an OK was sought from the president of Roche.

Neither the Annual Report for 1977 nor the one for 1978 mentions the two new permanent members. It was in line with policy that all members are members. Harald's transition was simply a change in the wording of his contract, while Georges' position was to provide him with ideal conditions for carrying out his ongoing, novel research on hybridoma technology. There is special mention (in Book 2) of the efforts made by the BII to persuade Georges to stay on as permanent member after winning the Nobel Prize and receiving an offer to become director of the Max Planck Institute in Freiburg, Germany.

QR1978_06 BII

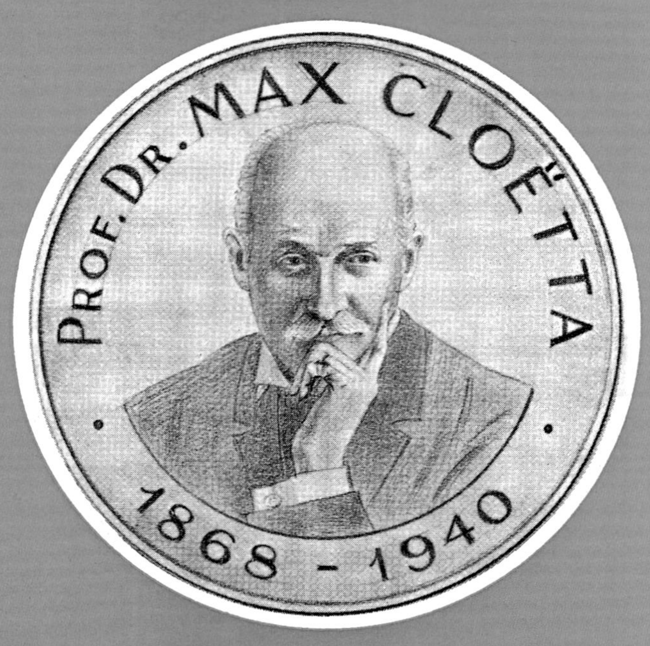

Preisverleihung 1978

STIFTUNG
PROFESSOR DR. MAX CLOËTTA

Heft Nr. 6

Cloning of Immunoglobulin Genes
(Klonierung von Immunglobulin-Genen)

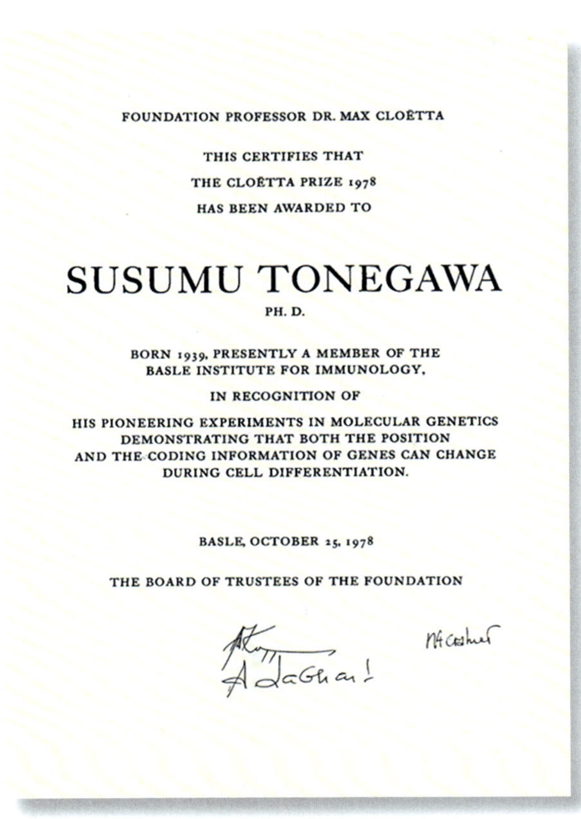
FOUNDATION PROFESSOR DR. MAX CLOËTTA

THIS CERTIFIES THAT
THE CLOËTTA PRIZE 1978
HAS BEEN AWARDED TO

SUSUMU TONEGAWA
PH. D.

BORN 1939, PRESENTLY A MEMBER OF THE
BASLE INSTITUTE FOR IMMUNOLOGY,
IN RECOGNITION OF
HIS PIONEERING EXPERIMENTS IN MOLECULAR GENETICS
DEMONSTRATING THAT BOTH THE POSITION
AND THE CODING INFORMATION OF GENES CAN CHANGE
DURING CELL DIFFERENTIATION.

BASLE, OCTOBER 25, 1978

THE BOARD OF TRUSTEES OF THE FOUNDATION

QR1978_07 BII

QR1978_08 BII

Max Cloëtta Prize for Susumu Tonegawa

The prestigious Max Cloëtta Prize, the highest scientific award in Switzerland, was given to Tonegawa for his "pioneering experiments in molecular genetics demonstrating that both the position and the coding information of genes can change during cell differentiation" [QR1978_07]. This prize is awarded in the month of October, the same month in which the Nobel Prize winners are announced. Nine years later Tonegawa receives the Nobel Prize.

Nobel Prize for Basel in 1978, but Not Yet for the BII

Werner Arber, together with Daniel Nathans and Hamilton Smith, was awarded the 1978 Nobel Prize for Medicine. Their discovery, the restriction enzyme, which cuts DNA strand molecules like a pair of scissors, is still one of the most important tools in molecular biology [QR1978_08]. Werner Arber was a valued member of the Advisory Board. The above caption "for Basel" is not entirely correct, since the work was done in Geneva, in Eduard Kellenberger's department.

Treasure Trove 1978

The database contains documents related to the BII in a broader context (lists, series of photographs, etc.).

QR1978_treasure BII

The Year 1979

Niels Jerne presented at the Advisory Board meeting his intention to retire in the foreseeable future. The Advisory Board and permanent members recommended that he continue holding the office. The Introduction to the Annual Report 1979 was the last one written by Jerne. It was his legacy, with issues close to his heart, such as "repertoire" and "idiotypic network". The book on immunological methods describing assay systems developed or used at the institute was published by Academic Press. Antonio Coutinho moved from Basel to Umeå and then to Paris.

Arrivals 1979 (15)
Fifteen scientists from various places in Europe, the USA and Canada joined the institute: *Vernon Alvarez, Kenneth Beh, George Bell, Rosa Bernabé, Jacques Chiller, Donald Gerson, Yoshikazu Kurosawa, Jean Langhorne, Maria Leptin, Carlos Martinez-A., John Reynolds, William Roeder, Carolyn Roitsch, Auli Toivanen, Paavo Toivanen.*

Came and Left in the Same Year (4)
Jack Haar, Claudia Henry, Maria Luisa Maccechini, Richard Smith.

Leavers 1979 (15)
Lucien Aarden, Sefik Alkan, Andrei Augustin, Robbert Benner, Claude Bernard, Ora Bernard, John Bywater, Antonio Coutinho, Stefanello de Petris, Christoph Heusser, Geoffrey Hoffmann, Claus Koch, Francis Loor, Alma Luzzati, Marc Shulman.

QR1979_01 BII

By Indirections Find Directions Out (Jerne Quoting Polonius)

Classical genetics dealt with the offspring of animals and plants. Classical immunology dealt with immunized animals and the variety of antibodies appearing in their blood serum. The cloning in bacteria of DNA segments containing immunoglobulin genes, the cloning of antibody-producing B lymphocytes by fusing them with immortal myeloma cells and the cloning of T lymphocytes retaining one specific function are all highly artificial procedures far removed from the unfolding of these elements in an intact animal. Nevertheless, these "indirections" will help us find "directions out".

Preparations for the Festschrift for Niels Jerne

Although Niels Jerne's round birthday was not yet an issue, his colleagues felt it would be appropriate to prepare a Festschrift for him – to be published in 1981 on his 70th birthday [QR1979_01]. Jerne might have been pleased even with a modest tribute, but the structure of the institute and the network of his friends and colleagues precluded a "narrow choice" of contributors. In an institute like the BII it would be out of place to hand-pick "a few" to make elitist presentations. From preliminary inquiries, it became obvious that "everybody" wanted to contribute.

Charley Steinberg and Ivan Lefkovits took it upon themselves to organize the volume, and they started to negotiate with publishers. The obvious choice was Karger, a prominent scientific publisher located in Basel. From the first round of negotiations it became clear that the institute would have to contribute towards the publishing costs (by purchasing a predetermined number of copies). The sum was of a magnitude that required approval by the director. Jerne of course was not supposed to know about the Festschrift, therefore he could not be asked for approval. Thus, the two editors (C.S. and I.L.) went directly to the president of Roche, who approved the project and had it financed from his special account.

Preparations started. Invited contributors received letters with standard instructions, and with a note that they would be charged for excess pages. The authors mostly kept to the page allowance, or paid the extra charges. Only one author declared that he was not willing to pay the charges or to shorten his manuscript. Thus, his paper was removed from the list and was not published.

The Manuscript of Linus Pauling

Linus Pauling was among the hundreds of people invited to contribute to the Festschrift. When the deadline for contributions came close, manuscripts kept arriving every day. Catherine Takacs, secretary for the Festschrift, collected them, and Charley Steinberg, when browsing through them, mentioned on a few occasions that he was curious as to whether or not Linus Pauling would contribute. This gave Dave Stewart (responsible for typing the manuscripts) the idea to play a hoax on Charley. It was agreed that Berry Kindred would write a "fake" paper having all the ingredients of a genuine paper, but which included hints that should make Charley suspicious. The paper was typed on US paper, sent to the USA in order to be mailed back to Basel from San Francisco. Charley was highly surprised to receive a paper written by Linus Pauling, and immediately started to read the manuscript. Every few minutes bursts of laughter came from his office, and comments like "he is absolutely crazy" and "that's incredible" were heard while he paced between his office and the cafeteria. After a while he called Catherine and demanded to see the envelope. She realized that Charley did not take the bite so easily and she brought the envelope; Charley checked the US format of the paper, the typing style, the margins, and again and again he exclaimed, "he is crazy". Then he went to Ivan Lefkovits and said, "we have to publish it, but he is nuts, everybody will realize that he has become crazy".

Then, and only then, did Steve, Catherine and Berry reveal the truth. Charley was relieved, but he was also in a very bad mood for the rest of the day.

Immunological Methods Volume 1 Published

The book was on the bestseller list of scientific publications for a considerable time.

Once the turnover of scientists at the BII reached a balance between scientists leaving and joining, a problem became evident: those leaving the BII took their methodological know-how with them. The impulse came from Maurice Landy [QR1979_02] to prepare a compendium of methodology developed and/or used at the BII, and to publish it with Academic Press, which he represented in Europe. This proposal fitted the prevailing mood at the BII very well, and Ivan Lefkovits and Ben Pernis took it upon themselves to assemble the methods used. In 1977 the preparation of the compendium started, and the book of methods was published 2 years later.

The book was on the bestseller list of scientific publications for a considerable time. The methodology book comprised the following chapters:

1. The Quality of Antibodies and Cellular Receptors (S. Fazekas de St. Groth)
2. The Isolation and Characterization of Immunoglobulins, Antibodies, and Their Constituent Polypeptide Chains (Jean-Claude Jaton, Daniel C. Brandt, Pierre Vassalli)
3. Peptide Mapping at the Nanomole Level (B.A. Moss)
4. Electrophoresis of Proteins in Polyacrylamide Slab Gels (Bela Takacs)
5. Resolution of Immunoglobulin Patterns by Analytical Isoelectric Focusing (Dietmar G. Braun, Kerstin Hild, Andreas Ziegler)
6. Isolation of Monoclonal Antibody by Preparative Isoelectric Focusing in Horizontal Layers of Sephadex G-75 (Wolfgang Schalch, Dietmar G. Braun)
7. Isotachophoresis of Immunoglobulins (Andreas Ziegler, Georges Köhler)
8. The Chemical Modification of Proteins, Haptens and Solid Supports (Hansruedi Kiefer)
9. Reagents for Immunofluorescence and Their Use for Studying Lymphoid Cell Products (Luciana Forni)
10. Radiolabeling and Immunoprecipitation of Cell Surface Macromolecules (J. Richard L. Pink, Andreas Ziegler)
11. Haptenation of Viable Biological Carriers (Helmut M. Pohlit, Werner Haas, Harald von Boehmer)
12. Production and Assay of Murine Anti-Allotype Antisera (Judith Johnson)
13. Preparation of Mouse Antisera against Histocompatibility Antigens (C. Garrison Fathman)
14. Technique of HLA Typing by Complement-Dependent Lympholysis (John W. Stocker, Domenico Bernoco)
15. The MLR Test in the Mouse (Tommaso Meo)
16. A Sensitive Method for the Separation of Rosette-Forming Cells (Bruce E. Elliott)
17. The Use of Protein A Rosettes to Detect Cell Surface Antigens (Judith Johnson)

QR1979_02 BII

18. Hapten-Gelatin Gels Used as Adsorbents for Separation of Hapten-Specific Lymphocytes (Werner Haas)
19. Assay for Plaque-Forming Cells (Ivan Lefkovits, Humberto Cosenza)
20. Plaquing and Recovery of Individual Antibody-Producing Cells (Marc Shulman)
21. Assay for Specific Alloantigen-Binding T Cells Activated in the Mixed Lymphocyte Reaction (Bruce E. Elliott, Zoltan Nagy, Markus Nabholz)
22. Assay for Antigen-Specific T-Cell Proliferation in Mice (Sefik S. Alkan)
23. Antigen-Specific Helper T-Cell Factor and Its Acceptor (Michael J. Taussig)
24. *In vitro* Immunization of Dissociated Murine Spleen Cells (Max H. Schreier)
25. Induction of a Secondary Antibody Response *in vitro* with Rabbit Peripheral Blood Lymphocytes (Alma L. Luzzati)
26. Induction of Immune Responses with Clonal Dominance at High Antibody Levels (Dietmar G. Braun)
27. Limiting Dilution Analysis (Ivan Lefkovits)
28. Establishment and Maintenance of Murine Lymphoid Cell Lines in Culture (Max H. Schreier, Bernd J. Weimann)
29. Clonal Growth of Cells in Semisolid or Viscous Medium (Norman N. Iscove, Max H. Schreier)
30. Preparation of Sendai Virus for Cell Fusion (Reet Tees)
31. Fusion of Lymphocytes (Georges Köhler)
32. Soft Agar Cloning of Lymphoid Tumor Lines: Detection of Hybrid Clones with Anti-SRBC Activity (Georges Köhler)
33. Isotope Laboratory (Helmut M. Pohlit, Jürg Widmer, Ruedi Frech)
34. Analysis of Immunological Data (Alberto Piazza)

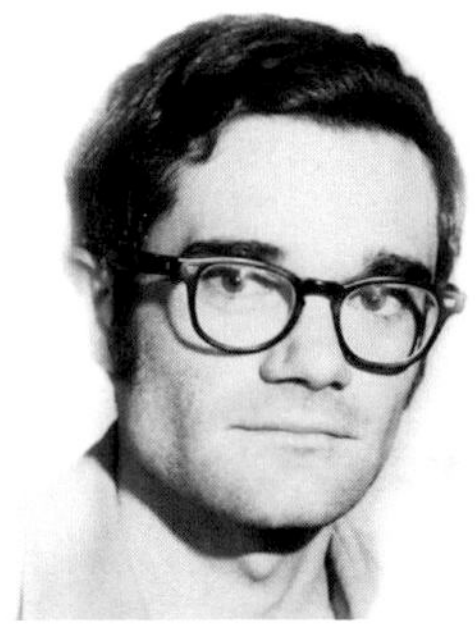

Bruce Elliott

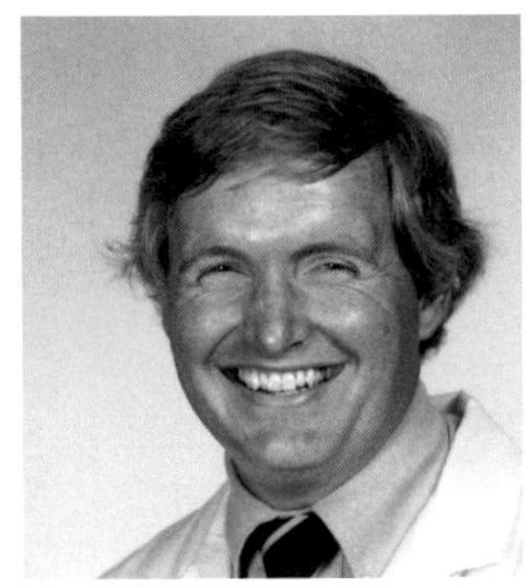

Garry Fathman

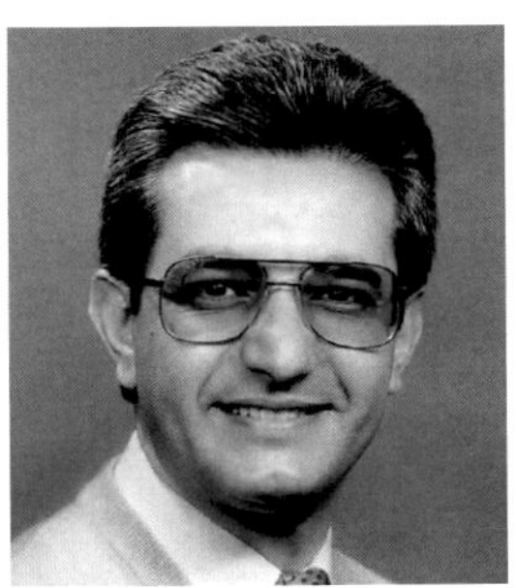

Sefik Alkan

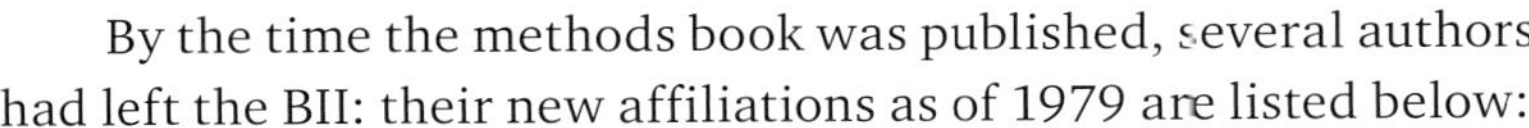

By the time the methods book was published, several authors had left the BII: their new affiliations as of 1979 are listed below:

- Domenico Bernoco, University of California, Los Angeles, Calif., USA
- Bruce E. Elliott, Queen's University, Kingston, Ont., Canada
- C. Garrison Fathman, Mayo Medical School, Rochester, Minn., USA
- Jean-Claude Jaton, University of Geneva, Geneva, Switzerland
- B.A. Moss, CSIRO Animal Genetics, North Ryde, N.S.W., Australia
- Markus Nabholz, ISREC, Lausanne, Switzerland
- Zoltan Nagy, Academy of Sciences, Budapest, Hungary
- J. Richard L. Pink, Department of Pathology, University of Geneva, Switzerland
- S. Fazekas de St. Groth, CSIRO Animal Genetics, North Ryde, N.S.W., Australia
- Bela Takacs, Hoffmann-La Roche, Basel, Switzerland
- Michael J. Taussig, ARC, Institute of Animal Physiology, Babraham, UK

Sefik Alkan to Novartis and Alba Therapeutics, 1979

After Sefik had concluded his appointment at the BII (1976–1980) he accepted a position at Ciba-Geigy Basel (which later upon fusion with Sandoz became Novartis). At Novartis Pharma Sefik worked for 18 years (1980–1998). He was in charge of studies on the human interferon α family. His research group produced monoclonal antibodies for epitope mapping and for assay development.

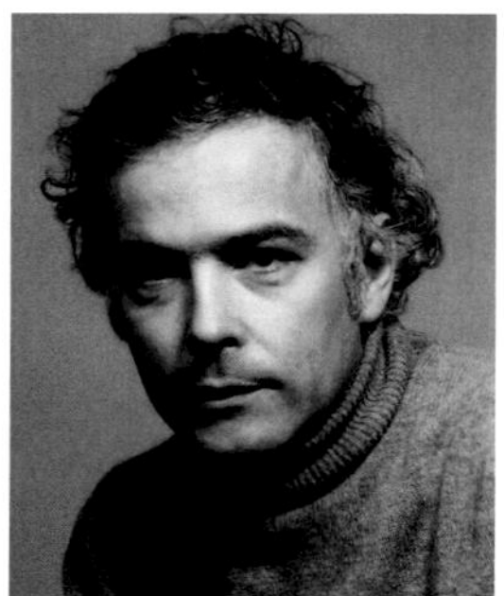

Werner Haas

During the course of his studies Sefik discovered that the extracellular matrix protein tenascin-W suppresses interactions between antigen-presenting cells and T cells. Sefik lists in his CV a number of low-molecular-weight immunosuppressive molecules, like calcineurin inhibitors, purine nucleoside phosphorylase inhibitors and different corticosteroids, rapamycin with various implications in basic and applied science.

Sefik Alkan was successful doing basic science, and he continued to be successful as a "drug discoverer" in the area of immunological diseases. Sefik always tried to bridge basic and applied science. He did so in several organizations like Novartis, Aventis, 3M Pharmaceuticals and Alba Therapeutics.

In Alba Therapeutics he rose to the function of Executive Vice-President with Preclinical Development Responsibilities. There he supported clinical development of peptidic and non-peptidic inhibitors for the treatment of autoimmune diseases.

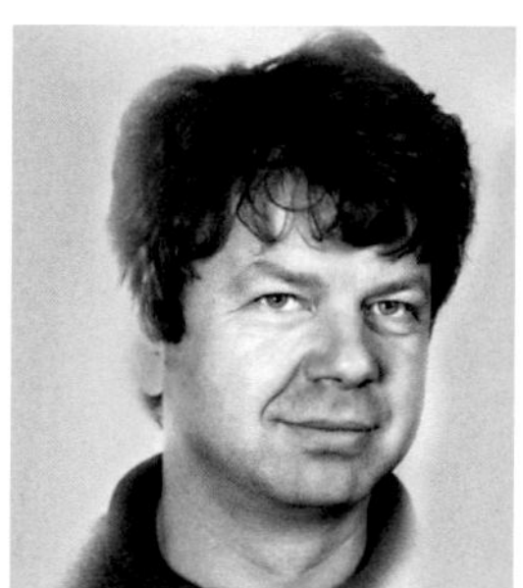

Harald von Boehmer

Werner Haas on His Scientific Alter Ego Harald von Boehmer

Werner Haas slowly but systematically acquired an encyclopedic knowledge in many science disciplines. With diffidence he stated that this can be a disadvantage. He expressed it so: *"In science it is neither possible nor desirable to know everything. Once Harald said to me: 'Werner, we are a great team, I remember the important papers, and you remember the non-important ones.' That sounds sort of arrogant from Harald, but he was right, and I knew that he was right. In fact he hit the weakest point, not only of my involvement in science, but also of my life in general. In medicine, I gave up, because I felt I didn't know everything. My approach to science has been encyclopedic. I read everything, always expecting to find something important, even in obviously very bad papers. Thus, I often couldn't see the wood for the trees. Thanks to Harald I did not get completely lost in the ocean of the literature. There is no doubt: Harald was 'Faust' while I was 'Wagner'."*

Antonio Coutinho Moves to Umeå and Then Paris, 1979

Antonio learned to ask questions in Stockholm and find the answers in Basel.

Antonio Coutinho's first scientific assignment – after completing his medical studies in Portugal – was a position with Göran Möller at the Karolinska Institute in Stockholm, where he worked towards his PhD in Medical Microbiology. He joined the BII in 1975 and spent 5 fruitful years there. Despite his international standing, Antonio is perceived as a "Portuguese" immunologist. In fact, up to 2010, he was the only Portuguese scientist belonging to the distinct group of "ISI highly cited researchers" [QR1979_03].

He left Basel (1979) for the University of Umeå, and a year later he was offered the prestigious position of Head of the Immunology Department of the Pasteur Institute, Paris. Then in 1998 he made his final move, becoming the director of the newly founded Gulbenkian Institute for Science, Oeiras, Portugal.

In his career, Antonio had two distinguished mentors: the young Swedish Göran Möller, and the senior world-famous Niels Jerne. There is no history-related speech of Antonio in which the two names do not occur. Antonio learned to ask questions in Stockholm and find the answers in Basel. In his own words: *"Moving to the Basel Institute was to come to the center of the world. And to be close to Niels Jerne. Niels and Göran shared many of their virtues and opinions how science should be done. But with a different style, at least in some details. Jerne was older and enjoyed surprise and provocation as a strategy to get his ideas through; but he talked from the high stand of being the father of modern immunology. Deservedly so, as he has introduced Darwinian principles in the field, against an overwhelming majority, and when it seemed impossible that his theory could possibly be true. Perhaps then, by the end of the 1950s, Jerne was like Möller when I met him, who could not help but be provocative, for his ideas were truly novel and frontally against the establishment."*

Antonio's main work in Basel was towards understanding the idiotypic network. Because of this, he was probably the closest person to Niels Jerne at that time. Antonio was impressed by Niels, and Niels was by Antonio. Antonio talked so often about Niels that one could become suspicious that this was only self-aggrandizing lip service. But later, when he became head of the Gulbenkian Institute, it became clear to every visitor who was acquainted with the Basel Institute, that Antonio was probably the only scientist who successfully transplanted the atmosphere of the BII to another part of the world.

A good day for me was when Werner and Harald actually understood what I said to them, and a great day was when I actually understood what they said to me.

Don Bellgrau

Mathematical Model of the Immune Network Theory

Geoff W. Hoffmann took upon himself the ambitious task of extending the network hypothesis to a *defined model*. While Jerne coined a careful term, "Towards the network theory", Geoff start-

QR1979_03 BII

ed a serious modeling attempt by formulating a pair of differential equations that reflect some of the main postulates of the "plus-minus" network theory of regulation. The equations exhibit 4 stable states that correspond to the virgin, the suppressed, the immune and the "anti-immune" states of the animal with respect to the particular antigen. While Jerne's hypothesis dealt with antibody, Geoff included in his analysis both cells and molecules. Geoff continued working on this theory in his new position in Vancouver, Canada [QR1979_04].

Niels Jerne's Resolution to Resign

At the Advisory Board meeting in 1979, Niels Jerne quite officially raised the question of his retirement and the search for a successor. It is probable that the Board members were already aware of Jerne's intention – it was Niels' style to prepare people in advance by conducting individual talks relating to future statements, instead of making "big", surprising announcements. The Board discussed this point and in the minutes of the meeting it was recorded that the Board recommended that he continue in his function as director [QR1979_05].

QR1979_04 BII

QR1979_05 BII

It is probable that Jerne was flattered with this endorsement, but he pointed out that he would not stay in office beyond December 1981, when he reached the age of 70. He mentioned that permanent members had also recommended that he continue holding office. Nevertheless, the names of possible candidates to succeed him were put forward and discussed, and it was not so different from 1977 (described above) when the name of Ben Pernis kept coming up. The statements of 1977 provide an important clue to the events that unfolded upon Jerne's decision to retire.

Treasure Trove 1979

The database contains documents related to the BII in a broader context (lists, series of photographs, etc.).

QR1979_treasure BII

The Year 1980

Several scientists, Salvatore Cammisuli, Jacques Chiller, Gianni Garotta, Sarah Howie and Hans Hengartner, completed their BII assignment and moved to other places: Jacques Chiller back to California, Hans Hengartner to University Hospital, Zurich. The president of Roche, Fritz Gerber, thanked Niels Jerne for his services and appointed Fritz Melchers as the new BII director. Roche established a tighter supervision over the institute by creating a supervisory council.

Georg Wick on a Sabbatical from Innsbruck

Georg Wick was a regular visitor to the BII, and he also spent several of his sabbaticals there. He always thought of it as a *Mecca of Immunology*, and he was full of praise for Hoffmann-La Roche's support of the institute. His interactions with the BII occurred both under the reins of Niels Jerne and Fritz Melchers. In a truly Austrian cordiality he expressed his gratitude for the opportunity given to him to broaden his scientific horizon and also getting acquainted with new techniques that were developed and used in Basel. He reciprocated all this by inviting BII members to Innsbruck. Especially the conferences in winter with skiing opportunities at Kühtai were highly appreciated by the friends of "immuno-skiing". There is another mention of Georg's cooperation with the BII in Book 2 [QR1980_01].

Hans Hengartner Moves to the University Hospital, Zurich, 1980

Hans Hengartner joined the BII in 1975 upon completing a postdoc position at the MRC Laboratory of Molecular Biology in Cambridge, UK. During his 6 years at the BII, Hans collaborated and published with Georges Köhler, Alma Luzzati, Max Schreier, Marc Shulman, Garry Fathman, Harald von Boehmer, Werner Haas, Markus Nabholz, Tommy Meo, Helmut Pohlit and Louis Du Pasquier. The subjects of his studies were: immunoglobulin production by hybridoma lines, cloning of alloreactive T cells, induction of antibody formation in peripheral blood lymphocytes, localization of κ and heavy chains on chromosomes 6 and 12, and also somatic cell hybrids between frog lymphocytes and mouse myeloma cells.

Arrivals 1980 (12)
Twelve scientists from various places in Europe, the USA and Canada arrived in 1980: *Donald Bellgrau, Jack Bennink, Catherine Corbel, Howard Etlinger, Ellen Hsu, Tauro Neri, Christopher Paige, Mary Jane Potash, Michael Ratcliffe, Martin Weigert, Jesper Zeuthen, Duzhang Zhu.*

Came and Left in the Same Year (3)
Marinus Lamers, Dennis Osmond, Georg Wick.

Leavers 1980 (12)
Kenneth Beh, George Bell, Ross Cahill, Salvatore Cammisuli, Jacques Chiller, Gianni Garotta, Hans Hengartner, Iver Heron, Sarah Howie, Auli Toivanen, Paavo Toivanen, Massimo Trucco.

QR1980_01 BII

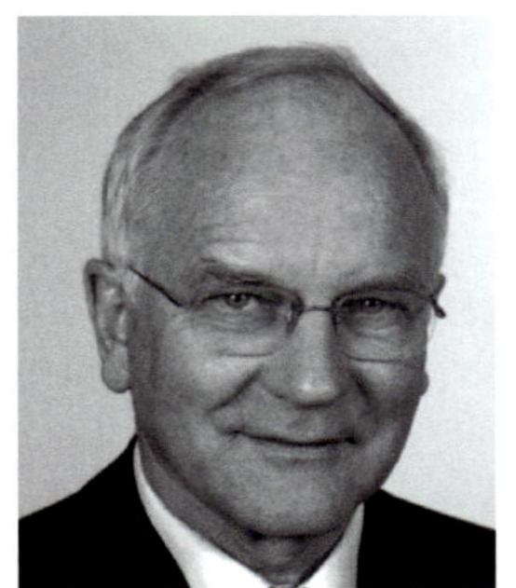
Hans Hengartner

In his new position in Zurich, he was head of the Institute of Experimental Immunology of the University Hospital (jointly with Rolf Zinkernagel). Among many important positions and prizes that awaited him in his career (professor ETH, member of Leopoldina) it is significant that he was chosen in the late 90s to be a member of the Swiss Board of Consultants, as one of the few consultants who knew the institute from the "inside" [QR1980_02].

Gianni Garotta to Roche, Basel, 1980

Upon completion of his appointment at the BII, Gianni Garotta was offered a position at Roche, Basel, with the responsibility for preclinical research on interferons, cytokines and monoclonal antibodies. His next position was at the Human Genome Sciences (Rockville, Md., USA), then Serono and RiboVax Biotechnologies (Geneva, Switzerland). At Serono he was the VP for Extramural Research and at RiboVax he was the CEO. Gianni pioneered the diagnostic application of monoclonal antibodies, discovered several molecules and characterized them as potential drugs. Seven of these drugs entered clinical trials, and one has been approved for therapy.

QR1980_02
BII

From Basel to Paris, 1980

The 4th International Congress of Immunology was held in Paris. The President of the Congress was Jean Dausset, and he made it

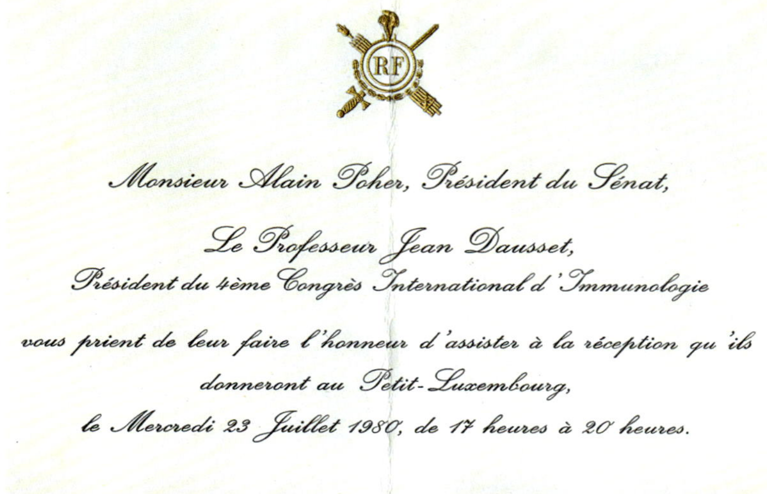
Monsieur Alain Poher, Président du Sénat,

Le Professeur Jean Dausset,
Président du 4ème Congrès International d'Immunologie

vous prient de leur faire l'honneur d'assister à la réception qu'ils donneront au Petit-Luxembourg,
le Mercredi 23 Juillet 1980, de 17 heures à 20 heures.

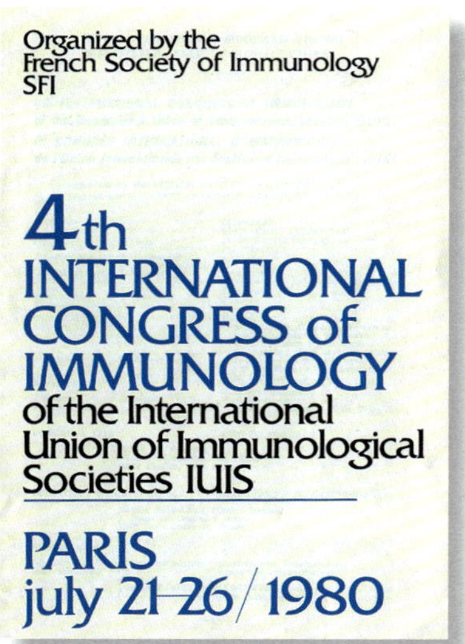
Organized by the
French Society of Immunology
SFI
4th
INTERNATIONAL
CONGRESS of
IMMUNOLOGY
of the International
Union of Immunological
Societies IUIS
PARIS
july 21-26/1980

into a special event, not only through high-quality scientific sessions, but also because of all the splendid receptions held in historical palaces of the *Grande Nation* [QR1980_03]. Again, several participants from the BII attended and presented their work, and dozens of the Paris attendees had previously given seminars in Basel.

Polly Matzinger, once when she was accused of being a narcissist, instead of denying it, said: "Everyone who loves to see his name on a publication is a narcissist."

How to Behave at Meetings and Seminars

Guests at the BII encountered a friendly and unpretentious atmosphere. Their seminars were less certain to pass in a polite and courteous manner. The lecturer did not need to say "Please interrupt me whenever there is something that is not understandable", since he/she was interrupted or stopped every so often. Some members, e.g. Charley Steinberg, Werner Haas and Polly Matzinger, loved to point out shortcomings or embarrass lecturers by aggressive remarks. There exists an entire collection of sarcastic comments by the members; here is an example given by Werner Haas from an extramural event in Sesimbra, Portugal: *"A scientist from the US, Steve Burakoff, gave a lecture on hapten-specific, cytotoxic T cells, a subject, which I believed to know better than anybody else. At a point when it was clear that he is being wrong, I shouted 'what do you think, that means?' and in an aggressive manner added 'absolutely nothing'. Later that day John Sprent reprimanded me, thus I decided to apologize. Unfortunately, when I did apologize, I addressed the wrong person (he didn't know what I was talking about). Some 20 years later I traveled with my boss at Roche, Juergen Drews, to Boston, to visit a group working at Harvard on diabetes. A man entered the room, approached me and said: Werner, do you remember Sesimbra? This man was Steve Burakoff."*

The Mary Jane Potash Memorial Seminars, 1980

In 1982 Howard Etlinger started a series of seminars, each called "The Mary Jane Potash Memorial Seminar". Seven were held, extending into the 1990s. Howard left the institute in 1983 but returned many times, sometimes to give a Mary Jane Potash seminar. Mary Jane Potash was a BII member between 1980 and 1982, and when she returned to the USA she worked mainly on AIDS research.

The topics of each seminar were diverse and intended to reflect aspects of the institute's ethos: to awaken curiosity, to ponder things that seem unrelated but end up to be related, to see worlds

QR1980_03 BII

I have never again in my whole life experienced an intellectually stimulating atmosphere that paralleled that encountered at the BII.

Georg Wick, Innsbruck

one had never imagined, like a fish that can't see water. For a while the seminars were half science and half all over the place. For example, the difference between heaven and hell which Howard called "memory". In the first seminar, Howard asked the audience whether fish drink water. Two voted "Yes", 3 voted "No", and about 35 didn't vote. (The answer is that some fish do and some don't.)

Charley Steinberg liked the seminars and occasionally when Howard, who was later working down the road at Roche, visited the institute, Charley would say: "When ya gonna give another Mary Jane Potash seminar?" On seminar days, Charley would write the announcement on the information board next to the ground floor elevator, and always draw a fish in water.

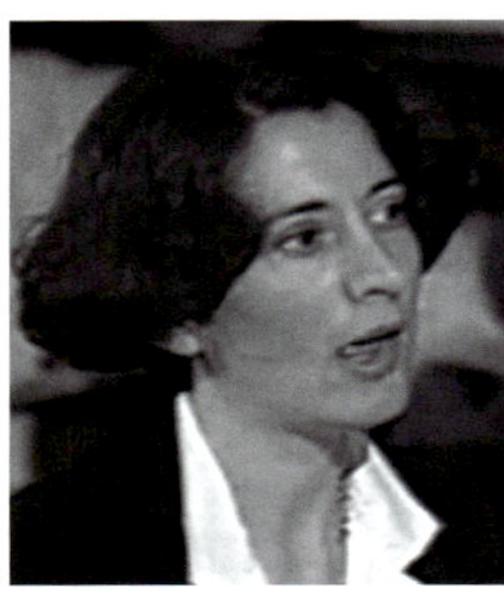

Mary Jane Potash

Charley is an example of the ethos that flowed from Jerne and touched and altered so many people for the better. As the years went by, Howard met ex-Basel institute scientists at gatherings and some spontaneously recalled the Mary Jane seminars with a smile. Howard doesn't explain the seminars' name; he feels that "we each need some mystery or else what's the point".

The Search for a New Director

In February 1980 Fritz Gerber, President of the Board of Directors of F. Hoffmann-La Roche, met Niels Jerne to inform him that Paul Sacher, co-owner of Roche, was concerned about the rumor regarding Jerne's intentions to resign the BII directorship. Jerne told Gerber that there was no urgency at present; it was only a precaution as he had had some health problems which now, fortunately, seemed to be resolved.

Gerber returned to the issue of the search for a new director [QR1980_04]. Jerne was surprised by the word, "search", as he assumed that Roche would be happy if the new director were chosen upon recommendation of the Advisory Board. Gerber bluntly said that it was not customary for the resigning director to choose his successor. He stressed that it was certainly not the way a commercial enterprise handles the issue. At that meeting (or perhaps earlier) Jerne handed over a list of potential successors. It comprised 5 names: Ben Pernis, Klaus Rajewsky, Gus Nossal, Ed Lennox and Fritz Melchers. The list was based on the preferences of the permanent members and by some members of the Advisory Board (the board never made a written recommendation).

QR1980_04 BII

Fritz Gerber thanked him for providing the list, glanced at the names and added, "I shall work with 4 names, Ben Pernis will not be among them". It was a gesture of trust towards Jerne that Gerber took up negotiations with Klaus Rajewsky, an eminent scientist from the University of Cologne. Rajewsky was offered the position of director and had several meetings with Gerber. In a VIP manner Rajewsky was chauffeur-driven from Zurich airport to Basel and after the negotiations returned to Cologne the same day. There are no written records but it is probable that Gerber was convinced that Rajewsky was the right choice. However, for reasons that were never fully clarified, the negotiations abruptly ended (Klaus probably let the final deadline for his decision pass). Two letters immediately followed: (1) Klaus Rajewsky was told that negotiations were terminated; (2) Fritz Melchers was offered the position of director. Fritz Gerber telephoned Niels Jerne to tell him that he – Fritz Gerber – accepted Jerne's wish to retire and had appointed Fritz Melchers in his place.

Although Niels Jerne was prepared to retire, this decision displeased him, as he had assumed that he himself would choose the time of handing over the position. It seems that parallel to the "late-stage" negotiations with Rajewsky, Gerber had already made up his mind to appoint Fritz Melchers as director. There is no exact record of the events, but perhaps the king-maker was Manfred Eigen, due to his special relationship with Paul Sacher. Eigen was a member of the Advisory Board, but did not stay in the hotel with the other board members – he stayed in Paul Sacher's home.

Immediately after Gerber's phone call, Niels Jerne arranged to meet several permanent members that same day to analyze the new situation.

Fritz Melchers: Primus inter Pares

Fritz Melchers informed the permanent members that he had received an offer from Fritz Gerber to become Niels Jerne's successor, and that he had accepted the offer. He said that he considered himself as *primus inter pares* and would not attempt to introduce any change in institute policy. Since he was aware that the institute was successful as it stood, and Jerne's vision had led to this success, there was no need to depart from the path Niels had set.

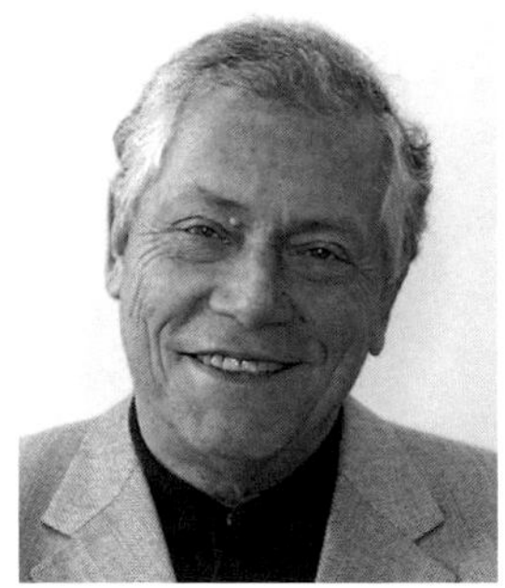
Fritz Melchers

Fritz concluded that he counted on the support of the permanent members. He moved into the office previously occupied by Jerne. Ingrid Schnurr resigned from her position of director's secretary, and 2 years later she left the institute for a prestigious job in the Paul Sacher Foundation for Twentieth Century Music on Münsterplatz, Basel. Melchers hired a new secretary, Mrs. Marguerite Jürgensen.

The Advisory Board (as well as the Board of Consultants) was of course informed about the change in the directorship. At the next board meeting, Fritz carefully outlined the future path of the institute, repeatedly stressing that there would be no departure from institute policy; thus, the board could continue functioning as it had in previous years. Fritz suggested, and the Advisory Board unanimously agreed, that Niels become its Honorary Chairman. Towards that end, Fritz informed the board that Niels was to be given a spacious office with a view of the Rhine, for him to use whenever he was in Basel. To enable good contact with Niels during his absence, the office would be maintained by Ingrid and later by Ivan Lefkovits.

Fritz Melchers had a good relationship with Fritz Gerber and Paul Sacher. Fritz felt, as did the permanent members, that the solid backing of Paul Sacher was crucial for the stability of the institute. Everything indicated that Fritz genuinely intended to keep the institute's path unchanged. There were, however, signs that Roche wished to exert a greater influence on the institute. Roche manifested this by establishing an additional board with the title "Scientific Council of the Board of Directors". In fact, this board rarely interfered with the running of the institute.

... Fritz genuinely intended to keep the institute's path unchanged.

In summary, Fritz handled all institute matters successfully and received unanimous acclaim from the Advisory Board. There was, however, a minor issue of concern: Niels had not headed a lab because he preferred to use his vast knowledge and experience in advising, when asked, any of the institute research groups. With Fritz as director the matter was different as he was an active researcher. None of Jerne's decisions were ever viewed from the angle of conflict of interest – and to some extent this was different with Melchers.

New Director with a Supervisory Council

Roche had used the opportunity of the change in directorship to gain (or at least to attempt to gain) a tighter control over the institute's activities. The gentleman's agreement between Jerne and Jann was never questioned, but the new constellation with Fritz Melchers as a director enabled Roche to establish tighter supervision of the institute by creating the "Scientific Council of the Board of Directors" [QR1980_05]. To some extent this did cut back certain rights of the director, but it did not create any impediment in the actual work carried out at the institute (and was not felt by the members). Mutual trust between Melchers and Roche remained

intact as the members of the Council, Manfred Eigen, Sidney Brenner, Walter Gehring, Jürgen Drews, Lukas Hoffmann, Jakob Oeri and Fritz Gerber, were respected personalities in science and commerce.

Farewell Party for Niels Jerne, October 1980

October meant for Niels the end of an era during which he had made the rules. The course of events had happened according to his ideas, but suddenly things changed. As mentioned in earlier chapters, Niels had intended for some time to step down from the directorship of the institute, but he had assumed that the change would happen in harmony with his wishes. He did not count on a "business call" from the Roche President telling him that a successor was now chosen and that this would be implemented immediately.

For most of the BII members this was a much less sensitive issue, just an anticipated "changing of the guard" – an expected one. True to the tradition of the institute, the moment had come to organize an adequate farewell party and to choose a good-bye present. As a special favor to Niels, Jean Tinguely agreed to build a small electrical tabletop machine reminiscent of his double helix sculpture which is now standing on the roof of the Basel Tinguely Museum. It was paid for by money collected from the scientific staff of the institute. As a surprise, the people from the workshop presented Niels with an exact miniature copy of the double helix standing in the institute's courtyard that they had constructed themselves.

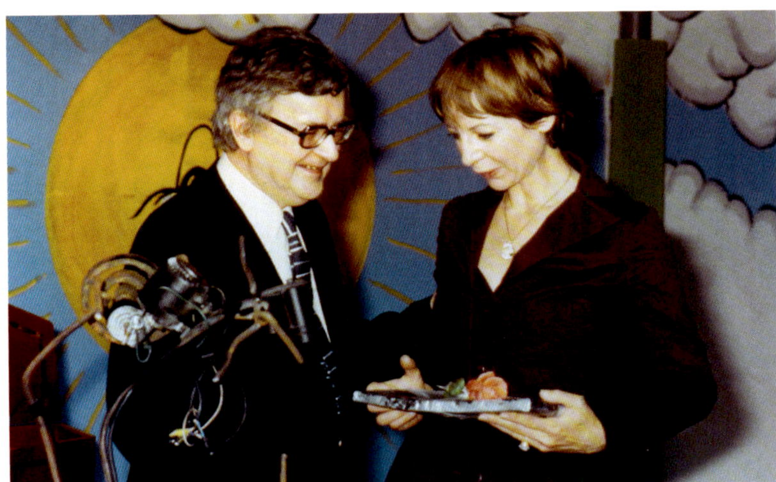

Niels and Alexandra Jerne

Many people helped organizing the festive party held in the beautifully decorated garage of the institute. There were a number of speeches. Also Niels said a few words. He certainly enjoyed the fine food and wine which was a 1971 Château Lafite-Rothschild, Pauillac. Two days later he traveled to his home in Castillon-du-Gard in France.

A Letter from Provence

Niels Jerne wrote an open letter to the staff of the BII dated November 11th, 1980:

TO

EVERY BODY

IN THE

BASEL INSTITU E R IMMUNOLOGY

Slowly recovering from the change in circumstances,
habits, tasks, and from the shock of suddenly being
divorced from , u all,
but unable to thank ea of you personally,
I should like all of you to know how grateful I feel
for your kindness, loyalty, and friendship
throughout ten years,
And wish to thank you all for arranging that
beautiful farewell party, five weeks ago, and for
your precious gifts:
The book with photographs and signatures has become
Alexandra's treasure; the ancient map of Basel
now hangs on the wall in my study room; and
Tingeley's motorized miniature double helix has found
a perfect spot above the cheminée of our dining room.
I send you all my very best wishes, and
au revoir perhaps in January.

Castillon-du-Gard
11 November 1980

Niels Jerne

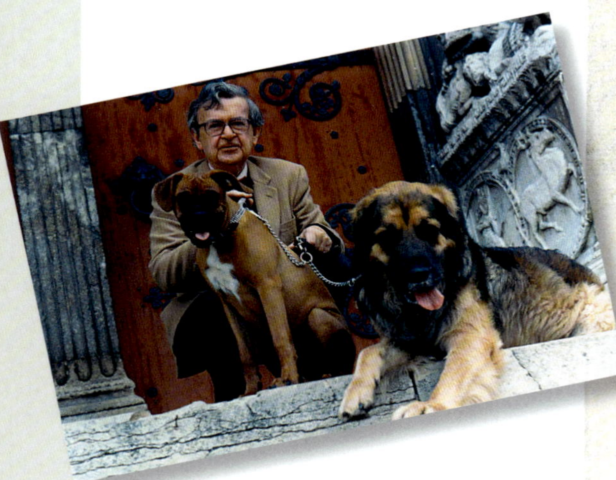

Niels Jerne with his dogs
in Castillon

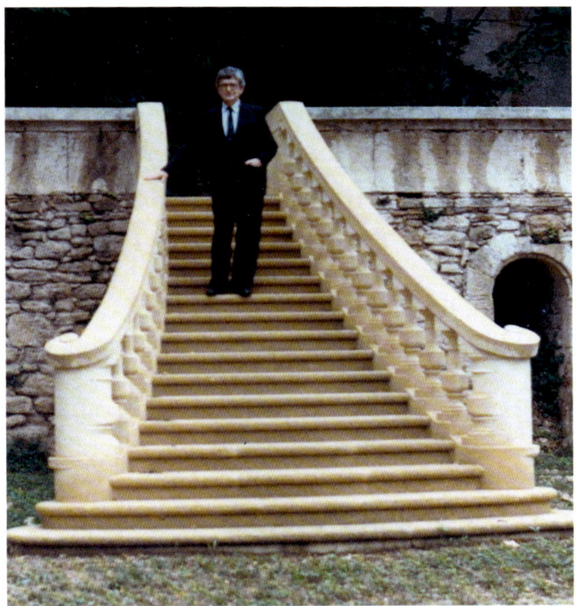

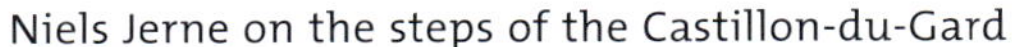
Niels Jerne on the steps of the Castillon-du-Gard

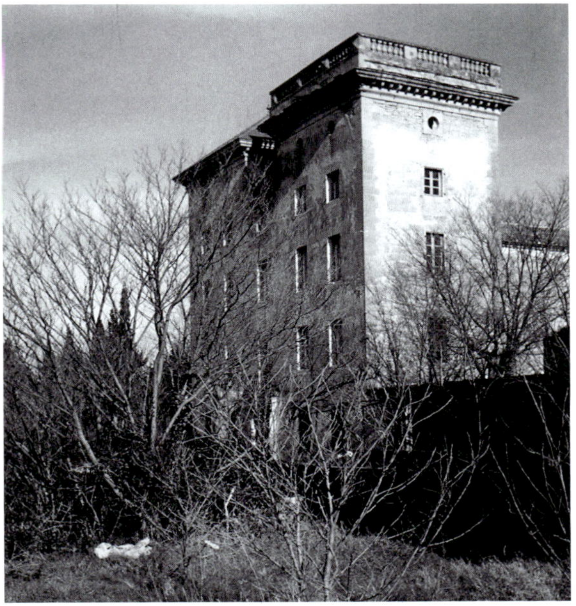
View of the Castillon from the garden

Nobel Prize to Former Members of the Advisory Board

Baruj Benacerraf, together with Jean Dausset and George Snell, was awarded the Nobel Prize for Medicine 1980 [QR1980_06]. Jean Dausset worked in the same field of research (histocompatibility antigens) as Ruggero Ceppellini.

Paul Berg, Walter Gilbert and Frederick Sanger were awarded the Nobel Prize for Chemistry in 1980 for the determination of DNA sequences (same QR code as Dausset).

Treasure Trove 1980

The database contains documents related to the BII in a broader context (lists, series of photographs, etc.).

The Year 1981

The celebration of the 10th anniversary of the institute was accompanied by a scientific symposium and by a major ballet performance of the BTA. The ballet was written and choreographed by Chris and Colleen Paige, Maria Leptin, Norman Iscove and others. A two-volume Festschrift on the occasion of Niels Jerne's 70th birthday was handed over to the septuagenarian. A conference on idiotypes was organized by Claudia Berek, Howard Etlinger and Michael Julius.

Arrivals 1981 (15)
Carol Conti, Franco Di Padova, Andrew Farr, Minoru Hirama, James Kaufman, Pawel Kisielow, Claus Koch, Martine Levy, Bernard Mély-Goubert, Masayuki Miyasaka, J. Richard Pink, Hung Sia Teh, Andreas Tsapis, Olli Vainio, R.C. von Borstel.

Came and Left in the Same Year (3)
Joachim Günther, Stefan Kaufmann, Kendall Smith.

Leavers 1981 (11)
Vernon Alvarez, Rosa Bernabé, Bonnie Blomberg, Johann Rudolf Frey, Yoshikazu Kurosawa, Jean Langhorne, Carlos Martinez-A., Albert Nordin, Susumu Tonegawa, Martin Weigert, Jesper Zeuthen.

QR1981_01 BII

10th Anniversary of the BII

The celebration of the institute's 10th anniversary provided the opportunity to look back at Niels Jerne's era and look forward to future scientific directions. The institute's seminar room did not have the capacity to hold the "main event", as the interest from the scientific community, as well as from the general public, was enormous. The venue thus chosen was Roche's large auditorium, and it was filled to the last seat.

As was customary for the BII, the celebratory speeches were kept to a minimum, leaving the stage for presenting highlights of scientific achievements. The speech of the President of the Board of Directors of F. Hoffmann-La Roche, Fritz Gerber, indicated that Roche considered the institute to be a valuable part of the company and promised to sponsor it in future years [QR1981_01].

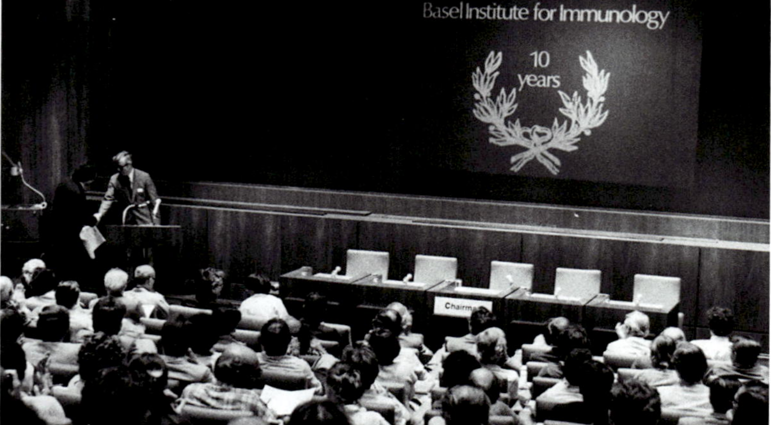

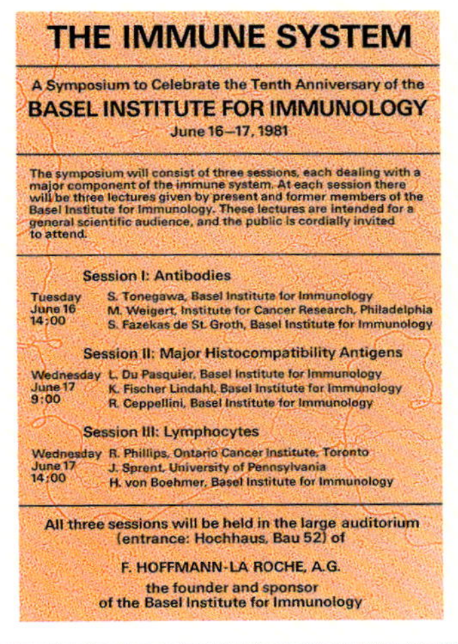

THE IMMUNE SYSTEM

A Symposium to Celebrate the Tenth Anniversary of the

BASEL INSTITUTE FOR IMMUNOLOGY

June 16–17, 1981

The symposium will consist of three sessions, each dealing with a major component of the immune system. At each session there will be three lectures given by present and former members of the Basel Institute for Immunology. These lectures are intended for a general scientific audience, and the public is cordially invited to attend.

Session I: Antibodies

Tuesday June 16 14:00
S. Tonegawa, Basel Institute for Immunology
M. Weigert, Institute for Cancer Research, Philadelphia
S. Fazekas de St. Groth, Basel Institute for Immunology

Session II: Major Histocompatibility Antigens

Wednesday June 17 9:00
L. Du Pasquier, Basel Institute for Immunology
K. Fischer Lindahl, Basel Institute for Immunology
R. Ceppellini, Basel Institute for Immunology

Session III: Lymphocytes

Wednesday June 17 14:00
R. Phillips, Ontario Cancer Institute, Toronto
J. Sprent, University of Pennsylvania
H. von Boehmer, Basel Institute for Immunology

All three sessions will be held in the large auditorium (entrance: Hochhaus, Bau 52) of

F. HOFFMANN-LA ROCHE, A.G.

the founder and sponsor of the Basel Institute for Immunology

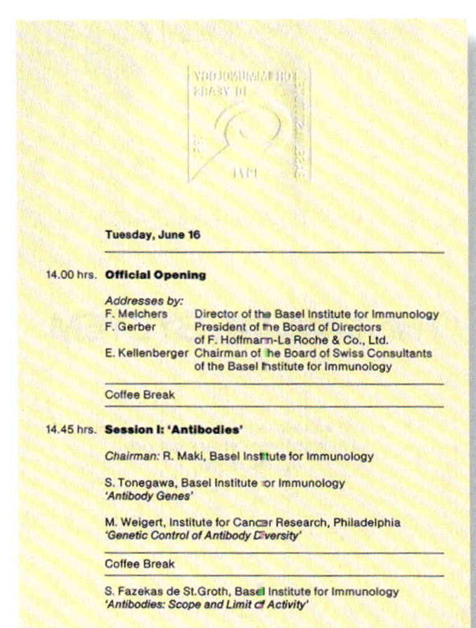

Tuesday, June 16

14.00 hrs. **Official Opening**

Addresses by:
F. Melchers — Director of the Basel Institute for Immunology
F. Gerber — President of the Board of Directors of F. Hoffmann-La Roche & Co., Ltd.
E. Kellenberger — Chairman of the Board of Swiss Consultants of the Basel Institute for Immunology

Coffee Break

14.45 hrs. **Session I: 'Antibodies'**

Chairman: R. Maki, Basel Institute for Immunology

S. Tonegawa, Basel Institute for Immunology
'Antibody Genes'

M. Weigert, Institute for Cancer Research, Philadelphia
'Genetic Control of Antibody Diversity'

Coffee Break

S. Fazekas de St.Groth, Basel Institute for Immunology
'Antibodies: Scope and Limit of Activity'

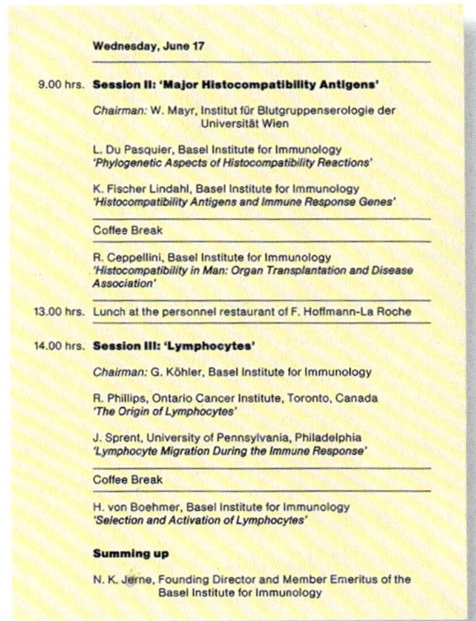

Wednesday, June 17

9.00 hrs. **Session II: 'Major Histocompatibility Antigens'**

Chairman: W. Mayr, Institut für Blutgruppenserologie der Universität Wien

L. Du Pasquier, Basel Institute for Immunology
'Phylogenetic Aspects of Histocompatibility Reactions'

K. Fischer Lindahl, Basel Institute for Immunology
'Histocompatibility Antigens and Immune Response Genes'

Coffee Break

R. Ceppellini, Basel Institute for Immunology
'Histocompatibility in Man: Organ Transplantation and Disease Association'

13.00 hrs. Lunch at the personnel restaurant of F. Hoffmann-La Roche

14.00 hrs. **Session III: 'Lymphocytes'**

Chairman: G. Köhler, Basel Institute for Immunology

R. Phillips, Ontario Cancer Institute, Toronto, Canada
'The Origin of Lymphocytes'

J. Sprent, University of Pennsylvania, Philadelphia
'Lymphocyte Migration During the Immune Response'

Coffee Break

H. von Boehmer, Basel Institute for Immunology
'Selection and Activation of Lymphocytes'

Summing up

N. K. Jerne, Founding Director and Member Emeritus of the Basel Institute for Immunology

Scientific presentations were given by Susumu Tonegawa, Martin Weigert, Louis Du Pasquier, Kirsten Fischer Lindahl, Ruggero Ceppellini, Bob Phillips, Jon Sprent and Harald von Boehmer.

Niels Jerne's talk was a "summing up", which provided a historical appraisal of events in the world of immunology.

Anniversary Celebration Continued at the BII

Ten years after Louis Du Pasquier had played the flute at the opening ceremony of the BII in 1971, with the same virtuosity he played again on this occasion. This time Christina Zeuthen accompanied him.

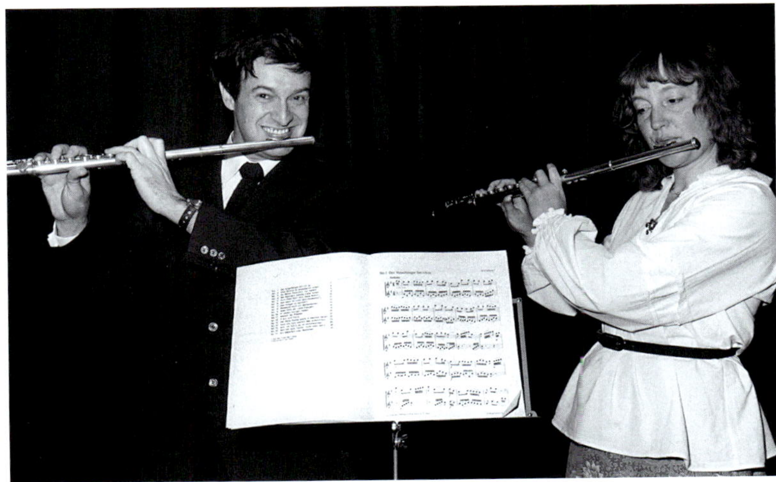

Louis Du Pasquier and Christina Zeuthen on the flute

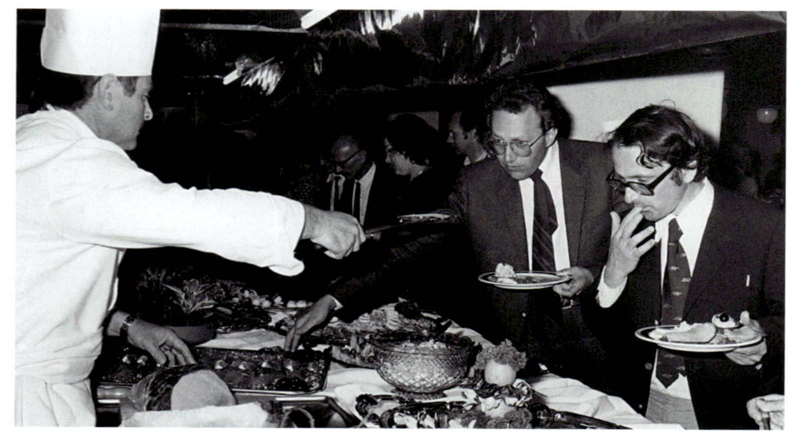

Wolfgang Mayr from Innsbruck and Ivan Lefkovits, BII

Haute Cuisine at the Anniversary Party

Fine food was served, though not the "finest" manners were noticeable at the buffet.

QR1981_02 BII

BTA 3: The Stem Cell Ballet

The high point of the celebration was a ballet on the immune system. It was written and choreographed by Chris and Colleen Paige, Maria Leptin, Norman Iscove, Rich Maki and Barbara Wernli, and performed by 38 dancers from the institute staff [QR1981_02].

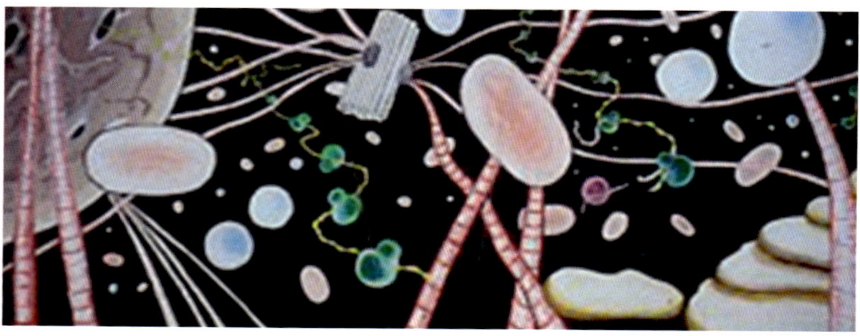

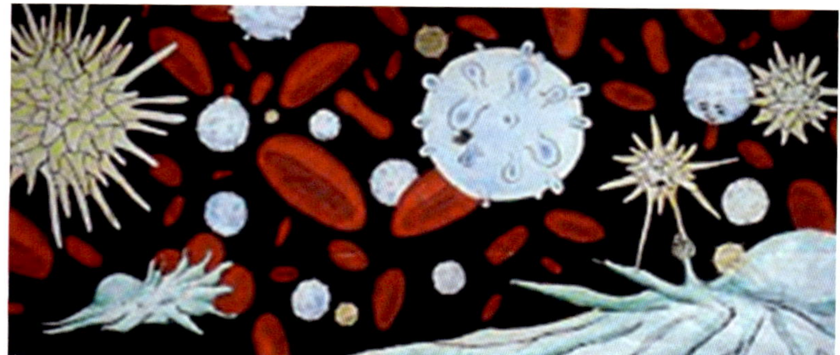

Stage decoration for the ballet

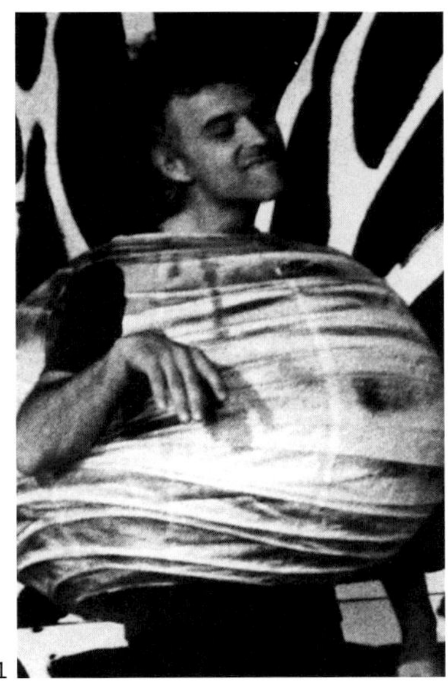
1

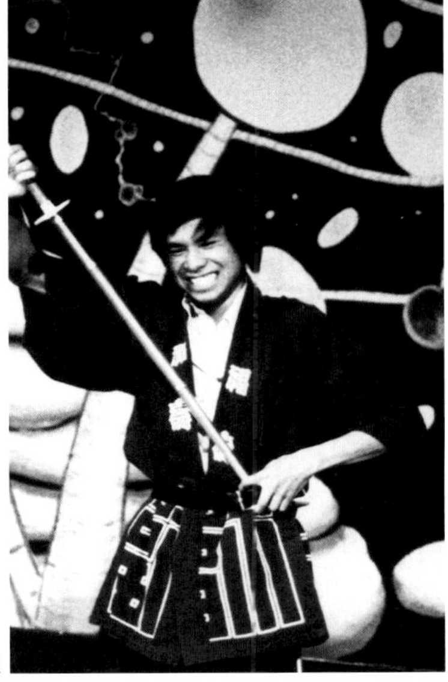
2

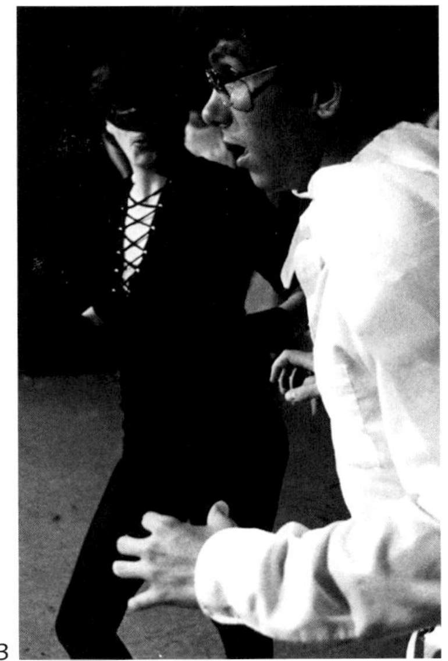
3

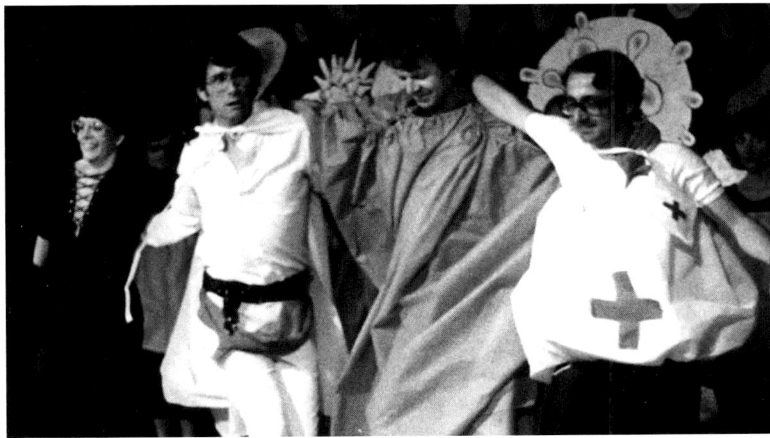
4

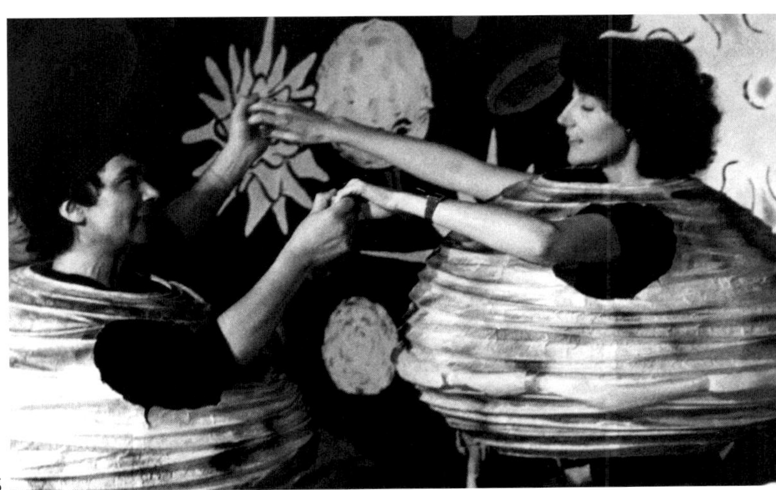
5

1 Those who knew him well can decipher Werner Haas' grimace

2 Of course there was never a shortage of Samurai at the institute

3 Only the cognoscenti recognize Kirsten Fischer Lindahl in disguise

4 From left: CTL, Antigen, Macrophage, Helper T cell

5 Poetic dance of cells, but competitive

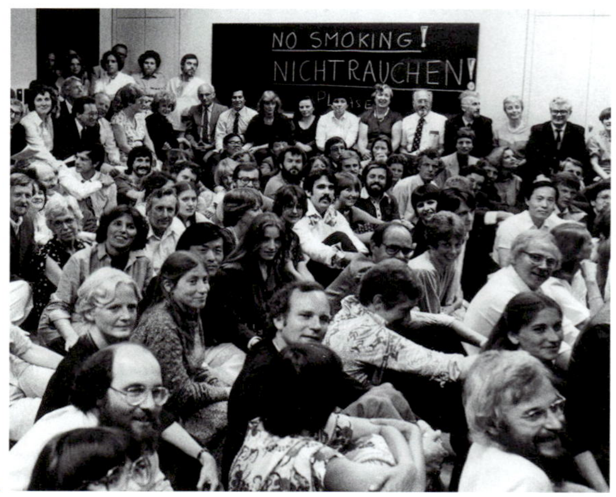

1

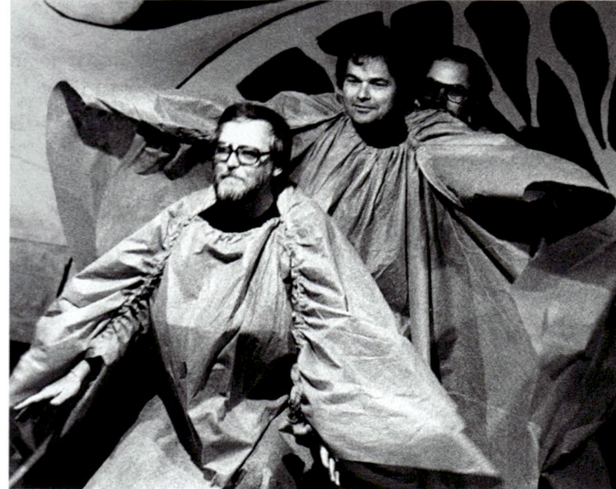

2

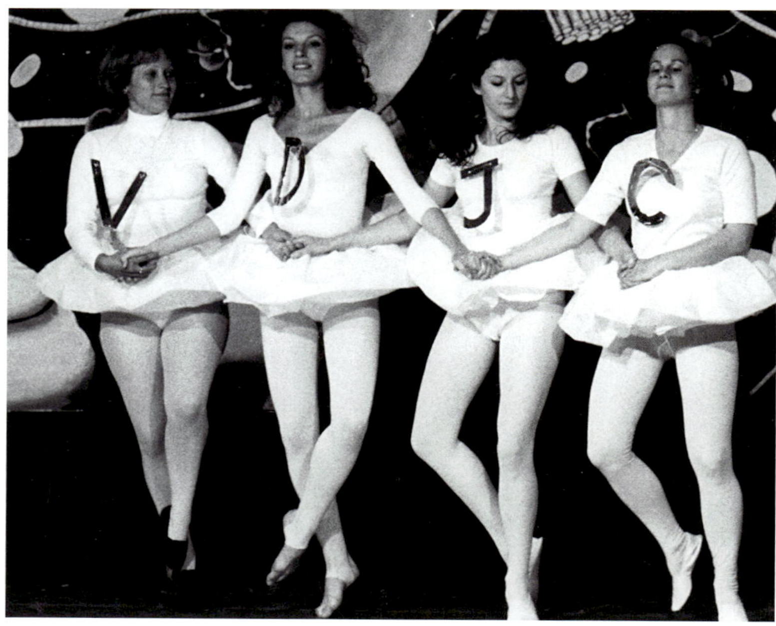

3

1 The audience shows its appreciation of the obviously successful performance

2 For what it is worth they are macrophages preparing to remove the foreign cells killed by the CTL – Harald von Boehmer is there too, his hand can be seen on the lower right. Al Nordin, Jesper Zeuthen and Don Gerson prepare to launch an attack

3 The most important scene – the clue to the entire story depicted by the four ladies V, D, J and C (V = variable gene segment, D = diversity gene segment, J = joining gene segment, C = constant gene)

Next page:
Scene from the Stem Cell Ballet performed by the BTA

QR1981_03 BII

The Origin of the Basel Theater for the Arts, BTA

The description of events relating to the plays performed at the BII does not seem a fit subject – at least at first glance – for inclusion in a history book on scientific achievements. But in the very first play, and in several that followed, the content was always science related. The actors (scientists and technicians) had fun planning, rehearsing and performing on stage, but the plays always had an underlying scientific context. This was sometimes "half-serious" and ironic, but somehow related to the scientific achievements of the institute [QR1981_03].

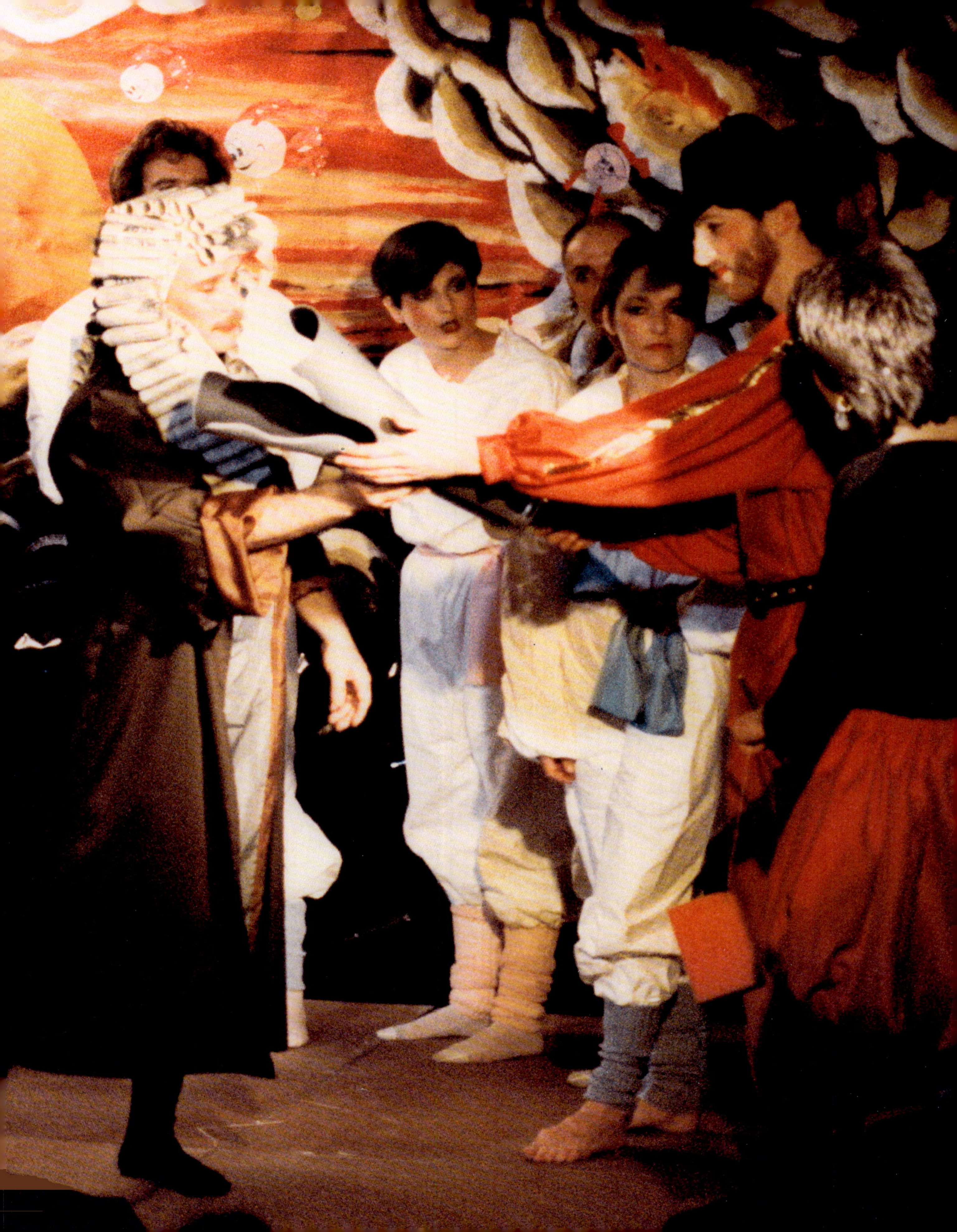

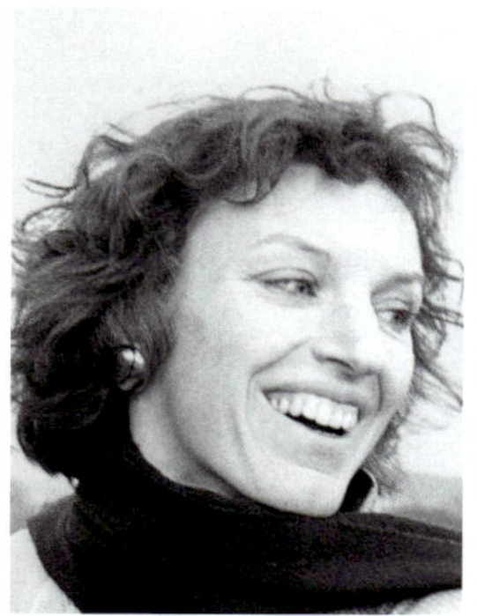

Maria Leptin

Chris Paige produced the *Stem Cell Ballet*. He and several colleagues wrote the script which was often changed during writing and also during rehearsal. The changes were always based on scientific or quasi-scientific arguments.

"If he is a T cell, then I want to be a macrophage."

"You are wrong, it is not the macrophage that releases this factor, it is the T cell that does it."

"But did you read the paper of Schimpl and Wecker?"
Surprisingly the actors started to devise an experiment to find out whether the factor is released during stimulatory events by macrophages or by T cells, as mentioned in the play.

The performance became known to the wider scientific community, due to the review in *Nature* (vol. 291, p. 606, 1981) by Miranda Robinson, which reads

... the ballet (was) performed with astounding verve ...

...the ballet (was) performed with astounding verve at the end of the celebration by respected scientific members of the institute and their technical staff, ingeniously costumed as a variety of lymphocytes and associated cells. Particularly notable were performances from Harald von Boehmer, benignly engulfing as a macrophage; Kirsten Fischer Lindahl, chilling as the malespecific T killer cell, Ivan Lefkovits clinically efficient as a T helper cell, and, at a more molecular level, Charles Wood as a Samurai recombinase cleaving a corps of nucleotides that athletically recombined to code for antibodies too numerous to mention...

RIMB, Nutley, Honors the BII's 10th Anniversary

Although the two institutes founded and supported by Roche functioned completely independently, there were always friendly contacts between Basel and Nutley. To commemorate the BII's 10th anniversary, the Roche Institute of Molecular Biology (RIMB) donated a brass plaque to the institute [QR1981_04].

QR1981_04 BII

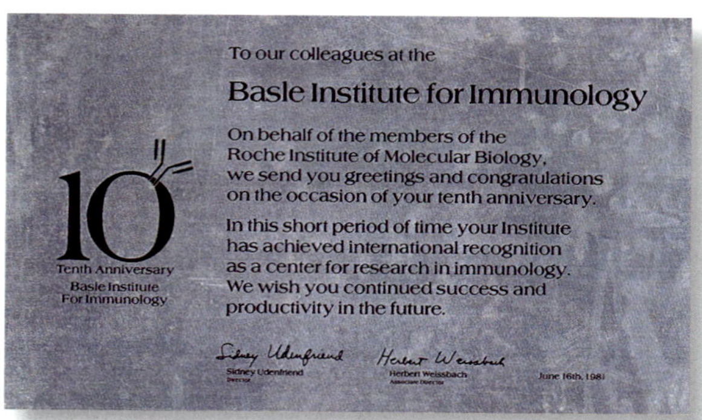

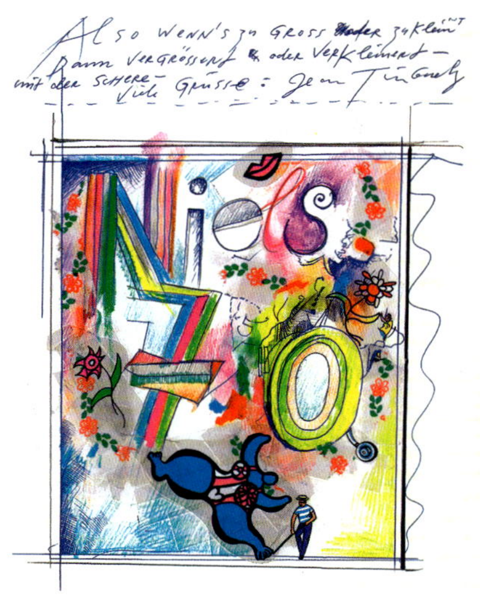

The Immune System: A Festschrift in Honor of Niels Kai Jerne on the Occasion of his 70th Birthday, Volume 1, "Past and Future", Volume 2, "The Present", edited by Charles M. Steinberg and Ivan Lefkovits, S. Karger, Basel, 1981.

A Festschrift in honor of Niels Jerne must be an event in the world of immunology. The reader expects to find in it the fruits of the prodigious scientific achievements of Jerne as reflected in modern immunology, and his expectations are more than fulfilled. The two volumes, published by S. Karger and edited with loving care and ingenuity by Charles M. Steinberg and Ivan Lefkovits, gather contributions from scientists who, at various points in time, happened to collaborate with Jerne, to witness the moments in which his thoughts erupted with clarity in the form of daring theories, or simply to obliquely cross the path of Jerne's scientific career.

The first volume, appropriately entitled "Past and Future", displays the vigor of good science and history blended in a series of magnificent articles. For whoever wants to understand how immunology emerged as a subtile and sophisticated science out of the boredom of blind serology, the perusal of these pages written by immunologists and non-immunologists will be both enlightening and delightful. The contributions of Stent, Maaløe, Mitchison, and Sato are probably the highlights of this volume, excelling in the clarity of ideas and the beauty of style. But there is a unity of the volume. We find it in a central question, present here in most contributions, a question so carefully avoided in conventional papers submitted to established scientific journals: "How does the scientific approach serve our understanding?" This question, which authors ask themselves here freely, with dedication and without fear, sounds like an echo to Jerne's famous "So what?" Titles like "Was an Idiotype Network Working in the Evolutionary Past" (Matsunaga and Ohno), "Specificity – or Why Immunology is Unlikely to Become Boring Soon" (Pohlit), or "The Joint Evolution of Antigens and Antibodies" (Fazekas de St. Groth) evoke only a few among a large set of contributions which together communicate to the reader the conviction that immunology today is healthy, with deep roots in experimental reality, and that it carries the weight of a good part of modern biological thinking. The general scholarly tone is refreshed by some good "boutades": "The Ideal Rabbit" (Kelus), "Le Têtard et l'Anticorps" (Du Pasquier), "Immuno-ornithological Conversations" (Pink and Ziegler).

The over 450 pages of the second volume cover so much science that we cannot review particular issues or cite outstanding articles. In order to connect the past with the future, the editors display here, in the most appropriate presentation, the elusive and evanescent "Present". In doing so they let a large group of leading scientists tell their story. They do it at the historical moment when primitive immunology switched to science. But primitive societies, as noted by Graham Greene, generate legends. The living legend in immunology is Niels Jerne, and confronted with it in these volumes our leading scientists, one by one, spontaneously, as if driven by some mysterious force, show us more about themselves than they probably ever did before.

B. Pernis and A. A. Augustin

Festschrift and Glazed Cake, 1981

Two volumes of a Festschrift were prepared for Niels Jerne's 70th birthday [QR1981_05]. The copy that was festively presented to Niels was leather-bound, and he was very pleased with it. On publication the book became a major *oeuvre* of scientific interest and has remained of historical value ever since, as summarized by Pernis and Augustin (shown above).

A group of scientists made an extra large chocolate cake with a glazed surface on which the Tinguely motif from the book cover was reproduced. Jerne was pleased but looked tired. The next day he took a train to Provence, where Alexandra expected him in time for Christmas Eve.

University of Basel Paid Reverence to Jerne, 1981

Niels Jerne received several honorary degrees from many universities, but the degree given by the University of Basel he accepted with great gratitude. The handwritten manuscript of his acceptance speech is given in [QR1981_06].

QR1981_05 BII

Idiotypes, 1981

In so far as the first conference on idiotypes in Les Baux-de-Provence, 1976, had been Niels Jerne's "private conference", in the meanwhile the field had become an experimentally active area and so the time was ripe to hold a workshop. Claudia Berek, How-

QR1981_06 BII

ard Etlinger and Michael Julius [QR1981_07] organized the meeting, and it was attended by some of the scientists involved in the initial empirical observations on idiotypy, and also by colleagues who had made fundamental theoretical contributions to this area. The subjects discussed included genetic and structural bases for idiotypes as well as the regulation of their expression. Work on DNA and protein sequencing had progressed, and idiotypes could now be defined structurally and serologically. Nevertheless, it was stated that the mechanisms of the network remained mysterious.

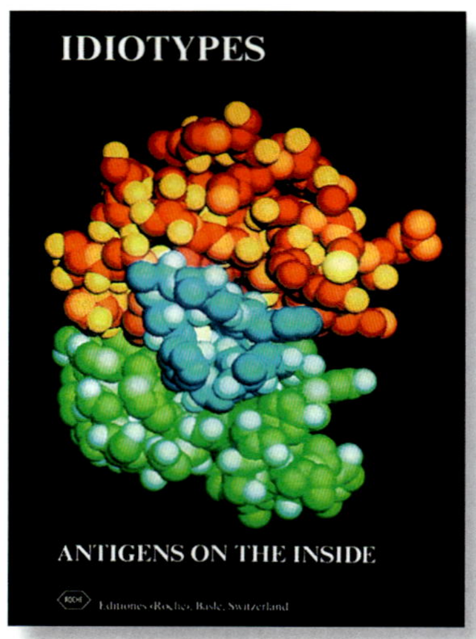

Niels Jerne gave the introduction to the workshop. This was followed by 3 sessions:

Session I: Genetics of idiotypes
Session II: Structure of idiotypes
Session III: Regulation of idiotype expression

Chairpersons of the sessions were Martin Weigert, Jacques Oudin and Klaus Rajewsky.

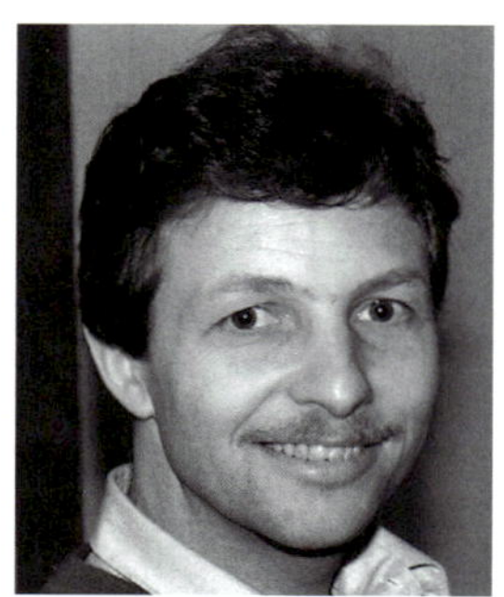

Chris Heusser

The fundamental importance attached to idiotype network regulation in 1981 was illustrated by 3 major talks:

- Eberhard Weiler, University of Konstanz, “Two types of immunological unresponsiveness: antigen-induced versus anti-idiotype induced”
- Pierre-André Cazenave, Pasteur Institute, Paris, “Idiotypic network: the internal images of allotypic determinants”
- Jacques Urbain, Free University of Brussels, “A functional idiotypic network in the immune system?”

Jacques Urbain used an interrogative title for his talk, to indicate uncertainty. This uncertainty was made explicit by Howard Etlinger in his talk showing results that questioned the idiotype network as fundamental to the immune system. In hindsight, this questioning by Urbain and Etlinger might have had validity because, at the present time (written 2015), most work on idiotype network regulation has been abandoned.

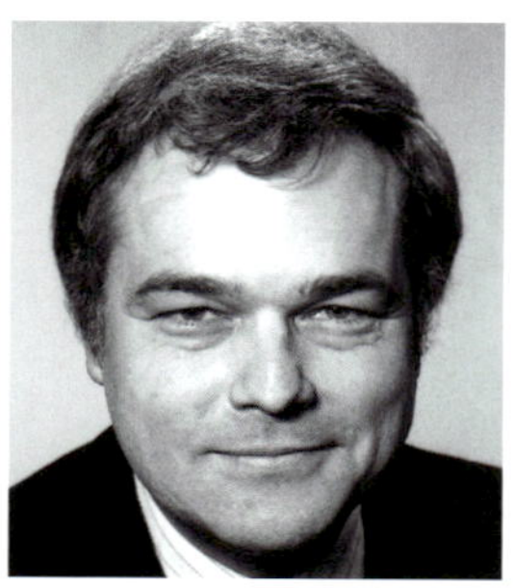

Jesper Zeuthen

Other speakers (besides the organizers) were: Sefik Alkan, B. Clevinger, Claudia Berek, Chris Heusser, Heinz Köhler, Klaus Eichmann, Antonio Coutinho, P.J. Gearhart, M.L. Gefter, L. Staudt and Michael Julius. The proceedings of this workshop were edited by Ingrid Schnurr and published by Editiones Roche.

QR1981_07 BII

Immunological Methods Volume 2 by Academic Press

Academic Press published the second volume of the methods developed and used at the BII, then the third, and finally in 1994 Volume 4. The books continued to be bestselling for Academic Press, and because of the rapid turnover of scientific staff at the BII they were indispensable as a source of continuity in methodology [QR1981_08].

Russian Translations: Методы исследований

There was a special agreement with Roald Nezlin that he translate the *Methods* books into Russian. Within a very short time the Russian edition was released. To start with it was not surprising that the Soviet scientific establishment was interested to obtain translations (they did not have hard currency resources to buy the original English language books), but what was really surprising was the swiftness of translation. This is described in the related QR documents [QR1981_09].

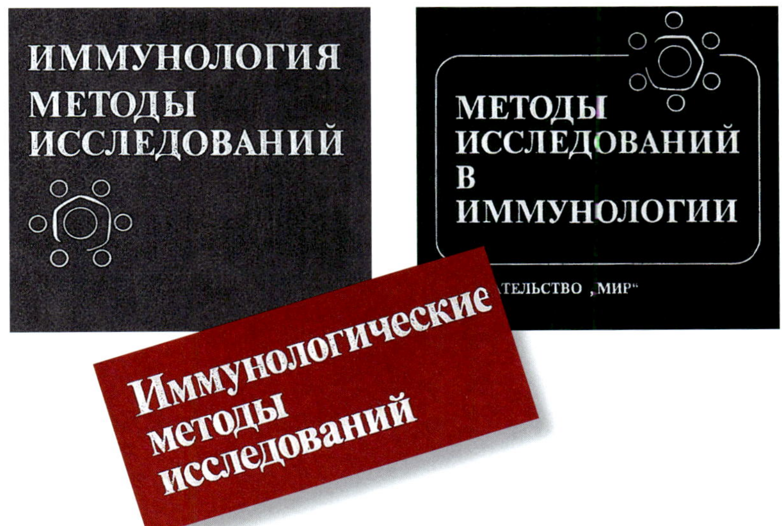

Treasure Trove 1981

The database contains documents related to the BII in a broader context (lists, series of photographs, etc.).

The Year 1982

Ruggero Ceppellini, a founding member of the BII, retired at the age of 65 years. A symposium on the major histocompatibility complex in man was organized in his honor. Theo Staehelin (former permanent member, affiliated with Roche since 1977) arranged a hybridoma course at the BII in order to spread hybridoma technology across the Swiss community. A course on B lymphocyte differentiation was organized by Chris Paige and Richard Pink. Kirsten Fischer Lindahl ran a workshop on class-I-like antigens.

Arrivals 1982 (10)
Manfred Brockhaus, Barbara Fagg, Roland Gisler, Geoffrey Henson, Olli Lassila, Bonnie Mathieson, James McCubrey, John McKearn, Ronald Palacios, Geronimo Terres.

Came and Left in the Same Year (2)
Kyung Jin Kim, Christine Petit.

Leavers 1982 (13)
Jack Bennink, Claudia Berek, Ruggero Ceppellini, Carol Conti, Andrew Farr, Donald Gerson, Ole Henriksen, Martine Levy, Mary Jane Potash, Hitoshi Sakano, Charles Sidman, Hung Sia Teh, R.C. von Borstel.

Ruggero Ceppellini's Retirement, 1982

The first BII permanent member to retire was Ruggero Ceppellini when he reached the retirement age of 65 years [QR1982_01]. The process did not go smoothly as Ruggero wanted to bend the retirement rules. For his extrovert personality, retirement made no sense, especially as he would be the first member of the institute to be "phased out" (apart from Niels Jerne, who was a special case).

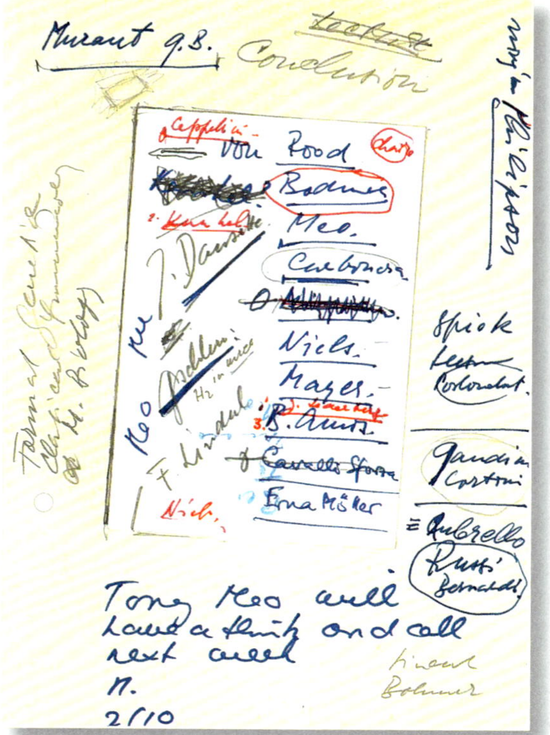
Tony Meo will have a think and call next week
M.
2/10

QR1982_01
BII

Finally Ruggero agreed that a goodbye symposium be organized for him. However, complications arose when the list of invited speakers and guests had to be drawn up. In the end, though, it was an acclaimed event and an excellent symposium.

Ruggero's fascination with the polymorphism and the biological function of the major histocompatibility complex in man (which he always insisted must have a physiological function and not exist just to harass transplantation surgeons) attracted a group of young scientists (many from Italy) to the institute, the majority of whom became prominent experts in their fields. Ruggero was a winner of numerous national and international awards (including the Feltrinelli Prize), and he was nominated several times for the Nobel Prize.

Earlier it was mentioned that he should have played an important role in the monoclonal antibody project initiated at Roche, but he backed out of it due to the consequences of the Seveso misfortune.

The Roche "Monoclonal Antibodies" Project Continues

Years previously, at the initiation of the BII, Roche expressed the hope that *"the presence of a highly qualified group of scientists dedicated to fundamental research and working in academic freedom may provide new knowledge and valuable stimulation to industrial research".*

This vision became true with the establishment of an applied immunology project within the Roche research facility, headed by a former permanent member of the institute, Theophil Staehelin, and supported by a group of scientists. By 1982, it had achieved significant breakthroughs [QR1982_02] and elevated Roche not only to become one of the first pharmaceutical companies in the world with knowledge in the field of hybridomas and monoclonal antibodies, but also to have the know-how to keep the lead.

A Work Permit for the Head of the Cell Sorter Facility

As already explained, there were quotas on the number of foreigners allowed to work in Switzerland. Contract negotiations had to take this fact into consideration. A residence permit was always issued for a year, and the prolongation was arranged through an office in Roche. The authorities were much more lenient with the BII than with other institutions, as the cantonal statistics showed that the BII was a "healthy" place, as people not only "came", but also "left" (after a while).

Therefore it was a surprise that when Billy Leiserson was to be hired as a replacement for Tim Knaak, the Cantonal *Arbeitsamt* declined to provide the work permit [QR1982_03]. Zdenek Trnka, the BII administrator, was puzzled that the few lines of justification (explaining that no suitable person for this job was available on the Swiss work market) were not sufficient – previously they always were – so he contacted the *Arbeitsamt* in order to explain the issue. The person responsible told Trnka that this job was not important enough for a work permit to be granted. Trnka was explicitly told that they do not read the justification in detail, they just look at the salary offered. The clerk said: "If this salary is offered, it cannot be an important job". Finally Billy Leiserson received a work permit.

The Basel Population and the Chauffeur of Bus 34

The acceptance of the institute by the neighborhood and by the general population was always exemplary. There was never a problem with noise, emissions or improper behavior. Quite to the contrary, the institute offered jobs, and the staff were friendly. The positive attitude was evident within the Basel population, although there was a memorable exception which the institute members referred to as the "bus 34 syndrome". The bus stop was such that the driver could see directly into Lab 07: on one occasion a celebration was taking place for a paper having been accepted in the prestigious journal *Nature*. The driver noticed the glasses of wine, and an hour later – on the second or third time round – he became irritated on seeing the half-empty bottles. On scrutinizing the scene the next time round – more empty bottles had accumulated – he felt it was his obligation to call the Personnel Department of Roche and complain.

Roaccutane, Bollag and Pletscher, 1982

QR1982_03 BII

QR1982_04 BII

Werner Bollag, a scientist at Roche, succeeded remaining in splendid isolation for decades, to pursue a research program to study vitamin A-like compounds. The result of his diligent work was the product Roaccutane (isotretinoin) against acne, launched in 1982. Bollag's project was by no means just a basic research project: he completed it from basic formula to final product, not least because of Alfred Pletscher's protective hand. The BII was certainly not involved in it, but with admiration was aware of how a personality such as Pletscher's ensured yet another Roche success [QR1982_04].

The BII Research Environment Forms Geniuses

The generation of antibody diversity (with Susumu Tonegawa), reverse genetics (with Georges Köhler), courses on immunological methods, films on the function of the immune system, and papers in *Nature*, *Science*, *PNAS* and *Cell*: what more could be subsumed under the name of André Traunecker?

André was involved in a wide spectrum of activities – pursued in his position as technician – without having a formal university education. He worked with two Nobel Prize winners, designed his own projects, and finally attained his doctorate years after the BII had been closed down.

His name will appear repeatedly: in descriptions of the Summer Schools, and in the production of the film for the 25th anniversary of the BII. All this speaks for André, and it also speaks for the BII and its research environment that fostered such success [QR1982_05].

ulp UNIVERSITÉ LOUIS PASTEUR STRASBOURG

ATTESTATION DE REUSSITE

DIPLÔME DU DOCTORAT

La Responsable de la Division de la Recherche et des Etudes Doctorales de l'Université Louis Pasteur de Strasbourg, certifie que :

M. André TRAUNECKER

Né(e) le : 13/11/1949 à SIERENTZ (68)

a obtenu le 18/09/2008 devant l'Université Louis Pasteur de Strasbourg, le grade de **DOCTEUR DE L'UNIVERSITE DE STRASBOURG I**, en **Aspects cellulaires et moléculaires de la biologie.**

En foi de quoi, le présent document lui est délivré.

Strasbourg, le 03/10/2008
Pour la Responsable de la Division de la Recherche
Et des Etudes Doctorales
La Responsable du Bureau des Etudes Doctorales

J. HUBE

Nota : Il n'est pas délivré de duplicata de ce certificat. Il appartient au titulaire d'établir lui-même et de faire certifier conformes par la Mairie de son domicile les copies qui peuvent lui être nécessaires.

Le Conseil Scientifique de l'Université Louis Pasteur de Strasbourg réuni le 21 novembre 2000 a décidé que les mentions " honorable - très honorable - très honorable avec les félicitations " ne seront plus attribuées par l'ULP pour les thèses soutenues à partir du 1er Janvier 2001.

The Horizontal Structure and "Laissez-Faire"

The horizontal structure – as exercised at the BII – meant not only the absence of hierarchy among scientists, but also what decades later was referred to as a "lean structure" or "lean management" in reducing the chain of commands (from top to the bottom) to a minimum. The horizontal structure of the BII was true to the idea of having minimal decision-making steps, but its main aspect was that the scientists would not be told "from above" what to do.

The succession of the directorship from Jerne to Melchers did not change the "mechanism" of the horizontal structure.

Scientists would pursue projects that they wished to pursue, and no authority told them what to do. Budget, lab space and team formation were the only constraints that had to be taken into consideration. There was always a strong propensity towards "laissez-faire", such as avoiding checks and controls when not truly necessary. Thus, participation at conferences, taking holidays, inviting colleagues for seminars – to name but a few – were at the discretion of the scientist.

There were, however, some limitations. The director intervened when it became known that a member had accepted an additional position. This was done without reprimanding the scientist, but simply by asking him to give up the position. Instead of having written rules, or imposing sanctions and censure, problems were solved ad hoc. This approach worked well, except in rare instances when a member had plainly misused the trust.

QR1982_05 BII

The following anecdotal event (about misusing the "let it be") was ingrained in the collective memory of the institute: a scientist entered the administrator's office, mentioning he was on his way to see the director to request approval of a collaborative visit for a joint project. He came out of the director's office, smiling, and told the administrator: "It is approved, here is the visitor's CV, please arrange a 1-month contract". The administrator did so, not realizing that for one reason or another the director had actually turned down the request. The visitor arrived in due course, and soon an unpleasant confrontation occurred when the "non-approved" visitor and the director met. A corrective measure was taken, and the aftertaste remained as corridor gossip. The basis for decision-making was not shaken by this event.

The Role of Gender

"No thanks, I want to talk to your boss."

A good scientist at the BII was a good scientist irrespective of gender. There were occasional male-female tensions; for instance, if a woman scientist refused to be helped into or out of her coat, or if she did not want the door to be held open for her. A young scientist from Poland, educated in the classical, conservative way, attempted to kiss the hand of a female scientist. He was heavily reprimanded for that. A scientist from Austria was giving a seminar and pointed out that the missing points on the graph shown on the slide were due to missing analyses because his technician was on pregnancy leave. This statement caused uproar, and several female scientists ostentatiously got up and left the seminar room.

The gender problem often came from without. Marie Kosco, an intelligent, ambitious, successful young scientist had a well-trained, handsome male technician, Bruno Fol. Once a salesman entered the lab, and when walking past Marie she asked him, "may I help you"? The salesman snorted, "no thanks, I want to talk to your boss", and went straight to Marie's technician, Bruno.

Irreproducible Results and Improper Scientific Conduct

The horizontal structure of the BII and the fact that there was no hierarchy of positions created a work atmosphere that was favorable to promote nothing less than diligent and solid work. Nevertheless, reports from other institutions about fabricated results, e.g. the famous case of painting a mouse's fur to mimic skin-grafting, prompted scientists at the BII to ask whether there could be cases of improper scientific conduct within the institute.

There never was a scientific scandal at the BII, which of course does not mean that an unnoticed fraud occurred. Obviously, over the years, many results were obtained that were irreproducible, which for a while created tensions or even distrust among colleagues. In most instances, these occurrences were self-correcting, as scientists abandoned projects that yielded irreproducible results – there was no pressure from a "boss" to continue something unsound.

Some reports – whether presented at the Monday lunch seminars or in the Annual Reports – turned out to be unsubstantiated, e.g. the claim that the T cell receptor was immunoglobulin or that the T cell factor was antigen-specific. And there were some instances when a double-blind control was not truly double-blind, and accusations of cheating were raised. There was no intentional cover-up of these rare instances, and no "whistle-blowing" was necessary.

It became apparent that cellular immunology was a "soft science" compared to molecular biology. Several reasons were given for this. Experimental animals were often not of the kind (genetic background, specific-pathogen-free status) expected. Tissue culture depended on the use of fetal calf serum, which in turn varied from batch to batch. In several instances, unnoticed infection spread in the animal colony, or the composition of the tissue culture medium (commercial or in-house) was faulty.

A highly sensitive method for detection of antibody has been imported from the Pasteur Institute to the BII. At Pasteur it was used for detecting antibody in rabbit serum, in Basel it was supposed to be used for bullfrog larvae. In this system the antibody responses measured by inactivation of the bacteriophage ΦX 174 failed to show specificity. Charley Steinberg looked at the titration curves and said: "I bet that something is wrong with the phage stock." Electron-microscopic examination (made by E. Kellenberger's group) showed that the "precious" phage stock from Paris was a mixture of various phages, aerial contaminants and "other stuff". Misconduct was prevented in Basel, but scientists from Pasteur had a few papers published with the same starting material (they could have checked their "phage stock" but did not).

Everything else that could be referred to as improper scientific conduct goes into the category of "selecting representative results" and ignoring experiments that did not fit the picture. Jerne's position was that science, as a reiterative, self-correcting process, would always come to the right conclusion.

B Hybridoma Course by Theo Staehelin's Group at Roche, 1982

Theo Staehelin took it upon himself not only to establish monoclonal antibody technology at Roche, but also to facilitate the spread of the hybridoma technology across the Swiss scientific community [QR1982_06]. The course was sponsored by the Schweizerische Kommission für Molekularbiologie (SKMB) and was held at the institute from September 6th to 17th, 1982. It was organized by Theophil Staehelin, John Stocker and Brigitte Durrer from the Roche Applied Immunology Group, greatly supported by Georges Köhler.

The techniques taught were: preparation of hybridoma cells, cloning of cells, testing of antibody specificity with special emphasis on a panel of anti-interferon antibodies, class and subclass determination of monoclonal antibodies, detection of antigen after protein blotting on nitrocellulose.

Seminars:

G. Köhler — "Production of monoclonal antibodies"
T. Staehelin, Roche — "Monoclonal antibodies against interferon"
J. Stocker, Roche — "Human monoclonal antibodies"
L. Du Pasquier — "Monoclonal antibodies in the frog system"
J.-P. Mach, Ludwig Institute, Epalinges — "*In vivo* tumor localization of radio-labeled monoclonal antibodies"
G. Schatz, Biozentrum, Basel — "Use of monoclonal antibodies for studying membrane biogenesis"

Students:

D. Fracheboud (Fribourg), B. Zanolari (Basel), M. Garavito (Basel), M. Southgate (Geneva), G. Danisi (Geneva), J. Kistler (Geneva), A. Meister (Riehen), M. Schwyzer (Geneva), C. England (Bern), H. Sigrist (Bern), A. Metzler (Zurich), F. Jay (Zurich).

QR1982_06 BII

Course and Workshop on B Lymphocyte Differentiation, 1982

QR1982_07 BII

An advanced study course (October 4th to 13th, 1982) and a workshop (October 15th to 17th, 1982) on B lymphocyte differentiation, sponsored by EMBO, were held at the institute. Christopher Paige and Richard Pink organized the course [QR1982_07]. The laboratory work carried out during the course included assays for B cells and their precursors, cell fractionation and biochemical analysis of immunoglobulin proteins. The program also included introductory lectures on hemopoiesis (N. Iscove), anatomy and embryology of the lymphoid system (R. Gisler, N. Le Douarin) and B cell development (F. Melchers).

The teaching staff comprised 27 scientists from the BII and elsewhere:

M. Coltey, M. Cooper, C. Corbel, A. Coutinho, F. Dieterlen, L. Forni, R. Gisler, T. Graf, M. Hirama, N. Iscove, J. Kaufman, P. Kincade, T. Kishimoto, N. Le Douarin, R. Maki, J. McKearn, F. Melchers, D. Osmond, C. Paige, R. Perry, R. Phillips, R. Pink, M. Ratcliffe, A. Toivanen, P. Toivanen, O. Vainio, M. Wabl.

The follow-up workshop consisted of 5 sessions, each attempting to answer a particular question on B cell differentiation:

M. Cooper	"Where do B cells come from?"
R. Perry	"How are Ig genes made and expressed?"
K. Rajewsky	"How are B cells selected?"
C. Paige	"What are B cell subpopulations?"
W. Haas	"How are B cells activated?"

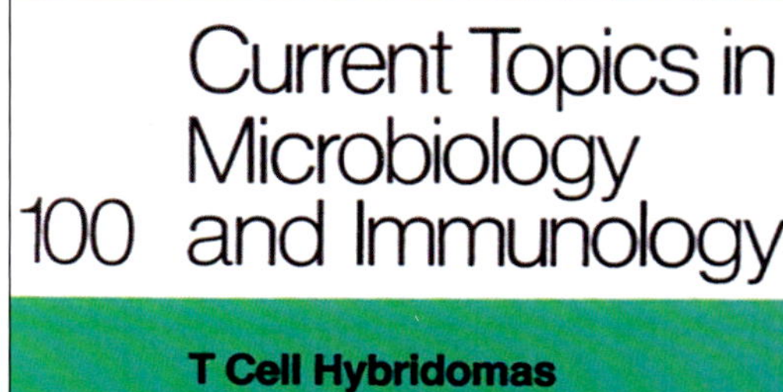

Monograph on T Cell Hybridomas, 1982

The proceedings of the workshop on T cell hybridomas were published in the 100th anniversary volume of *Current Topics in Microbiology and Immunology* [QR1982_08].

Kirsten Fischer Lindahl's Workshop on Class-I-Like Antigens

A workshop on murine class-I-like antigens (non-classical MHC class I) was organized by Kirsten Fischer Lindahl on October 25th,

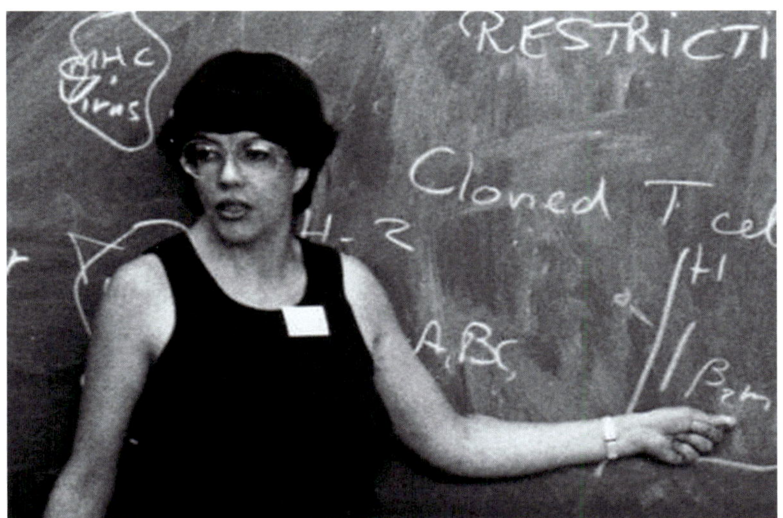

Kirsten Fischer Lindahl

QR1982_08 BII

1982 [QR1982_09]. The class-I-like antigens range in their degree of polymorphism from a single form (Qa-2) to 6 or more (Qed and TL). The interest in this subject came from the discovery that the majority of H-2-like genes are not encoded in the K and D regions of the H-2 complex. The main emphasis of the workshop was to try to attribute "a function" to these molecules. Only years later was the function unraveled when targets for unrestricted killing by T cells were defined.

The small format of the workshop led to stimulating discussions with the participation of K. Moriwaki from the National Institute of Genetics, Mishima, Japan, W.L. Maloy from the NIH, Bethesda, J. Michaelson from NYU Medical Center, L. Flaherty from the Kidney Disease Institute, Albany, N.Y., E. Günther from the Max Planck Institute for Immunobiology, Freiburg, and K. Wonigeit from the Medizinische Hochschule, Hannover.

Don Bellgrau's Work on Cytotoxic T Cell Precursors

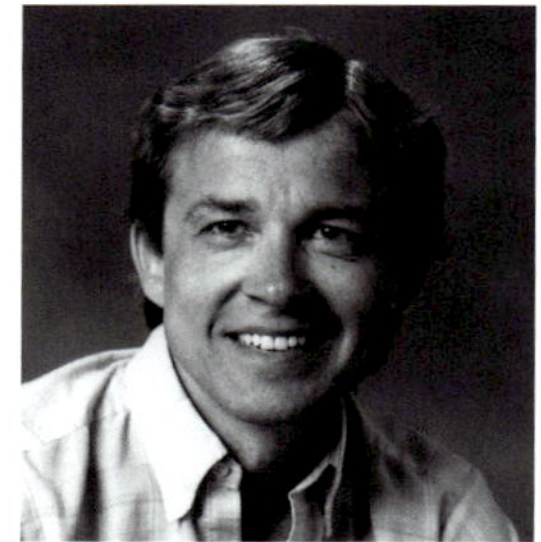
Donald Bellgrau

QR1982_09 BII

Don came to Basel from Darcy Wilson's laboratory at the University of Pennsylvania. Don (as well as several other research groups) was deeply interested in T cell receptor biology, using as a research tool an F1 anti-parental model first championed by Ramseier and Lindenmann. Don and Darcy struggled to make antibodies but were rewarded by discovering T cell anti-idiotypic responses.

In several studies Don demonstrated that activation of anti-tumor killer cells requires T helper lymphocytes, which in turn are activated by tumor antigens presented in an immunogenic form by Ia-positive accessory cells syngeneic to the CTL. He proposed that activation of CTL precursors in vivo depends on intimate contact between them and antigen-presenting accessory cells.

It was his "Basel experience" that made Don look for work opportunities in similar circumstances, i.e. somewhere with mountains, excellent research possibilities in immunology and enough financial reward. This is why he aimed for a position in Denver which opened up for him in 1983.

Treasure Trove 1982
The database contains documents related to the BII in a broader context (lists, series of photographs, etc.).

QR1982_treasure BII

Proteomic Laboratory

In collaboration with Leigh Anderson (Argonne National Laboratory, Chicago), Ivan Lefkovits established a laboratory for large-scale, two-dimensional gel electrophoresis. Anderson's system for simultaneous analysis of twenty samples was duplicated in the BII workshop.

The Year 1983

Antonio Lanzavecchia established a human immunology laboratory focusing on T and B cell biology. Klaus Karjalainen initiated a molecular biology group, related mainly to (soluble) TCR receptors. Prior to expiration of their limited contracts, both scientists became permanent members. Fritz Melchers organized a workshop on the Mechanisms of B Cell Neoplasia. Harald von Boehmer, Bonnie Mathieson and Werner Haas held a course on T lymphocyte differentiation. Christine Brack, who decisively contributed to the success of Tonegawa, moved to University Hospital Basel.

Antonio Lanzavecchia Starts a "Human Immunology" Laboratory, 1983

Antonio Lanzavecchia joined the institute in 1983 with a clear plan to introduce "human immunology" into the BII. Before him Ruggero Ceppellini, another Italian scientist, had already been exploring the "human immune system", but doing so within the highly competitive field of HLA analysis. Instead, Lanzavecchia focused on mainstream T and B cell immunology, just choosing a "species" new to the institute [QR1983_01].

When the institute was established, most of the research projects were geared towards the use of experimental animals. Jerne wanted a balance of species – mouse, chicken, frog, sheep and rabbit – but not including humans. Ceppellini, on the other hand, was interested in working with human beings, using volunteers, blood donors, etc., as in hospital laboratories. Later, when powerful experimental in vitro models had been developed, the scene became ripe for introducing the human model, but without the direct involvement of patients.

Thus, Lanzavecchia came to Basel at the right time: in vitro models were accessible, T and B immunology know-how was available, and his work was successful from the outset. Before his first contract expired, he was offered a permanent position, since Ceppellini, a founding member of the BII, had just retired. Antonio's research has covered several aspects of human immunology: antigen processing and presentation, dendritic cell biology, lymphocyte activation and circulation, and analysis of the cellular basis of T and B cell memory.

Arrivals 1983 (20)
Gerard Farmer, Antonio Iglesias, Klaus Karjalainen, Gordon Keller, Michael Kiefer, Antonio Lanzavecchia, Tomas Leanderson, Kenneth Marcu, Polly Matzinger, Janet McCarty, David Nemazee, Gerd Pluschke, Peter Robinson, Anthonius Rolink, Nancy Ruddle, Nobuo Sakaguchi, Ralph Snodgrass, Michael Steinmetz, Wilfried Weber, Siegfried Weiss.

Came and Left in the Same Year (2)
Georg Holländer, Kiyoshi Takatsu. ▶

QR1983_01 BII

▶ **Leavers 1983 (19)**
Donald Bellgrau, Christine Brack, Catherine Corbel, Franco Di Padova, Howard Etlinger, Maria Leptin, Richard Maki, Bonnie Mathieson, Bernard Mély-Goubert, Tauro Neri, Michael Ratcliffe, John Reynolds, William Roeder, Carolyn Roitsch, Max Schreier, Geronimo Terres, Andreas Tsapis, Olli Vainio, Duzhang Zhu.

Using clones of antigen-specific B and T cells, he demonstrated that B cells efficiently capture, via membrane immunoglobulins, the specific antigen which is then internalized and processed into peptides, which are presented to T helper cells in an extraordinarily efficient manner. This study uncovered a critical step in the process of T-B cell cooperation that is essential for high-affinity antibody production. Further he showed that antigens can be effectively targeted to surface molecules other than membrane immunoglobulins, a finding that has contributed to current strategies of antigen targeting to improve vaccination.

Antonio obtained his degree in medicine in 1976 at the University of Pavia where he specialized in pediatrics and infectious diseases. From 1983 to 1999 he was a member of the BII and in 1999 became the founding director of the Institute for Research in Biomedicine (IRB) in Bellinzona. Just a glimpse in the IRB Annual Report shows that he successfully set up his new institute along the lines of the BII, even adopting the format and style of the BII Annual Report. He holds teaching positions at several universities (University of Genoa, University of Siena and at the ETH Zurich; his title there, "Professor of Human Immunology", is a novum).

In mid 2014 Antonio was appointed President of the Fondazione Regionale per la Ricerca Biomedica of the Lombardy Region in Italy.

Polly Matzinger, the Clever Bunny, Arrives, 1983

Polly Matzinger completed her studies at the University of California, San Diego, and obtained her PhD in 1979. She did her postdoctoral work at the University of Cambridge (UK), and in 1983 joined the BII [QR1983_02]. Polly became an invaluable member due to her talent, intelligence, wit and social skills. Later in this book, her achievements and positions after leaving the BII are detailed. Many of her accomplishments are given in the above-mentioned QR code, but some of her more "unusual features" are given below (in part taken from the "oral history" of the BII and partly from various newspaper clips).

QR1983_02 BII

There can be few scientists in the world who count being a Playboy bunny among their favorite jobs and who can claim that they turned to science after getting picked up in a bar. Dubbed "the person least likely to succeed in life" by her schoolmates, Polly did indeed succeed. Her work has been published in the most respected science journals, such as *Nature* and *Science*, but she caused also irritations by her unconventional and extrovert char-

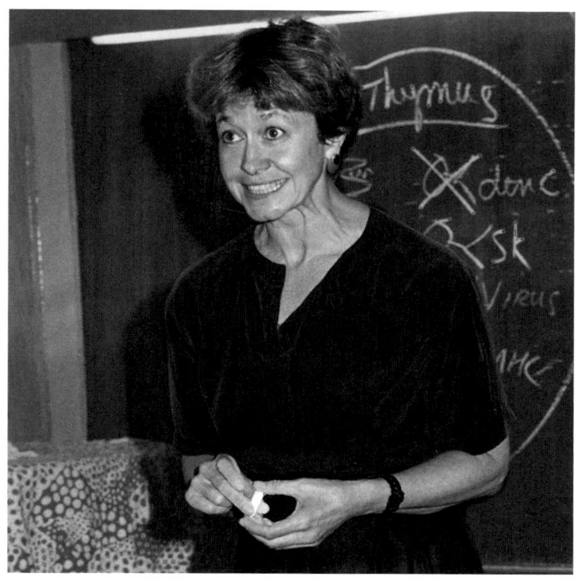

Polly Matzinger

acter. Her first published paper gave her dog as co-author, a fact that considerably annoyed the journal publishing it.

Before that she worked as a jazz musician, trained problem dogs, ironed shirts, cleaned bricks and worked as a cocktail waitress: "Then I worked as a pool bunny – a Playboy bunny playing billiards. It paid 40 cents an hour and I got to listen to a lot of great conversations. It was a great job. And then I got picked up in a bar", she says. "But not in the normal way that one gets picked up. I was serving two professors who would come in and talk science and I would listen. One day they were talking about mimicry – how one butterfly will mimic another butterfly and how a good tasting butterfly will mimic a bad tasting butterfly. So I asked them a question that I'd wondered about for years – why has no animal ever mimicked a skunk? A raccoon with a white stripe down its back would have a selective advantage. Their mouths fell open – a cocktail waitress asking this sort of question, and they didn't know how to answer it."

Thus, Polly turned to science and completed her studies. When she applied for a position at the BII, she presented the work she was doing in Cambridge. In order to avoid a politically incorrect description, nothing further can be said, other than that she made a staggering appearance in hot pants in her debut seminar. She proved her talent by explaining things in an extraordinarily clear and logical manner. She was accepted, and her arrival in Basel was a true enrichment of the institute.

She worked hard, always had time to talk to people, organize workshops, teach at courses (even taking it upon herself to help the secretaries understand very basic science) and open-endedly argue on any scientific issue, provided the subject was not boring. Her work and her "danger model of the immune system" will be discussed in Book 2.

Klaus Karjalainen Starts a Molecular Biology Group, 1983

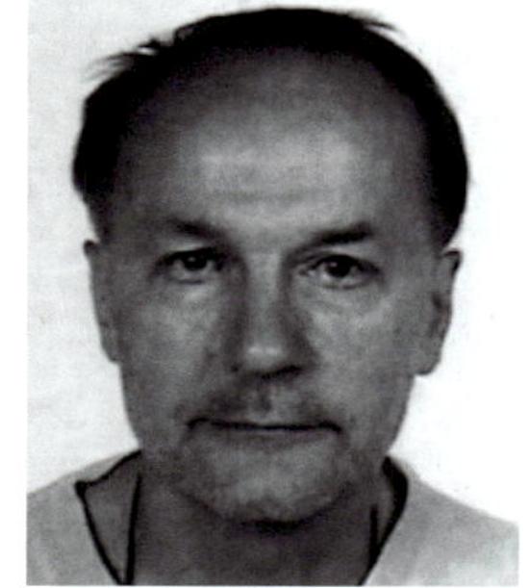

Klaus Karjalainen

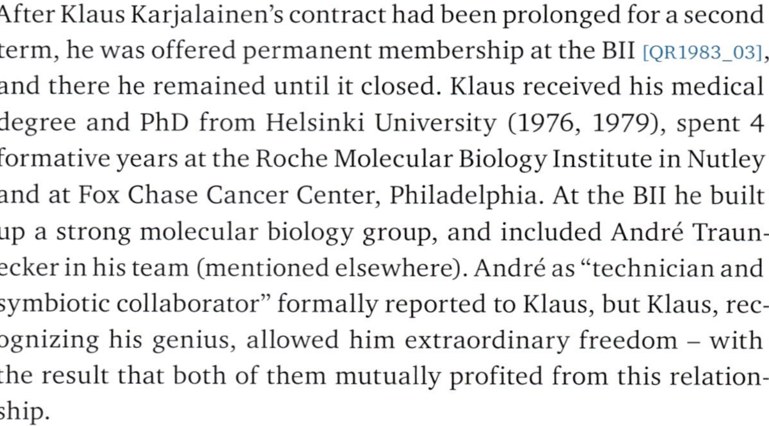

After Klaus Karjalainen's contract had been prolonged for a second term, he was offered permanent membership at the BII [QR1983_03], and there he remained until it closed. Klaus received his medical degree and PhD from Helsinki University (1976, 1979), spent 4 formative years at the Roche Molecular Biology Institute in Nutley and at Fox Chase Cancer Center, Philadelphia. At the BII he built up a strong molecular biology group, and included André Traunecker in his team (mentioned elsewhere). André as "technician and symbiotic collaborator" formally reported to Klaus, but Klaus, recognizing his genius, allowed him extraordinary freedom – with the result that both of them mutually profited from this relationship.

Karjalainen is remembered at the BII for his work on the soluble T cell receptor, and on specific low-affinity recognition of the major histocompatibility complex plus peptide by soluble T cell receptor. Klaus has contributed to the understanding of the so-called superantigens, which activate T cells by simultaneously binding the Vβ domain of the TCR and MHC class II molecules on antigen-presenting cells.

It was mainly André Traunecker's work which showed that soluble TCR is expressed, assembled and secreted as an αβ-heterodimer by a myeloma cell line transfected with the recombinant genes. It is biologically active: it specifically inhibits antigen-dependent activation of the relevant T cell clones and thus discriminates between proper and irrelevant peptides presented by major histocompatibility complex molecules.

In 2000 Karjalainen joined Antonio Lanzavecchia at the IRB, Bellinzona, and then moved to the Nanyang Technological University at the School of Biological Sciences in Singapore. Klaus describes himself as an immunologist with special interest in inflammation, hematopoiesis and stem cell research. On his Web page he states that he abhors the procedures leading to patenting, as well as patents, of which, paradoxically, he owns 4.

QR1983_03 BII

DNA Cloning and Transfection Become a Major Experimental Approach

Cloning techniques became more widely used and over 10 projects described in the 1983 Annual Report addressed projects related to gene transfer, as detailed in [QR1983_04]:

- A new mouse fibroblast line for DNA-mediated gene transfer
- Transfection of T cells with a gene for a class I MHC antigen
- Gene transfer of class II MHC molecules
- Introduction of the K and L genes from the hybridoma Sp6 into cells of various lineages
- Transfer of heavy and light chain genes into B cell lines
- Gene transfer of *in vitro* modified Ig genes into cultured B cells
- Transient expression and stable transformation of non-fibroblastic cells
- Cloning *Xenopus* genomic DNA fragments related to genes encoding the V-region of mammalian Igs
- Cloning of cDNA for multi-HGF from WEHI-3 cells
- Cloning of cDNA of inducible lymphokines from EL4
- Cloning of T cell-specific cDNA sequences

Workshop on the "Mechanisms of B Cell Neoplasia", 1983

B lymphocytes were extensively studied by Fritz Melchers at the BII and by a score of scientists at other institutions. Fritz Melchers, Michael Potter and Martin Weigert prepared a workshop to discuss 3 aspects of B lymphocytes: their normal development, the pathogenesis of B cell neoplasms and mechanisms of immunoglobulin gene rearrangement.

The workshop was divided into 5 sessions:

I: Development of mature B cells from stem cells
II: Development of Ig-secreting plasma cells from mature B cells
III: Tumors of B lymphocytes, and retroviruses
IV: Chromosome translocations associated with B cell tumors
V: Molecular biology of B lymphocyte tumors

Eighteen speakers from different institutions [QR1983_05] contributed to the workshop. Editiones Roche published the proceedings of the conference in 1983.

The meeting started with a review of the control of normal B lymphocyte proliferation and differentiation, as a basis for a discussion of the pathogenesis of available tumor model systems, and of the significance of the chromosomal translocations. It was

QR1983_04 BII

QR1983_05 BII

known that immunoglobulin gene complexes for κ light chains and heavy chains are located on chromosomes 6 and 12, respectively. Reports were given at the workshop on the findings of non-random translocations in mouse plasmacytomas, occurring at the mentioned chromosomes 6 and 12.

A similar finding had been described in Burkitt's lymphoma in man, where the non-random translocations occurred in most of the tumors. These non-random translocations suggested that the particular genes involved in chromosome breakage and rejoining might be of interest to growth regulation.

Course and Workshop on T Lymphocyte Differentiation, 1983

Stem cell invasion in the embryonic and early postnatal thymus of birds and mammals, and thymic regeneration after transplantation of hemopoietic progenitors were studied in many laboratories. Thus, a need arose to standardize and unify the experimental approaches. To follow up the EMBO course on B cell differentiation held at the BII a year earlier, a course on T cell differentiation was organized by Harald von Boehmer, Bonnie Mathieson and Werner Haas. The format of the course was similar to the previous one, in that the first part comprised laboratory work, and the last 2 days were of workshop character with an enlarged audience [QR1983_06].

The laboratory work included identification and removal of young avian and murine thymic rudiments, isolation of thymic endoderm, histology of the thymus, grafting of thymus lobes in adult mice, identification and separation of thymocyte subpopulations, detection of thymus migrants in peripheral organs, and thymus organ cultures, as well as limiting dilution cultures of T lymphocytes.

The teaching staff was: H. von Boehmer, W. Boersma, W. von Ewijk, W. Haas, E. Jenkinson, F. Jotereau, P. Kisielow, B. Mathieson, M. Nabholz, R. Scollay, K. Shortman and K. Smith. The workshop at the end of the course consisted of 4 sessions, chaired by K. Shortman, J. Sprent, W. Haas and H. von Boehmer.

QR1983_06 BII

Human Proteome Project, 1983

The first Human Proteome (HUPO) conference at Cold Spring Harbor was organized by Jim Watson in order to prepare a document for the US authorities which related to the initiative to explain how proteins function. The initiative was intended to be the "successor" project of the HUGO initiative. Watson was aware of the fact that Ivan Lefkovits was building up a major proteomic laboratory (at that time the expression "proteomics" was not used, it was called 2-DE), but it was in Watson's interest to include a strong European laboratory in the project [QR1983_07]. It has already been mentioned that Lefkovits' facilities at the BII duplicated those in Leigh Anderson's laboratory; nevertheless, it turned out that Watson preferred to have the BII involved rather than the Argonne National Laboratory. Fritz Melchers did not support this idea, fearing that the balance of the horizontal structure would be at stake, as participation in the HUPO project would require a large operation. Therefore, collaboration on the HUPO project was tuned down to the extent that Lefkovits could participate at HUPO conferences, but not share any of the responsibilities.

Christine Brack Moves to University Hospital Basel, 1983

In 1977 Christine Brack came to the BII from the Biozentrum, Basel, and after 6 years of successful work on a number of projects, especially those in collaboration with Susumu Tonegawa, she moved to the University Hospital Basel, where a Laboratory for Molecular Gerontology of the Psychiatry Clinics had been newly established.

Before joining the institute and while she worked there, Christine collaborated with a number of high-profile scientists, such as Eduard Kellenberger, Tom Bickle, Walter Gehring and Charles Weissmann. This was on a number of diverse projects (interferon α, trypanosome), but nevertheless her most important contribution was related to the work for which Tonegawa was awarded the Nobel Prize in 1987.

In QR code [QR1983_08], reference is made to the 8 seminal papers that she co-authored with Tonegawa. Most of them are based on her own specialty: electron microscopy of DNA. In her electron micrographs she was able to distinguish between DNA double strands and DNA single strands, loops of introns, and portions of exons, all which was needed for understanding the mechanisms of the Ig gene rearrangements.

QR1983_07 BII

Christine Brack's contribution to Susumu Tonegawa's discoveries was truly appreciated by her colleagues at the BII. A research report from an earlier period (Annual Report 1979) reveals the profound impact Christine Brack's work had on Tonegawa's project for which he was awarded the Nobel Prize.

QR1983_08 BII

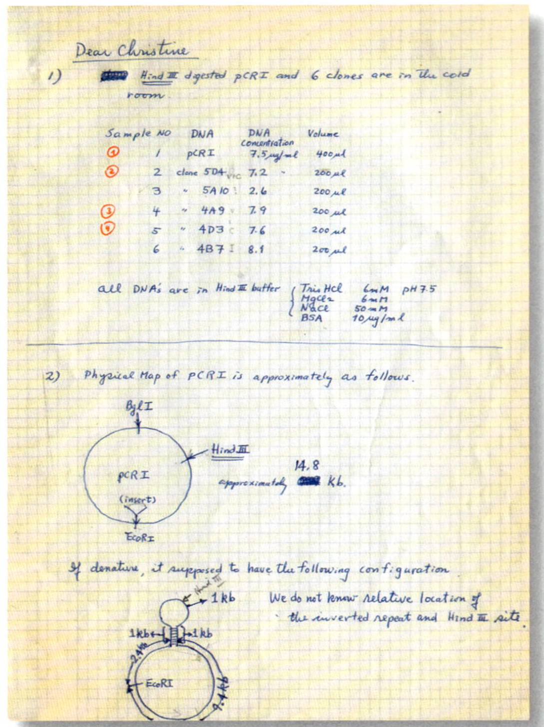

Dear Christine

1) Hind III digested pCRI and 6 clones are in the cold room.

Sample NO	DNA	DNA concentration	Volume
1	pCRI	7.5 μg/ml	400 μl
2	clone 5D4	7.2	200 μl
3	" 5A10	2.6	200 μl
4	" 4A9	7.9	200 μl
5	" 4D3	7.6	200 μl
6	" 4B7	8.1	200 μl

all DNA's are in Hind III buffer { Tris HCl 6 mM pH 7.5, MgCl2 6 mM, NaCl 50 mM, BSA 10 μg/ml

2) Physical Map of pCRI is approximately as follows.

If denature, it supposed to have the following configuration

We do not know relative location of the inverted repeat and Hind III site.

Hand drawing of DNA strands to distinguish single strands from double strands, and indicating the position of loops

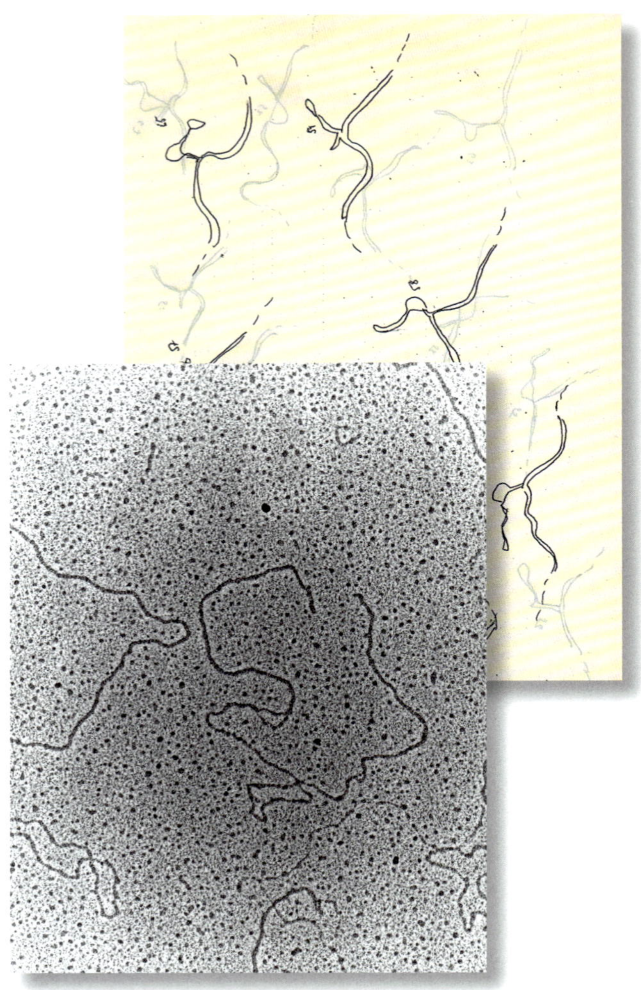

Electron-Microscopic Analysis of Transcription

Member: C. Brack

Technician: U. Baumgartner

A new electron microscope technique has been developed for rapid characterization of transcription in vitro. DNA is transcribed with E. coli *RNA polymerase in vitro, and the RNA is hybridized to its template. Measurement of the resulting transcription R-loop molecules allows accurate mapping of transcription initiation sites (promoter sites) and analysis of the direction and rate of transcription from each initiation site. A number of known prokaryotic promoters on phage X DNA have been mapped to within 100–300 nucleotides. Transcription initiation sites were also mapped on several bacterial plasmids that were used as vectors for DNA cloning (pBR322, pSF2124). At present we are trying to adapt this method to eukaryotic systems, hoping to identify transcription initiation sites on cloned DNA fragments carrying specific eukaryotic genes (e.g. mouse immunoglobulin genes).*

Charley Steinberg made a seminal contribution towards guiding Tonegawa's initial research in Basel. This is mentioned later in this volume. Protocols of Christine Brack's work are stored in the Roche archives. Three pages of her protocols are shown above.

From Basel to Kyoto, 1983

The 5th International Congress of Immunology (after the ones held in Washington, Brighton, Melbourne and Paris) was held in Kyoto. Several participants from the BII attended and presented their work there [QR1983_09].

Committee on Ethics and Conditions of Experimentation with Animals

The public carefully watched the use of experimental animals and the conditions under which mice, rabbits, chickens and sheep were maintained. The BII was less the focus of attention than the "big" pharmaceutical industries; nevertheless, the BII adopted a thorough policy to adhere meticulously to the rules, in order to avoid conflict or criticism. A special cantonal office regulated the use of experimental animals, and permission for each "prototype experiment" had to be obtained (the authorization was valid for a year, for multiple experiments within the year). Throughout the years there were some problems with the authorities who sometimes requested more detailed applications and justifications, but in most instances approval was granted. It was definitely not the case that "academic freedom" would be *carte blanche* for any kind of animal experimentation. For some types of experiment, such as for the induction of peritoneal exudate, or for thoracic duct canulation, it was difficult to obtain permission; some other experiments were simply banned.

In December 1983, a Committee on Ethics and Conditions of Experimentation with Animals was established at the BII [QR1983_10]. It convened for the first time on December 20th, 1983. The members of the committee were: L. Du Pasquier, K. Fischer Lindahl, R. Gisler, M. Miyasaka and R. Pink from the BII, and P. Thomann from the University of Zurich.

QR1983_09 BII

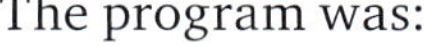

The program was:

- Topic 1: Visit to the animal facilities
- Topic 2: Methods employed in animal experimentation
- Topic 3: Internal guidelines for experimentation with animals

QR1983_10 BII

Excerpts from the minutes describe the situation in 1983: "With respect to the animal facilities a barrier system is used, which has been adapted to the needs of the scientist. To make it more stringent, some mice are also kept in isolators, but this limits the number of animals that can be kept. According to Dr. Thomann it is acceptable to keep sheep in house for 3–4 weeks, and in metabolism cages for 4–5 days." There was a detailed discussion on the anesthesia methods to be used in different animal species.

Short guidelines were issued and given to the scientists and technicians in the institute. They contain a translation of the relevant paragraphs from the *Swiss Bill for the Protection of Animals* (1978 version) and from the Ethical Principles for Scientific Experimentation on Animals.

Seveso Oak Forest Park

In the chapter for 1976, the Seveso disaster was described and the consequences for the BII were mentioned. The waste from the clean-up of the plant was packed into barrels that were supposed to be disposed of in a legal manner. Mannesmann Italiana was contracted to dispose of the content of the barrels. Investigative journalists found that en route to the destination, the barrels "disappeared". It turned out that Mannesmann Italiana had hired two subcontractors to get rid of the toxic waste. Finally, over 9 years after the disaster, the 41 barrels were found in an unused abattoir in Anguilcourt-le-Sart, a village in northern France. Roche took over the procedure and on November 25th, 1983, issued a statement declaring that the toxic waste had been incinerated in Switzerland – in Basel – closely watched by Greenpeace activists. They climbed up the chimney of the incinerator and found that the exhaust emitted was cleaner than the air entering the incinerator.

QR1983_11 BII

Treatment of the soil in the affected area of Seveso was so comprehensive that the dioxin level is now below that which is normally found. The whole site has been turned into a public park, *The Seveso Oak Forest Park*, and it is said that Seveso is now the least polluted place in Italy [QR1983_11]. Although the Seveso issue and the clean-up seemed not part of the BII history, in fact the influence was there, since BII members were confronted with the issue on the homefront ("How can you work for a company that is polluting our country?"). The thorough clean-up was an adequate answer.

Treasure Trove 1983
The database contains documents related to the BII in a broader context (lists, series of photographs, etc.).

QR1983_treasure BII

The Year 1984

Zdenek Trnka, administrative director of the BII, retired at the age of 65 years. A symposium organized by Fritz Melchers, Roland Gisler and Bede Morris, "Sheep as an Experimental Model in Immunology", was held in his honor. Fritz Melchers and Roland Gisler organized a course on the microanatomy of the immune system. Manfred Brockhaus and Richard Pink completed their term at the BII and were hired by the Research Department of Roche. Peter Robinson left for the German Cancer Research Centre, Heidelberg; Stephen Fazekas returned to Australia. Niels Jerne and Georges Köhler were awarded the Nobel Prize for Medicine (shared with César Milstein from Cambridge).

New Approaches: In situ Hybridization, cDNA Libraries, FACS

Research projects that had been started in previous years continued, but due to the availability of new methods, the emphases on some projects shifted. As the institute had modernized its cell sorting facilities, the fluorescence-activated cell sorting (FACS) approach became the standard technique for analyzing cell subpopulations; several research groups reported results on subpopulations of cells involved in the immune response, using FACS approaches. It became possible to visualize by in situ hybridization the expression of mRNA for IgM or IgG in a single resting B lymphocyte. As studies on Ig gene structures, both in terms of studying rearrangements of portions of genes and of controlling elements, became feasible, projects were initiated in species other than the mouse, especially in chickens and frogs. Studies of soluble mediators of various immune functions, especially IL-1, IL-2 and IL-3, became the focus of interest of several research groups.

Studies of cell differentiation using both in vitro and in vivo approaches were among the largest types of research projects. cDNA libraries of genes expressed at different stages in the differentiation of T and B lymphocytes were constructed and extensively used [QR1984_01].

Research at the institute on the TCR was as much the center of interest as it was in many immunological institutes worldwide. In particular, the most successful team was in Canada, where Tak

Arrivals 1984 (10)
Jan Andersson, John Cambier, Zlatko Dembic, Taichi Ezaki, Martin Flajnik, Dario Grossberger, Hajime Karasuyama, Jukka Pelkonen, Akiko Takeda, Gillian Wu.

Leavers 1984 (9)
Manfred Brockhaus, Stephen Fazekas de St. Groth, Ellen Hsu, Kenneth Marcu, J. Richard Pink, Peter Robinson, Nancy Ruddle, Zdenek Trnka, Wilfried Weber.

QR1984_01 BII

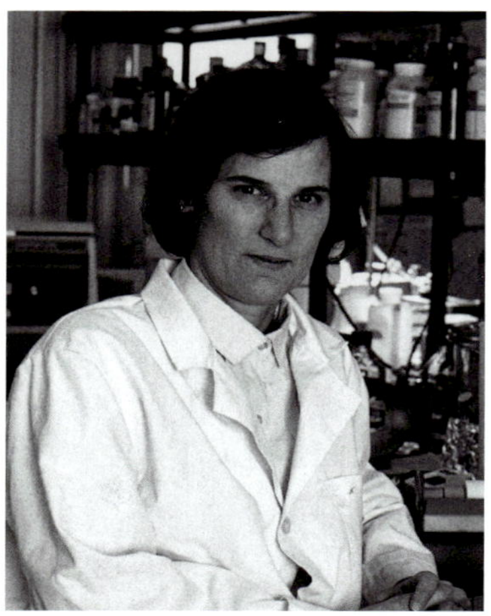

Nancy Ruddle

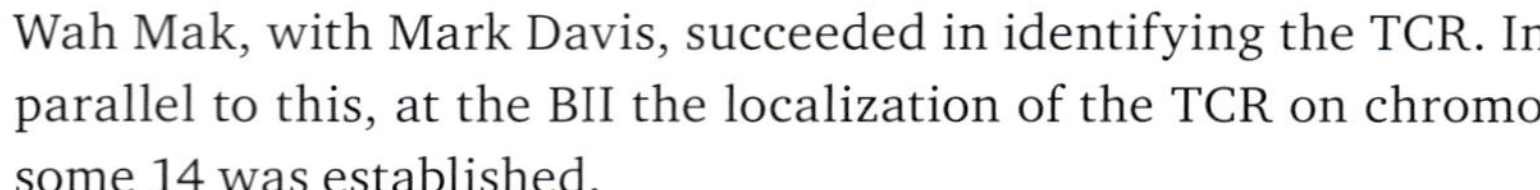

Wah Mak, with Mark Davis, succeeded in identifying the TCR. In parallel to this, at the BII the localization of the TCR on chromosome 14 was established.

Manfred Brockhaus and Richard Pink to Roche Basel

Manfred Brockhaus, TNF, Alzheimer

Manfred Brockhaus, after several years at the BII, joined the research facilities of Hoffmann-La Roche in Basel. At the institute the main emphasis of his research had been on glycoproteins and their role in the modulation of clonal proliferation of IL-3-dependent clones. He performed collaborative experiments with Klaus Karjalainen, Zlatko Dembic and Harald von Boehmer on the functional properties of bone marrow T lymphocyte progenitor clones. At Roche, Manfred became involved in the project on the tumor necrosis factor which resulted in more than 30 papers; at the end of his Roche career he worked on the Alzheimer project.

Brockhaus' work prior to joining the institute was with Hilary Koprowski at the Wistar Institute in Philadelphia, with whom he co-authored 6 papers, mainly on gastrointestinal cancer-associated antigens [QR1984_02].

Richard Pink, Chicken Immunology

In 1984 J. Richard Pink completed his second assignment at the BII. He worked there from 1971 to 1977 and again from 1981 to 1984. These years were dedicated to chicken immunology [QR1984_03]. He had powerful allies at other places in Europe, where chicken immunology was prominently pursued: Georg Wick and Karel Hala in Innsbruck, Paavo Toivanen in Turku, Morten Simonsen in Copenhagen, Tomas Hraba and Juraj Ivanyi in Prague and London. Georg Wick had produced the worldwide first specific anti-B anti-T cell antibodies by immunization of turkeys with chicken bursa and thymus cells, respectively, followed by exhaustive cross-absorption. He brought these reagents to the BII in order to confirm their specificity using the new FACS technology. He then acquired the first FACS machine in Austria for his lab in Innsbruck.

QR1984_02 BII

QR1984_03 BII

In his first period at the BII, Richard Pink (with Vincenzo Miggiano and PhD student Andreas Ziegler) characterized genes and antigens of the chicken MHC, in collaboration with the Prague group, who provided inbred chicken strains for this purpose. Richard left the institute in 1977 for Pierre Vassalli's lab in Geneva, where he studied mouse lymphocyte membrane proteins using the newly described two-dimensional gel electrophoresis technique. However, he had not lost interest in the chicken model and returned to the BII in 1981, partly to maintain the valuable colony of inbred birds. During the next 3 years, he developed methods of studying clones of developing B lymphocytes in single bursal follicles. Initial work carried out with Olli Vainio, Olli Lassila and Mike Ratcliffe led to fruitful collaborations with the groups of Jean-Claude Weill and Paavo Toivanen, and to recognition of the different ways that B lymphocytes can develop in different species. The results were reported in some 20 papers. The chicken colony at the BII later served for further studies of the chicken MHC and B cell biology. It was maintained by the above-mentioned scientists and by other colleagues (including J. Kaufman and J. Salomonsen) until the institute closed.

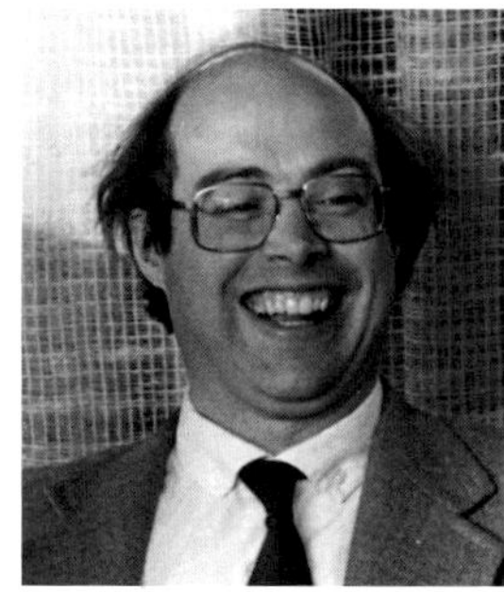
Richard Pink

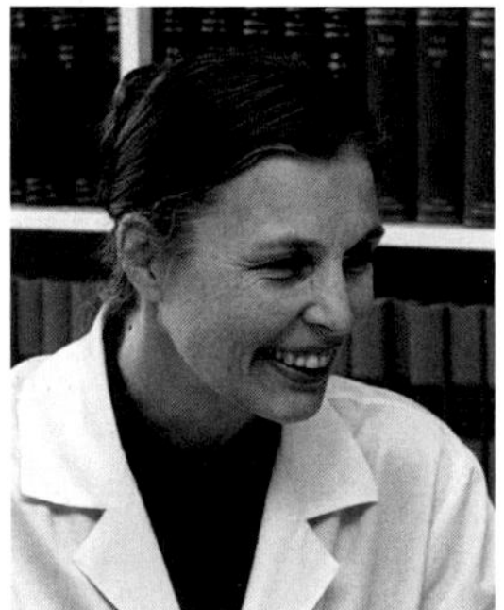
Auli Toivanen

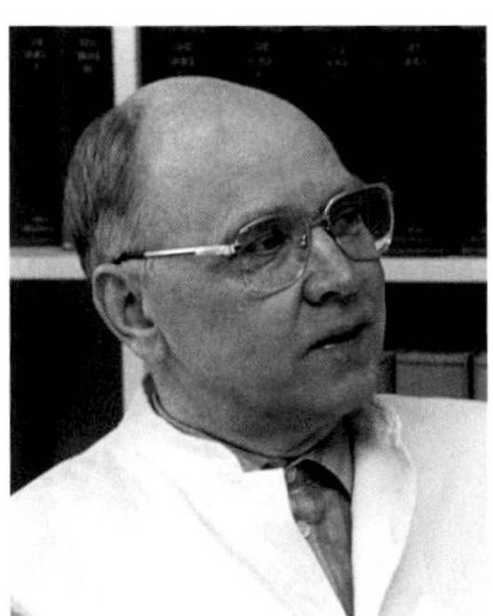
Paavo Toivanen

Roche Malaria Vaccine

In 1984 Richard moved to Gianni Garotta's lab at the Roche Central Research Unit, Basel. He and Francesco Sinigaglia started work on human T cell responses to malaria antigens and soon joined the Roche Malaria Vaccine project. The role of ex-BII members in this project was important, starting with the support of John Stocker and Theo Staehelin in the early 1980s. Working on the project were two other ex-BII members, Howard Etlinger and Bela Takacs, also in the Central Research Biology Unit, then headed by Michael Steinmetz. Don Gerson, then VP Manufacturing at Connaught Labs in Canada, supplied the tetanus toxin to be used as a carrier protein for the malaria antigens of this vaccine. With various colleagues, Richard published over 20 papers on malaria and headed the malaria preclinical work from 1986. The project was stopped in 1994 because no malaria antigen, from Roche or elsewhere, had fulfilled criteria for development as an effective vaccine. Richard's later work at Roche was on gene therapy in the nervous system. In 1998 he left Roche and worked with the WHO Tropical Disease Research Programme in Geneva to help organize meetings on new adjuvant development and establish a high-throughput screening program for the discovery of new antiparasitic drugs.

Richard's junior years in immunology were with César Milstein (co-authoring 5 papers) and with Hugh Fudenberg (co-authoring 4 papers). In Fudenberg's laboratory in the early seventies, he co-authored and published a monograph entitled, *Basic Immu-*

nogenetics. He modestly stated to his friends that he knew so little that he had to learn more by writing things down. For many years the book was a bestseller.

Peter Robinson, Complexity of Qa-2 Antigens

Peter Robinson left the BII to join the German Cancer Research Centre in Heidelberg. In Basel he collaborated with several research groups, predominantly with Kirsten Fischer Lindahl and Ivan Lefkovits. One of his preferred projects was the study of the restricted recognition of β_2-microglobulin by cytotoxic T lymphocytes.

Furthermore, he unraveled the molecular complexity of Qa-2 antigens employing protein spot identification by two-dimensional gel electrophoresis. He was an excellent experimenter, ready to give competent advice to all [QR1984_04].

Advances in Monoclonal Antibodies

The skill in preparing monoclonal antibodies kept increasing, and the resulting reagents became invaluable tools for experiments that were previously not feasible to perform. During 1984, monoclonal antibodies with specificities for MHC-encoded H-2 antigens, for minor antigens in connection with the MHC, for murine T lymphocytes, for the polar fraction of cellular lipids, for sheep blood cell surface antigens as differentiation markers and for various autoantigens were established at the BII. In earlier years, monoclonal antibodies could only be made in mouse-mouse combination; some time later the production of human-human hybridomas, which secrete antibody in quantities comparable to murine or rat hybridomas, became available [QR1984_05].

QR1984_04 BII

QR1984_05 BII

Zlatko Dembic Dropped Cells on the Floor

Zlatko Dembic, then working with Michael Steinmetz at the BII, wanted to transfer MHC restricted specificity to a T cell line by transferring α- and β-TCR genes. Zlatko needed a very large number of cells for these experiments. Jacqueline Mathur and Werner Haas cultured T cell clones in many liters of conditioned media. Upon handing over to Zlatko the precious enriched cell population, Zlatko dropped them on the floor. Werner and Harald got very angry and called Michael Steinmetz. Michael joined the excited participants, listened to aggressive complaints for an endless

10 minutes, and then said with a very calm voice: "I think, the best is, you grow the cells again." That was Michael – a master of containment.

Storage of Embryos in Liquid Nitrogen

As mentioned in the chapter for 1983, cantonal authorities strictly controlled the use of experimental animals. Maintaining 6–10 strains of mice was conveniently handled by the animal breeding facilities of the institute. With the advent of transgenic animals (and with the need for animals expressing variants of genes) it was necessary to accommodate a much larger number of different strains. Thus, the process was introduced to store embryos in liquid nitrogen so that mouse strains could be made "on demand" (by thawing the embryos and implanting them into female mice). This procedure was introduced at the BII with the side benefit that it allowed the valuable strains to be protected from disease or fire [QR1984_06].

Seminars at the Meetings of the Board of Advisors and the Board of Swiss Consultants, 1984

It became customary that the board meetings would be accompanied by a scientific session. It was enlightening for board members to listen, for instance, to Werner Haas and Georges Köhler. Werner explained the latest findings on the T cell receptor, identified in 1984 by Tak Wah Mak and Mark Davies in Canada. Georges gave an insight into the usefulness of transgenic mice for studying the properties of monoclonal antibodies.

W. Haas	"T cell receptor for antigen"
R. Palacios	"IL3-dependent murine cell clones representing three states of B cell development"
J.R.L. Pink	"Big bang versus steady models of B cell creation"
J. McCubrey	"Transfection of lymphoid cells of different lineages with TNP-specific Ig genes"
A. Iglesias	"*In vitro* modifications of Ig genes"
G. Köhler	"Transgenic mice carrying genes for heavy and light chains of monoclonal antibodies"

Stephen Fazekas Returns to Australia, 1984

Stephen Fazekas' entrée into science was decades before most of the scientists mentioned in this book wrote their first paper. Stephen published a paper in *Nature* (1948;162:294) with the title "Viropexis, the Mechanism of Influenza Virus Infection". He

remained true to this subject of study, although adjusting always to the most modern and innovative approaches, including automated production of monoclonal antibodies in a cytostat (*J Immunol Methods* 1983;57:121–136). Incidentally, he was one of the few who had a chance to see the original apparatus of Aaron Novick and Leo Szilard described in *Science* (1950;112:715). At that time, a cytostat was called chemostat.

It is not entirely clear whether or not Jerne considered Fazekas for a permanent position (no written documents exist), but Fazekas made a point that because no double-taxation treaty existed between Australia and Switzerland, he could not live in Switzerland permanently [QR1984_07]. Indeed, he came to the BII twice (and in an interim period he was a visitor). Among his scientific achievements was the proposal "that the first encounter with antigen is decisive for all the future reactivity of the organism", which he dubbed "original antigenic sin".

Stephen descended from Hungarian nobility and he insisted that the epitheton ornans, "de St. Groth", was always used. His full name, Stephen Nicholas Emery Egon Fazekas de St. Groth, is given on Web pages. He was born in 1919, and in 1984 at the age of 65 he left the BII. His departure was extremely modest, just a cup of espresso and a glass of champagne. On his final day at the institute, Stephen still set up his last experiment that was to be analyzed (if it ever was) in his absence 4 days after his retirement. It could well be that his last experiment refers to Martin Luther's words: "Even if it were the last day on earth, plant a tree".

Nobody remembers any longer that it was Stephen who invented the visualization of proteins by Coomassie brilliant blue staining (Fazekas de St. Groth et al., *Biochim Biophys Acta* 1963; 71:377–391).

Microanatomy of the Immune System, 1984

QR1984_07 BII

QR1984_08 BII

Once again an EMBO practical course took place and was held in November 1984. It was entitled "The Physiology and Microanatomy of the Immune System". The aim of the course was to bring together scientists from the BII and other places (Holland, UK, Japan, Australia) to learn state-of-the-art methodology related to the architecture of those organs where lymphocytes function, home and exert their activity [QR1984_08].

A broad range of animal species (mouse, rabbit, guinea pig, chicken and sheep) were considered. Lectures, round-table discussions and experimental work were on the main part of the program, with speakers Dennis Osmond, John Reynolds, Bede Morris, Masayuki Miyasaka, John Humphrey, Robbert Benner, Jon Sprent and Harald von Boehmer. The experimental work was demonstrated by Richard Pink, Olli Lassila, Roland Gisler, Louis Du Pasquier, Ellen Hsu and Martin Flajnik. The use of transgenic animals in evaluating lymphocyte development was explained by Gordon Keller and Georges Köhler.

The methodology for the isolation of cells from bone marrow, thymus, spleen, lymph nodes and fetal liver was dealt with on the introductory days.

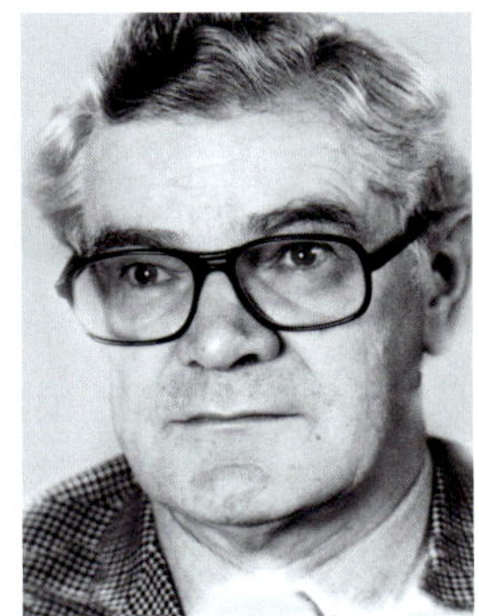

Zdenek Trnka

Retirement of Zdenek Trnka, 1984

Zdenek Trnka, a permanent member of the institute, celebrated his 65th birthday on December 22nd, 1984, and he retired at the end of the year. This was an occasion for a group of his friends and collaborators – from within the institute as well as from abroad – to organize a symposium in his honor from November 25th to 27th, 1984. In this symposium entitled "The Sheep as an Experimental Model in Immunology", the potential use of adult, neonatal and fetal sheep for studying immunological phenomena was discussed. The presentations at the meeting focused on those aspects of immunity, which, like fetal immune responsiveness, can only be studied from a physiological standpoint in large animals. There was an attempt to assess these developments with regard to the direction research in immunology might take in the future, and the role that large animal immunology may play in these developments. The symposium was organized by Fritz Melchers, Roland Gisler and Bede Morris. The speakers in the three sessions were B. Morris, M. Brandon, R.N.P. Cahill, P. McCullagh, J. Reynolds, R. Pabst, J. McConnell, M. Miyasaka, T. Ezaki, W. Kimpton, J.B. Hay and T.C. Moore [QR1984_09].

IMMUNOLOGY OF THE SHEEP
Edited by B. Morris and M. Miyasaka
Editiones ‹Roche›, Basle, Switzerland

QR1984_09 BII

Roland Gisler, Head of Administration

On Zdenek Trnka's retirement a new head of administration was appointed, to start on January 1st, 1985. Roland Gisler (whom Fritz Melchers recruited from Ciba-Geigy) was chosen to take this position. Roland was one of the few scientists who successfully changed back to academia from applied pharma research. Roland became a valued member of the BII; besides research he loved teaching, and as head of administration he could utilize his excellent connections to Swiss scientific and social circles [QR1984_10].

QR1984_10 BII

The Nobel Prize 1984

The Phone Call from Stockholm

When Niels Jerne retired, his status changed from "member" to "honorary member". On the days and weeks he occasionally spent in Basel, he used a small office on the top floor of the BII, which, when he was absent, was maintained first by Ingrid Schnurr and later by Ivan Lefkovits. Jerne used it for his editorial work (*PNAS*, *European Journal of Immunology*), and it continued to be the place where friends and colleagues joined him to discuss science and everything else. He happened to be in Basel when he received the telephone call from Stockholm.

Phone calls and cables of congratulation continued for hours. It was the same for Georges Köhler. A spontaneous celebration started minutes after the calls. There was never a shortage of champagne in the institute cold rooms, but within hours all the Veuve Clicquot and Dom Pérignon bottles were empty.

The institute returned to its normal scientific activities but preparations for the Stockholm celebration started. For the Stockholm ceremony the number of invitees is always limited, but Georges Köhler managed to make a special arrangement that allowed all the members of his laboratory – scientists and technicians alike – to participate. Georges generously funded everything for them all. For Georges this was the "point" when present and future merged.

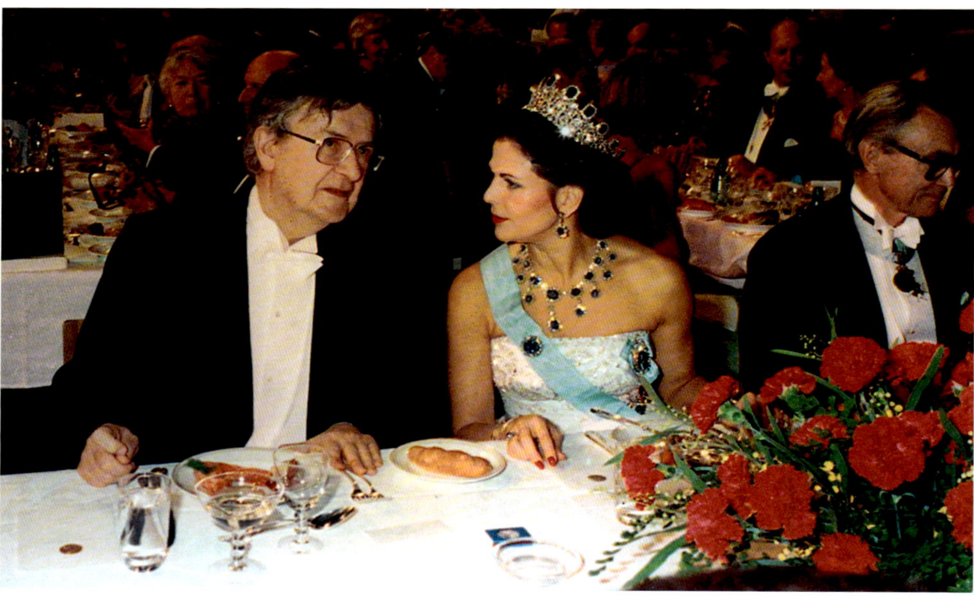

Her Majesty Queen Sylvia with Niels K. Jerne

Niels Jerne did it differently: he invited friends who had played a decisive role in his scientific life; prominently among them were Gunther and Inga Stent, and Ole Maaloe. From his research coworkers he invited Claudia Henry and Ivan Lefkovits with his wife Hana; Ingrid Westen-Schnurr, his secretary throughout his Basel years, and her husband Hannes, were invited as well.

Apart from the ceremony and the Nobel Prize speeches, the highlight of the events was the dinner in the Blue Hall of Stockholm City Hall with His and Her Majesties King Carl Gustaf and Queen Silvia, and with 1,320 invited guests. The dinner was served by 660 lay waiters (thousands of waiters-to-be applied and 660 were chosen). The clue for that number is that all 1,320 guests were served simultaneously: each waiter carried a platter with plates for two people, they entered the hall in a long queue and placed the plates in front of the guests at the sound of a gong. This of course ensured that neither the King nor the Queen had to wait, or that eating would commence while the waiters moved from table to table.

At the table with the King and Queen were Niels and Alexandra Jerne, Georges and Claudia Köhler, César and Celia Milstein, and also Carlo Rubbia, Simon van der Meer and Bruce Merrifield with their wives. Jaroslav Seifert could not attend, and Jana Seifertova took his seat.

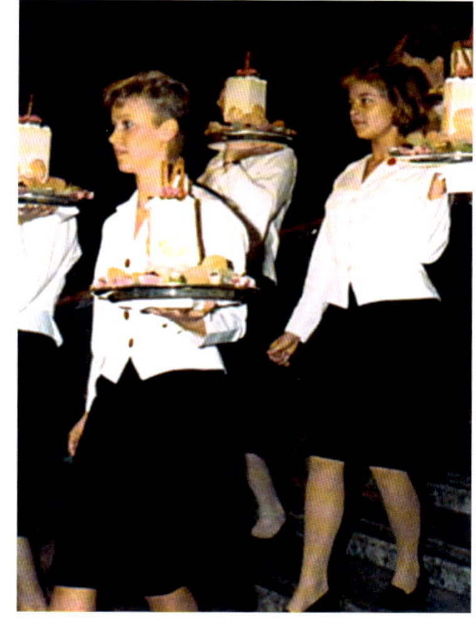

MENU

Saumon mariné aux genièvres
Pâté aux morilles, sauce moutarde

▪

Canard sauvage rôti, sauce aux cassis
Gâteau aux pommes de terre et carottes

▪

Parfait Glace Nobel
Petits fours

VINS
Moët et Chandon, Brut Impérial
Château Vieille Tour, 1979
Eau minérale Ramlösa

Café

BUFFET
The Famous Grouse
Queen Anne
Gordon´s Dry Gin
Carpano Punt e Mes
Boissons de Spendrup

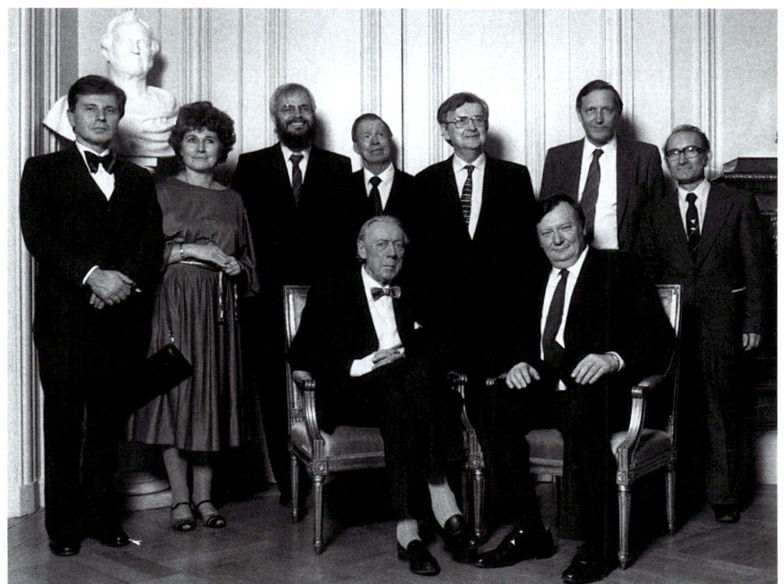

From left: Mr. and Mrs. Seifert, Georges Köhler, Bruce Merrifield, Niels Jerne, Simon van der Meer, César Milstein. In front: Robert Stone and Carlo Rubbia

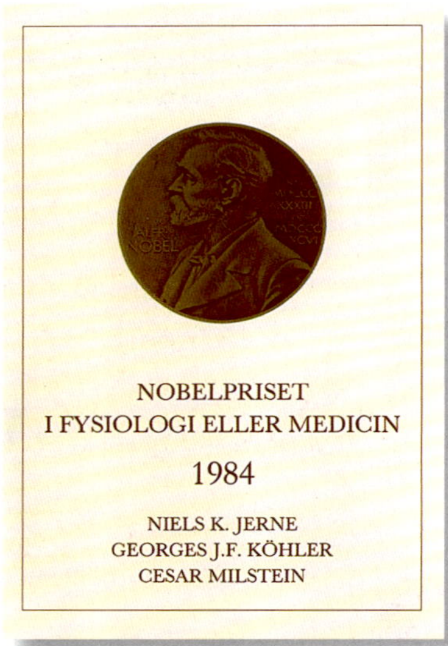

By his theories Jerne has outlined the development of modern immunology.

Press Release from the Nobel Assembly at the Karolinska Institute: Nobel Prize for Niels K. Jerne, Georges Köhler and César Milstein

The Nobel Assembly of Karolinska Institutet has today decided to award the Nobel Prize in Physiology or Medicine for 1984 jointly to Niels K. Jerne [QR1984_11], Georges J.F. Köhler [QR1984_12] and César Milstein [QR1984_13] for theories concerning "the specificity in development and control of the immune system" and the discovery of "the principle for production of monoclonal antibodies".

Summary

Niels K. Jerne is the great theoretician in immunology. In three main theories he has in a visionary way elucidated essential questions concerning specificity, development and regulation of the immune response. The natural selection theory regarding antibody formation breaks with old views on the immune response and is a starting point of modern cellular immunology. His second theory explains how the cells of the immune system, which mature in the thymus gland, develop under the influence of the transplantation antigens of the host. The third, and most important theory, predicts how the immune response is regulated by a complicated network consisting of antibodies and anti-antibodies. The principles of the network theory are beginning to be exploited in prevention, diagnosis and treatment of disease. The hybridoma technique for the production of monoclonal antibodies represents one of the most important methodological advances in biomedicine during the 1970s. An antibody producing cell and all its daughter cells produce an identical antibody molecule (monoclonal antibody). Since long scientists nourished the hope that it would become possible to produce monoclonal antibodies with predetermined specificities. This dream became a reality in 1975 when Georges J.F. Köhler and César Milstein described the hybridoma technique for production of monoclonal antibodies. They immortalized antibody producing cells by fusing them with tumour cells. The method allows unlimited production of monoclonal antibodies with predetermined specificity. Monoclonal antibodies have opened up completely new fields for theoretical and applied biomedical research and allow precise diagnosis and also treatment of disease.

QR1984_11 BII

QR1984_12 BII

QR1984_13 BII

An Explanation of the Diversity of the Immune System

The most important task for the immune system is to defend the body against bacteria, virus and other microorganisms. The spe-

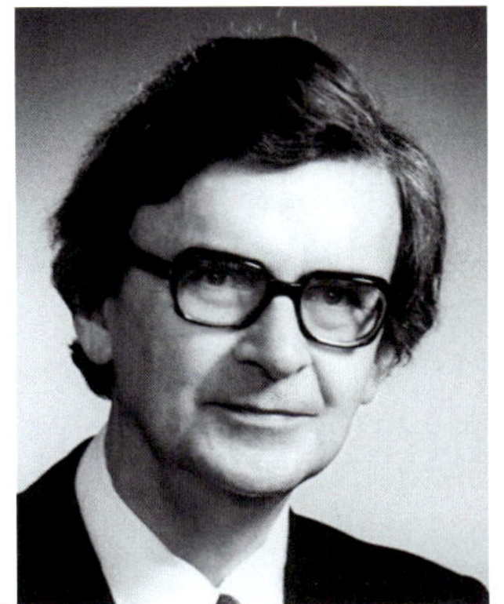

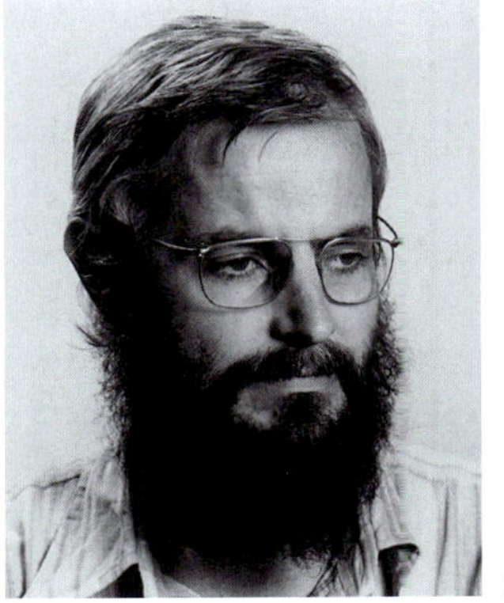

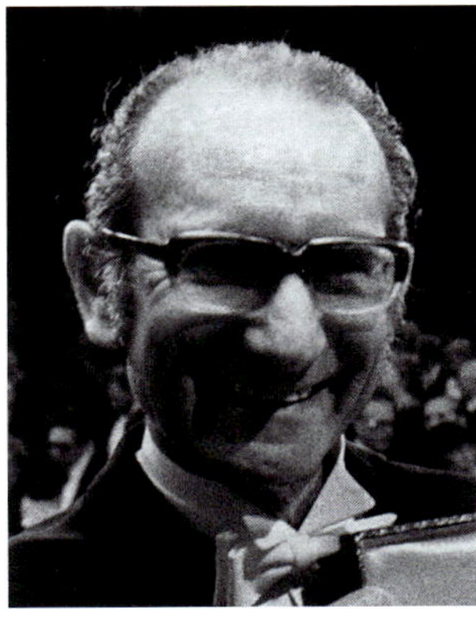

1 Niels Jerne
Prize share: 1/3

2 Georges J.F. Köhler
Prize share: 1/3

3 César Milstein
Prize share: 1/3

cific defense is exerted by a subgroup of white blood cells (lymphocytes). The immune system needs to recognize and react specifically with a large number of foreign substances (antigens). How the lymphocytes develop these vital properties and how they build up the highly specialized recognition system of the immune apparatus has long been an area of intensive research. Niels K. Jerne is the leading theoretician in immunology during the last 30 years. In three main theories he has elucidated central issues concerning specificity, development and regulation of the immune system in a comprehensive and convincing way. By his theories Jerne has outlined the development of modern immunology.

Theory 1: Specificity Is Predetermined

In his *Natural Selection Theory of Antibody Formation* from 1955 Jerne explains the development of a specific antibody response in the following way. Each individual has a large number of natural antibodies with specificities for all antigens towards which the individual can respond. These antibodies develop already during fetal life in the absence of external antigens. The foreign antigen then selects the antibody molecule, which has the best fit. The antigen-antibody binding stimulates the production of this particular antibody specificity. Jerne's natural selection theory contrasted to the dogmatic views of the antibody response as formulated in the instruction theories which were prevailing at that time. According to these theories the antigen serves a template for the production of antibodies. In Jerne's natural selection theory it is implied that the generation of the enormous number of antibody specificities is independent of exogenous antigens. This view on the nature of the immune system constitutes the basis for modern immunology.

For the Nobel ceremony the number of invitees is always limited, but Georges Köhler managed to make a special arrangement that allowed all the members of his laboratory – scientists and technicians alike – to participate. Georges generously funded everything for them all.

Theory 2: Reactivity against Self-Antigens Creates Diversity

The natural selection theory is mainly concerned with the maturation of the immune system after it has acquired the ability to react with antigen. In the second theory on the *Somatic Generation of Immune Recognition* set forth in 1971 Jerne explains how the immune system develops from stem cells to mature lymphocytes which can react with antigen. He presupposes that every individual possesses all genes needed for the production of antibodies, and antibody-like molecules, which can bind all strong transplantation antigens of the species. Jerne suggests that lymphocytes mature in the thymus gland and in other lymphoid organs where they are exposed to the transplantation antigens of the individual. Cells which recognize the antigens are stimulated and enter cell division. As mutations accumulate in rapidly dividing cells new immunological specificities may develop. At the same time the specificities of the lymphocytes for self transplantation antigens are weakened. The mature lymphocytes will recognize foreign antigen associated with transplantation antigens. The theory explains how the immune system normally matures through the influence of self antigens. It also offers an explanation for the regulation of immunological specificity by genes belonging to the transplantation system.

Theory 3: Antibodies, Anti-Antibodies ...

In his third main theory, the *Network Theory* from 1974, Jerne explains how the specific immune response is regulated. The theory has greatly stimulated research and led to new insights into the immune system. Recently its principles have been applied to diagnosis and treatment of disease. A basis for the network theory was the observation that antibodies can elicit anti-antibodies directed against antigen binding structures on the first antibody (Figure 1). Moreover, anti-antibodies can stimulate the production of still another generation of antibodies, anti-anti-antibodies. Essentially, this antibody cascade is endless successively adding new specific properties to the immune system. The various antibody generations either stimulate or suppress the production of one another. Under normal conditions the network is balanced. When an antigen is introduced the equilibrium is disturbed. The immune system tries to restore balance which leads to an immune response against the antigen.

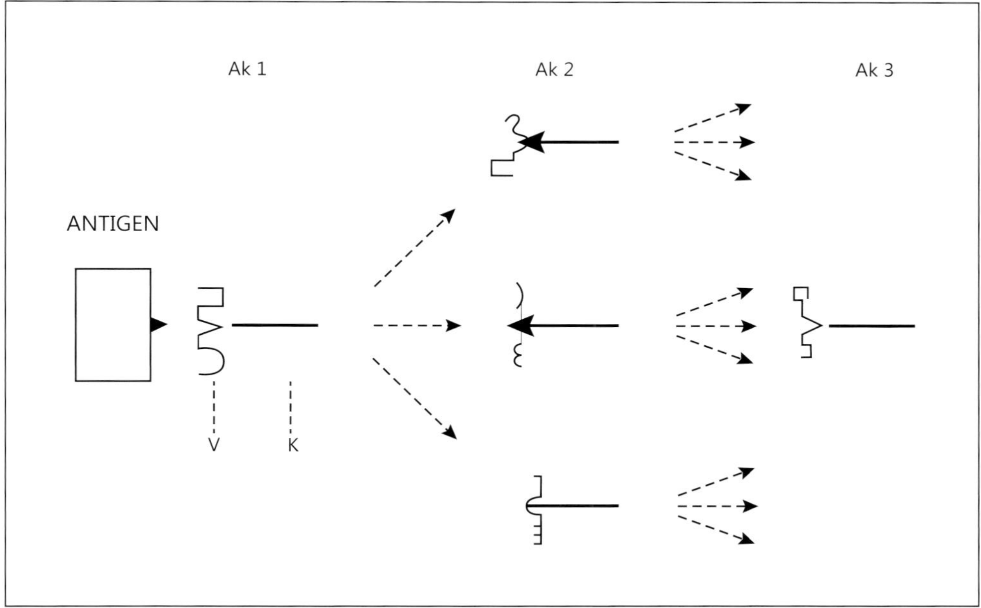

Figure 1. *The Network Theory*. Antibody 1 (Ak-1) has a structure in its variable (V) region which can bind the antigen. The V-region of Ak-1 contains unique structures which stimulate the production of various anti-antibodies (Ak-2). Some Ak-2 express V-region structures which mimic the antigen and which therefore can stimulate Ak-1 production. Each antibody generation induces the production of still another and larger set of anti-antibodies in a cascade-like manner. The various sets of antibodies stimulate or suppress the production of each other in a complex network. Under normal conditions the network is balanced. However, the equilibrium is disturbed when an antigen is introduced and binds to Ak-1. The immune system attempts to restore the balance, i.e. it leads to an immune response. Some examples where the network theory has been applied to experimental and clinical medicine are given in the following. 1. *Infectious diseases*. Anti-antibodies have been used in animals as a kind of vaccine against parasitic infections (trypanosomiasis), urinary tract infections, hepatitis and other infectious diseases. 2. *Allergy*. Anti-pollen antibodies may elicit allergic symptoms when an allergic person is exposed to pollen. The production of anti-pollen antibodies has been prevented in animals by anti-antibodies. 3. *Autoimmune disease*. Autoimmune disease may be caused by antibodies directed against the body's own tissues. Experimental autoimmune disease has been successfully treated with anti-antibodies. 4. *Transplantation*. Anti-antiimmunity may be important in organ transplantation by contributing to immunological tolerance against antigen on the foreign graft. 5. *Endocrinology*. Anti-antibodies against hormones and hormone receptors may prevent binding of the hormone to the receptors. This has been described for insulin and its receptor. 6. *Tumours*. Anti-antibodies have been attempted as treatment of certain tumours of the human immune system.

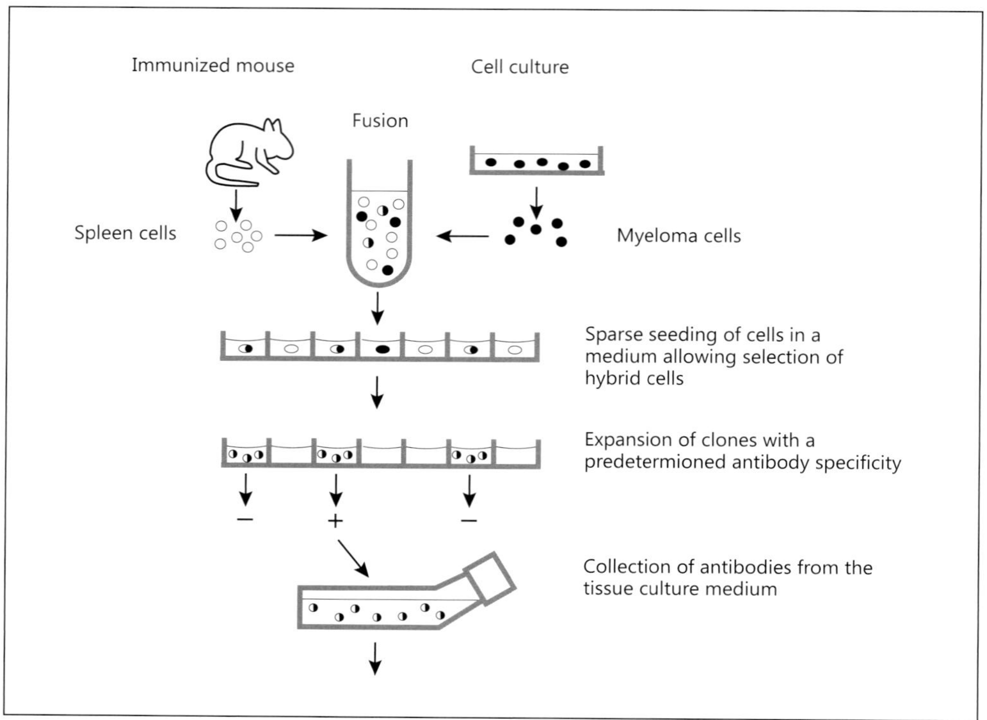

Figure 2. Principal steps in the production of a hybridoma. Spleen cells are prepared from animals, usually mice, which have been immunized with a selected antigen. These cells are then fused with myeloma cells maintained in culture in the laboratory. The product of this fusion is referred to as a hybridoma. Surprisingly, a hybrid of two cells can survive and also continue to divide. In this particular hybrid the myeloma cells contribute the capacity for survival, whereas the spleen cells direct the synthesis of antibodies with the preselected specificity. By special arrangements it is possible to achieve a multiplication of hybridoma cells but not of isolated myeloma cells. The hybrids obtained are propagated in a highly diluted state so that colonies deriving from single hybrid cells can be isolated. By use of a sensitive method the clones which produce the specific antibodies are identified. A particular hybridoma can then be used for future, unlimited production of a highly specific antibody. The availability of monoclonal antibodies has opened completely new possibilities for basic as well as applied biomedical research. The following examples of the use of monoclonal antibodies can be given. 1. *Detailed studies of the distribution of different functions in different parts of antigen molecules.* These studies may concern building elements of infectious agents; cell products such as enzymes and hormones; surface structures of cells etc. The mapping of variations in the surface components of influenza virus which explain the occurrence of repeated infections is one example. 2. *High degree purification of substances,* e.g. interferon, by taking advantage of the unique capacity displayed by a particular monoclonal antibody to bind to a certain antigen. In this case one uses a technique referred to as affinity chromatography. 3. *Diagnostic characterization of diseases* by identification of special structures on the surface or on the inside of cells. Hereby it is possible to distinguish between different forms of tumours and follow the development of tumours. Furthermore, it is possible to distinguish between different kinds of normal white blood cells. This is of importance for the characterization of certain immune deficiency conditions as seen e.g. in connection with the disease AIDS (acquired immune deficiency syndrome). Diseases caused by infectious agents can also be diagnosed by use of monoclonal antibodies. Thus, virus infected cells and bacteria or parasites inside or outside cells can be identified with a unique degree of specificity. 4. *Treatment of diseases.* Monoclonal antibodies against specialized white blood cells have been used with some success in connection with transplantation. There may also be possibilities to use monoclonal antibodies for treatment of tumours.

Hybridoma – A Technique for Eternal Production of Monoclonal Antibodies in Cell Cultures

Besides gene technology, which has already been honoured by several Nobel Prizes, the hybridoma technique represents the most important methodological advance within the field of biomedicine during the 1970s. The development of this technique is based on several observations concerning basic biological phenomena. There are cells in the body – immune lymphocytes – which can produce millions of different antibodies. However, each single cell can only produce antibodies with a certain predetermined specificity. A prerequisite for the formation of a multitude of antibodies is, therefore, the existence of an excess of lymphocytes. If the body is exposed to a certain foreign antigen there may be stimulation of a lymphocyte which fortuitously has been endowed with the capacity to identify this particular antigen. This lymphocyte then starts to divide and forms a clone of cells which produces identical – monoclonal – antibodies. The development of a clone of cells in connection with a normal immune response occurs under carefully controlled conditions. In rare cases, however, the body loses control over a clone of antibody producing cells. This may lead to formation of a special type of tumour (myeloma). Myeloma cells usually retain their capacity to produce a certain antibody, but because of the accidental emergence of the tumour one normally does not know with which antigen this antibody reacts. White blood cells responsible for producing antibodies are highly specialized cells. As a consequence they lack the capacity to survive for a longer time if they are removed from the body and incubated in a tissue culture medium. In contrast, myeloma cells can occasionally be cultivated continuously. Since long, biomedical research workers have nourished the dream to be able to propagate clones of cells which produce antibodies with predetermined specificity. This dream materialized when Georges J.F. Köhler and César Milstein in 1975 introduced the so-called hybridoma technology for production of monoclonal antibodies. The principal features of the hybridoma technology are shown in Figure 2 on the previous page.

Treasure Trove 1984

The database contains documents related to the BII in a broader context (lists, series of photographs, etc.).

QR1984_treasure BII

The Year 1985

The year started routinely and uneventfully. There was no indication that in less than 8 weeks a major disaster would hit the institute. As was the case for all previous years, new members started to arrive.

Arrivals 1985 (14)
Bjärne Bogen, Susan Carson, Christopher Coleclough, David Gray, Wayne Hein, Julia Hurwitz-Coleclough, John Kearney, Susan McClure, Lucia Mori, Hans-Georg Rammensee, Brigitta Stockinger, James Turpen, Yasushi Uematsu, Gayle D. (Monte) Wetzel.
The number of scientists arriving during 1985 was lower than in previous years because – as described below – a devastating fire prevented the smooth functioning of the laboratories throughout the year.

Came and Left in the Same Year (3)
Sabine Fleischer, Bede Morris, Roland Scollay.

Leavers 1985 (16)
John Cambier, Taichi Ezaki, Barbara Fagg, Gerard Farmer, Kirsten Fischer Lindahl, Werner Haas, Geoffrey Henson, Minoru Hirama, Antonio Iglesias, Norman Iscove, Michael Kiefer, Pawel Kisielow, Georges Köhler, James McCubrey, John McKearn, James Turpen.

QR1985_01 BII

Less than a month after the Stockholm dinner, science was back to normal. This was the case for everybody except those who were moving to new positions – among them Georges Köhler, who was offered a position as Director of the Max Planck Institute in Freiburg.

BTA 4: "Reflections", the Goodbye Performance for Georges Köhler

Although the horizontal structure ensured equal working conditions and social status for all members, certain differences became apparent, at the latest when scientists were about to leave. In as far as an ovation can be long or short, a goodbye to a former colleague can be cordial or just a polite gesture. Georges Köhler's disposition was such that he would have preferred to move to his new position in Freiburg without great ado. But in spite of his modesty, he was too much of a celebrity to let it happen that way. And he was a likeable person.

Chris Paige, Norman Iscove and some other coworkers prepared the BTA's production – unfortunately the full groundwork was not adequately recorded. The performance was staged in the third week of January 1985 [QR1985_01]. As an undertone of the play, a certain sadness became apparent because Georges was about to leave. It also became clear (from the play as well as through the grapevine) that Georges hesitated; he would rather have stayed. The institute tried to make arrangements with Roche, but the Roche management could not work out a proposal. In "Reflections", it was only hinted that if Roche had offered Georges an option for early retirement (to give him a chance to compensate for the "early" Nobel award), then Georges would have stayed.

When the applause stopped, people left cheerfully without any premonition that a disastrous event would soon hit the institute.

The Fire, February 27th, 1985

February 27th was a Wednesday, and this year it was the special Basel Carnival (Fasnacht) Wednesday [QR1985_02]. At 14.15 the fire alarm rang out throughout the institute, shrill and frighteningly loud, and for so long that it became clear that this was not a drill but a real evacuation order. The staff curiously assembled at the entrance and when, 5 or 6 minutes later, the Roche fire brigade siren was heard, huge fire engines blocked the street and fire fighters started to unroll the hoses, it was obvious that the institute was on fire.

The city fire brigade arrived a few minutes later as the carnival procession had compelled them to make a detour. The BII staff assembled on the opposite pavement of the Grenzacherstrasse, and watched. Flames were pouring out of an air duct on the roof of the institute. At 14.26, the institute's main clock stopped.

QR1985_02 BII

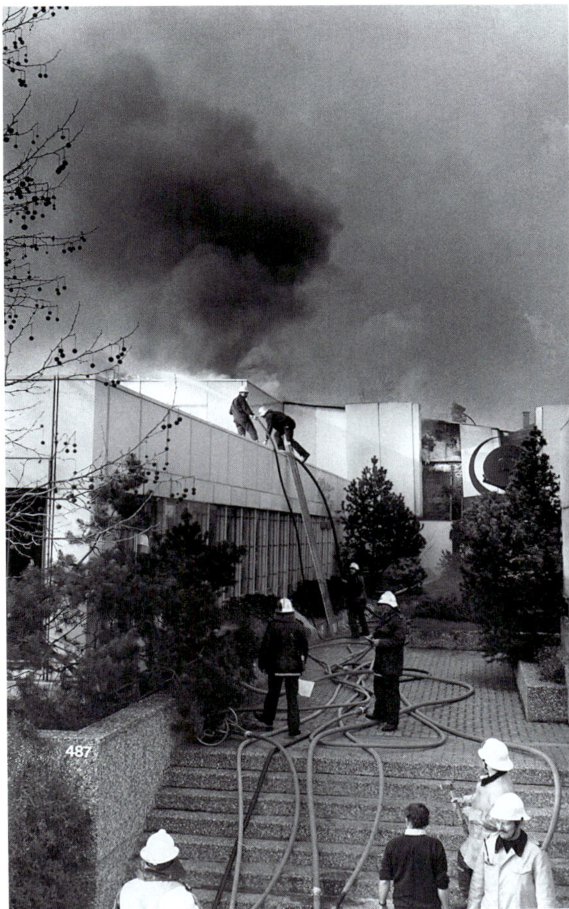

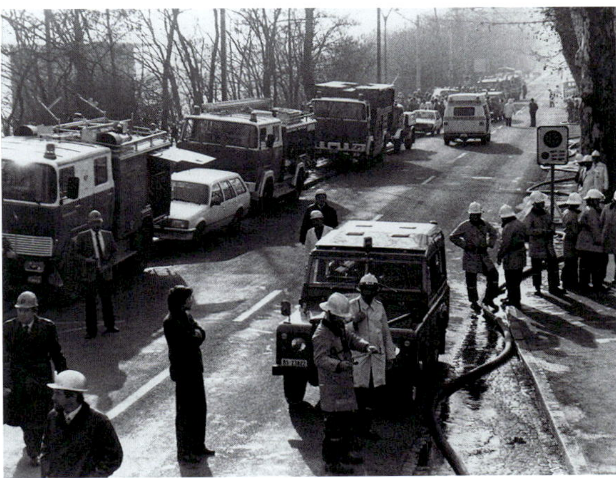

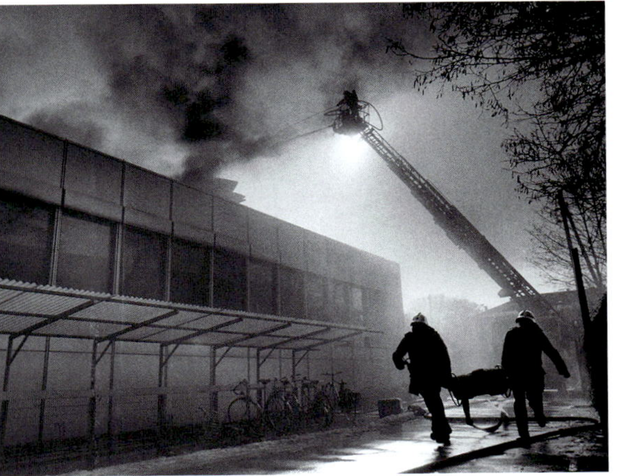

Girafe en Feu/Phoenix Arises from the Ashes

When the sun set on the last day of Fasnacht 1985, it was not known whether the sun had also set on the institute. But the rescue operation started immediately. Although the metaphor of Phoenix arising from the ashes is a powerful image, Dali's "Girafe en feu" is more appropriate: the giraffe is burning, but the drawers in the body of the woman contain knowledge that has to be saved and disseminated.

The BII was renowned for furthering the growth of knowledge, and one purpose of this narrative is to examine the past and learn from its legacy. The book itself contains many "drawers" that the reader is encouraged to delve into and explore [QR1985_03].

QR1985_03 BII

Acknowledgment
Louis Du Pasquier is thanked for his suggestion to conclude Book 1 with this picture. What followed after the fire is described in Book 2.

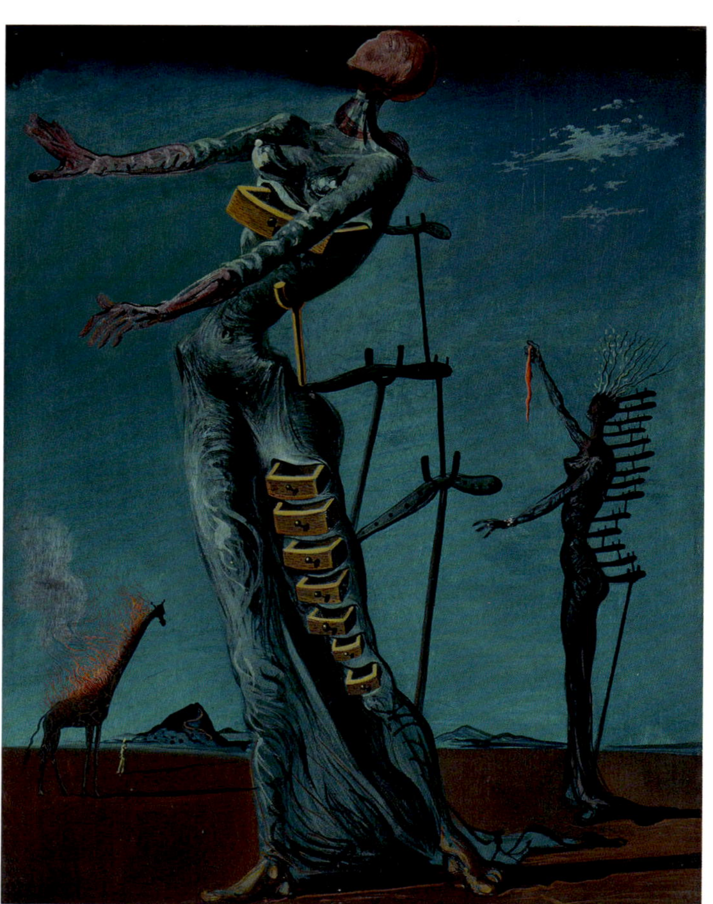

Salvador Dalí: Girafe en feu, um 1936/1937, Öl auf Holz 35 × 27 cm, Emanuel Hoffmann Stiftung, Depositum in der Öffentlichen Kunstsammlung Basel.
Foto: Öffentliche Kunstsammlung Basel, Martin P. Bühler

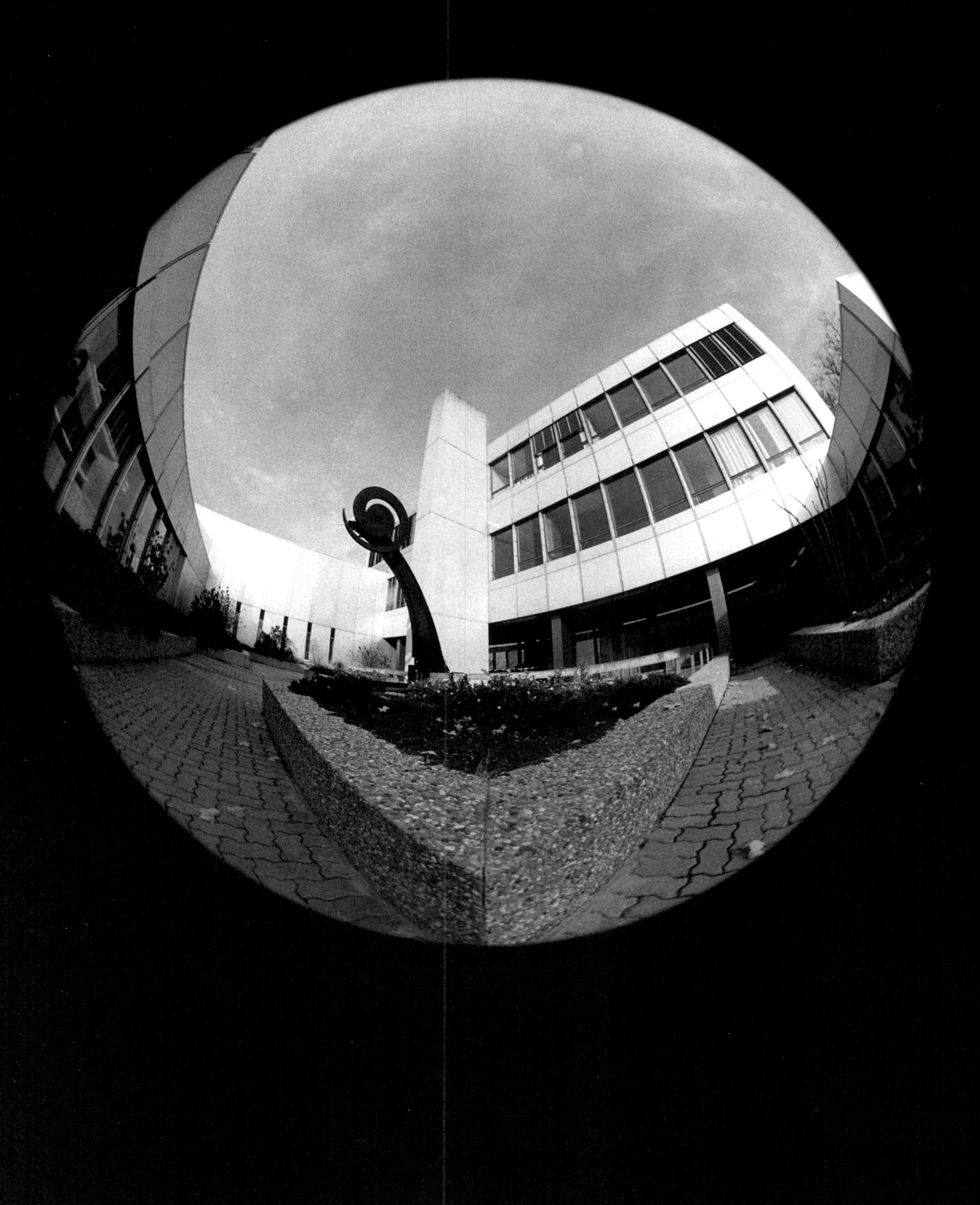

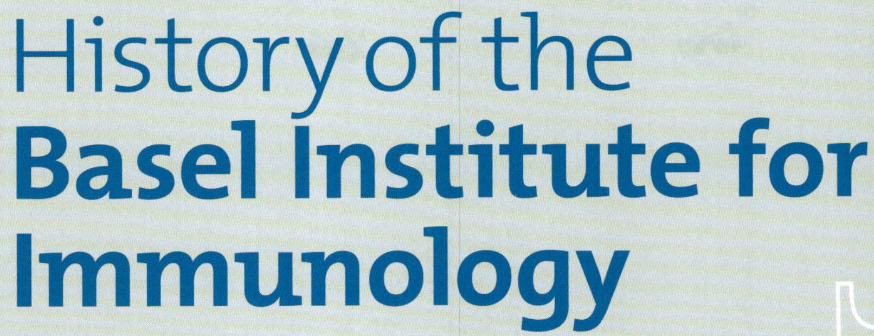

History of the **Basel Institute for Immunology**

Book 2

1985–2001

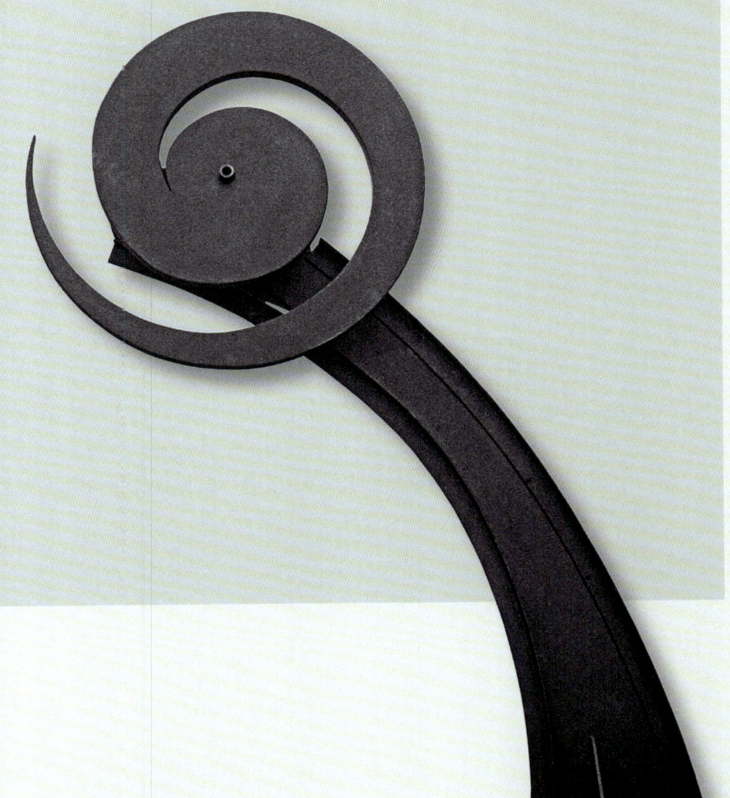

Beyond Jerne's Mind

In Niels Jerne's mind, as well as in the opinion of the prevailing scientific community of the late sixties of the last century, the concept "what immunology is about" was well established, although greatly oversimplified: it was about the *specific antibody response to antigens*. In a lecture in France in early 1970 [QR1985_04], Jerne used the slogan "no antibody, no immunology". Today nobody would use this phrase, but at the time the institute was founded Jerne's narrow definition was of a decisive importance. The distinction between innate and acquired immune systems was accepted, but rarely discussed. Jerne did not deny that something like the "first and second line of defense" existed, but his main standpoint was that without understanding the origin and function of specific antibody response, none of the accessory functions could ever be understood.

Now, decades later, nobody would engage in an argument on "whether the innate or the acquired immune system is more important". But it is highly probable that Jerne's decision to concentrate on elucidating the origin of antibody specificity was the key to the success of the Basel Institute: it is likely that had the BII had all-encompassing research programs, it would have failed to make the discoveries that it did make.

Antibody Response versus Immune Response

In the very beginning, when Jerne defined his program as "the origin and the function of specific antibody response", it was already known that antibody is produced by lymphocytes, but the distinction between T and B cells had not yet been established. As soon as the role of T lymphocytes became known, both as helper cells for antibody response and as key players in transplantation, cell interaction theories were incorporated into core research at the BII. The B cell-T cell dichotomy made it necessary to adjust the terminology, and instead of specific *antibody* response (B cells), the wording changed to "specific *immune* response" (B and T cells). *Immune* response was somewhat broader than *antibody* response; nonetheless what remained was the term "specific".

QR1985_04 BII

Innate Immunity and Acquired Immune System

The BII was certainly not antagonistic towards the emerging field of innate immunity, but research on it – for better or worse – was not carried out there. As there was "academic freedom" at the BII, projects concerning "innate immunity" would not have been stopped or prevented (also see below Antonio Coutinho's view on this subject). The reason why many research directions only remained "niches" was because of the selection procedure for hiring new members. This has been mentioned elsewhere, but to reiterate, scientists who had already successfully accomplished their training, and perhaps completed their "first postdoc work" elsewhere, applied to the institute with a description of a project they wanted to pursue. An applicant with a solid project (whether risky or not) had a good chance to be accepted, provided it suited the main research direction of the institute.

... it is highly probable that Jerne's decision to concentrate on elucidating the origin of antibody specificity was the key to the success of the Basel Institute ...

The unique feature of the BII was that the newly arriving scientist could initiate the research project that he meant to perform, but he could switch to any other project when he felt that the altered one would be more promising or more interesting than the original one. As with any project, there was a certain risk of failure, but this was well compensated by the chance to lift the lid of a completely intact treasure box. For the institute, the risk of a scientist behaving erratically was negligible, because of the limited time contract.

Among the applicants there were only a few, if any, who were interested in innate immunity and who for that matter would be able to devise a promising project.

Antonio Coutinho on Innate Immunity and Mitogen Receptors

Mitogenic activation of B cells and T cells, because it is "nonspecific" and independent of antigen reactivity of the responding lymphocytes, was, naturally, not within Jerne's concerns. "Mitogen receptors" are today central to innate immunity (Toll-like receptors). Yet it represented the central research interest of Möller, and it was extensively pursued at the BII, first by Möller's group (Sjöberg and Andersson), later by Coutinho and Melchers. Eventually Jerne paid due attention to this approach because of the perspectives it opened for quantitative immunology.

Major Histocompatibility Complex

For Jerne, the world of immunology would have been a more amiable one if the major histocompatibility complex (MHC) could have been disregarded. MHC is a genetic region encoded by a large gene family that controls many aspects of the immune system [QR1985_05]. Many genes, among others those controlling class I and class II molecules, are involved and are essential for a functional immune system. Nevertheless, once Jerne recognized that the issue of histocompatibility and cell surface recognition could not be ignored, he succeeded to incorporate the MHC notions into his immunological *Weltanschauung* and in his hypothesis of self-nonself discrimination.

Jerne's Nobel Prize came just in time to enable him to call the era of elucidation of antibody specificity as "concluded" and to promote opening up new vistas. Although Fritz Melchers, Niels Jerne's successor, was a "B cell researcher", he was prepared to support projects that had previously been omitted, and he ensured that such projects would receive due attention.

Natural Killer Cells

Research projects on natural killer cells were one of the neglected issues. There is some controversy about the early work on natural killer cells, but now it is accepted that the discovery was made in the early seventies of the last century at the Karolinska Institute, Stockholm, in the laboratory of Eva Klein and Hans Wigzell [QR1985_06]. Natural killer cells typically do not fall in the category of cells participating in *specific* immune responses, since they provide a fast and efficient response to virus-infected cells, and they do so in the absence of antibodies and without MHC recognition. This is exactly the delineation that distinguishes the first from the second line of defense. The BII was ready to follow this new research direction, and once it was taken up at the BII, it resulted in excellent research.

QR1985_05 BII

Jerne, in his function as honorary chairman of the Advisory Board, continued to follow the changing arena of research, and he wisely – though not always whole-heartedly – approved of the new approaches. There was however an important development which he considered with open disbelief. It was the interplay of T cells and the MHC. Decades earlier Jerne had introduced the term "epitope", which was meant to be a more precise definition of an "antigenic determinant". The portion of the antigen that fitted the antibody-combining site was defined as an epitope. Epitope meant

QR1985_06 BII

to be both a physical entity and a "shape". The entire repertoire of antibodies was an arena of shapes (of the combining sites), in that a fitting counterpart to each combining site could exist. The portion of the combining site of antibody was termed *paratope*, while the portion of the antigen was the *epitope*. All this was about shapes, and about the affinity of epitope-paratope fitting.

This was the case in B cell immunology, and the starting assumption in T cell immunology was – how else could it be – that the T cell receptor recognizes antigen in a similar fashion. As a result of many years of research, it turned out (as shown in countless reports in this book) that instead of the above-mentioned proposition, T cell receptors detect the "inner" structure of the antigen, in the form of "their" peptides. For those who were around at that time, it was fascinating to follow the unraveling of the three-dimensional structure of the MHC molecule containing a longitudinal groove capable of accommodating the peptide. Thereupon it is the peptide-MHC combination that is recognized by the T cells. Jerne was delighted by the solution, but irritated that the peptides were called T cell epitopes.

Antonio Coutinho Summarizes the Dilemma

"*Immunology came of age with the selective principles of antibody formation (Jerne 1955) and the clonal selection theory (Burnet 1957). The theory was clear and amenable to direct test, promoting considerable progress in cellular and molecular immunology. It posed the central question as to the genetic origin of antibody diversity, settled 20 years later when progress in molecular biology allowed for the study of eukaryotic genes. It is as if everything has been solved, and good people start leaving the field. It seems to me, however, that we are just at the end of one particular period of development in the discipline. Thus, while we can today manipulate genes, engineer molecules and control cellular behaviours, we are quite disarmed when trying to manipulate the system. Surprisingly, perhaps, we continue to treat allergy as we did before IgE was known, we have no specific therapy for autoimmune diseases, we are unable to tolerize the recipient of an organ to the tissues of the donor, and we seem incompetent to derive vaccines to protect the larger part of the world population from parasite infections.*

There are at least two ways of dealing with this paradox. One, more often found, maintains that all we need is more information on details and to continue to invest in the description of genes, molecules and cells. Another, more provocatively, claims that those kinds of

problems cannot be solved in the same framework, which was appropriate to address other levels of organization and description. It is argued that we must move from molecular and cellular immunology to 'system immunology', for the good reason that properties such as tolerance and self-nonself distinctions are complex, and cannot be 'reduced' to isolated components." [QR1985_07].

Autoradiograph of a protein pattern on a two-dimensional polyacrylamide gel electrophoretogram

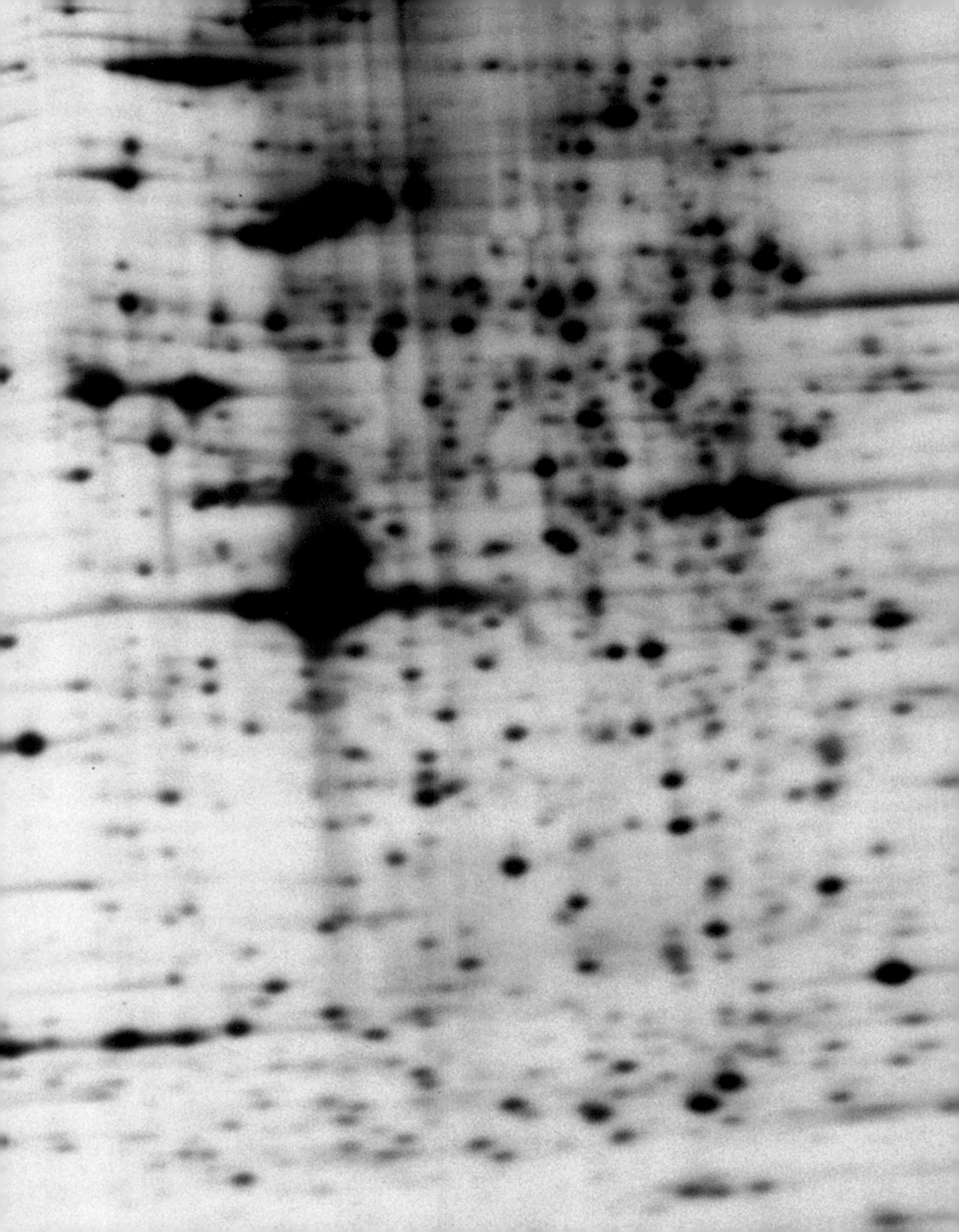

Spring 1985

A major fire following an explosion in the ventilation system damaged about one third of the institute, fortunately without human casualties and without harm to the animal stock. Scientists from the damaged portion of the institute "squeezed" into the intact laboratories, and for the rest of the year restoration and reconstruction work went on. Several planned courses were postponed to the following year(s). Only the B Cell Neoplasia conference and a workshop on the Role of Interleukin-2 in B Cell Physiology were held as planned. Many contracts for new members were deferred as well. Publication success did not diminish.

Chiaroscuro, February 27th, 1985

The fire was extinguished in the night of February 27th/28th, and the extent of devastation became visible at daylight. The fire brigade of Basel City had left, while the Roche fire brigade patrolled the site. Some of the institute's staff stayed throughout the night, only going home in the late morning. The main concerns were to ensure that no human casualties occurred, no animals were hurt, and that live biological material (cell lines) was saved (see also the QR1985_02 of Book 1).

All this was achieved. Several hundred cages were removed from the animal units during the hours when the fire raged, and not a single mouse died. For several hours it was not sure whether anybody was trapped in the elevator – fortunately this was not the case.

On the same day a formal "Rescue Committee" was established, comprising Chris Paige, Charley Steinberg and Ivan Lefkovits [QR1985_08]. Later Fritz Melchers (who was abroad at the time of the fire) was co-opted. One of the Rescue Committee members arranged with the Migros food retailer to send a "refrigerator truck" with deep freeze compartments to the institute, in which to store the biologicals retrieved from the out-of-function deep freezers. This turned out to be a crucial step towards saving invaluable experimental material so that it could be used immediately.

QR1985_08 BII

The Roche fire brigade, whose function was to secure the damaged site, helped to move the deep freezers to a place where electricity from a generator was temporarily made available. Designated members and technicians then transferred the material

(Photographs: Dario Grossberger)

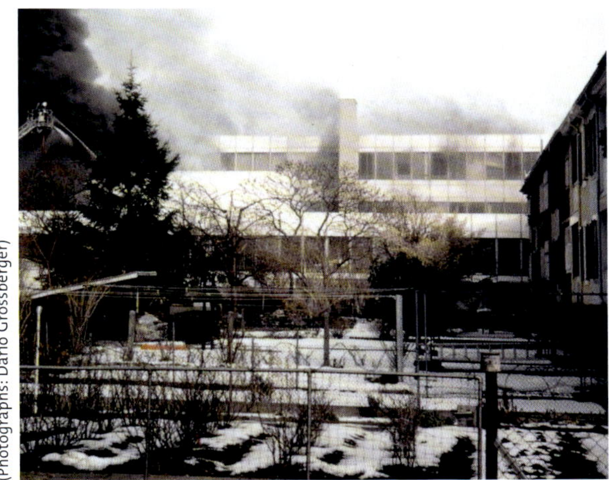

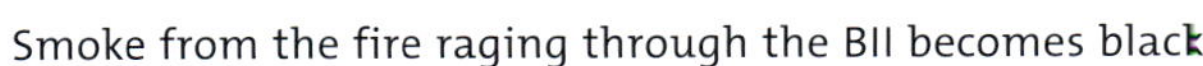

Smoke from the fire raging through the BII becomes black

IF YOU HAVE ANY SUGGESTIONS FOR GETTING THE INSTITUTE RUNNING AGAIN OR IF YOU HAVE ANY PROBLEMS CONTACT ONE OF THE MEMBERS OF THE RESTORATION COMMITTEE

from the freezers to the Migros refrigerated truck; the word "designated" refers to the fact that nobody else was allowed to enter the building as the conditions – darkness, slippery floors – were dangerous. Out of 18 (–70°C) deep freezers, 16 retained the frozen condition of the biologicals, even when the outside mantle melted and/or the cooling system was damaged; the insulation was satisfactory. Alfred Benz from the Roche fire brigade played a pivotal role in this rescue operation.

For many hours after the fire had been extinguished, it was not clear whether the institute would ever be able to continue functioning in its premises. Once a 3 m × 3 m sterile environment (with curtains separating clean/unclean areas) was created (by Chris Paige), and when the first growing cell lines were placed in the incubators, it was time to rename the Rescue Committee "Restoration Committee".

For many hours after the fire had been extinguished, it was not clear whether the institute would ever be able to continue functioning on its premises.

The priorities of the restoration procedure were to

- maintain safety throughout the clean-up,
- define the basic functions that had to be maintained (keeping cell lines and cell cultures alive; reinstalling liquid nitrogen tanks and deep freezers), and
- perform the clean-up without interfering with basic functions.

As mentioned above, the content of the deep freezers (–70°C) remained unharmed. But there was another place where the damage was minimal, and that was surprising. The bulk of 28 liquid nitrogen tanks (containing vials of frozen cells and other tissues) remained intact, such that even the surroundings (the walls and

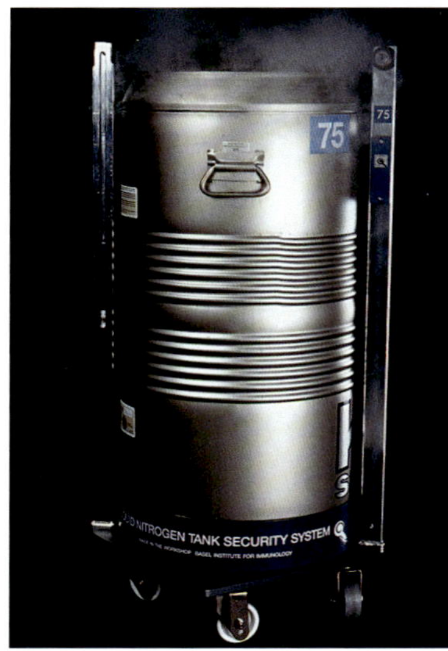

A liquid nitrogen tank for storing the cells

the ceiling) were undamaged. At closer inspection it became clear that during the fire – when the local temperature increased beyond the critical point – liquid nitrogen started to evaporate, and the "huge bubble" of the oxygen-free area prevented the fire reaching the N2 tanks. At the time of inspection, 16 tanks contained residual liquid nitrogen, and the material was transferred to new tanks and was usable.

The clean-up of the debris was a prerequisite for starting the restoration, and it was a major logistic task with the aim to achieve 90% clean-up within 10 days. To this end, all available cleaning companies in Basel were summoned to the site; the 7 companies under contract were: ARC, Arnosti, Bach, Civatti, Jeggi, SPC and Wettstein. During the first days up to 160 people were involved.

On each floor a different company worked. It so happened that the staff of each company wore uniforms of different color and style. This turned out to be of great value in supervising the workers, and see that they were at their right place on the correct floor. This ad hoc accidental color coding worked very well.

The institute bought every doormat (several hundred of them) available in supermarkets and shops and a mat was placed at the entrance to each lab and office. On the 11th day after the start of the clean-up (i.e. the 17th day after the fire), the institute was cleared of debris and damaged furniture. The walls were black from burned-on soot, but otherwise clean.

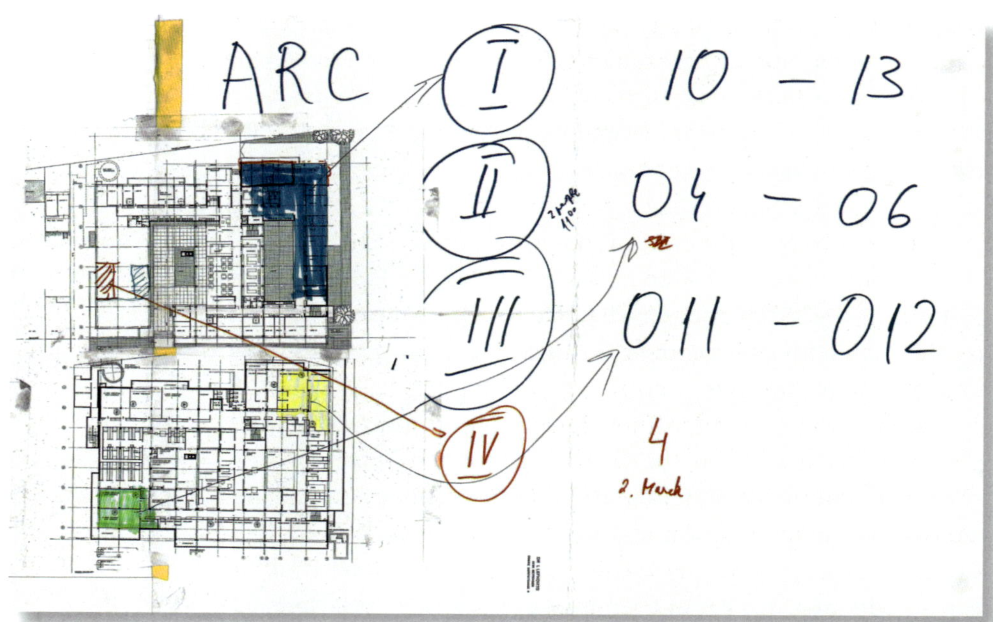

Cleaning schedule

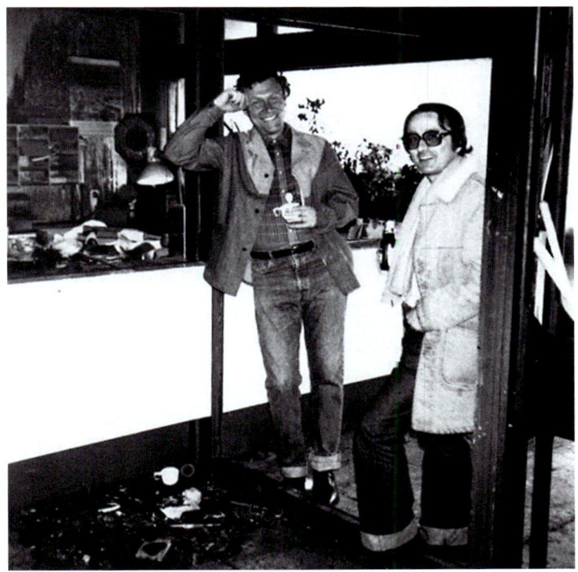

Fritz Melchers and Ivan Lefkovits at the fire-demolished entrance to the institute

Technicians and scientists worked on thoroughly cleaning their labs. The ones which were less damaged provided asylum for staff from labs which had to be closed down.

In the entire clean-up period there was a single incident, and it was socially relevant. One worker, a young woman, approached a BII Restoration Committee member to ask if she could work in cleaning the library. This request was of course granted, but on the third day the person in question did not turn up. Upon enquiry, the boss of the cleaning company said that she had been made redundant. The reason being that through her request to work cleaning the library, they found out that she had a higher education (Matura), and by the rules of the company she was overqualified. After heated discussion (threatening the company that their services would be discontinued) she was reemployed – to the full satisfaction of the BII and to the relief of the young lady.

The first laboratory which received the status "clean" was Lab 9, under Chris Paige's supervision, where all sterile work (re-inoculation of cell lines) was done [QR1985_09].

Although there were no major problems during the reconstruction, there were many hindrances. The insurance wished to have a list of instruments that were to be replaced. It was the task of the company RAG to check and label the instruments. Thus, the lab work was often interrupted because an instrument (centrifuge, vortex, balance, pH-meter) was removed by "RAG people" and replaced later by one with an OK label.

QR1985_09 BII

Jacques Bron, the person in charge of technical administration from the beginning of the institute – so much needed during the reconstruction – could not help. He became terminally ill and died on August 1st, 1985 [QR1985_10]. Quoting from the obituary: "Despite his serious illness, he kept coming back to the institute until just a few days before his life ended, because he wanted to help rebuild it after the fire."

Jacques Bron came to the institute in 1970 to help Ivan Lefkovits organize the institute's infrastructure while the building was under construction. After the institute had been completed, he was responsible for equipping all the laboratories and general facilities, and for keeping them running. He fulfilled all requests made by new scientists and met the needs of the over 300 scientists who passed through the institute's doors. Jacques Bron was replaced by Peter Balzarini, who then continued Jacques' work.

Legally Speaking

It was the responsibility of the Restoration Committee to oversee the entire reconstruction procedure. Although the birth of the Rescue Committee had been an ad hoc decision of 3 members, the committee remained "in power" throughout the entire restoration period.

Legally speaking, the decision on any of these matters was supposed to lie in Roche hands. Roche – as any big company – had a thorough, vertically organized chain of command, and for many of their offices the Restoration Committee was certainly not the most comfortable "negotiation" partner. Before the Rescue Committee renamed itself Restoration Committee, there were issues on which the committee decided to ignore instructions that undermined the rescue procedure. It is beyond the scope of this book to go into further detail, but one of the things that the Rescue Committee successfully prevented (with Fritz Melchers' full support) was the idea of some non-specified Roche officials to close down the institute for a period of 18 months, transfer all activities to Roche premises (and maybe rented space elsewhere in the city) and then reopen a fully renovated institute. It was obvious to BII members that such a decision would mean the end of the institute.

It was practical of Fritz Melchers to recognize that the "impetus of reconstruction" was well placed in the hands of the team Paige, Steinberg and Lefkovits, while the formal managers (head of administration, safety officer) would not be needed for organizing the reconstruction.

For completeness sake, it is worth mentioning that the insurance of Canton Basel covered all the damage. The only item they criticized was the cost of the cleaning. The requirement of 7 cleaning companies was considered excessive – but the insurance company finally agreed to cover this cost too. A detailed report on the entire fire episode is deposited in the Roche Historical Archive.

A Migros deep-freeze storage room, rented by the Rescue Committee, was used beyond 1985. There was a daily commuting service to bring material needed to the institute.

The "famous" self-service of the prefire era was not available for several months. While cooperation and sharing amongst colleagues remained the norm, a few unfortunate examples of hoarding material came to light. For the narrator of this story it was an unpleasant déjà vu of the not fully forgotten past in a "socialist country" where everything (including toilet paper) was a scarce commodity.

Hundreds of Letters from all over the World

A decade and a half previously the main subject among immunologists was the new institute. Now the immunology community was shaken up by the news of the fire. Phone calls did not go through, but cables arrived, letters came, and offers of help from near and far poured in.

Some of the documents which show this concern are given in the [QR1985_11]. A touching letter from Canada (Cinader and friends) is reproduced below:

Please accept our best wishes for the rapid restoration of the ravages of the fire of 26 February. The Basel Institute for Immunology has a very important place in the affection and in the conceptual thinking of our as in the scientific consciousness of Immunologists all over the world. We are delighted to learn that your work of restoration is rapidly progressing.

With best regards,

Yours sincerely,

S. Dubiski B. Cinader R.H. Painter
G. Carayanniotis Barbara M.S. Pulleyblank B. H. Barber
Shin Komatsubara Atsushi Kohno Usha Ponnappan

QR1985_11 BII

Special Arrival of a New Member at a Special Time

In the last chapter of Book 1, members joining the institute during 1985 are listed. Besides them, one arrival is worthy of special mention in this chapter [QR1985_12]. On Friday March 1st, 1985, Hans-Georg Rammensee was supposed to start work at the BII. Hans-Georg arrived from Tübingen, turning up in front of the institute carrying a black attaché case: he could not believe his eyes (as he told later). He was standing at the devastated entrance of the institute, rooted to the spot. A BII member observed him, little needed to be explained, and upon mutual agreement with the director, his starting date in Basel was rescheduled. In the 1987 chapter, his achievements at the BII are summarized and his further career is outlined.

Kirsten Fischer Lindahl Leaves for Dallas, 1985

Kirsten graduated from the University of Wisconsin, Madison, in 1975. Her mentor and co-author of a number of publications was Fritz Bach, one of the most prominent scientists in the field of transplant immunology. Kirsten spent more than 7 years at the BII. Then she was offered a position at the University of Texas South Western in Dallas as a group leader, and soon she became a fellow of the prestigious Howard Hughes Medical Institute (HHMI), a position which she held until her retirement in 2003. The HHMI was founded by the American businessman Howard Hughes back in 1953; it is one of the largest funding organizations for biological and medical research in the United States.

Kirsten was a mouse geneticist, and for a considerable part of her career she was interested in maternally inherited cell surface antigens [QR1985_13]. She studied mitochondrial inheritance in mice, and compared the chromosomal and extrachromosomal genes in both inbred and wild mice. One of the examples of her work is the finding that the same MHC recombinational hot spots are active in crossing-over between *wild/wild* and *wild/inbred* mouse chromosomes. Several of her work projects were related to mouse chromosome 17.

QR1985_12 BII

During her years at the institute, she collaborated and published with Antonio Coutinho, Andrei Augustin, Eva-Lotte Larsson, Jean Langhorne, Peter Robinson, Ivan Lefkovits, Charlie Sidman, Luciana Forni, Michael Steinmetz and Yasushi Uematsu. She loved to discuss scientific matters with Charley Steinberg and Stephen Fazekas.

QR1985_13 BII

An ad hoc mention is made here that Kirsten co-authored a paper entitled "Crystal Structure of the MHC Class Ib Molecule H2-M3" with her husband Johann Deisenhofer, some years after he was awarded the Nobel Prize for chemistry.

Werner Haas Accepts a Position at Roche, 1985

Werner enjoyed collaborating with Harald von Boehmer, elevating it into an extraordinarily efficient and successful teamwork. Nevertheless, Werner knew that one day he would leave the BII, as it was not consistent with BII rules that two scientists working on the same problems could be permanent members. So there was never a conflict on this between Harald and Werner. After 10 years working at the BII, it was obviously not easy for Werner to go out into the "real world". He applied to many places worldwide: Paris, Umea, Edmonton and others. In the end, he was offered a position in Roche because of a recommendation by Fritz Melchers. Fritz arranged a meeting with the newly appointed Roche research head, Hermann Bujard, whom Werner liked as soon as he met him for the first time.

The move to Roche took place in 1985, and according to Werner's memory it was when Zlatko Dembic succeeded in transferring both antigen specificity and MHC restriction specificity by the transfer of the genes encoding the two TCR chains. Thus, Werner's dream of the concept of two independent receptors (one for the antigen and one for the MHC restriction element) was destroyed once and for all. He felt that the loss of this dream ended his desire to have a career as a basic research scientist.

Bujard let Werner do whatever he wanted, as long as he agreed to be his consultant in immunology. After a short stay in the monoclonal antibody lab, Werner began some molecular biology work with Willi Hunziker, but soon he became a "full-time" consultant to Bujard and thereafter to Jürgen Drews.

Norman N. Iscove Moves to Heidelberg and Then to Toronto

After spending years at the Friedrich Miescher Institute and at the BII, Norman Iscove moved some 200 km north to Heidelberg, which turned out to be a stepping stone for his return to Canada [QR1985_14].

QR1985_14 BII

Norman has made significant and pioneering contributions to hemopoietic stem cell research that advanced the field in both methodology and concept. His laboratory has concentrated on identifying genes that specify the sustained capacity for self-renewal that uniquely characterizes the long-term reconstituting stem cells.

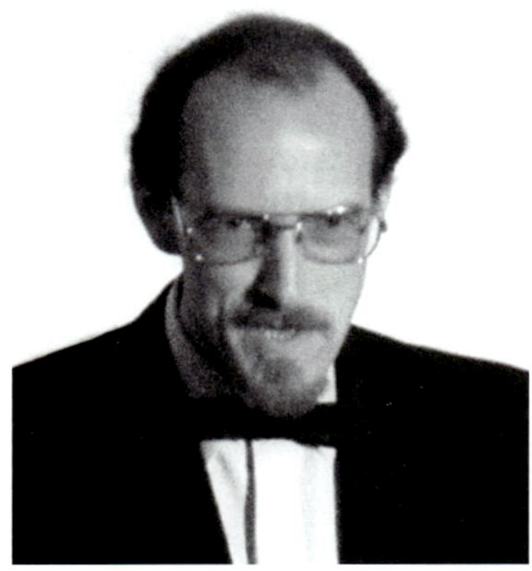
Norman Iscove

He has held the following positions:

Junior rotating internship, New Mount Sinai Hospital, Toronto
PhD student, Ontario Cancer Institute
Postdoctoral fellow, Friedrich Miescher Institute, Basel
Member, Basel Institute for Immunology, Basel
Visiting scientist, European Molecular Biology Laboratory, Heidelberg
Senior scientist, Ontario Cancer Institute, Toronto
Professor, Departments of Medical Biophysics, Immunology, Medicine, OCI, Toronto

During the reconstruction efforts, neither scientific activity nor the Basel Theater for the Arts plans were reined in, although the BII stage was not available for performances. "Urgent need" arose when the time drew closer to Norman Iscove's move to his next position (Heidelberg). Norman had been involved in all previous performances, and it was unacceptable to skip a goodbye event just because of a missing stage.

BTA 5: "Diary", the Goodbye Performance for Norman Iscove

The performance took place in a forest clearing in Basel-Land, but of course the self-aggrandizing language of the script (Chris Paige and volunteers) referred to the "Prestigious Theatre in the Woods", and stated that it was the first time the BTA had taken its act on the road [QR1985_15].

The plot was based on the fictitious discovery of Norman Iscove's diary, which listed decisions related to his future:

- The decision to do research
- The rejection of marriage
- The discovery of serum-free medium
- To publish or not to publish

The play referred to Norman's CV, which reads:

Norman Nelson Iscove, a Canadian, was born in Canada to his mother in a hospital. This apparently positive experience resulted in this early decision to dedicate his life to humanity with special emphasis on poor, young women. Although initially he attempted to fulfil his desires through a career in Medicine, he found that the acquisition of a Medical Diploma did little to relieve his pent-up needs. A brief period in Surgery convinced him that his clinical talents were limited to the examination room. After briefly contemplating a stint on the

QR1985_15 BII

Psychiatrists couch, Dr. Iscove flung himself full force on the Research Bench. Pursuing his goals first in Toronto at the OCI and later in Basel at both the FMI and BII Dr. Iscove has left his mark the world over.

The BTA performance for Iscove took place in a forest clearing in Basel-Land, the "Prestigious Theatre in the Woods".

The main character in the play is of course Norman, played by 5 BII actors (Ruedi Frech, Michael Julius, Martin Flajnik, David Gray and Charley Steinberg):

- The Norman Faust
- The Norman Figaro
- The Norman McBeth
- The Norman Hamlet
- The Norman Moses

The play, full of irony, insider jokes and scientific undertones, met with great applause.

Susan Carson Comes from Sir Walter Bodmer's Laboratory

One of the scientists arriving at the institute just at the end of the clean-up and at the fresh start after reconstruction was Susan Carson [QR1985_16]. She came to Basel upon the suggestion of Michael Steinmetz, who had met her on his visit to the HLA Laboratory of Sir Walter Bodmer at the Imperial Cancer Research Fund, London.

Susan came to Basel as an experienced neurotransmitter receptor biologist, earning her reputation in the Neurobiology Laboratory of the ENS in Paris, and in the Department of Pharmacology at the University of Oxford. In Basel she focused on the expression of specific immunologically relevant proteins (of class II MHC family), trying to answer the question of what controlled the sequential expression of proteins at a particular stage in B cell lineage development. Her specific scientific interest was the analysis of long-range control of gene expression in particular, before it was expressed at the mRNA or protein level, i.e. at the chromatin level.

Susan entered into a collaboration with Gill Wu, mapping the mouse immunoglobulin λ-locus, using the long-range gene mapping technique that she set up with Michael Steinmetz.

Upon completion of her work at the BII she moved to the Molecular Immunology Department of the MRC, Mill Hill, London.

Conference on the Mechanisms of B Cell Neoplasia, 1985

QR1985_16 BII

A workshop on the Mechanisms of B Cell Neoplasia, organized by Fritz Melchers and Michael Potter, was held at the institute from January 7th to 9th, 1985. This meeting brought together investiga-

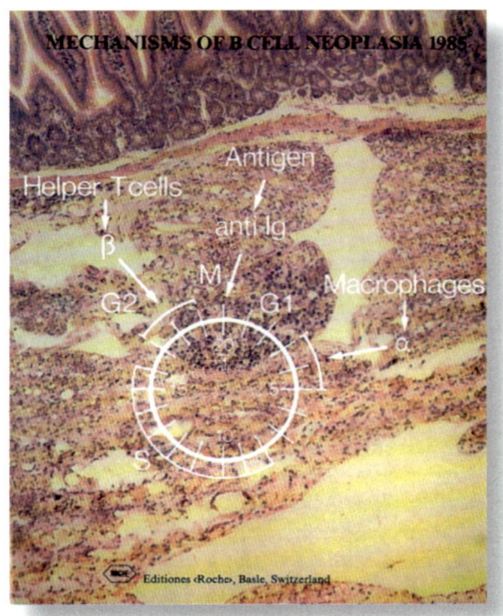

tors studying the growth and development of normal B cells, the characterization, pathogenesis and molecular genetics of B cell neoplasms, the relationship of immunoglobulin genes and oncogenes in chromosomal translocations, and the induction of neoplasms by infection or transfection with viruses carrying such oncogenes.

The conference was divided into 3 sessions:

- Cell cycle and its regulation and deregulation
- Progression models for deregulation of controls
- Role of viruses in B cell neoplasia, transfection, transgenic mice

Workshop on the Role of IL-2 in B Cell Physiology, 1985

A workshop on the role of IL-2 in B cell physiology was held at the institute on October 14th and 15th, 1985. Many investigators had reported that IL-2 plays a prominent role in B cell growth and differentiation. Although this conclusion had been elevated to the level of scientific dogma, an increasing number of reports to the contrary suggested that a closer look at the question might be in order. The workshop included investigators supporting the majority opinion as well as those having the opposing view [QR1985_17].

The proponents thought that mitogen preactivation of B cells was required to elicit responsiveness to IL-2. The arguments forwarded by the opponents concerned the caveat that a small proportion of non-B IL-2-responsive cells could mediate indirectly an effect on B cells. All conditions resulting in B cell populations responsive to IL-2 were also demonstrably contaminated with 1–10% T cells. On closing, neither protagonists nor opponents had moved from their original positions.

QR1985_17 BII

Treasure Trove 1985
The database contains documents related to the BII in a broader context (lists, series of photographs, etc.).

QR1985_treasure BII

The Year 1986

Michael Steinmetz, a permanent member of the BII, accepted an offer from Roche to become head of the Roche Biology Department. This marked an era of closer collaboration with Roche: Jürgen Drews, in his double function as head of Pharma Research and head of Roche Corporate Research, tried to attract BII members to join Roche, but without interfering with BII activities. Werner Haas, John Stocker, Michael Steinmetz and Zlatko Dembic accepted the call. Theo Staehelin had gone to Roche a decade earlier. BII members became involved in the TNF project. Further, a major event was to open the reconstructed institute to the Basel public. Part of this open day was a theater play performed by the members of the BII: "La Notte della Battaglia". The Chernobyl disaster caused major concern at the institute. An EMBO course on the MHC (with practical laboratory work) was organized, as well as a major workshop on tolerance. Sensitized by the fire (with no casualties), the animal committee considered improvements on the use of animals.

New Head of Roche Pharmaceutical Research

There were several changes that directly influenced the relationship of the BII with Roche management. Jürgen Drews became head of Pharma Research (1985) and head of Roche Corporate Research (1986). He fully understood the aim of the BII and helped to defend its independence, wherever and whenever needed.

Jürgen Drews regularly visited the institute, and a very cordial relationship developed with its director, Fritz Melchers, and with the permanent members. When Werner Haas' work contract at the BII terminated, after several prolongations, Drews offered Haas a "special" position in the Roche headquarters in which Haas was to evaluate critically the decision-making of Drews' office. This was a unique constellation, and Werner Haas thoroughly enjoyed the role of the King's fool and jester. Drews retired in 1998.

Michael Steinmetz, Permanent Member, Leaves for Roche, 1986

Michael Steinmetz made a profound impact on the BII, but as the restrictions of the size of research groups were seriously limiting his horizons, he accepted an offer from Roche Basel to become head of the Roche Biology Department. To recapitulate, Michael

Arrivals 1986 (17)
Jochem Alsenz, Steven Bauer, Christoph Berger, Una Chen, Akira Kudo, John Lambris, Harald Prahl, Robert Pytela, Eddy Roosnek, Richard Scheuermann, Joseph Schwager, Maria Luisa Sensi, Paschalis Sideras, Karsten Skjoedt, Uwe Staerz, Olli Vainio, Judy Ways.

Came and Left in the Same Year (2)
Ellen Hsu, Suzanne Kennedy-Stoskopf.

Leavers 1986 (9)
Zlatko Dembic, Michael Julius, John Kearney, Tomas Leanderson, Janet McCarty, Masayuki Miyasaka, Lucia Mori, Nobuo Sakaguchi, Michael Steinmetz.

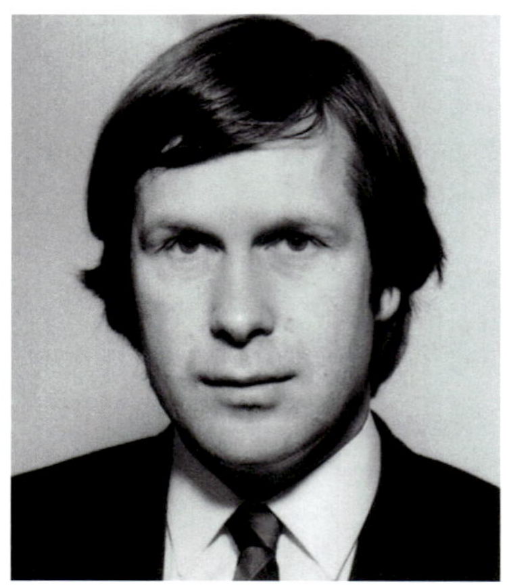

Michael Steinmetz

received his academic education in chemistry at the University of Hamburg, and before joining the BII he held academic positions at the University of Munich and the California Institute of Technology [QR1986_01]. His research focused primarily on histone/DNA interactions, antibody genes, genes of the MHC and the structure and function of TCR genes. He published dozens of scientific papers in leading journals, such as *Nature*, *Science*, *Cell* and *PNAS*.

Tumor Necrosis Factor and Cachectin

Decades ago a soluble product of lymphocytes and macrophages was identified that caused the lysis of certain types of cells, including tumor cells. Soon it was discovered that cachectin, a protein known to cause fever and wasting in tumor patients, was identical to this factor. In hindsight, the misconceived name "tumor necrosis factor" (TNF) refers to a group of proteins with mostly inflammatory functions. Later the cell membrane structures responsible for binding TNF molecules were identified and named TNF receptors.

While TNF and its receptors provided many interesting tools to basic biology researchers for studying the signaling pathways of host defense, they soon became also a drug target for pharmaceutical research and a way to establish the role of TNF in human diseases. A race began to develop new pharmaceuticals that eventually led to new medicines against recalcitrant inflammatory conditions such as rheumatoid arthritis (RA) and other autoimmune diseases. In addition, it was hoped to develop therapies against widespread human diseases such as atherosclerosis, osteoporosis, allograft rejection and cancer.

Involvement of BII Members and Former BII Members in the TNF Project

Genentech scientists had cloned TNF-α in 1985 at a time when Genentech was still independent. Michael Steinmetz, who moved from the BII to Roche, became the head of the Biology Central Research Unit of Roche. He gave the TNF project his full support, despite the fact that no therapeutic use was yet in sight.

Scientists at Roche (Hansruedi Lötscher and Werner Lesslauer) and former BII members (Manfred Brockhaus and Zlatko Dembic) purified and cloned the first 2 TNF-α receptors, later called CD120a and CD120b, and participated in the study of their biological functions (Lucia Mori). André Traunecker at the BII was the first to suggest an artificial receptor construct, and indeed a

QR1986_01 BII

joint Roche-BII project began with the help of Klaus Karjalainen. The resulting product became the first anti-TNF-α used in a clinical trial, where it turned out to be a strikingly effective medicine to help RA patients [QR1986_02].

Nevertheless, Roche management decided to terminate the project based on market considerations. The clinical scientist responsible for the RA project joined another company and developed the anti-TNF-α antibody Humira for the same indications, RA and inflammatory bowel diseases. It has a shared market volume of above USD 10 billion per year, together with several other anti-TNF-α agents. It is fair to say that the anti-TNF-α medicines were the greatest therapeutic innovation in rheumatic disease for decades. In the QR code, Manfred Brockhaus describes the difficult course of developing this drug at Roche. His account sheds light not only on the fruitful interactions between BII members and Roche scientists, and on the fact that Roche attracted first-class scientists from the BII, but also that Roche failed to bring a powerful immunology product to the market because of incorrect business predictions.

Zlatko Dembic to Roche, and Then to Norway

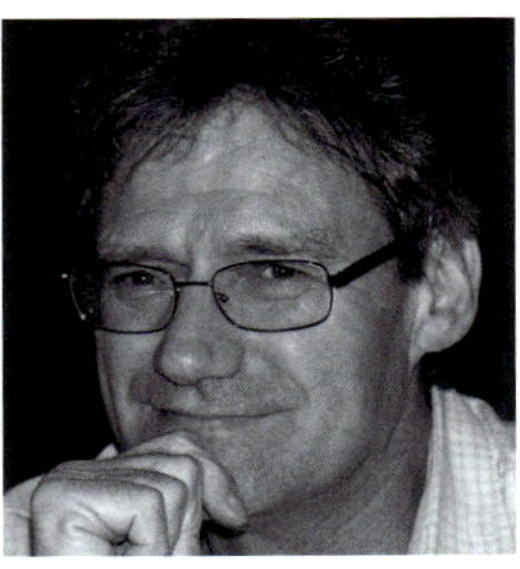

Zlatko Dembic

Zlatko Dembic, upon completing his contract at the BII, received an offer from Roche to take up a position as "senior scientist" with the assignment to develop a project related to molecular biology of cytokine receptors. Several other former BII members were already at Roche, and Zlatko initiated collaborations with Manfred Brockhaus, Michael Steinmetz, Werner Haas and others. His work on molecular cloning and expression of human IFN-γ receptor (published in *Cell*) and his work showing that 2 human TNF receptors have similar extracellular but distinct intracellular domain sequences (published in *Cytokine*) established his reputation as a scientist who could provide important input into pharmaceutical research.

QR1986_02 BII

During his Roche time – where Zlatko became a group leader – he continued collaborating with BII members, especially with Harald von Boehmer, Charles Mackay and Yasushi Uematsu.

In [QR1986_03] a list of his publications is provided – some of which became highly influential. In his future career he continued publishing in *Cell*, *Nature*, *PNAS*, *Blood*, and, last but not least, in the *Scandinavian Journal of Immunology,* of which he became Editor-in-Chief. In addition, a number of documents and photographs are linked to the QR code.

QR1986_03 BII

The highlights of Zlatko's work at the BII were: (i) characterization of TCR genes, (ii) identifying the chromosomal location of TCR α-chain gene in mice, (iii) identification of the function of the CD8 coreceptor molecule, (iv) discovery of the TCR β-chain gene enhancer.

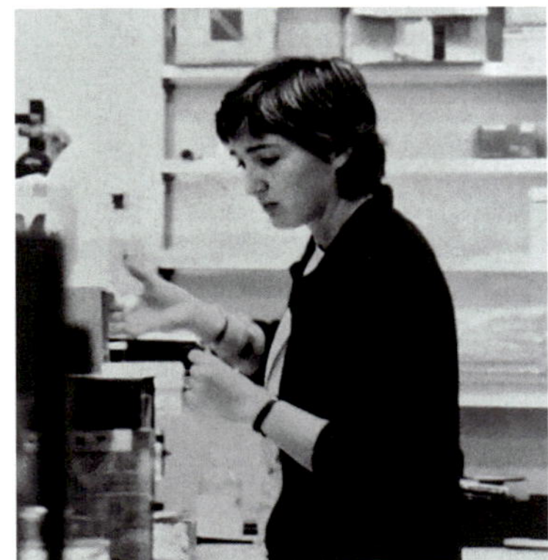

Lucia Mori

Lucia Mori and Her Studies on T Cell Receptors

In 1985, Lucia was among the young scientists who joined the large group of Michael Steinmetz, attracted by the molecular work on TCRs, when only a few such genes were known. The atmosphere of the Lab 012 was of great excitement in performing novel TCR gene transfer experiments. By cloning the TCR genes of the putative "T suppressor cells" Lucia convincingly showed that the TCR could not be involved in "antigen-specific suppression". When Michael Steinmetz became director of ZFE/Bio, Lucia joined his Department at Roche where she established a new experimental model to investigate the role of TCR genes in the induction of autoimmunity. From 1994, at the Department of Biomedicine of the Basel University Hospital, alongside Gennaro De Libero, her husband, she decisively contributed to the discovery of self-metabolites stimulating human TCR γδ cells, and of self-lipid antigens stimulating TCR αβ cells, including natural killer T cells. From 2010 to 2016 she was head of a research group at the Singapore Immunology Network, Agency for Science, Technology and Research (A*STAR) in Singapore, where her studies focused on the TCR repertoire of human innate-like T cells. Back to Basel, she became involved in translational immunology projects exploiting the unique properties of innate-like T cells.

Masayuki Miyasaka and Lymphocyte Circulation

Masayuki Miyasaka worked at the BII for 6 years (1981–1986), and upon completion of his appointment he returned to Japan to become a "principal investigator" at the Department of Immunology, Tokyo Metropolitan Institute of Medical Sciences [QR1986_04]. His research in Basel was geared towards studying lymphocyte migration in experiments that were performed in Zdenek Trnka's group. Masa met Zdenek at the 4th International Congress of Immunology in Paris (1980), flew to Basel for an interview and received an offer on the spot. Less than a year later he joined the BII and became a pillar of Trnka's research activity. His relationship with Zdenek and his wife Eva lasted long beyond his time at the BII.

Back in Japan – with his experience of making monoclonal antibodies – his group succeeded in generating monoclonal antibodies against the human IL-2 receptor β-chain (*PNAS*, 1989) and cloned its gene (*Science*, 1989).

In the QR code a description of Masa's continuing career is outlined, especially his success in establishing a number of novel monoclonal antibodies against rat adhesion molecules. Masa's career continued in Osaka (as a full professor at Osaka University Medical School) until his retirement in 2012.

The QR code also details his function as president of the Japanese Society for Immunology and his role as Secretary-General of the 14th International Congress of Immunology in Kobe (2010); besides that, his collaboration (as a visiting professor at University of Turku, Finland) with his long-term colleagues Sirpa Jalkanen and Marko Salmi is mentioned.

After 12 Years in Basel Michael Julius Accepted an Appointment in Montreal

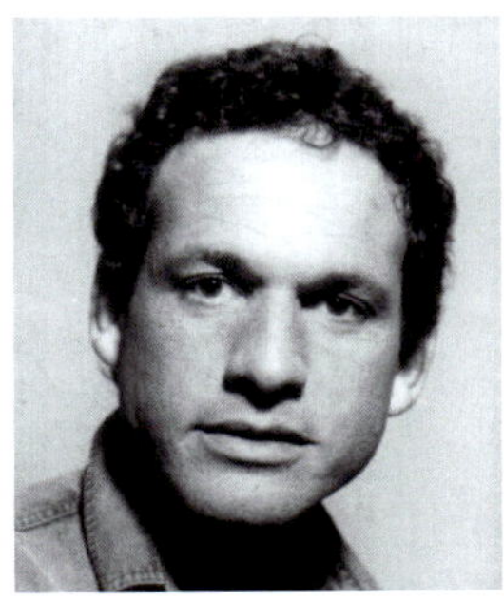

Michael Julius

Michael came from Stanford University just at the right time (1975) to be a prime contributor to the intense and energetic atmosphere of the BII. He became one of the pillars of the institute: his move to Montreal was a great leap for him but a loss for the BII. At McGill University in Montreal, he assumed an associate professorship in the Department of Microbiology and Immunology. A few years later he received a chair of the Department of Immunology at the University of Toronto [QR1986_05]. Under his stewardship the department achieved special ranking as the "pre-eminent academic immunology initiative in Canada". Throughout his career his work was geared towards understanding the biochemistry of lymphocyte activation, and the cellular and molecular interactions culminating in protective immunity. Although in Basel he only focused on "basic research" issues, in Canada he developed an interest in autoimmune diseases and illnesses resulting from a dysregulated immune system. Besides his scientific and administrative activities, he became an editor of the highly cited Seminars in Immunology.

QR1986_05 BII

Members Move to Sweden, the USA and Japan

QR1986_06 BII

Besides the above-mentioned scientists, several members left the BII to continue careers in Lund (Sweden), Birmingham (Alabama, USA) and Kumamoto (Japan) [QR1986_06]. Tomas Leanderson

Professor Werner Arber
Dr. David Baltimore
Professor Baruj Benacerraf
Professor Paul Berg
Professor W. Boguth
Professor Valentin Bonifas
Dr. Sydney Brenner
Dr. T. Brunner
Dr. Jean-Charles Cerottini
Professor H. Cottier
Dr. R. Dulbecco
Professor Gerald Edelman
Professor Manfred Eigen
Professor W. Gehring
Dr. Fritz Gerber
Dr. René von Graffenried
Professor François Gros
Professor A. Haessig
Professor Bernhard Hirt
Professor Albert Huerlimann
Dr. John Humphrey
Professor Karl Illmensee
Professor Henri Isliker
Professor François Jacob
Professor Niels K. Jerne
Professor Robert Keller
Professor Eduard Kellenberger
Sir John Kendrew
Professor J. Lindenmann
Professor H. Loeffler
Dr. S.F. Luria
Professor Ole Maaloe
Professor P.A. Miescher
Professor N. Avrion Mitchison
Professor G.J.V. Nossal
Professor Lennart Philipson
Professor Dr. A. Pletscher
Dr. Guido Richterich
Professor Robert Schwyzer
Professor Gottfried Schatz
Dr. M. Sela
Professor E. Sorkin
Professor Gunther Stent
Professor Alfred Tissieres
Professor P. Vassalli
Professor J.D. Watson
Professor A. de Weck
Professor Charles Weissmann
Dr. O. Westphal
Dr. Rolf M. Zinkernagel

A small selection of the participants

became a lecturer in molecular immunology and was appointed professor of Immunology at Lund University. He became president and CEO of Active Biotech in Lund. His last project completed at the BII was on characterization of activities inducing polyclonal maturation of activated B lymphocytes to immunoglobulin secretion. Nobuo Sakaguchi became professor of Immunology at the Department of Immunology of the Kumamoto University, Japan. John Kearney became professor of Microbiology at the University of Alabama at Birmingham, Alabama. He is a recipient of the American Association of Immunologists career award.

Festivities on Completion of the BII Restoration

The reconstruction of the BII to its original glory was marked by a combination of various activities – from an official ceremony and concert to a theater production, a dinner and a party. For the institute it was such an important event that scientists from Switzerland and abroad were invited, and attendance was indeed remarkable.

Two days (Saturday and Sunday, April the 26th and 27th, 1986) were allotted to the festivities. The starting point was the Open House to commemorate the special occasion (*Tag der offenen Tür*) for visitors from Basel and surroundings. Each laboratory pre-

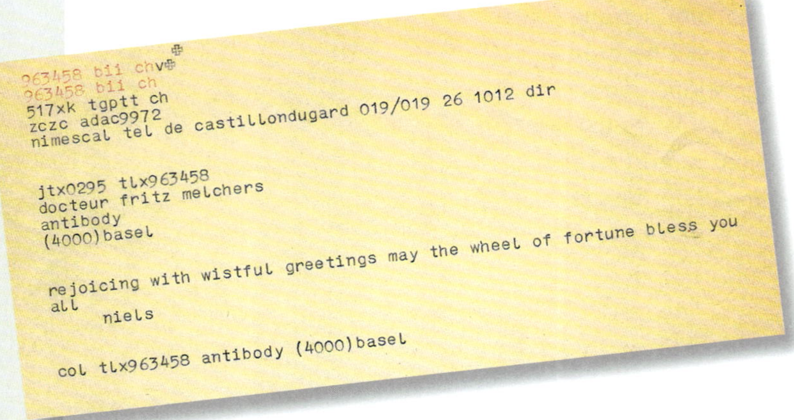

963458 bii ch
963458 bii ch
517xk tgptt ch
zczc adac9972
nimescal tel de castillondugard 019/019 26 1012 dir

jtx0295 tlx963458
docteur fritz melchers
antibody
(4000)basel

rejoicing with wistful greetings may the wheel of fortune bless you
all
niels

col tlx963458 antibody (4000)basel

Niels Jerne sent a cable from Castillon

Basel Institut für Immunologie
Grenzacherstrasse 487

Tag der offenen Tür

Samstag, 26. April 1986
von 9 bis 16 Uhr

Jedermann
ist herzlich eingeladen

Wir bitten die Besucher, das öffentliche Verkehrsmittel (Buslinie 31, Haltestelle Allmendstrasse) zu benützen, weil keine Parkplätze in der Nähe des Instituts vorhanden sind.

pared a poster or a short movie, directed at the layman, on the research work pursued. The next day the local press was very positive about the event.

Some 1,600 visitors came to look round the institute [QR1986_07]. They were interested in everything: instruments, animal facilities, isotope laboratory, mechanical workshop and of course video clips from the Nobel ceremony of Niels Jerne and Georges Köhler.

On Sunday April 27th, the celebrations started with a concert of works by Johannes Brahms (1833–1897) given by the soloists Anne-Sophie Mutter and Gérard Wyss. The program included the sonata in A major, op. 100, and the sonata in D minor, op. 108.

QR1986_07 BII

KONZERT

zur Feier der Wiederherstellung des Basel Instituts
für Immunologie

Solisten:
Anne-Sophie Mutter – Violine
Gérard Wyss – Klavier

PROGRAMM

Johannes Brahms
1833–1897

Sonate A-dur
für Klavier und Violine, op. 100
Allegro amabile /
Andante tranquillo /
Allegretto grazioso (quasi andante)

Sonate d-moll
für Klavier und Violine, op. 108
Allegro / Adagio / Un poco presto e
con sentimento / Presto agitato

Sonntag, 27. April 1986

Several speeches and addresses followed:
Fritz Gerber, president F. Hoffmann-La Roche and Zurich Insurance
Hans Rudolf Striebel, Regierungsratspräsident Basel-Stadt
Jürgen Drews, director Roche Research
Walter Gehring, Biozentrum Basel
Fritz Melchers, director BII

Thereafter there was a plentiful buffet dinner, followed by a party and the opera "La Notte della Battaglia", performed by the Basel Theater for the Arts.

BTA 6: "La Notte della Battaglia"

At the end of the Open House day, the members of the institute performed a theater play with the title "La Notte della Battaglia" [QR1986_08]. It took weeks to rehearse, and to prepare the stage and the costumes of the "artists".

QR1986_08 BII

Polly Matzinger, Billy Leiserson, Janet McCarthy, André Traunecker, Fritz Melchers and Monte Wetzel were among the performers.

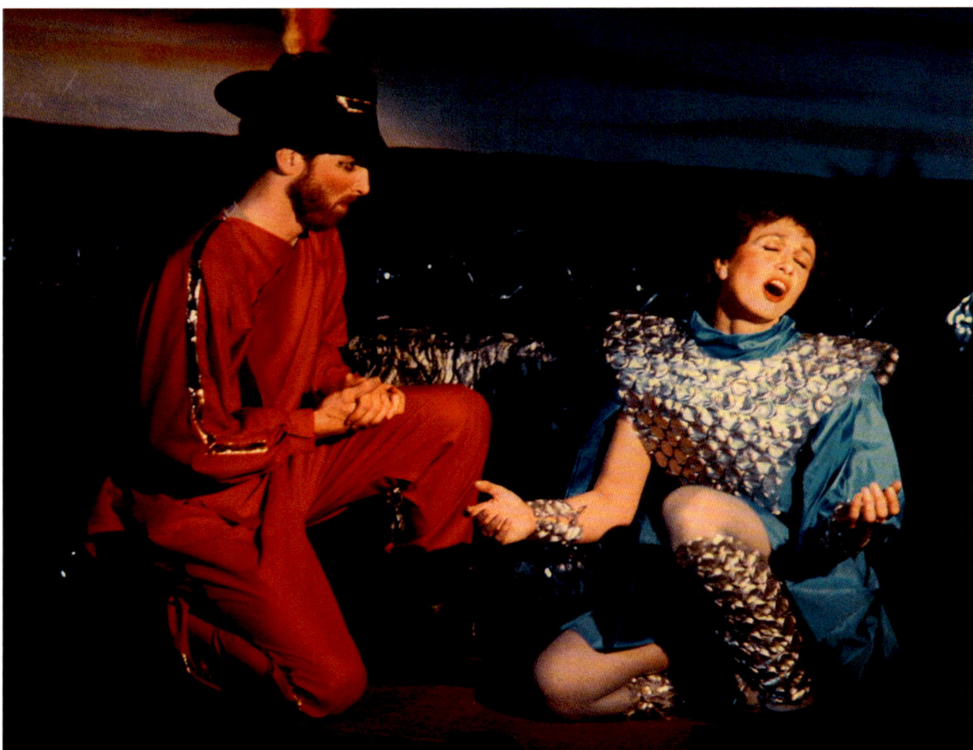
Billy Leiserson and Polly Matzinger

Monte Wetzel and the BTA

Monte succeeded in keeping a good balance between scientific and epicurean pleasures. His start at the BII coincided with the culmination of the restoration efforts after the fire, and it did not take long before he developed the same empathy and love that everyone felt for the institute. Monte became instrumental in preparing a theater play under the umbrella of the BTA to mark the reopening of the refurbished institute. When it became known that in addition to food, music, dancing and speeches, not just a few sketches but rather a grand spectacle might be "needed", the conception of the opera "La Notte della Battaglia" befell. Monte quickly recognized the importance and scale of these efforts and volunteered his theatrical and operatic talents, *be they as they may have been*, for "The Opera". Monte assumed the role of the Sage of T Cells, well traveled along the lymphatics of life and as a teacher of newly hatched and tweener thymocytes as they learned of themselves, and others. This role was demanding but very satisfying for Monte, and – as he stressed in follow-up interviews – he thoroughly enjoyed playing it in "The Opera". It is fair to say that his efforts were met with stunning acclaim and approval from an audience who appreciated the entire experience of "The Opera" and associated libations, perhaps the libations as much as "The Opera" itself.

Monte participated in several more productions with the same actors, often in farewell performances for members on their way to their "after-the-institute futures".

Monte assumed the role of the Sage of T Cells, well traveled along the lymphatics of life ...

The BTA and Self-Aggrandizement

An excerpt from the leaflet issued for the performance is given below. Irony, sarcasm and self-aggrandizement were intentional – people were mocking themselves.

"The Basel Theater for the Arts reaches new depths tonight in their presentation of LA NOTTE DELLA BATTAGLIA. This work was created for the reopening of the Basel Theater itself which was destroyed by fire sometime in the past. Tonight's performance demonstrates not only that the Theater is intact, but also that this versatile troupe retains its unique ability to portray science in the Arts. Although their last two productions, DIARY and REFLECTIONS, both received reviews, the critics wondered whether the BTA had lost its interest in science on stage. LA NOTTE emphatically dispels this notion. Cells, Receptors, Factors, Terrible Viruses, not only appear on stage, but also sing in a manner never before heard. THIS IS OPERA

The opera reflected the spirit of the BII – the immune system relies on diverse elements to cooperate to produce immunity – and diverse members at the BII often found cooperation to be the key – whether advancing their science or producing an opera or recovering from fire.

Of course, the best part of the opera was giving Anne-Sophie Mutter (then still in her teens) a backstage tour before the event!

C. Paige

MAGNIFICA. The critics are astounded. How could such a production be achieved? What drives this troupe to these levels? How can they live normal lives after what they have done? The director was asked recently 'Why? Why did you do it?' Unfortunately, his answer was erased. In a second interview the director was asked why he chose to use so many languages in LA NOTTE. He replied 'to appreciate Opera Magnifica, one requires a certain je ne sais quoi, waisch? Besides we perform at a level which cannot be described in words – the audience must be brought to that level – that's one reason we perform so late'.

The director was further asked to comment on the unique use of overtures in LA NOTTE: He replied, 'the lack of voice in overture has often disturbed me. Scholars the world over have searched and to date not one word of voice has been found in operatic overtures – in this respect they resemble the preludes to many well known arias which are also lacking vocal sections. I believe this startling discovery can be attributed to a pressure to publish which led to the premature presentation of many of these works. Sadly, they may also have had little to say – think of Wagner's Ring – 21 years of work and he could hardly think of anything to say – thousands of those little notes written around monosyllabic sounds. Or Verdi with his 'La' fixation. LA NOTTE represents the first serious attempt to overcome three hundred years of word deprivation'."

Chernobyl the Same Day

While the institute was happily celebrating the completion of the reconstruction after the devastating fire in 1985, some 2,000 km eastwards – in Chernobyl, Ukraine, a place difficult to find on a map – a devastating explosion and a nuclear meltdown occurred [QR1986_09]. The festivities at the BII absorbed the attention of the members to such an extent that they only realized what had happened from visitors that day. Luca Piali – later a member of the BII but at that time a 20-year-old student – remembers that he received news of the Chernobyl explosion at the very moment he entered the BII building. For Luca the two events remained forever intermixed, imprinted on his memory as a reminder of the transitoriness of life.

QR1986_09 BII

Another Fire in the Basel Area

On November 1st, 1986, a fire broke out in an agrochemical warehouse of a Sandoz factory in the Schweizerhalle industrial zone on the outskirts of Basel. As fire fighters battled the blaze, around 20 tons of insecticides, fungicides and herbicides leaked out into the river Rhine. It turned into a major environmental disaster which was followed by an unprecedented decontamination of the Rhine. At the time of writing, the Rhine in the Basel area is one of the cleanest rivers in Europe.

Polly, Mel and the Model of "Danger"

The narrator of this volume explicitly asked Polly about the use of the description "clever bunny". Although she did not object, a doubt remains: would one look for some distinct attribute when referring to a "male" rather than a "female"?

Instead of analyzing the pros and cons, here is a comparison of two very different and still very similar scientists – one is "macho male", and the other is a "refined female": Mel Cohn and Polly Matzinger. As mentioned in the chapter for 1977, Mel started a series of seminars at the BII to promote discussion on any interesting issue in immunology (mainly, of course, on two-signal-theory). Polly arrived some 10 years later, and in a very similar extrovert fashion induced discussions on any interesting issue (mainly of course on tolerance). Both Polly and Mel liked and provoked disagreement, and tried to win the debate.

Both Polly and Mel were available at any time to discuss anything. Polly's Tolerance Workshop with its three-volume transcript is a phenomenal document of such an exercise. Polly's teaching abilities became known to all, especially to the participants of the Summer Schools in Czechoslovakia. Polly counteracted male chauvinism by being cleverer and more alert than any male counterpart. Once she was accused of being a narcissist, and instead of denying it she said, "Everyone who loves to see his name on a publication is a narcissist" [QR1986_10].

The Danger Model – A Preview

In the meantime Polly Matzinger developed a model of "danger", influencing a generation of young immunologists. This model is described in the 1994 chapter, and here, as a "preview", a short synopsis is given: the immune system does not distinguish between self and nonself, but discriminates between "dangerous" and "safe" by recognition of pathogens or alarm signals from injured or stressed cells and tissues. When tissue cells are distressed because of injury, infection or oncogenic transformation, they start

QR1986_10 BII

to secrete or express on their surface so-called "danger signals". Such signals are also released to extracellular space in the case that a stressed cell dies by necrosis or pyroptosis (as opposed to apoptosis, controlled cell death). "Danger signals" include DNA, RNA, heat shock proteins, hyaluronic acid, serum amyloid A protein, ATP, uric acid and also cytokines like interferon-α, interleukin-1β, CD40L and so on.

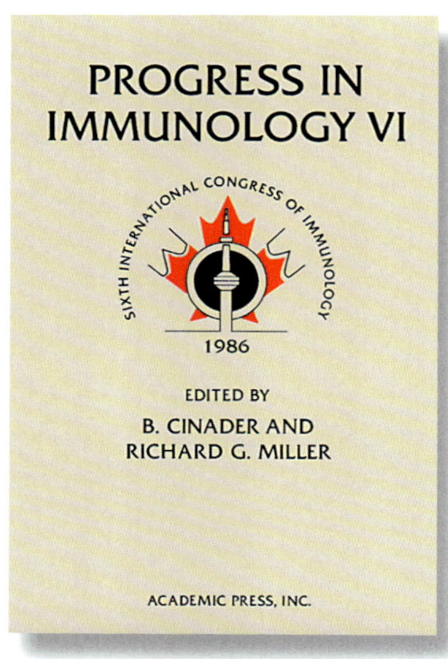

6th International Congress of Immunology in Toronto, 1986

Similarly to all previous International Congresses of Immunology (which started in 1971), the 6th International Congress of Immunology in Toronto was an interesting event for the mere fact that the first major party for the "alumni" of the BII took place there. People who had once worked at the BII wanted to meet up and chat, as if they were in the courtyard of the institute [QR1986_11].

Institute members gave 7 major presentations:

A. Takeda — "Variation of LFA-1 structure which reflects lymphocyte differentiation"
M. Miyasaka — "Lymphocyte emigration from the thymus"
W.R. Hein — "Monoclonal antibodies to sheep hemopoietic cells"
J.F. Kearney — "Idiotype-directed interactions during B cell ontogeny"
H. von Boehmer — "Ontogeny of T cell receptors for antigen"
G.E. Wu — "Development of the VH repertoire in mouse B cell colonies"
L. Du Pasquier — "Ontogeny of the immune system in *Xenopus*"

EMBO Practical Course on "Evolution and the MHC", 1986

QR1986_11 BII

QR1986_12 BII

At this course, Jim Kaufman, Martin Flajnik and Louis Du Pasquier organized practical laboratory work for the 18 students [QR1986_12]. It involved molecular and functional approaches designed to identify and define various aspects related to the mammalian MHC in the amphibian *Xenopus*, the cyclostome *Petromyzon*, the tunicate *Botryllus* and the sponge *Ephydatia*.

The practical work covered, among other things, immunoprecipitation and DNA cross-hybridization. Supporting lectures and discussions concerned the definition and evolution of the MHC, the immunoglobulin superfamily and their relationships to other aspects of evolution and development.

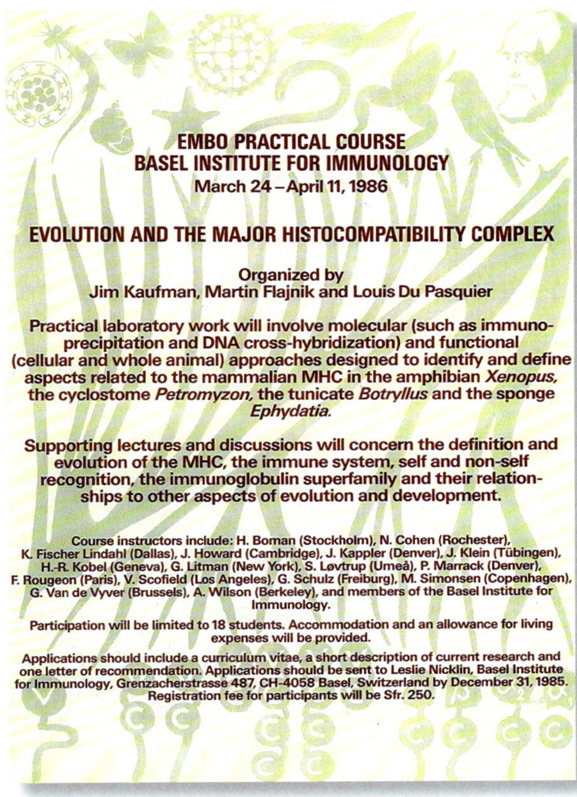
EMBO PRACTICAL COURSE
BASEL INSTITUTE FOR IMMUNOLOGY
March 24 – April 11, 1986
EVOLUTION AND THE MAJOR HISTOCOMPATIBILITY COMPLEX
Organized by
Jim Kaufman, Martin Flajnik and Louis Du Pasquier
Practical laboratory work will involve molecular (such as immunoprecipitation and DNA cross-hybridization) and functional (cellular and whole animal) approaches designed to identify and define aspects related to the mammalian MHC in the amphibian *Xenopus*, the cyclostome *Petromyzon*, the tunicate *Botryllus* and the sponge *Ephydatia*.
Supporting lectures and discussions will concern the definition and evolution of the MHC, the immune system, self and non-self recognition, the immunoglobulin superfamily and their relationships to other aspects of evolution and development.
Course instructors include: H. Boman (Stockholm), N. Cohen (Rochester), K. Fischer Lindahl (Dallas), J. Howard (Cambridge), J. Kappler (Denver), J. Klein (Tübingen), H.-R. Kobel (Geneva), G. Litman (New York), S. Løvtrup (Umeå), P. Marrack (Denver), F. Rougeon (Paris), V. Scofield (Los Angeles), G. Schulz (Freiburg), M. Simonsen (Copenhagen), G. Van de Vyver (Brussels), A. Wilson (Berkeley), and members of the Basel Institute for Immunology.
Participation will be limited to 18 students. Accommodation and an allowance for living expenses will be provided.
Applications should include a curriculum vitae, a short description of current research and one letter of recommendation. Applications should be sent to Leslie Nicklin, Basel Institute for Immunology, Grenzacherstrasse 487, CH-4058 Basel, Switzerland by December 31, 1985.
Registration fee for participants will be Sfr. 250.

Besides the members of the BII, the course instructors were: N. Cohen, K. Fischer Lindahl, J. Howard, J. Kappler, J. Klein, H.-R. Kobel, G. Litman, S. Løvtrup, P. Marrack, F. Rougeon, V. Scofield, G. Schulz, M. Simonsen, G. van de Vyver and A. Wilson.

EMBO Workshop on "Tolerance, the Rules, the Strategies and the Mechanisms", 1986

A workshop on Immunological Tolerance, sponsored by EMBO, was held at the institute from October 20th to 25th, 1986. Polly Matzinger, Martin Flajnik, David Nemazee, Hans-Georg Rammensee, Ton Rolink and Brigitta Stockinger organized it [QR1986_13].

Presentations were short and discussions long, leading in several instances to the establishment of new collaborative interactions among the participants. At the outset of the meeting, Mel Cohn set two goals:

(1) to present the essence of as many experiments as possible and understand them as best possible;

(2) to refine the mechanism of the self/nonself discrimination.

QR1986_13 BII

The first goal was achieved in long hours discussing all relevant issues and experiments, ranging from philosophy and mathematical models of tolerance to whole animal research. The second goal was not achieved; nevertheless, an important viewpoint emerged, namely that there will not be one mechanism but several. Tolerance is not strictly mediated by deletion or suppression, or by networks, or by the availability of T cell help or lymphokines. The animal, like any intricate machine, has backup systems to prevent autodestruction by the immune system.

A sample of the program is given below:

M. Cohn	"Comments on the self/nonself discrimination"
R. Scollay	"Development of T lymphocytes"
F. Melchers	"Development of B lymphocytes"
N.R. Klinman	"Is the presence and persistence of Ag required for the induction and maintenance of tolerance?"
J. Robinson	"What cells present the antigen and where?"
P. Matzinger	"How do the cells react to tolerogen?"
M. Weigert	"Evidence for and against deletion of autoreactive cells"
M. Cohn	"Is T cell help involved in establishment of tolerance?"

The full program and list of participants are included in the QR code.

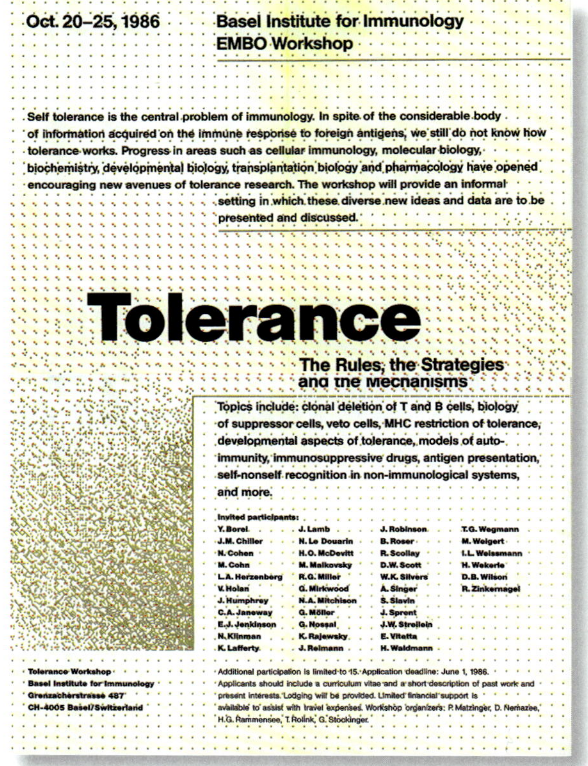

Coupling of Synthetic Antigens to Carriers for Antibody Production

A course on coupling of synthetic antigens to carriers for antibody production, sponsored by the Swiss Committee for Molecular Biology, was held at the institute in late October 1986. A series of 5 lectures was given during the course, and 5 experiments were performed in the laboratory. The course was organized and taught by Hansruedi Kiefer.

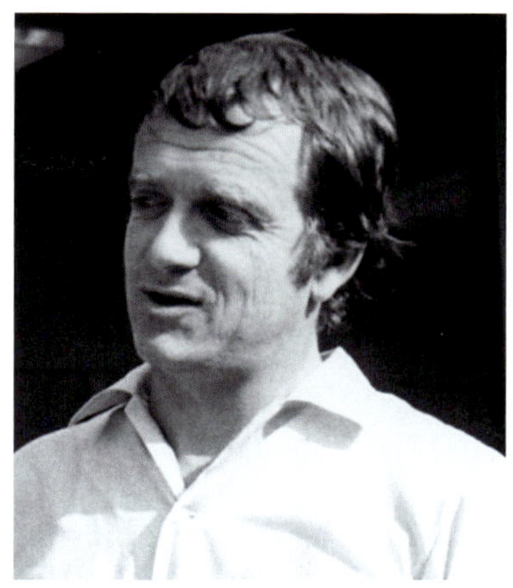

Hansruedi Kiefer

Animal Committee 1986

As described in Book 1, since 1983 a Committee on Ethics and Conditions of Experimentation with Animals had existed. The committee convened regularly, and its decisions were accepted routinely. This was clearly perceptible when new developments in scientific techniques could be of concern for society. It was also the case when new technologies were "imported" by newly arriving scientists at the BII. For most animal experimentation work, licenses from the Cantonal Government were required [QR1986_14].

An excerpt from the minutes of the 7th Meeting, held on December 11th, 1986, reads as follows: *"The application for a license to produce transgenic mice has been approved by governmental authorities. In license Nr. 25400 (immunization of rabbits) the number of animals that can be used should be increased from 100 to 300 per year. There is an increase in demands for polyclonal rabbit antisera by several scientists at the institute. Uwe Staerz asked for a modification of license Nr. 11011 (immunization of hamsters), allowing him to immunize Armenian as well as Syrian hamsters with murine cells.*

Jim Kaufman will have a visitor from Egypt who plans to bring snakes to the institute. Measures have to be taken to prepare appropriate cages (P. Balzarini). We will also contact a specialist at the Swiss Tropical Institute to gain advice. A request for a license allowing injection, bleeding and euthanasia of snakes has to be filed. Peter Thomann pointed out that we might need a certificate indicating that the snakes are laboratory bred and not captured wild reptiles."

That this precaution was necessary is shown by the case of Roland Jost, who was bitten by a snake and suffered a swollen arm for weeks (fortunately without consequences).

The chicken breeding in Oberfrick was found to be "inconspicuous" and should be kept that way. It was decided to replace the door in the rabbit-breeding unit in Rodersdorf by a more solid one, and install an alarm system.

Seminars by BII Members during the Meetings of the Advisory Board and the Board of Consultants

In the chronology of the scientific activities there were always two fixed dates: one for the Meeting of the Advisory Board and the other for the Meeting of the Board of Consultants. Each meeting also served to present some research highlights to the Boards, but also to the BII members. Listed below are contributions from several years up to 1986.

1977

B. Kindred, "Requirements for an immune response in athymic mice"
H. von Boehmer, "Tolerance and cell cooperation in bone marrow chimeras"
H. Cosenza, "A network of T and B cells in the immune response"

1978

T. Meo and H. Hengartner, "Chromosomes controlling antibody expression"
C. Brack and H. Sakano, "Structural genes for antibody"
W. Haas and H. von Boehmer, "T-killer lymphocytes"
M. Julius and A. Augustin, "T-helper lymphocytes"
A. Coutinho and S. Cammisuli, "B lymphocytes"

1979

C. Brack, "Organization of immunoglobulin κ light chain genes"
R. Maki, "Structure of immunoglobulin heavy chain genes"
S. Tonegawa, "Mode of somatic recombination of immunoglobulin genes"
L. Du Pasquier, "Introducing the immune system of *Xenopus*"
B. Blomberg, "The major histocompatibility complex and antibody diversity in natural and laboratory-made polyploid *Xenopus*"

1980

M. Schreier, "Functional characteristics of cloned helper T cells"
S. Fazekas de St. Groth, "The antibody repertoire, as reflected by monoclonal antibodies"
R. Maki, "The organization of genes for immunoglobulin heavy chains"
W. Roeder, "Structure and expression of immunoglobulin heavy chain genes"
G. Köhler, "Immunoglobulin M mutants"
C. Sidman, "Control and biosynthesis of IgM polypeptides"

1981

N. Iscove, "Burst promoting factor: evidence for action on early cells in several hemopoietic lineages"
C. Paige, "Analysis of B cell progenitors in fetal and adult mice"
J. Reynolds, "The production, migration, and fate of B lymphocytes"

1982

J.R.L. Pink, "Monoclonal antibodies against chicken lymphocyte differentiation antigens"

M. Leptin, "Monoclonal antibodies against IgM: their fine specificity and effect on B cell function"

S. Fazekas de St. Groth, "Automatic production of monoclonal antibodies"

1983

N. Iscove, "The multi-lineage hemopoietic growth factor from WEHI-3 cells"

R. Palacios, "Long-term culture of factor dependent murine B cell precursors"

G. Keller, "Generation of hemopoietic blast cell colonies *in vitro*"

1984

J. McCubrey, "Transfection of lymphoid cells of different lineages with TNP-specific Ig genes"

A. Iglesias, "*In vitro* modifications of Ig genes"

G. Köhler, "Transgenic mice carrying genes for heavy and light chains of monoclonal antibodies"

1985

J.F. Kaufman, "Evolution of the major histocompatibility complex"

K. Fischer Lindahl, "Hmt – a far-out member of the MHC"

M. Steinmetz, "Molecular organization of murine MHC genes"

1986

J. Schwager, "*Xenopus* immunoglobulin genes"

G.E. Wu, "Inheritance of VH gene usage in mice"

J.F. Kearney, "Idiotype-directed interactions and development of B cell diversity"

G. Keller, "Gene transfer as a means of analysing hemopoietic stem cell development *in vivo*"

H. Karasuyama, "Establishment of cell lines which constitutively secrete mouse IL-2 in large quantities using a cDNA expression vector"

J.D. Lambris, "Structural basis of C3 interactions with other complement components"

Research Categories in the Annual Report

1986 was the first fully functional year after the devastating fire. The Annual Report contained 146 reports, and they fall into 20 research categories (the grouping here and in all previous reports was done by Charley Steinberg). It shows a definite shift towards work on surface antigens and lymphokines, and also on complement components:

T cell receptor genes and products (9 reports)
Antibody diversity (6 reports)
Ig gene structure and rearrangement (12 reports)
MHC genes and products (12 reports)
Genetic recombination (2 reports)
Structure and synthesis of various surface antigens (8 reports)
Complement (10 reports)
Lymphokines and their receptors (8 reports)
Antigen processing (4 reports)
Lymphocyte activation (11 reports)
Helper T cells (4 reports)
Cytotoxic cells and lines (6 reports)
B cell differentiation (11 reports)
T cell differentiation (6 reports)
Hemopoietic cell differentiation (3 reports)
Infection, inflammation and serum proteins (4 reports)
Autoimmunity (8 reports)
Tolerance and self/nonself discrimination (10 reports)
Lymphocyte physiology (3 reports)
Methods and equipment (9 reports)

A Nobel Prize for Work on Nerve Growth Factor

Stanley Cohen and Rita Levi-Montalcini, friends of the BII, were awarded the Nobel Prize for Medicine 1986. They worked at Washington University in St. Louis in the 1950s, later they isolated nerve growth factor and went on to discover epidermal growth factor. Their research on cellular growth factors has proven fundamental to understanding the development of cancer and designing anticancer drugs.

Paul Sacher Celebrates His 80th Birthday

QR1986_15 BII

On 28th April, 1986, Paul Sacher, the conductor and patron of 20th century music, celebrated his 80th birthday with a concert of the Basel Chamber Orchestra that he had founded in 1926 [QR1986_15]. The program, conducted by Sacher himself, included some of his own commissions with soloists Mstislav Rostropovitch, Anne-

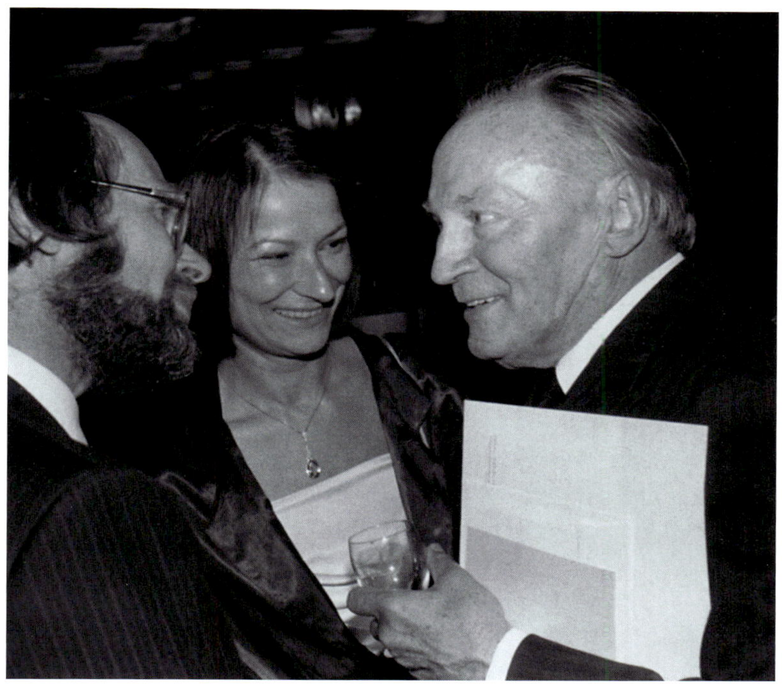

Paul Sacher with Ingrid and Hannes Westen

Sophie Mutter and Aurèle Nicolet. At dinner afterwards Paul Sacher sat surrounded by composers, such as Luciano Berio, Pierre Boulez, Elliott Carter, Henri Dutilleux and Witold Lutoslawski, with whom he maintained close personal ties. At the same time the official opening of the Paul Sacher Foundation for 20th Century Music was celebrated. Sacher had placed more than 200 commissions for musical scores. Those together with more than over 100 complete musical estates by composers from all over the world are now available for research to musicologists and musicians. The Foundation's statement of purpose reads as follows:

The Foundation shall serve to safeguard the musical estate of its founder and its other holdings in the fields of cultural, intellectual, art, and above all music history. It shall seek to complete and enlarge its archival inventory within the means at its command. With its own research facilities and employees, the Foundation shall care for its archival materials and make them accessible to the scholarly community. It is also empowered to grant research, publication, and similar commissions to outside persons. Its activities shall be international in scale.

Treasure Trove 1986
The database contains documents related to the BII in a broader context (lists, series of photographs, etc.).

QR1986_treasure BII

The Year 1987

Chris Paige followed a call to Canada. During his 8 years at the BII he decisively shaped the institute. He did so not only with his scientific achievements, but also as a stage director of the "Basel Theater for the Arts" and as a member of the Rescue Committee after the fire at the BII. In his honor a BTA performance, "Linear-B", was given on the new "Christopher J. Paige Memorial Stage". The institute was pleased to congratulate Alfred Pletscher on the anniversary of the creation of the "Zentrum für Lehre und Forschung", which Pletscher successfully headed for 10 years. Another celebrated event was the 20th anniversary of the "Roche Institute of Molecular Biology" in Nutley, N.J., USA. The most important event for the institute's reputation in science was the Nobel Prize awarded to Susumu Tonegawa.

Arrivals 1987 (11)
Lawrence D'Hoostelaere, Antonio de la Hera, Laura Lee Gill, Charles Mackay, Claude-Agnès Reynaud, Catherine Servis, Hans-Jürgen Thiesen, Alan Tunnacliffe, Judith Varner, R.C. von Borstel, Jean-Claude Weill.

Leavers 1987 (10)
Christoph Berger, Bjarne Bogen, Hajime Karasuyama, Susan McClure, Christopher Paige, Hans-Georg Rammensee, Marialuisa Sensi, Paschalis Sideras, Karsten Skjoedt, Akiko Takeda.

QR1987_01 BII

QR1987_02 BII

Jean-Claude Weill and Claude-Agnès Reynaud, from Paris, 1987

Jean-Claude Weill was one of the few members who were offered a permanent member position when joining the institute [QR1987_01]. Previously, only the founding members were in possession of a permanent contract from the start. Susumu Tonegawa became a permanent member once his achievements made it clear that the offer of a permanent member status was overdue. Georges Köhler received a permanent position upon returning from Cambridge.

The matter of "permanent" positions is dealt with in other sections of this book. The Orwellian issue of *all members being equal* was kept understated, in that nowhere in BII documents (Annual Reports or BII Booklets) was it mentioned who from the scientific staff was on a "permanent" and who on a "time-limited" contract. Here it suffices to say that Jean-Claude Weill received this offer as recognition of his high scientific standing, and probably because he would "not be available" by other means.

Claude-Agnès Reynaud joined his group as a member [QR1987_02]. Both Jean-Claude and Claude-Agnès remained at the BII for 5 years (1987–1991).

Prior to their arrival, Jean-Claude Weill and Claude-Agnès Reynaud were working on the gene rearrangement events in the chicken, with the major finding that gene conversion generates most of the chicken immunoglobulin light chain diversity. At the institute, Jean-Claude's team continued to work on the preimmune

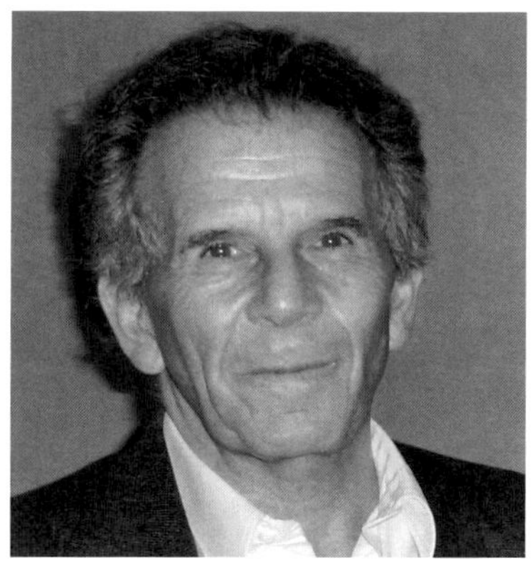

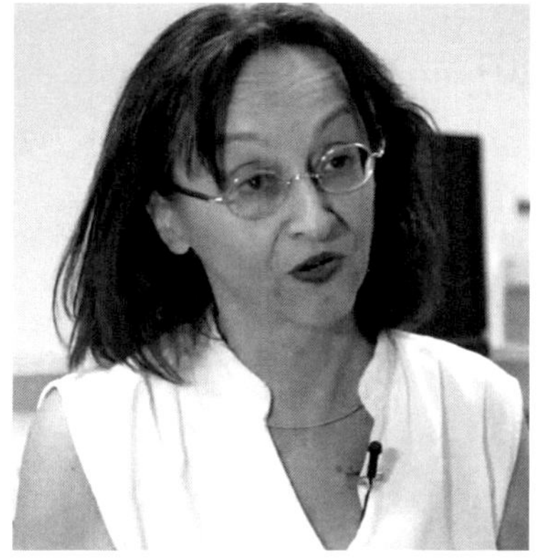

Jean-Claude Weill,
Claude-Agnès Reynaud

repertoire of the chicken, discovering a hyperconversion mechanism that is involved in these processes. They refined the work by introducing chicken Ig genes into mouse transgenic lines, revealing that Ig receptor genes and T cell antigen receptor genes rearrange through identical heptamer-nonamer recognition sequences. A similar enzymatic machinery performs these events in both types of lymphoid cells.

At the time of writing, Jean-Claude Weill and Claude-Agnès Reynaud are scientific codirectors of the Inserm Unit "Développement du système immunitaire" in Paris. Their work continued along the research lines of their BII achievements, extending it to studies of negative regulation of Ig gene rearrangement by transcriptional silencers.

Chris Paige Leaves for Canada, 1987

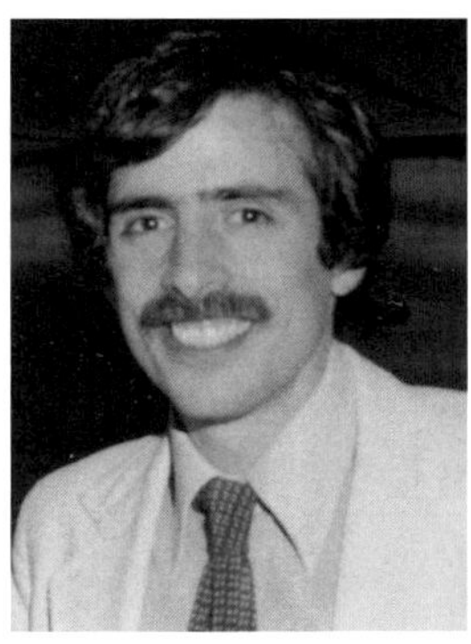

Chris Paige

Chris Paige worked at the BII from 1980 to 1987. He decisively shaped the life of the institute – not only through his achievements in experimental work, but also with two additional tasks: (a) as a stage director of the Basel Theater for the Arts, and (b) as a member of the Rescue Committee after the fire at the BII.

Chris received a PhD in Immunology at the Sloan-Kettering Division of Cornell University Graduate School of Medical Sciences in 1979. His early work with Paul Kincade shaped the research direction that he then pursued at the BII. It was work on colony-forming B cells, and on the fate of fetal and adult B cell progenitors. During the years at the BII, Chris published 33 papers (his first paper at the institute was with Susumu Tonegawa et al. in *Science* on immunoglobulin gene rearrangement in immature B cells).

On leaving Basel, Chris joined the Ontario Cancer Institute as a senior scientist. In 1990, he became the founding director of the

Arthritis and Autoimmunity Research Centre as well as director of Research at the Wellesley Hospital. His further outstanding career is outlined in [QR1987_03].

(a) Stage director: of 13 performances Chris Paige directed 5, and for several of them he wrote the script (jointly with others):

The Stem Cell Ballet (1981)
Reflections (1985) (for Georges Köhler)
Diary (1985) (for the departure of Norman Iscove)
La Notte della Battaglia (1986)
Susumuli, Prince de Bâle (1988)

Chris traveled from Toronto to Basel especially to direct the play "Susumuli, Prince de Bâle". At the last performance Chris was given a standing ovation and, as a present, a special folding chair inscribed "Stage Director".

(b) Chris' function on the Rescue Committee has already been mentioned; in this context it is worth noting that the ease and talent of directing a theater performance was also displayed in his work for the Rescue Committee. Without his perseverance and organizational talent in clearing a place to perform sterile work (not for experimentation but merely for reinoculation of growing cell lines) none of the precious cell lines would have survived.

BTA 7: World Premiere of "Linear-B" Performed by the BTA, Dedicated to Chris Paige

The tradition of performing a theater play continued after "La Notte della Battaglia", which had attracted considerable attention within and outside the institute. The new play was entitled "Linear-B" and was complete with *Lokalkolorit* connotations full of irony and sarcasm. It contained criticism and self-criticism, especially about the "self-aggrandizement" of some scientists. This was put in the mouth of the 19th century Russian mathematician Nicolai Lobachevski. The title itself (Linear-B) comes from Greek syllabic script (1450 BC) with the connotation of B lymphocytes [QR1987_04].

QR1987_03 BII

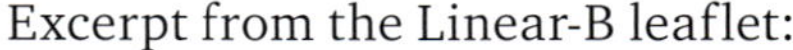

Excerpt from the Linear-B leaflet:

"The world premiere of a between-the-acts musical play in which all of the dialogue is between the lines, and which examines the cosmological basis of science. The Basel Theater for the Arts celebrates its 10th anniversary this year. With LA NOTTE DELLA BATTAGLIA (1986), the BTA reached the pinnacle of success, and as one critic said, 'There is no way now for the BTA to go but down'. The company of the BTA accepted the inexorable logic of this comment – it fired the direc-

QR1987_04 BII

THE PLOT

There is no plot. The entire play is a lecture by Professor emeritus Seymour B. Less, B.A., B.C.G.F., M.Sc., T.R.F., Ph.D., at the National Academy of the dwarf planet Linear-B. Prof. Less is presenting the results of his long-term, ongoing, inconclusive experiment to produce a transgenic human being, an odd species on the planet Earth. Like scientists everywhere, Prof. Less attempts to relieve the tedium of his ponderous lecture with slides. These slides are somewhat more animated than is customary.

Slide I shows how the gene is transfected. Three B-cells from Linear-B crash-land on the farm of Mr. Pagliucca and his pregnant wife in southern Italy. After many attempts to find a common language, they succeed in communicating in Linear-B. Mrs. Pagliucca is offered a "Gene & Tonic" to transfect the child she is carrying. The male descendants of the transfected child carry the transgene on their Y chromosomes, but it does not function. It needs to be activated. The B-cells seek out a descendent, now called Paige, in New York. Slide II shows how they feed a transacting factor to a gang of ferocious mosquitos, who in turn will transmit the factor to Paige by biting him. The remaining slides show the astounding talents conferred on Chris Paige by the activated gene.

tor, and this production of LINEAR-B is the result. It is an attempt to explore the depths of science. Here we see on the stage not science itself, but the co(s)mic forces that are the fundament of science.

LINEAR-B will be performed on the new 'Christopher J. Paige Memorial Stage'. The dedication speech was made by the famous mathematician and theatrical critic, N. Lobachevski: "One score minus ten years ago our mothers and fathers brought forth in this institute a new theatre, conceived without talent and dedicated to the proposition that none is really necessary. Now we are engaged in a great new performance, testing whether that theatre, or any theatre, so conceived and so dedicated, can long endure. We are met in a great auditorium of that theatre. We have come to dedicate its stage as a final memorial for those who here gave their memberships that that theatre might live. It is altogether fitting and proper that we should do this. But in a larger sense we cannot dedicate, we cannot consecrate, we cannot hallow this stage. The brave women and men, present and departed, who struggled here, have consecrated it far above our poor power to add or to detract. The world will little note nor long remember what we write here, but it can never forget what they did here. It is for those of us still present, rather, to be dedicated to the great task remaining before us – that from these honored departed we take increased devotion to that cause for which they here gave the last full measure of devotion – that we here highly resolve that these

Linear-B was brilliant – both in design and execution – the highlight of course was when my two leading ladies, Maria of the Ballet and Polly of the Opera, who, for various reasons, were not best of friends, embraced on stage – a BTA moment for the ages.

C. Paige

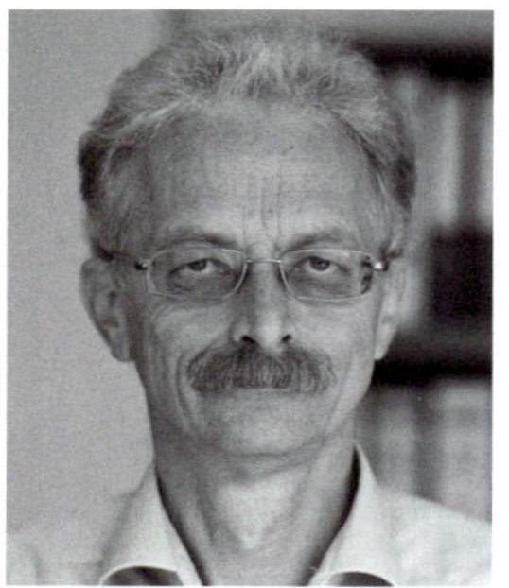

Hans-Georg Rammensee

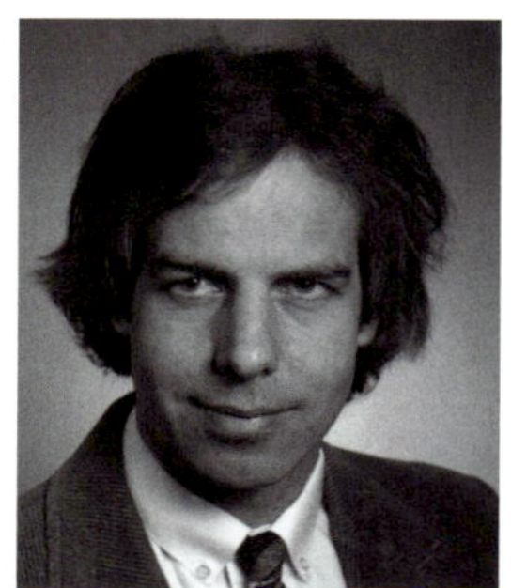

Bjarne Bogen

departed shall not have gone in vain, that this theatre, under its director, whoever he or she may be, shall have a new birth of mindless enthusiasm and that extravaganzas of the unmentionable, by the untalented, for the insensitive shall not perish from this institute'."

Hans-Georg Rammensee Leaves for Tübingen and Heidelberg

Hans-Georg Rammensee was offered a position by the Max Planck Institute in Tübingen as Head of the Immunology Unit. He moved some 6 years later to the German Cancer Institute in Heidelberg to form the new "Abteilung Tumorvirus-Immunologie". His years in Heidelberg were only an interim before he received an offer to return to Tübingen, not back to the Max Planck Institute but to head the Institute of Cell Biology of the University of Tübingen.

In the QR code [QR1987_05] his entire career including awards and prizes are described, and documents attached. The BII years were the years of his major discoveries related to peptide binding (deposition) into the groove of MHC molecules, which allowed a new interpretation of T cells recognizing the primary structure of antigens rather than their shape. Thus, the T cell epitope was clarified. During his time at the BII he published 15 papers.

Other Scientists Leave the BII

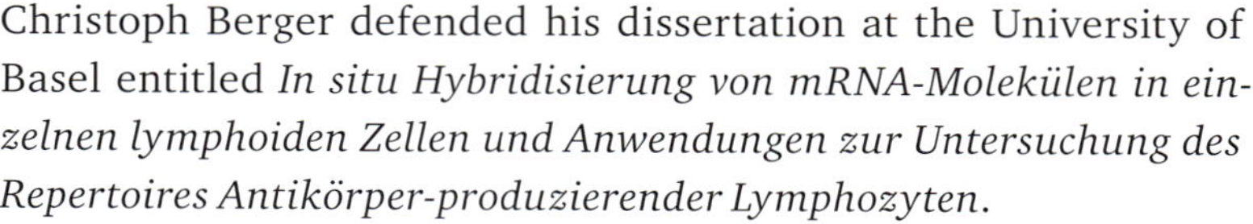

Christoph Berger defended his dissertation at the University of Basel entitled *In situ Hybridisierung von mRNA-Molekülen in einzelnen lymphoiden Zellen und Anwendungen zur Untersuchung des Repertoires Antikörper-produzierender Lymphozyten*.

QR1987_05 BII

Bjarne Bogen, a Norwegian immunologist, after spending several years at the BII, continued his career as a professor of Immunology at the University of Oslo.

QR1987_06 BII

Beside Christoph and Bjarne there were other scientists leaving the BII in the same year, like Hajime Karasuyama, Susan McClure, Marialuisa Sensi, Paschalis Sideras, Karsten Skjoedt and Akiko Takeda, and they are also cited in the QR code [QR1987_06].

The Roche Institute of Molecular Biology after 20 Years

QR1987_07 BII

Herbert Weissbach [QR1987_07], Roche Institute of Molecular Biology, Nutley, wrote the following report:

"The Roche Institute of Molecular Biology celebrated its 20th anniversary in 1987. It was a memorable occasion with many of our

former staff and members of the Board of Scientific Advisors participating in the two-day symposium. During that event, I couldn't help but to reminisce about those early days in 1967 when this 'experiment' was begun, and reflect on the past two decades. Initially, this chapter was going to concentrate only on the inter-relationship between the Institute and the Company. However, I realized that to fully appreciate the role and nature of this unique institute, it is necessary to understand how it came into being and the historical factors that set the foundation for where we are today. In going back to whatever records I could find, it became apparent that many of the facts and events are not recorded anywhere. Fortunately, there are still people here, especially Sidney Udenfriend and John Burns, who have aided me in filling in some of the 'holes', but much of the account is from my own memory and is obviously tempered by my personal views and reflections. There are only three of us, Udenfriend, Burns and myself who were intimately involved in the events in 1967 that led to the Roche Institute of Molecular Biology. At that time, I was a member of Udenfriend's laboratory at the National Institutes of Health (NIH) and Burns had recently become Vice President and Director of Research at Hoffmann-La Roche in Nutley. I should note that in the late '50s we all had been together in Bernard Brodie's laboratory at the NIH. In March 1967, Udenfriend told me of seeing…" (continued and extended in the above-mentioned QR note).

Herbert Weissbach also wrote about the Basel "sister" institute:

"Although I am in no position to speak for our sister institute, the Basel Institute for Immunology, I suspect that it faces a similar problem. The solution depends on an institute-company relationship that requires considerable effort by both partners. The institute must not only be respected by all for its scientific excellence, but should be sensitive to the research efforts of the company. This requires, where appropriate, for institute scientists to act as consultants, to participate in research collaborations and, in general, care about the company. The institute director and other senior scientists should act as bridges between the institute and scientists in other research areas. All of this can be done without sacrificing or violating the principles on which the institute functions as stated in the charter. If this is not done, the institute will slowly become isolated, and hostility surely will develop with other groups in the research division. However, Roche management must do their part also. They must believe and express openly their views that the institute is an integral part of the research centre, despite the fact that its immediate goals are different. Any doubt should be laid to rest. For reasons that now make little

sense to me, this remains a chronic problem that continually has to be addressed. Perhaps, even after 2 decades, there is a need for education in this area."

The 10th Anniversary of the Zentrum für Lehre und Forschung

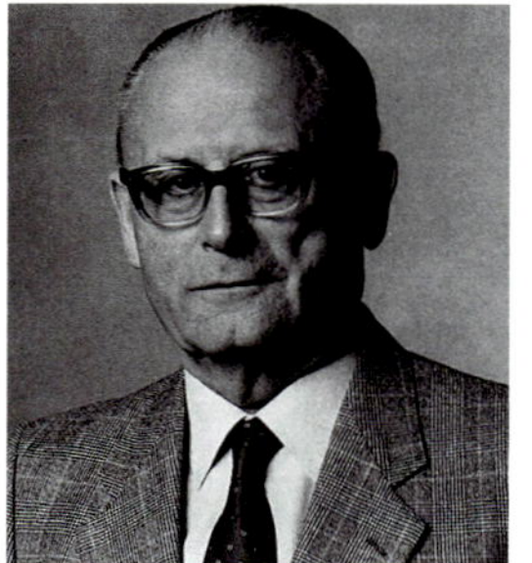

Alfred Pletscher

There was a special relationship between the BII and the Zentrum für Lehre und Forschung (ZLF). Alfred Pletscher, when he was still a powerful representative of pharma research in Roche, realized that medical institutions (hospitals and clinics) had different requirements than research institutes devoted to basic research, and he also realized that the research facilities of the medical research laboratories in Basel were scattered over too many small locations, often places that could not afford sophisticated instrumentation, and even if they could, the instruments would not be fully used by the isolated small work groups. Pletscher succeeded in acquiring

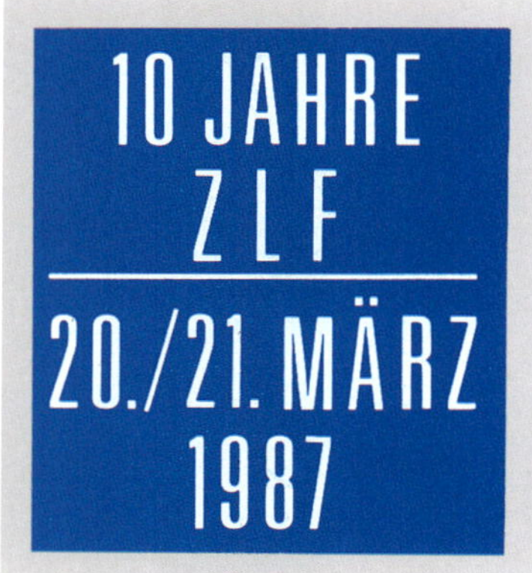

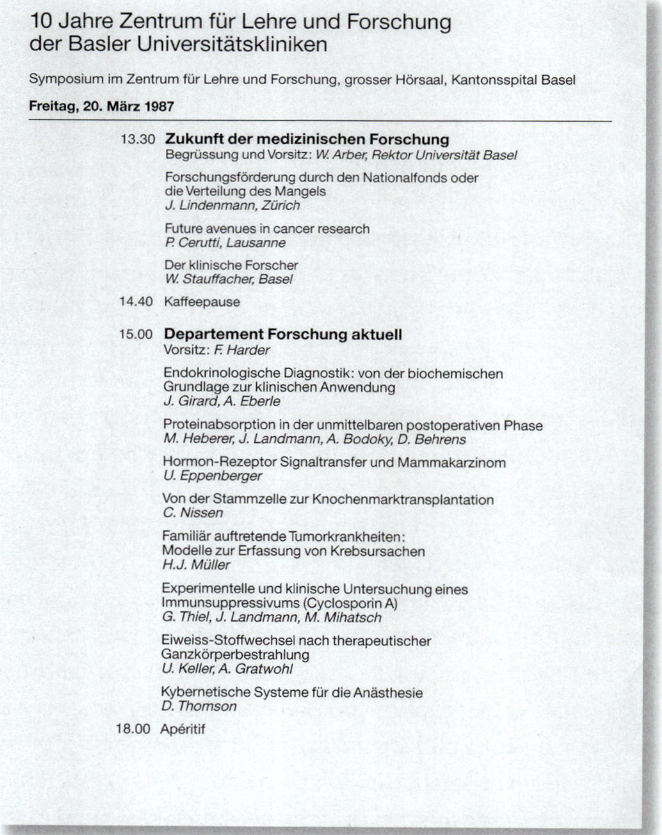

10 Jahre Zentrum für Lehre und Forschung
der Basler Universitätskliniken

Symposium im Zentrum für Lehre und Forschung, grosser Hörsaal, Kantonsspital Basel

Freitag, 20. März 1987

13.30 **Zukunft der medizinischen Forschung**
Begrüssung und Vorsitz: *W. Arber, Rektor Universität Basel*

Forschungsförderung durch den Nationalfonds oder die Verteilung des Mangels
J. Lindenmann, Zürich

Future avenues in cancer research
P. Cerutti, Lausanne

Der klinische Forscher
W. Stauffacher, Basel

14.40 Kaffeepause

15.00 **Departement Forschung aktuell**
Vorsitz: *F. Harder*

Endokrinologische Diagnostik: von der biochemischen Grundlage zur klinischen Anwendung
J. Girard, A. Eberle

Proteinabsorption in der unmittelbaren postoperativen Phase
M. Heberer, J. Landmann, A. Bodoky, D. Behrens

Hormon-Rezeptor Signaltransfer und Mammakarzinom
U. Eppenberger

Von der Stammzelle zur Knochenmarktransplantation
C. Nissen

Familiär auftretende Tumorkrankheiten: Modelle zur Erfassung von Krebsursachen
H.J. Müller

Experimentelle und klinische Untersuchung eines Immunsuppressivums (Cyclosporin A)
G. Thiel, J. Landmann, M. Mihatsch

Eiweiss-Stoffwechsel nach therapeutischer Ganzkörperbestrahlung
U. Keller, A. Gratwohl

Kybernetische Systeme für die Anästhesie
D. Thomson

18.00 Apéritif

money from industry, canton and private sponsors to create an institute in which all these small laboratories could unite, share state-of-the-art equipment and enjoy adequate laboratory conditions. This became the ZLF, and in 1987 it celebrated its 10th anniversary [QR1987_08].

Strictly speaking, this does not belong in a history of the BII, but in fact it does, because, due to Alfred Pletscher's exceptional personality, he is one of the "fathers" of the BII.

The Swiss National Science Foundation and Prof. Alfred Pletscher

Prof. Pletscher visited the BII regularly over the years, especially for all the interesting events held there. As he often said, for him the institute was an inspiration for much of his decision-making as president of the Swiss National Foundation (1980–1987). The BII did not have to apply for funds from the Swiss National Science Foundation but offered advice and expertise whenever needed. Pletscher was an important go-between for establishing scientific contacts between all the institutions with which he was involved [QR1987_09].

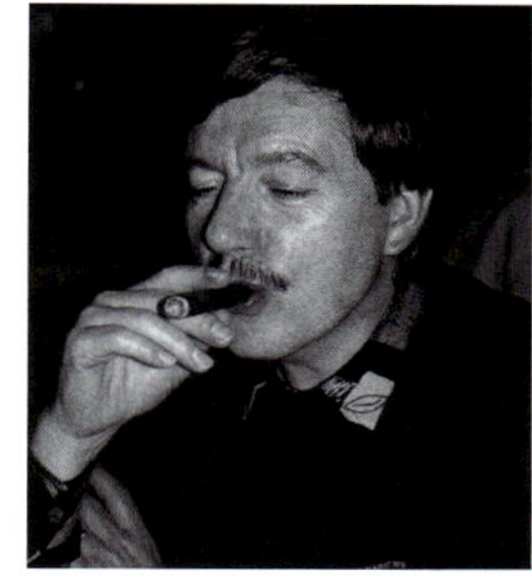

Toni Heinis

Additional Services and Facilities due to Retirements

Several services were introduced or reorganized, such as peptide synthesis headed by David Avila, and oligonucleotide synthesis supervised by Hansruedi Kiefer. Peter Balzarini was head of infrastructure at that time, Peter Thommen was head of the purchasing department, and Bert Temminck, Jerome Aarden and Randy Baron ran the computer facilities. The librarian, Zdena Joukl, retired and was replaced by Rachel Looser. Otto Kamber, head of the workshop for many years, also retired, and he was replaced by Toni Heinis [QR1987_10].

What Was Studied in 1987?

Although the diversity of projects at the BII was always broad, the focus remained on "specificity". This emphasis was never imposed on BII members, instead, scientists selected to join the institute (from the world-wide reservoir of applicants) well fitted the existing framework. The Annual Reports summarized the range of experimentation (see previous chapter), shown by the headings of the grouped reports. Below is another list, taken from the subhead-

ings of the Introduction to the 1987 Annual Report, which by somewhat different criteria – chosen by Fritz Melchers – provided an adequate overview of the development of BII research:

- The invasion of the immune system
- The preexisting repertoire of natural antibodies
- The repertoires of antigen-recognizing cells
- T cell-independent B cell stimulation – the rapid expansion of "natural" antigen-specific IgM antibodies
- The interactions of T cells with antigen on A cells: T cells do not see native antigen
- MHC polymorphism – one genetic basis for the immunological individuality of the host
- T cell stimulation
- Helper T cell-dependent B cell stimulation: how to make better-fitting antibodies and change their defence strategy
- How is an antigen accepted to be self, not foreign?
- The generation of an endless repertoire of lymphocytes
- B cell development
- T cell development
- Selection of α/β-expressing T cells in the thymus
- Tolerance – and how to break it

1987 Nobel Prize for Susumu Tonegawa

Susumu Tonegawa was awarded the Nobel Prize for Medicine in 1987 for his discovery of the genetic mechanism that produces antibody diversity [QR1987_11]. He describes the problem that he approached as follows:

"After I arrived in Basel, I initially attempted to continue the project of my days in Dulbecco's laboratory, namely, the transcriptional control of the simian virus 40 genes. However, I soon realized that this was not a subject that aroused great interest in an institute almost entirely staffed by immunologists, nor one that allowed me to take full advantage of my many talented colleagues. I therefore decided to learn immunology by talking to them, reading papers, and asking questions. An immunologist, Ita Askonas, and a geneticist, Charley Steinberg, became my tutors and were most helpful to me in getting into a new field. It was during this process that I was introduced to the problem of the origin of antibody diversity.

QR1987_11 BII

Immunologists agreed that an individual vertebrate synthesizes many millions of structurally different forms of antibody molecules even before it encounters an antigen. A typical antibody molecule is composed of two identical light chains and two identical heavy chains. Each of these two types of chain exhibits great sequence variability in the amino terminal regions among the antibody molecules. However, immunologists and geneticists were divided for many years into two schools of thought with respect to the issue of whether the genetic diversity required for the synthesis of these proteins is generated during evolution and is carried in the germ line or during development of the organism in which case it would be present in somatic but not germ line cells. In this germ line theory, antibody or immunoglobulin genes are expressed in exactly the same way as those for any other protein, and no special gene-processing mechanisms are needed. On the other hand, the model requires an enormous number of immunoglobulin genes inherited from the parents. One major difficulty for germ line theories of antibody diversity was the observa-

1987 Nobel Prize to Susumu Tonegawa

"If he is brilliant, tell him to come", was Prof. Niels K. Jerne's answer to Prof. Renato Dulbecco's suggestion that one of his team members would fit into the Basel Institute for Immunology. As a consequence Susumu Tonegawa joined the Institute in 1971 and remained a member until the end of 1981, when he was appointed professor of biology at the Cancer Research Centre of MIT.

Prof. Tonegawa, born in Nagoya, Japan on September 5, 1939 began his studies in biochemistry at Kyoto University and received his doctorate 1968 under Prof. M. Hayashi at the University of California in San Diego for his investigations on the regulation of gene translation in bacteriophages. He then joined the team of Prof. R. Dulbecco at the Salk Institute in La Jolla and worked on the SV40 monkey virus until his move to Basle.

Inspired by the ideas of Prof. Jerne, Dr. Tonegawa conducted pioneering experiments in Basle between 1972 and 1981 which for the first time clarified the structure and organization of the antibody genes. He was able to explain how the B-cells of the immune system, using no more than a few hundred genes, construct tens of millions of different antibodies and thus find the 'right' immune response to an almost infinite number of antigens. Starting in 1975, Dr. Tonegawa and his colleagues at the Basel Institute for Immunology demonstrated that the immunoglobulin genes in the germ line do not consist of a coherent piece of information, i.e. a single gene, but rather of three or four different genes.

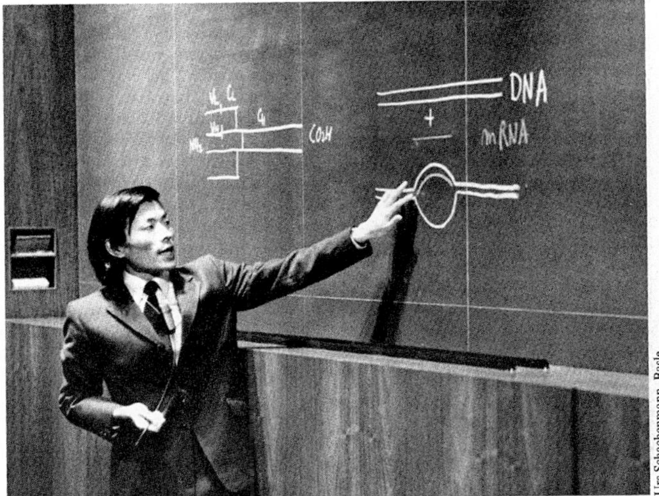

Prof. Tonegawa at the time of his work in Basle.

When a new B-lymphocyte clone develops, the pieces of DNA are reordered and joined with each other. Tonegawa's studies on the structure of individual genes showed that each element itself consists of a group of adjacent pieces of information. The possible combinations for the immunoglobulin genes are numerous. The large number of antibody structures, formed by genetic recombination, is further increased by somatic mutations, i.e. changes which take place in the DNA of antibody-forming cells. Somatic mutations are not included in the genetic information handed down from generation to generation.

Susumu Tonegawa is still well remembered in Basle for his habit of showing up in late afternoon and working for the sake of quiet all night through. His well-deserved Nobel Prize could therefore be linked to the old roman expression 'post tenebras lux'.

On January 18, 1988 a honorary symposium was held at Roche Basle under the title 'The genetic basis of the diversity of recognition in the immune system'.

Many BII scientists contributed to Susumu's work but three of them deserve special mention: Charley Steinberg, Christine Brack and André Traunecker.

tion that all antibody polypeptide chains of a given type share a common genetic marker (allotype) that segregates as a single Mendelian gene. If there were many thousands of light and heavy chain genes, how could the same genetic marker in all of these genes have been maintained?"

The above is an excerpt from Susumu's Nobel lecture, the full text of which is given in the QR code.

Many BII scientists contributed to Susumu's work but three of them deserve special mention: Charley Steinberg, Christine Brack and André Traunecker.

Nineteen papers were co-authored by these three scientists, and further papers were co-authored by Nobumichi Hozumi, Rita Schuller, Ora Bernard, Bonnie Blomberg, Hiroshi Sakano, Gaston Matthyssens and Armando Bernardini. The list is only of historical interest; nevertheless, it raises the question as to which one of the coworkers mentioned would share the Nobel Prize if, according to the rules, it were not limited to 3 people.

In the 1988 chapter, the celebration of Susumu's Nobel Prize and the performance of a theater play by the BTA will be described.

Treasure Trove 1987

The database contains documents related to the BII in a broader context (lists, series of photographs, etc.).

THE BASEL THEATER FOR THE ARTS

presents

L I N E A R - B

The world premiere of a between-the-acts musical play in which all of the dialog is between the lines, and which examines the cosmological basis of science.

The Basel Theater for the Arts celebrates its tenth anniversary this year. Starting with the intellectually demanding SNOW WHITE (1977), each new production - THE STEM CELL BALLET (1981), REFLECTIONS (1985), DIARY (1985) - reached an ever higher level of artistic achievement. With LA NOTTE DE LA BATTAGLIA (1986), the BTA reached the pinnacle of success, and as one critic said, "There is no way now for the BTA to go but down". The company of the BTA accepted the inexorable logic of this comment - it fired the director, and this production of LINEAR-B is the result. It is an attempt to explore the depths of science. Here we see on the stage, not science itself, but the co(s)mic forces that are the fundament of science.

LINEAR-B will be performed on the new "Christopher J. Paige Memorial Stage". The dedication speech was made by the famous mathematician and theatrical critic, A. Lobachevski:

"Onescore minus ten years ago our mothers and fathers, brought forth in this Institute a new theater, conceived without talent and dedicated to the proposition that none is really necessary. Now we are engaged in a great new performance, testing whether that theater, or any theater, so conceived and so dedicated, can long endure. We are met in a great auditorium of that theater. We have come to dedicate its stage as a final memorial for those who here gave their memberships that that theater might live. It is altogether fitting and proper that we should do this. But in a larger sense we cannot dedicate, we cannot consecrate, we cannot hallow this stage. The brave women and men, present and departed, who struggled here, have consecrated it far above our poor power to add or to detract. The world will little note nor long remember what we write here, but it can never forget what they did here. It is for those of us still present, rather, to be dedicated to the great task remaining before us - that from these honored departed we take increased devotion to that cause for which they here gave the last full measure of devotion - that we here highly resolve that these departed shall not have gone in vain, that this theater, under its director, whoever he or she may be, shall have a new birth of mindless enthusiasm and that extravaganzas of the unmentionable, by the untalented, for the insensitive shall not perish from this Institute".

The Year 1988

The start of the year was marked by the preparation of a BTA performance in honor of Susumu Tonegawa with the title "Susumuli, Prince de Bâle". The play was preceded by a conference: "The Genetic Basis of Diversity of Recognition in the Immune System". It was a year when the turnover accelerated and several members who for years had shaped the research direction of the institute left.

Arrivals 1988 (18)
Jean-Marie Buerstedde, Giulia Casorati, Gennaro De Libero, Anna Erdei, Dimitrios Goundis, Beat Imhof, Hiroyuki Kishi, Paola Panina, Hitoshi Sakano, Jan Salomonsen, Walter Schuler, Bernadette Scott, Gek-Kee Sim, Andreas Strasser, Shunichi Takeda, Damir Vidovic, Michael Wiles, Thomas Wirth.

Came and Left in the Same Year (3)
Anna Lassila, Helmut Sauter, Hung-Sia The.

Leavers 1988 (13)
Martin Flajnik, Dario Grossberger, Julia Hurwitz, Gordon Keller, Olli Lassila, Jukka Pelkonen, Gerd Pluschke, Robert Pytela, Catherine Servis, Ralph Snodgrass, Judith Varner, Judy Ways, Gillian Wu.

QR1988_01 BII

The year 1988 was an "easy" time. Apart from the Nobel Prize celebration there was nothing to distract the institute staff from working diligently and well. The irregularities and shortcomings that occurred during the year of the fire and at the time of the reconstruction were already forgotten. Through regular turnover 13 members left the BII, all of them finding positions where their career wishes were generally fulfilled – whether they became professors or joined pharmaceutical companies, anything was possible. There were some exceptions; one of them for instance left science and became highly successful in a somewhat unrelated field, see further below (Dario Grossberger).

Most Cited Swiss Papers, 1973–1988

One third of all citations of scientific papers published in Switzerland was shared by the University of Zurich and the BII, 14 and 13.8%, respectively. This impact should be considered from the standpoint that the number of scientists at the BII was less than 1% of the total number of scientists in Switzerland.

100 Most Cited Swiss Papers of 1973-1988: Percentage Share By Institutions

1	University of Zurich	14.0%
2	Basle Inst. Immunology	13.8%
3	University of Geneva	12.2%
4	ETH, Zurich	7.7%
5	University of Basle	6.3%
6	University of Bern	5.3%
7	Hoffmann-La Roche, Basle	4.5%
8	F. Miescher Inst., Basle	4.0%
9	Swiss Inst. Exp. Cancer Research, Lausanne	3.3%
10	IBM Corp., Ruschlikon Sandoz Ltd., Basle	2.0% 2.0%

NB. Owing to a higher average rate of citation in the life sciences than in the physical sciences, this list favors institutes that conduct biological and medical research. SOURCE: ISI's Science Indicators

Thirteen Species and More to Come

Decades earlier, when Niels Jerne described the 5 species that he intended to include in the studies performed at the Basel Institute, he said roughly this:

"We want to study the Immune System in (a) the mouse species, since it is easy to work with mice, and there exist many different strains, each one good for some defined aspect of the system, in (b) rabbits, since there are well-defined allotypes and idiotypes, and one can obtain a good amount of blood, in (c) birds, since the ontogeny of the Immune System occurs outside of the mother, in (d) frogs, since there is a complete rebuilding of the Immune System from tadpole to adult organism, in (e) sheep, since it is a large animal, by the size the closest to human, and one can study recirculation."

And he added: *"We exclude experiments on humans, except of using blood for analysing serum components."*

This makes "5 + 1" species, and that was the starting point. On the cover page of the Annual Report for 1988 there is an evolution tree that depicts species in which the BII became successively interested. Instead of "5 + 1" there are 13 species, and it shows the widened scope of the immune system investigation.

Thirteen species: primates, rodents, rabbits, sheep, birds, crocodilians, snakes, turtles, frogs, salamanders, bony fish, sharks, lampreys.

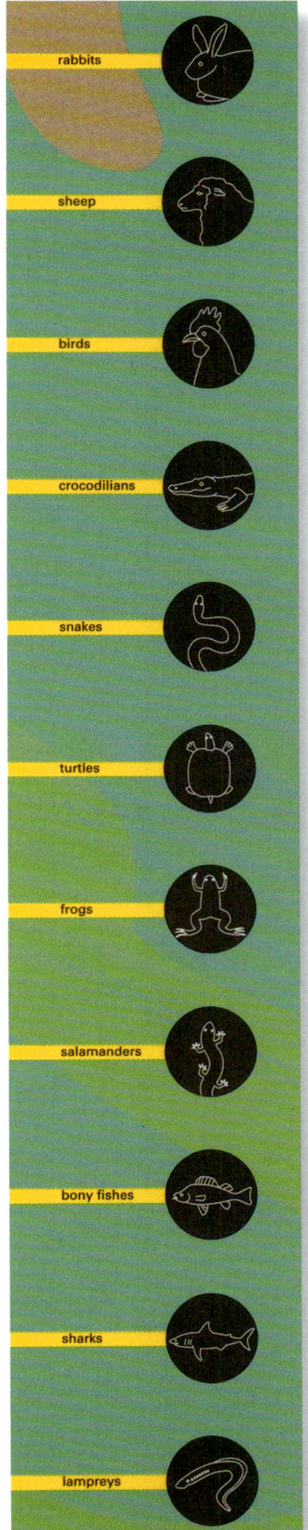

Martin Flajnik Leaves for Miami and Then Baltimore, USA

Martin Flajnik was a former student and a close collaborator of Louis Du Pasquier. When he was at the BII he worked primarily on the immune system of the amphibian *Xenopus* and together with Jim Kaufman developed various research programs regarding the ontogeny and phylogeny of class I and class II MHC molecules. He left the institute in 1988 to join the Department of Microbiology, University of Miami, where he established his own research group which worked mostly on sharks, and after several years there he became a full professor [QR1988_01].

In 1992 he moved to the University of Maryland at Baltimore, USA. His publication record shows that he collaborated with scientists from the BII and for many years continued to make short visits there. His work centered on the evolution of the immune system, in order to discern the origins of adaptive immunity. Through his work it became known that adaptive immune systems are present in jawed and jawless vertebrates, even if they use different protein families to build up the repertoire of their antigen receptors.

Martin had shown that cartilaginous fish possesses all the building blocks of an adaptive immune system similar to that of humans; nevertheless, it exhibits in addition some unusual "heavy chain only" receptors, analogous to those of the camel, that allow the build-up of a totally different repertoire of B cells. Martin's general interest for the evolution of the immune system in Metazoa led him to survey studies made in many different groups of animals, in order to conclude in a paper with Louis Du Pasquier that "immune features being found in animals previously believed only to have innate immunity have prompted us to revisit the artificial dichotomy between adaptive and innate immune systems" *(Evolution of innate and adaptive immunity: can we draw a line?)*.

Julia Hurwitz and Chris Coleclough Accepted Positions in Memphis

Julia Hurwitz and Chris Coleclough, a married couple with 2 children, were an unusual and uncommon constellation at the BII, as scientific positions were usually not offered to husband and wife. However, Julia and Chris applied to the BII independently, and the staff selection committee approved each application separately (the rule of not employing husband and wife at the same place might be considered today as politically incorrect, but then it was the case, with some exceptions, e.g. sabbaticals). Below, the research directions of Julia in her new position at the St. Jude Children's Research Hospital in Memphis, Tenn., USA, are briefly described, while Chris' move is mentioned in the chapter for 1997 as he came to the BII as a visitor (many times) working with Ivan Lefkovits.

Julia describes her work as follows: "Respiratory syncytial virus (RSV) and the human parainfluenza viruses (hPIV) are the leading causes of hospitalizations for viral respiratory tract diseases in infants and young children. Sendai virus (SeV) is a mouse respiratory virus that merits consideration as a Jennerian vaccine for hPIV-1 due to its similarity with hPIV-1 in terms of sequence, structure and antigenicity. The SeV backbone can also be manipulated using reverse genetics to create SeV-based RSV and hPIV-3 vaccines. An important research direction opened upon discovery that a single intranasal vaccination with the combined recombinant SeV protected cotton rats from challenges with hPIV-1, hPIV-3 and RSV. This made a compelling case for the advanced development of the SeV-based vaccine." Further information is given in the QR code [QR1988_02].

QR1988_02 BII

Gordon Keller to Denver, New York and Toronto

Gordon Keller spent 3 years at the BII working on stem cells, collaborating and publishing with several other members (Norman Iscove, Chris Paige, Ralph Snodgrass, Michael Wiles and Bob Phillips), and after completing his appointment at the BII he moved to the National Jewish Centre for Immunology and Respiratory Medicine in Denver, Colorado, and later to the Mount Sinai School of Medicine in New York City. In 2007, Gordon returned to Canada to establish a laboratory at the Medical and Related Sciences Centre in Toronto (known as the MaRS Centre).

Gordon Keller is highly respected for his pioneering research on applying developmental biology findings to in vitro pluripotent stem cell differentiations. One of his last publications at the BII (with Ralph Snodgrass) dealt with "Clonal fluctuation within the haematopoietic system of mice reconstituted with retrovirus-infected stem cells" (*EMBO Journal* 1987). His studies documented profound clonal changes, occurring for a long time following reconstitution, and highlighted the difficulties in establishing lineage-specific stem cells.

Olli Lassila to Turku

Olli Lassila carried out successful research at the BII, analyzing the early events in the initiation of an immune response. With Olli Vainio and Polly Matzinger he published an authoritative paper, "Can B cells turn on virgin T cells?" (*Nature* 1988), which was on capturing and presenting antigen to T cells. Such a presentation involves two distinct steps: (1) display of the antigen, which requires uptake, processing and reexpression of the antigen in association with MHC molecules on the presenting cell surface, and (2) triggering, in which the presenting cell provides signals leading to the activation of the responding T cell. By exploiting the unique properties of the avian hematopoietic system, he examined the presenting capacity of B cells in vivo and found that resting B cells are unable to activate resting T cells. With several projects he continued in Turku, and also he maintained collaboration with various members of the BII.

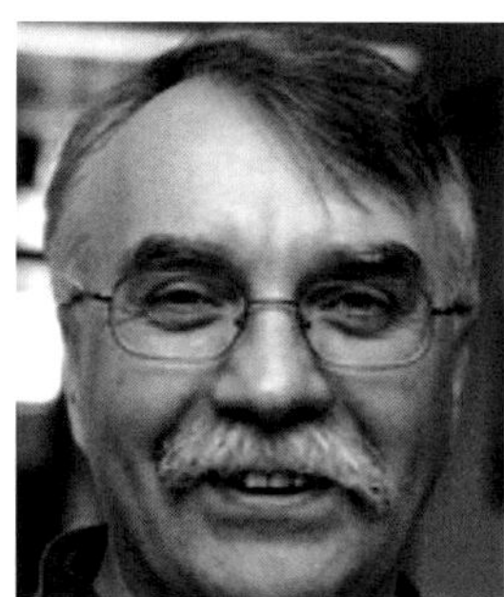

Olli Lassila

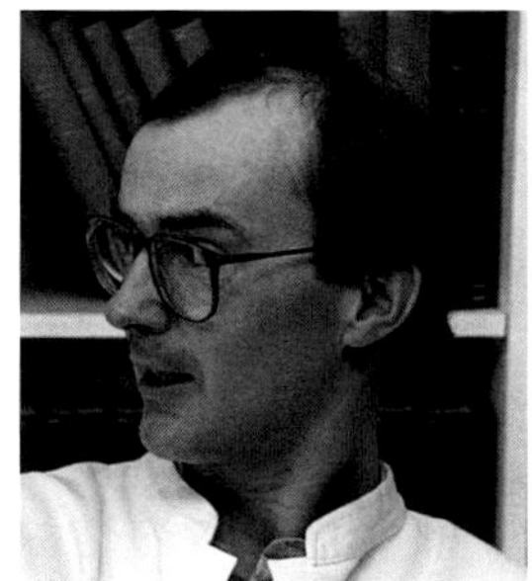

Olli Vainio

Gerd Pluschke Remained in Basel

Gerd Pluschke was one of the few immunologists at the BII with interests in host–pathogen interactions, approaching this topic by studying the molecular mechanisms of disease protections. His move to the Swiss Tropical Institute in Basel was auspicious for him in order that he could continue his earlier BII studies on the resistance of newborn mice to K1 *Escherichia coli* infection, and in an attempt to elucidate the protective properties of antilipopolysaccharide antibodies in *E. coli* infection. He describes his research interests as "infection biology focusing on host–pathogen interactions, molecular epidemiology, immunology and vaccine design". In the QR code his joint papers with various members of the BII, among them S. Pelkonen, M. Achtman, L. Jenni, L. van Alpen and I. Lefkovits, are described.

Ralph Snodgrass to Chapel Hill, North Carolina

Ralph Snodgrass, after 3 years at the BII, accepted a position at the Lineberger Comprehensive Cancer Center, University of North Carolina Chapel Hill School of Medicine. In Basel he published several papers in *Nature*, resulting from a productive collaboration with Michael Steinmetz and Harald von Boehmer. The main emphasis of his work was on the ontogeny of TCR in the thymus.

Years later Ralph became a co-founder of the company VistaGen, mentioned in the section on biotech companies.

Gillian Wu Left but Kept Ties with the BII

Gill Wu came from Canada, and after several years of successful work, and establishing many friendships (especially with the late Charley Steinberg), she returned to Canada. Although the BII Annual Report lists her departure twice, 1986 and 1988, she remained a regular visitor for more than a decade. The Basel environment (in Gill's own words) left a lasting impression in terms of gaining the conviction that anything doable can be done, and that studying V(D)J recombination, repertoire, locus mapping and B cell development goes very well with developing the ability to discriminate between wines. Gill is proud that her sons flourished in the Swiss culture – this and other aspects of Gill's career (and her life in general) are given in the QR code [QR1988_03].

Dario Grossberger Left the BII and Soon After Gave Up Science

Dario owns and manages an orchard of semitropical fruit in Ventura County, north of Los Angeles, California. He produces mostly cherimoya. The fruit has a green skin and a creamy white, sweet pulp, with moderate acid. The fruit typically has many large, black seeds. Cherimoya (*Annona cheirimola*) is native to southern Ecuador and northern Peru, and is related to some fruits in the same genus which grow in more tropical areas. Cherimoya was probably taken to other parts of the world hundreds of years ago. It is produced in commercial plantings in semitropical areas of Spain, Chile, Peru, California, New Zealand, Australia and Israel.

Symposium in Honor of Susumu Tonegawa

On January 18th, 1988, in the large Roche auditorium, the BII and Roche celebrated the awarding of the 1987 Nobel Prize in Medicine to Susumu Tonegawa of the Massachusetts Institute of Technology [QR1988_04]. The celebration, with addresses by Raymond Probst, Niels Kaj Jerne and Hans-Rudolf Striebel, was followed by a symposium entitled "The Genetic Basis of Diversity of Recognition in the Immune System" with talks by present and former members of the institute:

Louis Du Pasquier	"Immunoglobulin genes in lower vertebrates"
Jean-Claude Weill	"Avian immunoglobulin genes"
Christine Brack	"Proteins interacting with regulatory sequences of Ig genes"
Martin Weigert	"Somatic hypermutation of Ig genes"
Matthias Wabl	"Hypermutation and selection"
Michael Steinmetz	"T cell receptor genes"
Harald von Boehmer	"T cell development in TCR transgenic mice"

BTA 8: Performance of "Susumuli, Prince de Bâle" for Susumu Tonegawa

In the evening there was a party at the institute with a stage production entitled "Susumuli, Prince de Bâle", directed by Chris Paige, former director of the Basel Theater for the Arts (BTA), and since 1987 a member of the Ontario Cancer Institute, Toronto. The cast included the entire company of the BTA and guest stars Renato Dulbecco, Matthias Wabl and Martin Weigert [QR1988_05].

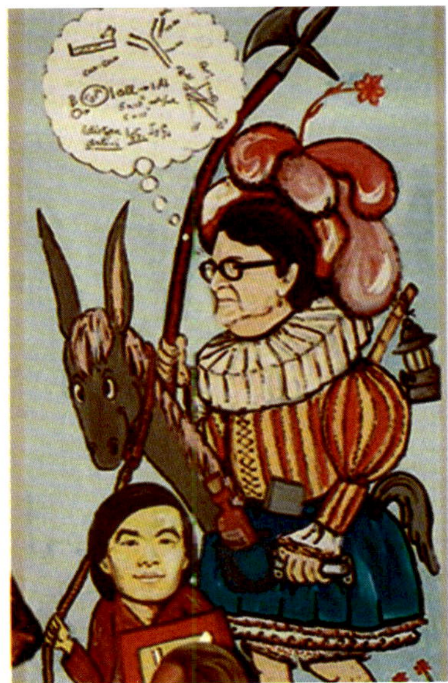

The Sancho Panza picture with the likenesses of Jerne and Tonegawa is from another BTA production but is fittingly placed here

QR1988_04 BII

QR1988_05 BII

PEOPLE

Susumuli, Prince of Bale

If one compares the newspaper articles on the success story of Susumu Tonegawa, it is apparent that the information is quite 'normalized' and except some amusing mistakes, all reports are similar. Not so, if one enters more unconventional information sources.

It is a ten years old tradition of the Basel Institute for Immunology to celebrate special events in the life of the Institute with a theatrical performance. The range is wide: a fairy tale in honour of Niels K. Jerne's 65th birthday, a ballet for the 10th Anniversary of the Institute (that was even mentioned in 'Nature') an opera for the re-inauguration after the fire. For the Nobel Prize Award to Susumu Tonegawa, the Basel Theater for the Arts has presented 'Susumuli, Prince of Bale', defined in the programme as 'a somewhat dramatic portrayal of the life and times of Susumuli'.

Nearly all scientists, technicians and administrative personnel at the Institute at the various times have been participating to the productions of the BTA. For 'Susumuli', an important guest actor has been the Nobel Prize winner Renato Dulbecco, to whom was given the role 'of imparting the wisdom of the ages to the young Susumuli'.

No better words than those used in the programme could give an idea of the 'drama'. Here they are.

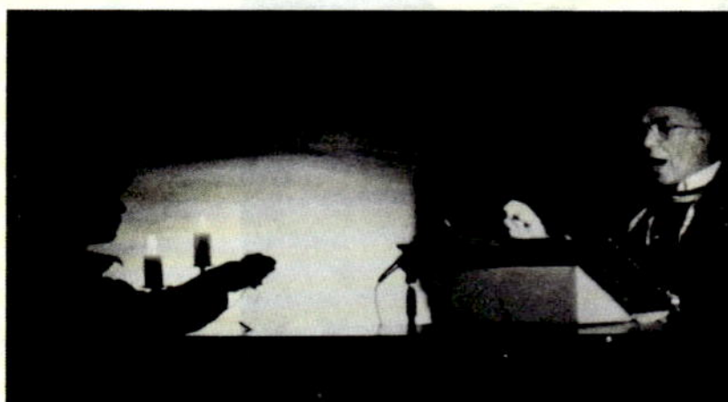

The wise monk (Renato Dulbecco) talking to the Susumuli supplicant (Vrene Stauffer) (relates to scene 1)

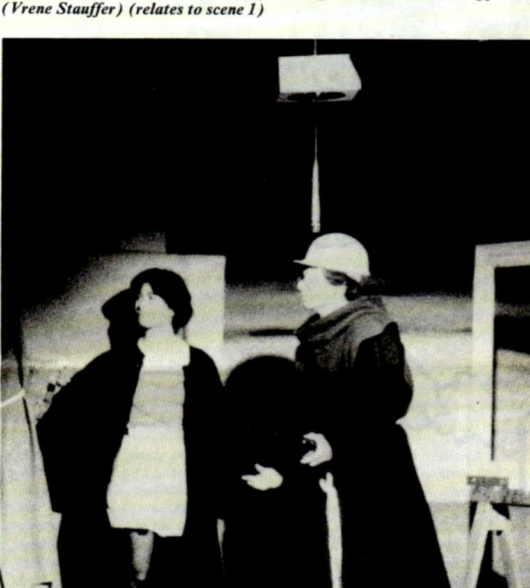

The horrified colleagues of the Susumuli industrious (Peter Balzarini, Diana Thorpe, Andreas Strasser) (relates to scene 2)

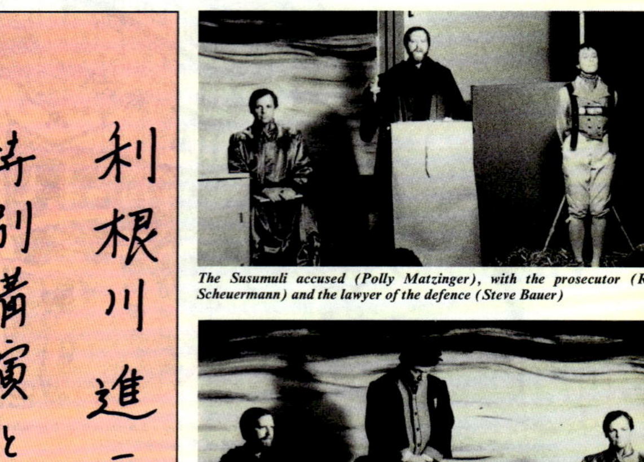

The Susumuli accused (Polly Matzinger), with the prosecutor (Rich Scheuermann) and the lawyer of the defence (Steve Bauer)

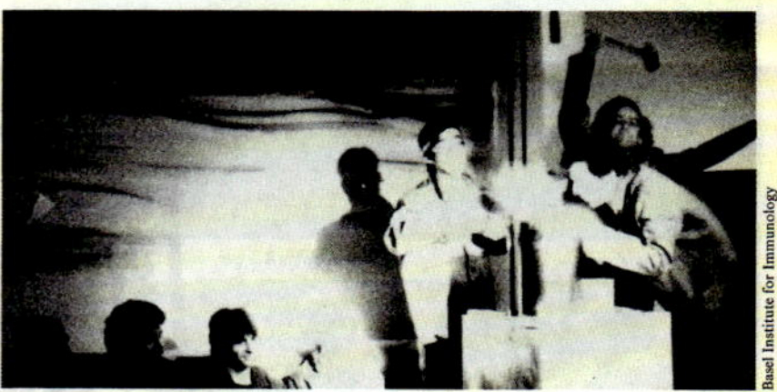

The Judge (Fritz Melchers) (figures 3 and 4 relate to scene 3)

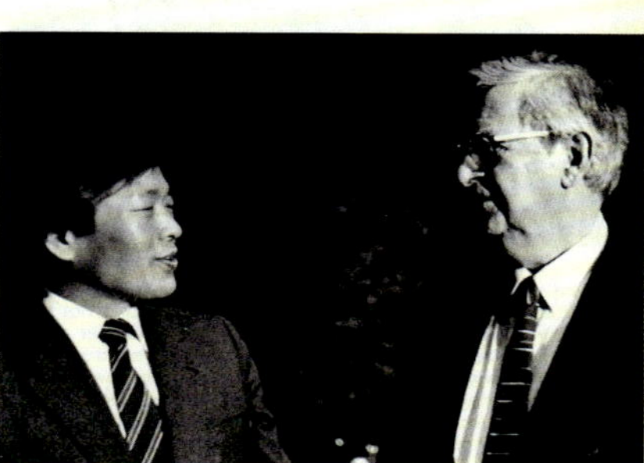

The Susumuli Nobel (Pat Riegert) discussing with the postdocs (standing: Yas Uematsu, Matthias Wabl, Jean-Claude Weill) (relates to scene 4)

The Plot

'Susumuli, Prince of Bale' is apparently a true story. It is based upon a manuscript unearthed recently in an ongoing excavation in the new world city of Toronto. How such a valuable document ended up in Toronto ... and why any excavations should have been ongoing in such a place ... these are questions which scholars still debate. At least one has pointed out that other ancient artifacts from Bale have also turned up in Toronto indicating perhaps an unknown trading link established in those dark days of history which have as yet not been illuminated. The mystery surrounding the discovery of the manuscript is no less than that concerning what it says. Here, however, the BTA has been fortunate in having a team of antiquarians well versed in making something out of nothing, creating constructs from fragments of evidence, unhindered by restrictions based on a pre- ... result. And so the docu- ... constructed and is ... miere perfor- ... r, in any

... in his present circumstances but to go off to Bale where fame awaits. As a token of his love he gives Susumuli a magic rock – a rock which, if properly refined, will yield fundamental knowledge. Susumuli, not a little bit puzzled, heeds the advice and goes off to Bale with his rock.

Scene 2

The next scene finds the young Susumuli working in his lab. We think his mind is occupied only with the thoughts of his rock and how to refine it – but man does not live by thoughts alone. Having recently left the director's office, some of Susumuli's colleagues happen by and notice, to their total horror, a strange glow emitted from Susumuli's lab which is accompanied by even stranger sounds. Clever fellows, they take the reasonable action of calling for help, and Picasso, hero of the Tower, enters to investigate the problem. Confronting Susumuli he demands that the witchcraft be stopped and judged by the people.

Sc...

... really carried much weight in these sorts of affairs ... and he goes free.

Scene 4

In the finale we see the culmination of Susumuli's quest. Now the master of a happy team of helpers he narrows in on the final technique to refine the rock. Pondering various approaches he succeeds in extracting what he wants and his glorious goal is realized. Happiness abounds and the story ends ... eh?

Prior to this dramatic presentation there was a more formal symposium in the Roche auditorium in Basle. After the presentation of the String Quartet Nr. 1 in C-major by Franz Xaver Richter (1709–1789) the vice-chairman of the board of directors of the Roche ...

... applied and project-oriented research at Roche. The Basle institute has become a valuable Roche family member with worldwide recognition.

... Prof. Niels Kaj ... itute ...

In his own address, Prof. Tonegawa first remembered his time in Basle, the longest and most beautiful period of his scientific career, as also the at times very close collaboration ...

Roche Started Cooperating with Amgen and Cetus, 1988

Amgen is an American multinational biopharmaceutical company headquartered in Thousand Oaks, California. The first major product was Epogen, a recombinant human erythropoietin product for the treatment of anemia associated with chronic kidney failure.

Cetus is a biotech company established in Berkeley, California. The cooperation was established as a consequence of intense competition to clone the gene for IL-2. Cetus created a proprietary recombinant version of IL-2. The drug showed promising results in treating renal cancer, but patients also developed significant side effects. Later IL-2 was approved and is now distributed by Novartis under the name Proleukin.

Several BII members worked in these and other follow-up companies.

Ruggero Ceppellini, Ole Maaloe and Bede Morris Died in 1988

Ruggero Ceppellini, permanent and founding member of the institute, died on June 5th, 1988. He was fascinated by population genetics of the genes of the major histocompatibility complex in humans, and by the mysteries that the incredibly high polymorphism held for their biological functions. He infected his colleagues with this fascination, many of whom became members of the institute and helped him establish the Turin-Basel connection. In his honor the "Ruggero Ceppellini Advanced School of Immunology" was founded.

Ole Maaloe, founding member of the Board of Advisors of the institute, died on May 21st, 1988. Ole had been Niels Jerne's doctoral adviser. With his life-long experience in quantitative biology and molecular genetics, he endorsed and encouraged the creation of an institute devoted to quantitative immunology.

Bede Morris, an Australian immunologist, member of the John Curtin School of Medical Research, Canberra, and a long-standing collaborator of the BII, died on July 2nd, 1988, in a car accident in France in the midst of doing collaborative work at the institute. Bede made the immune system of sheep his life-long center of interest, and his students continued this field of research at the institute.

Treasure Trove 1988

The database contains documents related to the BII in a broader context (lists, series of photographs, etc.).

QR1988_treasure BII

The Year 1989

Several (previously neglected) research directions were emphasized, such as complement-related projects. Special aspects of T cell receptor biology (γ/δ) attracted attention. Two workshops, one on "Severe-combined immunodeficient (SCID) mice" and another on "The mechanisms of B cell neoplasia", were held. The 7th International Congress of Immunology took place in Berlin with a large cohort of participants from the BII. The Velvet Revolution started in Czechoslovakia, and it received great support from the BII that was upheld for many years. The BTA performed "Pollygon" as a tribute to Polly Matzinger, who left the BII. Maja Sacher died at the age of 100 years.

Arrivals (8)
Dominique Dunon, Seiji Inui, Marie Kosco-Vilbois, Roland Lauster, Alexandra Livingstone, Lill Martensson, Mark Miller, Melanie Wilson.

Came and Left in the Same Year (3)
Inmaculada Esparza, Tomas Hraba, R.C. von Borstel.

Leavers (14)
Susan Carson, Christopher Coleclough, Anna Erdei, Laura Lee Gill, Polly Matzinger, David Nemazee, Harald Prahl, Uwe Staerz, Andreas Strasser, Yasushi Uematsu, Olli Vainio, Siegfried Weiss, Gayle D. (Monte) Wetzel, Thomas Wirth.

Immunology Was Changing in Small but Steady Steps

Just a superficial examination of the titles of the BII research projects indicates a substantial shift from earlier projects. Jernean questions were resolved, and immunology became increasingly intertwined with cell and molecular biology. Considering the achievements of Tonegawa and the follow-up of his work towards elucidating the T cell receptor structure, one can confidently say that the sharpest tools of molecular biology were developed precisely for solving immunology-related questions.

The institute itself became aware that the Jernean statement "no antibody – no immunology" needed to be redefined. In many institutes complement had been studied for decades, but that was not the case at the BII. The arguments were (and they were indeed valid) that complement had nothing to do with specificity. The 1989 Annual Report lists 11 complement-related projects – obviously not because of the specificity of response, but because of the response itself:

- Common binding domains in C3b for H, B, CR1 and CR2
- C3b binding sites for HSV-1 gC
- Multiple sites of interaction in C3 for CR2/EBV receptor
- Role of factor H and properdin in fluid phase C' activation
- Analysis of C3 from various species
- Expression of CR2 on human T cells
- Antigenic sites on C3 α- and β-chains
- Localization of neoantigenic epitopes in C3b and iC3b
- C1q receptor on mouse cells
- Alternate C3 gene product with possible BCGF activity

- Functional analysis of the thrombospondin motif

Although the description of the "shifts" belongs to the history of the BII, details can be found in the primary literature, or at least in individual research reports of the BII.

α/β as well as γ/δ T Cell Receptor

The issue concerning the two forms of the T cell receptor also became a focus of interest. For some time it was not known that besides the "standard" type of TCR containing α/β-chains, there was another type of T cell expressing γ/δ TCR. How could one be sure that such a detail (α/β vs. γ/δ) is worth studying? In 1989 it was not yet clear, but the puzzle was there, and members willing to explore it were there as well.

- An invariant TCR δ VDJ in BALB/c mice
- Resident pulmonary cells expressing the γ/δ TCR
- Sheep TCR gene expression
- Extrathymic self-renewal of α/β and γ/δ T cells
- Distinctive features of γ/δ T cells in ungulates
- Compartmentalization of human γ/δ T cells

Fourteen Members Left the BII in 1989

Chris Coleclough to Memphis

Chris Coleclough joined Klaus Karjalainen in 1985 to study diversification of the repertoire of λ light chains. Two influential papers (*Nature*, 1985) resulted, and thereafter Chris Coleclough worked with Ivan Lefkovits on cell-free translation products (from cDNA libraries) analyzed by two-dimensional gel electrophoresis. Because of his long-lasting collaboration with Ivan, his departure from Basel is listed later than that of his wife Julia. Chris, back in Memphis, published several papers with Peter Doherty, one of them on the Sendai virus and HIV glycoproteins.

Polly Matzinger's New Affiliation at the NIH, Washington

Polly Matzinger's new affiliation was the NIH, but in her heart – for many years – she was still at the BII: organizing conferences, teaching at courses and lecturing at Summer Schools. Her career after the BII is summarized in the documents in the QR codes.

Siegfried Weiss to the University of Oslo

Siegfried Weiss left the BII for the University of Oslo and later went

This process was called "receptor editing", and it gained prominence as the main mechanism of B cell tolerance.

on to the German Biotechnology Research Institute (GBF) in Bochum. He spent a considerable part of his scientific career at the BII, first working towards his PhD (1970–1978) and then between 1983 and 1989 as a member. In the years in between his two stays, he worked at the Salk Institute in San Diego and at the Max Planck Institute in Tübingen. (Note: the GBF was renamed as Helmholtz Centre for Infection Research.)

David Nemazee to Denver and La Jolla

David Nemazee, after spending several years at the BII, moved to the National Jewish Center in Denver, Colorado, and later to the Scripps Research Institute, La Jolla. Almost his entire career revolved around clonal deletion of autoreactive B lymphocytes (*Nature* 1989, *PNAS* 1989), and later he (and independently Martin Weigert) showed that autoreactive B cells could proofread, alter and re-express modified receptors to become non-autoreactive. This process was called "receptor editing", and it gained prominence as the main mechanism of B cell tolerance.

It has been shown that B cells' heavy-chain genes are rearranged first, then the light-chain genes. Checkpoints ensure that each B cell expresses only 1 receptor. Further details on this fascinating work are given in the QR code.

Monte Wetzel Leaves for the NIH, to Bayer, to Roche

Monte Wetzel's epicurean "talents" were mentioned earlier, and they well matched his work on the influence of various interleukins on B cell activation, cell cycle progression, proliferation and Ig secretion. One aspect that grew out of this research was the development of autoantibody secretion in response to various cytokines.

After Monte had left Basel, he continued this research in his new position at the NIH, Bethesda. Two years later, once he had concluded his work on autoantibodies and B cell subsets, he accepted an offer from the Biotechnology Division of Bayer Healthcare to lead the monoclonal antibody research unit.

As head of Immunobiology he contributed towards exploring and developing modified interleukins for the treatment of various diseases including asthma, allergy, autoimmunity, sepsis and cancer. Monte's research and experience at the Basel Institute were formative and prepared him intellectually for pursuing business aspects as well. His move to Roche Molecular Systems, in Pleasanton, California, is mentioned in the section on BII members choosing careers in Roche.

Anna Erdei, Yasushi Uematsu, Andreas Strasser

Anna Erdei, after 2 years at the BII, returned to Eötvös Loránd University, Budapest, where she became professor of immunology. Her main interest was in the regulation of B cell functions by complement receptors, and she also became interested in the role of innate immunity.

Yasushi Uematsu's career ladder was quite exceptional. He joined the BII from Chiba University, Japan, was a member for 4 years, moved to Hoffmann-La Roche where he researched autoimmune diseases, then he moved to the Zentrum für Lehre und Forschung, Basel, where he continued the work on autoimmune diseases. Later he became a senior scientist at Chiron Vaccines in Siena, Italy, and after that he rose to the position of research manager at Novartis Vaccines and Diagnostics.

Andreas Strasser, after several years at the BII (first as a PhD student, then as a member), moved to the Walter and Eliza Hall Institute, Melbourne, contributing to the understanding of the molecular mechanisms of apoptosis. The main question he addressed was how apoptosis regulation is disrupted during development of hematopoietic and epithelial tumors.

EMBO Workshop on the SCID Mouse, 1989

A workshop on the SCID mouse, sponsored by EMBO, was held at the institute from February 20th to 22nd, 1989. Walter Schuler, Mel Bosma and Bob Phillips organized it [QR1989_01].

The mouse mutant SCID impairs the rearrangement of antigen receptor genes, and as a consequence, SCID mice lack functional T and B cells. Since they lack functional lymphocytes, SCID mice can be grafted with all kinds of normal and genetically altered cells, even human cells. The SCID mouse is particularly interesting as a model for investigating both normal and abnormal cell differentiation. SCID is also studied by molecular biologists working on mechanisms of antigen receptor gene rearrangement.

A section of the program is given below; the complete program is included in the QR code:

M. Bosma	"The SCID mutation: occurrence and general effect on lymphoid system"
R. Phillips	"Functional characterization of lymphoid and myeloid systems"
R. Hardy	"FACS analysis of B and T cell deficiency: early lymphoid progenitors"
P. Kincade	"Characteristics and growth requirements of B lineage cells"

S.I. Nishikawa	"Growth and differentiation of B lineage cells"
V. Kumar	"Natural killer cell function"
W. Schuler	"Status of Ig and TCR genes: transcription and rearrangement"
A. Carroll	"TCR-δ rearrangement in thymocytes"
M. Gellert	"Joining of signal sequences in VDJ recombination"
D. Weaver	"Rearrangement of retrovirus vectors"
K. Blackwell	"PreB cells that rearrange κ light chain genes"
H. Sakano	"Molecular analysis of B cells from LTBM cultures"

Mechanisms of B Cell Neoplasia, 1989

The 7th workshop on B cell development and regulation, and the use of this knowledge to elucidate mechanisms of abnormal regulation in malignancy, was held in Basel from March 29th to 31st, 1989.

The techniques described for characterizing the various types of malignancies are useful in the diagnosis, prognosis and treatment of B cell malignancies. In this workshop, human malignancies were compared with animal models at the molecular and cellular levels, and the roles of different oncogenes were discussed with respect to modification of known oncogenes.

It was divided into 3 sessions:

Session 1: Pro- and Pre-B Cells

a) Avian: bursal lymphomas (myc, rel, myb)

b) Mammalian: Abelson, B-ALL (abl, cbl)

Session 2: B Cells

a) Endemic Burkitt's (myc), sporadic Burkitt's, AIDS lymphomas

b) Follicular lymphoma (bcl-2)

Session 3: Ig-Secreting Cells

a) B-CLL, multiple myelomas, benign monoclonal gammopathies

b) Expression and function of myc and other oncogenes

The program in full is reproduced in the QR code.

7th International Congress of Immunology in Berlin, 1989

The 7th International Congress of Immunology (the first one was in 1971) was held in Berlin; it was a historically unique congress, being the last major scientific event before the fall of the Berlin wall a few months later.

Fritz Melchers was responsible for the scientific program. Eighteen BII members presented their work; 5 of them were chairpersons of symposia or workshops [QR1989_02].

J. Kaufman “Phylogeny of MHC and cell interaction molecules: evolution of the Ig superfamily”

H. von Boehmer “Self-nonself discrimination by the immune system”

R. Palacios “Cytokines and lymphocyte progenitors; monoclonal antibodies recognizing pro-T cells and lineage-uncommitted cell precursors”

A.G. Rolink “Experimental models for autoimmune diseases”

D. Gray “T cell memory is short-lived in the absence of antigen”

D. Vidovic “Self-tolerance can cripple the immune system and Qa-1 restricted recognition of foreign antigen by afl T cell hybridoma”

G.D. Wetzel “Regulation of peritoneal Ly-1 B cell proliferation and differentiation by IL-5”

M. Kosco “Germinal center formation *in vitro*: requirement for FDCY”

W. Schuler “Animal models for primary and acquired immunodeficiencies”

H. Kishi “A TCR molecule that is associated with P but not A chain”

H. Prahl “Regulative function of CD5 (Ly-1) in T cell activation and differentiation”

L. Du Pasquier “Evolutions of the immune system”

C.-A. Reynaud “Evolution of Ig loci in different species”

O. Vainio “Functional and molecular characterization of avian analog of CD2”

G. De Libero “Establishment of human double positive thymocyte clones”

P. Panina “Degeneracy of human class II recognition”

S.R. Bauer “Characterization of the human Vpren protein”

U. Chen “The B cell cycle”

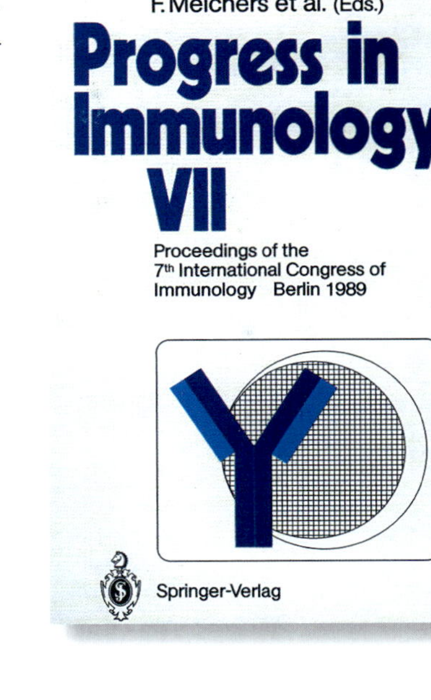

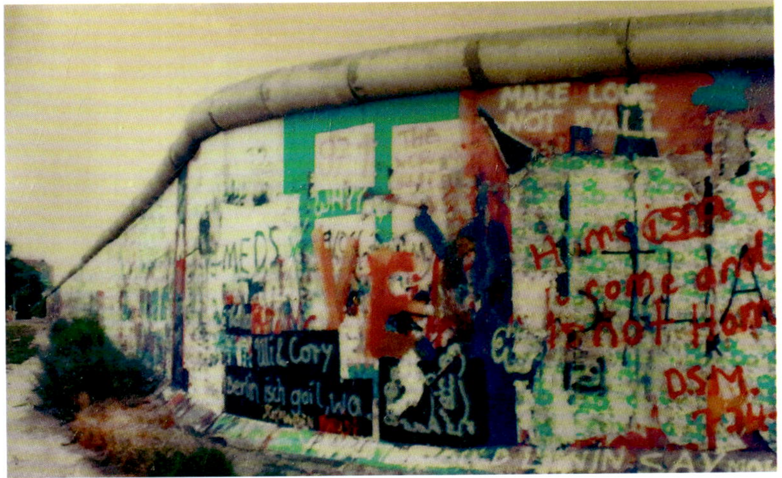

QR1989_02 BII

I have received a telephone call from Czechoslovak Academy of Science Prague, asking for support of student demonstrations in Prague. Yesterday the police remained in the background, today however, a strong police intervention is expected. They are asking us (at present they are telephoning all the academic Institutions all over the world) to support the Czechoslovakian students' cause by <u>sending a telegram</u>. Please give your signature below (the cable will be sent at 2 pm if 25 signatures collected).

Ivan Lefkovits

Signatures of BII members who offered their support

Support for the Velvet Revolution in Czechoslovakia

In November 1989 the Velvet Revolution started in Prague. Members of the BII supported the revolution wholeheartedly [QR1989_03]. Immediately after the old system had been overthrown, BII members started to provide help to Czechoslovakia.

BTA 9: "Pollygon", a Goodbye Tribute to Polly Matzinger

The 9th BTA play, "Pollygon", was staged to recreate Polly Matzinger's scientific and social impact on the BII. Polly's entire career, distorted through the BTA-specific lens, was reported in 8 acts. Both her scientific achievements and some outlandish stories recounted at parties were included in the plot, for example in Act 2 her interaction with the Basel police in "Pollyce Story" and in Act 5, "Driftwood and the Fleas", her co-authorship with her famous dog. The difficulty that the BTA crew encountered in establishing the plot was due to there being too many "Polly" stories to choose from, occurring during her time in Basel and earlier [QR1989_04]. Polly's extrovert character made her an ideal performer in many previous BTA plays, and in one of them she was supposed to die. This was taken up in "Pollygon" with the words: *Polly has written, sung, danced, acted, directed and even died for the BTA.*

Maja Sacher Died, 1989

Maja Sacher died on August 8th, 1989. Her life-long dedication to furthering modern art brought her fame internationally. She was important not just for the city of Basel, where she created the Museum of Contemporary Art, and Switzerland, but also for the world. She made donations to art whenever the need occurred. A square in Basel is named after her. Maja Sacher's gift of the Double Helix sculpture, created by her close friend Jean Tinguely, became the hallmark of the BII. For many years she and her husband Paul Sacher graciously invited the members of the Advisory Board to their home on the Schönenberg, which provided an ideal atmosphere for the exchange of experiences and opinions between the advisors and Roche management.

Nobel Prizes, 1989

Michael Bishop and Harold Varmus were awarded the Nobel Prize for Medicine 1989 for the discovery of the origin of retroviral oncogenes.

Michael Bishop was a member of the Advisory Board and a long-standing friend of the BII. His work on the human oncogene c-Src influenced several research projects at the institute.

Thomas Cech and Sidney Altman were awarded the Nobel Prize for Chemistry 1989 for their discovery of the catalytic properties of RNA.

QR1989_04 BII

Treasure Trove 1989
The database contains documents related to the BII in a broader context (lists, series of photographs, etc.).

QR1989_treasure BII

The Year 1990

The turnover continued – the arrivals and departures were in a harmonious balance. Departing scientists left a mark of their activities, while the newcomers could only show their potential. Roche purchased Genentech, which had just commercialized its first breakthrough product: human insulin produced from bacteria. Interferon-α_2 became thereafter the emblem of Genentech. The ENII workshop on retroviruses in autoimmune disease took place at the BII. Instruments to the value of several millions of Swiss francs were sent to "former socialist countries".

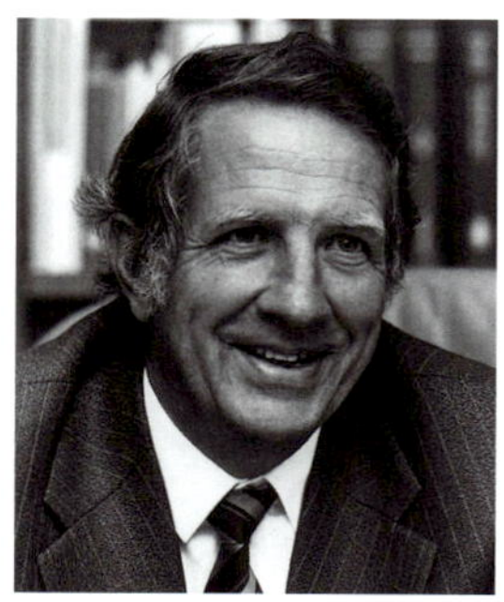

Jürgen Drews

Genentech Purchased by Roche

Jürgen Drews [QR1990_01] strongly believed in the power of research, and during his time at Roche a majority holding of the biotech company Genentech was acquired (1990), and the option for purchasing the rest was exercised less than 10 years later. Genentech was founded in 1976 by venture capitalist Robert A. Swanson and biochemist Herbert Boyer. The company had all the modern tools of molecular biology, in fact the same ones that were available at the BII and at the RIMB in Nutley, but Genentech had proven itself by making commercial products. Human insulin produced from bacteria was its first big breakthrough product (making insulin cheap and plentiful for those suffering from insulin-dependent diabetes).

One of Genentech's most important products was interferon-α-2a (approved by the FDA for the treatment of hairy cell leukemia); former scientists from the BII and RIMB, Nutley (Theo Staehelin and Sidney Pestka), were involved in the development of this product.

QR1990_01 BII

Help for Former "Socialist" Countries

The BII had a rich store of instruments that were in very good working condition but had been decommissioned due to the constant turnover of scientists. Several trucks left for Czechoslovakia, Latvia and Romania with instruments that were unavailable in those countries and could be put to immediate use.

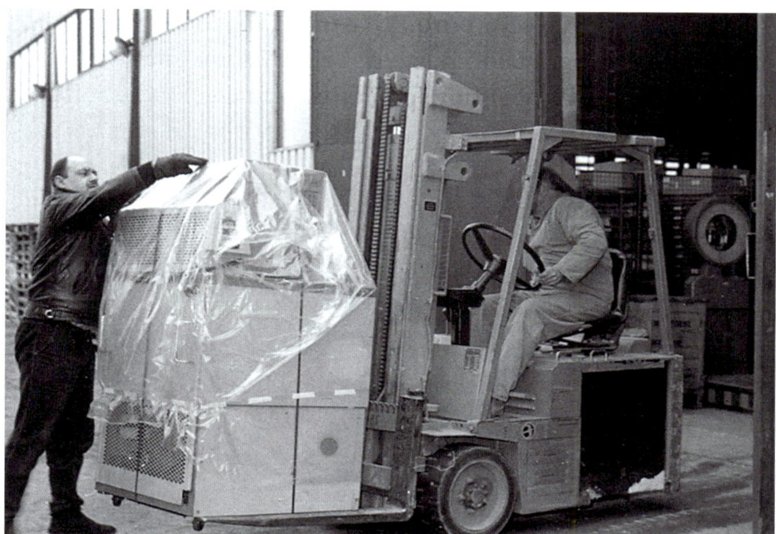

Scintillation counters, centrifuges and incubators were delivered to the Czechoslovak Academy of Sciences in Prague

Arrivals 1990 (10)
Agnes Baron, Paolo Dellabona, Shigeo Ekino, Gillian Griffiths, José Carlos Gutierrez-Ramos, Hajime Karasuyama, Insoo Park, Luc Reininger, Jacques Robert, Franca Ronchese.

Came and Left in the Same Year (5)
Ellen Hsu, Mark Miller, Ed Palmer (sabbatical), *Maria-Louisa Toribio, Georg Wick* (sabbatical).

Leavers 1990 (12)
Jochem Alsenz, Lawrence D'Hoostelaere, Gennaro De Libero, Dimitrios Goundis, Hiroyuki Kishi, John Lambris, Paola Panina, Eddy Roosnek, Hitoshi Sakano, Joseph Schwager, Alan Tunnacliffe, Damir Vidovic.

Ed Palmer Arrives for a Sabbatical

After 7 intensive years in Denver, Ed Palmer joined the BII for a sabbatical year [QR1990_02]. Ed's lab worked on understanding T cell recognition of antigens, alloreactivity, thymic selection and self-tolerance. In his first seminar after he had arrived in Basel, he explained his newest discovery that mouse mammary tumor proviruses encode a protein (superantigen) that is recognized by the T cell receptor. Thymocytes expressing TCR of this specificity are deleted in the thymus. Discussions with BII members, especially with Charley Steinberg, on the repertoire of T cells, marked Ed's sabbatical and led him to design experiments that were continued after his stay. It is probable that Ed's wish to spend his sabbatical in Basel was not only a science-oriented issue, but also a chance to offer his wife, Kathrin, a year in her "home country". Ed had met Kathrin Lehmann, a former BII technician, years earlier in California; they fell in love and married in 1982.

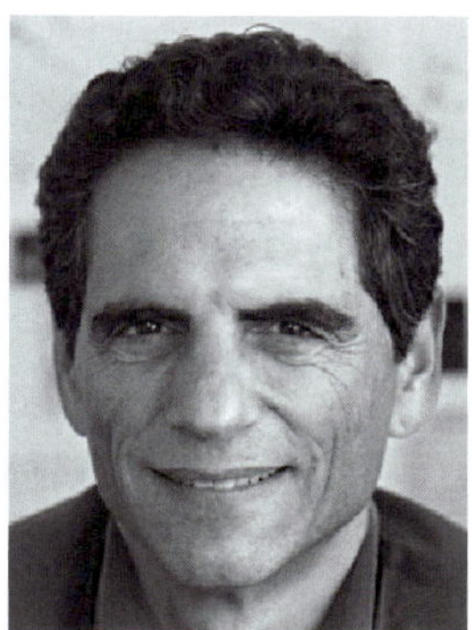

Ed Palmer

Roland Gisler, a Passionate Teacher

Beside his administrative duties and scientific collaborations (mainly with Beat Imhof), Roland took on teaching responsibilities at the University of Basel. This had already started before he joined the institute, but it became an important part of his working life, not only to give university courses but also to teach at summer

QR1990_02 BII

schools and extramural courses. His slides (in the pre-PowerPoint era) were sought after and eagerly copied by the students for their further education [QR1990_03].

After the BII had closed, he and Fritz Melchers continued teaching at the University of Basel.

Lectures for Students from Marburg and Prague

As mentioned elsewhere, students from Prof. Klaus Hartmann's Immunology Department at Philipps University Marburg were hosted each year for a series of lectures given by BII members. In 1990 the lectures accommodated a "newly emerging" group of medical students from Charles University, Prague, who for the first time after the fall of the iron curtain were given the opportunity to travel abroad.

The schedule was as follows:

BASEL INSTITUTE FOR IMMUNOLOGY

LECTURES FOR THE STUDENTS FROM PHILIPP'S UNIVERSITY, MARBURG AND CHARLES UNIVERSITY, PRAGUE

Friday, June 22, 1990	18:00 - 20:00	**IVAN LEFKOVITS** Introduction for the students from Prague
Sunday, June 24, 1990	18:00 - 20:00	**IVAN LEFKOVITS** Introduction for the students from Marburg
Monday, June 25, 1990	8:30 - 10:00	**ROLAND GISLER** B cell development
	10:00 - 11:30	**HARALD VON BOEHMER** T cell development
	LUNCH	
	12:30 - 14:00	**HANSREUDI KIEFER** Oligonucloetide synthesis
	14:30 - 16:00	**MICHAEL STEINMETZ** Genetic engineering in health care
	16:30 - 18:00	**DAVID GRAY** Immunological memory
Tuesday, June 26, 1990	9:00 - 10:30	**WALTER SCHULER** Severe combined immune deficiency
	10:30 - 12:00	**LOUIS DU PASQUIER** Evolution of the immune system
	12:00 - 12:30	visit the vivarium
	LUNCH	
	14:00 - 15:30	**GITTA STOCKINGER** Antigen presentation
	16:00 - 17:30	**HANS-GEORG RAMMENSEE** Peptides and MHC
	18:00 - 19:30	**IVAN LEFKOVITS** Summary session

QR1990_03 BII

ENII Workshop on Retroviruses in Autoimmune Diseases

This workshop, sponsored by the European Network of Immunology Institutes (ENII) and the German Society of Immunology (GSI), was organized (October 1990) by Ton Rolink, Joachim Kalden and Fritz Melchers. The idea that retroviral components are involved in autoimmune diseases had received renewed attention. Antibodies and T cells specific for retroviral gp70 and gag proteins were shown to recognize xenotropic and polytropic viruses rather than ecotropic viruses, and some of the antibodies cross-react with DNA. This raised many fundamental questions:

How is immunity to these retroviral elements induced?

Are the retroviral elements hidden self-antigens to which the immune system is not tolerant?

Are the retroviral elements encoded by infectious viruses?

The workshop addressed these questions in 7 sessions (detailed in the QR code):

Session 1: Retroviruses
Session 2: Expression of retroviruses
Session 3: Tolerance
Session 4: Is it all retroviral?
Session 5: Molecular mimicry
Session 6: Induction of autoimmune disease by exogenous retroviruses
Session 7: Endogenous retrovirus and disease

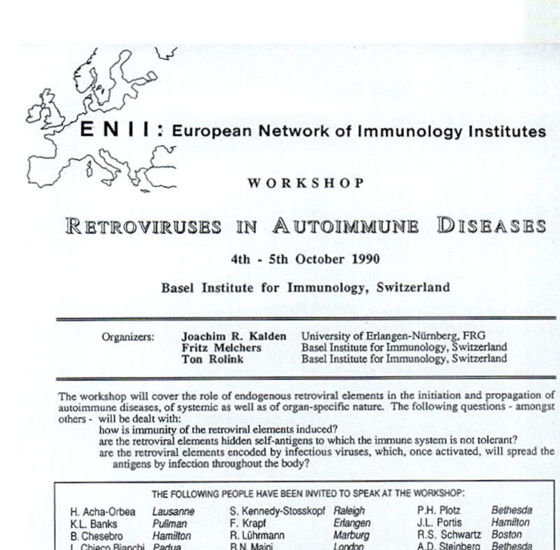

E N I I : European Network of Immunology Institutes

WORKSHOP

RETROVIRUSES IN AUTOIMMUNE DISEASES

4th - 5th October 1990

Basel Institute for Immunology, Switzerland

Organizers:	**Joachim R. Kalden**	University of Erlangen-Nürnberg, FRG
	Fritz Melchers	Basel Institute for Immunology, Switzerland
	Ton Rolink	Basel Institute for Immunology, Switzerland

The workshop will cover the role of endogenous retroviral elements in the initiation and propagation of autoimmune diseases, of systemic as well as of organ-specific nature. The following questions - amongst others - will be dealt with:
how is immunity of the retroviral elements induced?
are the retroviral elements hidden self-antigens to which the immune system is not tolerant?
are the retroviral elements encoded by infectious viruses, which, once activated, will spread the antigens by infection throughout the body?

THE FOLLOWING PEOPLE HAVE BEEN INVITED TO SPEAK AT THE WORKSHOP:

H. Acha-Orbea	*Lausanne*	S. Kennedy-Stosskopf	*Raleigh*	P.H. Plotz	*Bethesda*
K.L. Banks	*Pullman*	F. Krapf	*Erlangen*	J.L. Portis	*Hamilton*
B. Chesebro	*Hamilton*	R. Lührmann	*Marburg*	R.S. Schwartz	*Boston*
L. Chieco Bianchi	*Padua*	R.N. Maini	*London*	A.D. Steinberg	*Bethesda*
B. Fleckenstein	*Erlangen*	C. Moroni	*Basel*	J. P. Stoye	*London*
J.W. Hartley	*Bethesda*	H.C. Morse III	*Bethesda*	M. Weigert	*Philadelphia*
W. A. Haseltine	*Boston*	A.L. Notkins	*Bethesda*	I. L. Weissman	*Stanford*
S. Izui	*Geneva*	M.B.A. Oldstone	*La Jolla*	H. Will	*Martinsried*
J.D. Keene	*Durham*				

In addition to the speakers, **20-30** participants will be accepted. Hotel accommodation will be provided; travel and staying expenses to be covered by the applicants.
Applications - including curriculum vitae, list of publications, and a short letter indicating main scientific interests, in particular those related to the workshop topics - to be sent to:

Dr Ton Rolink
Basel Institute for Immunology
Postfach
CH-4005 Basel, Switzerland

DEADLINE FOR APPLICATIONS: 15 JULY 1990

Gennaro De Libero Moved to the ZLF, Basel

Gennaro De Libero [QR1990_04] left the BII but remained in Basel, joining the Zentrum für Lehre und Forschung of the University Hospital, which was later renamed Department of Biomedicine (DBM). There he established the first research group in immunology, paving the way for the migration of other BII members to the DBM. He is now professor of Tumor Immunology at the Faculty of Medicine of the University of Basel. His publication record shows over 150 papers. A continuing theme of his research has been T cell antigen recognition in human diseases with emphasis on cells recognizing "non-conventional" antigens. His studies led to the identification of phosphorylated mevalonate metabolites as the major tumor ligands stimulating human TCR $\gamma\delta$ cells, to the description of self-glycolipids as autoantigens and of tumor-associated lipid antigens, as well as to the discovery of novel mycobacterial lipid antigens.

QR1990_04 BII

John Lambris Moved to Philadelphia

John Lambris was offered a position at the University of Pennsylvania, where he soon became full professor. Using complement as a model system, John applied ideas embodied in engineering, computer science and biomedicine to study the structure and functions of the complement system. He and his coworkers elucidated the critical sites of complement component C3 responsible for its diverse functions, and contributed to the development of complement-based anti-inflammatory therapeutics through the discovery of the first small-size complement inhibitor, termed compstatin, which has exhibited consistent efficacy in clinical tests.

He established a unique association of complement components with non-inflammatory pathways by demonstrating the involvement of complement in the developmental processes, including liver and limb regeneration. More is given in the QR code, although one aspect might be mentioned here: he is one of the best-funded scientists, with some USD 50 millions from the NSF and NIH.

Paola Panina to Brescia and Then to Milan

Paola Panina left the BII for the University of Brescia, from where she moved to the San Raffaele Scientific Institute, Milan, Italy. She became a group leader in Reproductive Sciences. Her research was aimed at studying the physiopathology of gynecological and reproductive diseases, especially attempting to define infertility risk factors and ovarian reserve biomarkers.

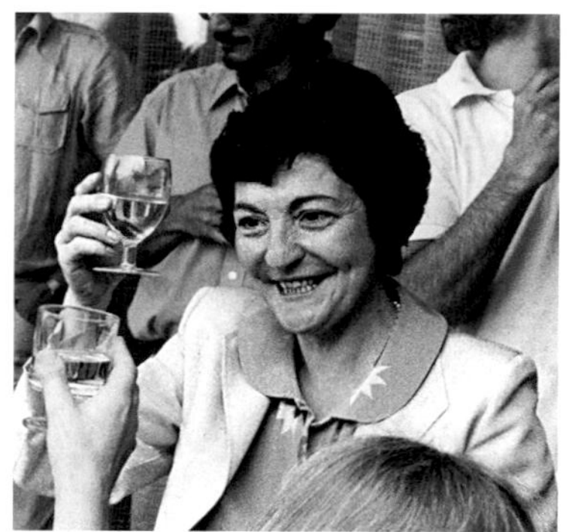

Luciana Forni

Luciana Forni, Special Status for a Special Technician

As mentioned elsewhere, scientists (except for a handful of permanent members) worked at the BII on the basis of time-limited contracts. After 2 or 3 years they moved on. This turnover was a feature of the institute that kept it young and competitive. Technicians had unlimited contracts, and most of them were very good and highly motivated, and they stayed at the BII for many years. Luciana Forni came to the BII to work with Ben Pernis, and when he left for the USA Luciana stayed on and collaborated with various scientists, most productively with Antonio Coutinho. She became more and more independent, started her own projects, published papers, and participated in scientific life. Although she became a scientist, she was still on the list of technicians (that was her formal "job description").

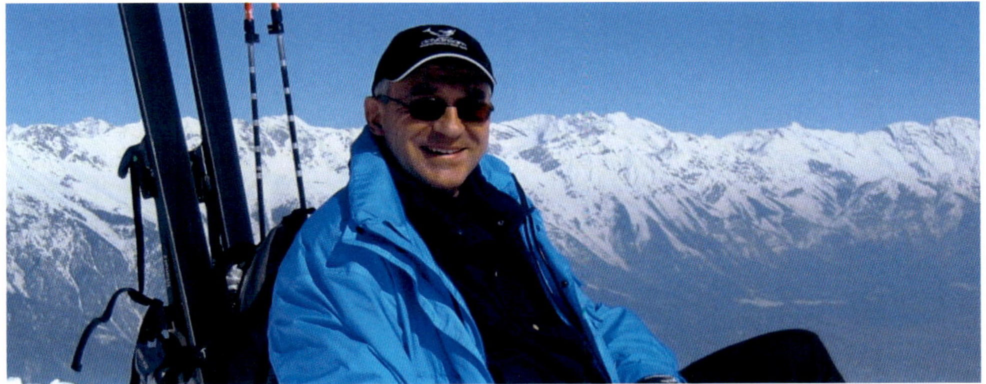

Georg Wick in the Alps

Then came the special "twist". Luciana wrote her doctoral thesis and earned her doctoral degree. She kept quiet about it and remained on the list of technicians. She could have presented her diploma, and her name would have been moved to the list of scientists. But then she would receive a 2-year contract and when it was up, she would have to leave the BII, as was the case for all the other scientists. For Luciana, the BII was so much her home that she preferred to stay on as a technician until her retirement. Luciana died in 2006 [QR1990_05].

Georg Wick Cooperates with the BII

Cooperation with Georg Wick continued well into the early nineties, beyond the period dealt with in Book 1. Georg and Ivan Lefkovits carried out extensive discussions on the use of limiting dilution analysis, and one of their first proteomic projects (when two-dimensional gel electrophoretic separation had not yet been included under the umbrella of proteomics) was the identification of protein patterns of thyroid glands from OS and normal chickens as a basis for target organ susceptibility. Interestingly, this set of experiments (published in *Immunobiology*, 1990, under the title "Molecular analysis of genetically determined target organ abnormalities in spontaneous autoimmune thyroiditis"), was Georg's introduction to proteomics, a field of research that had increasingly become the center of interest in his lab.

There was a third period of interaction with the BII when Georg joined Louis Du Pasquier's laboratory, where he completed morphological assessments of thymic nurse cells (comparing chickens, mice, humans and frogs). Back in Innsbruck, one of his students, Josef Penninger, then wrote an extensive thesis on the role of thymic nurse cells in positive T cell selection.

QR1990_05 BII

Treasure Trove 1990

The database contains documents related to the BII in a broader context (lists, series of photographs, etc.).

QR1990_treasure BII

The Year 1991

Research projects on T cell receptors and on the major histocompatibility complex remained the focus of attention. An immunology course in Prague was organized. The cell sorter facilities were refurbished and modernized. The opening of the new facilities was celebrated by a BTA performance, "A Musical Portrait of the Institute". Another play, "The Network Killers", on scientific fraud and its consequences was performed by the BTA. A workshop on B cell neoplasia took place in a similar format as in previous years. A symposium to honor the retirement of Andrew Kelus took place in the institute, and the 80th birthday of Niels Jerne was celebrated in Geneva.

Arrivals 1991 (12)
Yair Argon, Stéphane Demotz, Ulrich Deuschle, Hans Jörg Fehling, Johann Rudolf Frey, José A. Garcia-Sanz, Philip Griebel, Ursula Günthert, Peter Lane, Sabine Mai, Fiona McConnell, Eva-Susanne Strobel.

Came and Left in the Same Year (3)
Stephen Anderson, Martin Flajnik, Colin Watts.

Leavers 1991 (12)
Steven Bauer, Antonio de la Hera, David Gray, Andrew Kelus, Roland Lauster, Luc Reininger, Claude-Agnès Reynaud, Richard Scheuermann, Walter Schuler, Bernadette Scott, Brigitta Stockinger, Jean-Claude Weill.

Generation of Antibody Diversity Solved, What Next?

The solution of the generation of antibody diversity opened new vistas towards clarifying the role of the major histocompatibility complex (MHC) in the immune system, and its involvement in T cell biology. But the road was less clearly delineated than it was with antibody diversity. As Fritz Melchers puts it in the Introduction to the 1991 Annual Report: "*Scientific discovery is unpredictable, sudden, enormously surprising. As much as we try to describe the immune system as we know it … we are stupefied by the unexpected experimental results that hit the prepared mind like lightning. All of a sudden, our understanding changes and we acquire a new vision. If that is called scientific success, then it is habit-forming for those who experience it. The short moment of success, the excitement of being on top of the mountain of a problem is quickly over; we discover that while we have solved one problem, we have uncovered many more. And so we begin again, searching with plans describing the new situation as accurately as possible, not knowing where, or whether, enlightenment will come again*" [QR1991_01].

QR1991_01 BII

T Cell Receptors

The elucidation of the structural and functional aspects of T cell receptor (TCR) was the last great puzzle of the "specificity problem". The TCR progress reports are emphasized here, not only because of the importance of the TCR in the immune system, but for several other reasons as well. The BII played a special role in solving this problem as it was the only research facility where the TCR could be probed against the immune systems of several species (mice, birds, sheep, frogs) and which was needed to understand the T cell recognition system.

The TCR is a molecule found on the surface of T lymphocytes that is responsible for recognizing fragments of antigen as peptides bound to MHC molecules. The binding between TCR and peptide-MHC complexes is of relatively low affinity and is degenerate: that is, many TCR molecules recognize the same peptide antigen and many peptide antigens are recognized by the same TCR.

The TCR is composed of two different protein chains (it is a heterodimer). In humans, in 95% of circulating T cells, the TCR consists of an α- and β-chain, whereas in 5% of T cells, the TCR consists of γ- and δ-chains. This ratio changes during ontogeny and in diseased states, as well as in different tissues and in different species.

When the TCR engages with antigenic peptide and MHC (peptide/MHC), the T lymphocyte is activated through signal transduction, that is, a series of biochemical events mediated by associated enzymes, coreceptors, specialized adaptor molecules and activated transcription factors.

Immunology Course in Prague, 1991

The institute members recognized the importance of the events related to the fall of the "Iron Curtain" (November 1989), and soon thereafter contacts were established with scientists from various "former socialist" countries, especially with Czechoslovakia. After initial ad hoc help, a concerted effort with the Swiss Society of Immunology, the German Immunological Society and the European Network of Immunology Institutes was launched to provide aid and support – mainly in the form of teaching courses. The responsibility for these courses was placed in the hands of Ivan Lefkovits. Although the BII regularly organized courses in Basel, it was felt that the format of the intended courses should be such that instead of bringing a few "representatives" to Basel to teach them things that might be impracticable to implement because of their local conditions, the reverse should be attempted: teachers from the BII and from other centers of excellence should travel to those institutions and provide help locally under conditions that were implementable there [QR1991_02].

QR1991_02 BII

In 5 years (1991–1995) 1 theoretical course and 4 Summer Schools were organized in Czechia and Slovakia for students from Czechoslovakia, Hungary, Poland, Ukraine, Russia and Belarus. In the chapters for these years, the courses are briefly mentioned, and in the 1995 chapter all 5 of them are summarized.

At the course in Prague (1991), 28 lectures for the students of Charles University, and for colleagues of the Czechoslovak Academy of Sciences, were given by the following speakers:

Paavo Toivanen	"Function of Bursa of Fabricius"
Paavo Toivanen	"Cellular and Molecular Mechanisms in Avian B Cell Differentiation"
Hans Hengartner	"Antiviral Immunity"
Hans Hengartner	"Autoimmunity and Tolerance in Transgenic Mice"
Peter Lachmann	"Biology of Complement"
Peter Lachmann	"Protection against Complement Lysis"
Auli Toivanen	"Reactive Arthritis – An HLA-B27 Associated Disease"
Auli Toivanen	"Reactive vs. Rheumatoid Arthritis: What Can Be Learned?"
Roland Gisler	"Role of the Cell Adhesion Molecules in the Immune System"
Roland Gisler	"Microenvironments of B Lymphopoiesis"
Günther Hämmerling	"Peripheral Tolerance"
Jack Kettman	"Molecular Analysis of T Cell Clones"
Jack Kettman	"HIV Infection and Cytopathogenicity"
Jean-Marie Buerstedde	"Generation of Antibody Diversity"
Jean-Marie Buerstedde	"Gene Conversion"
Ole Werdelin	"Antigen Processing and Presentation"
Antonio Coutinho	"An Organism-Centered View of the Immune System"
Antonio Coutinho	"Genetic Determination and Ontogenic Selection of Ab Repertoire"
Hans-Georg Rammensee	"Trimolecular Complexes of MHC, Peptide, TCR"
Hans-Georg Rammensee	"Peptides Presented by MHC Class I"
Ivan Lefkovits	"The Ideal Lymphocyte"
Ivan Lefkovits	"Lymphocyte Gene Catalogue: Are Rare Genes Included?"
Lucien Aarden	"Cytokine Network"
Lucien Aarden	"Activation of Human T and B Cells"
Klaus Hartmann	"Ontogeny of the Thymus"
Klaus Hartmann	"Maturation of Lymphocytes in Autoimmune-Prone Mice"
Richard Pink	"From Genes to Vaccines"
Richard Pink	"Immunity against Malaria"

Excerpt from the course manual:

"Since the iron curtain has disappeared, we all savour the fact that distances are measured in kilometres and miles instead of permissions, stamps and visas. But the breakthrough of isolation has yet to come. The Czech and Slovak scientists are diligent readers of literature and reprint collectors. In the times of persecution and oppression, this was the best way to stay fit and to remain informed about the world. I suggest that we stop this old-fashioned approach and, instead, start to interact directly. We should not see each other through printed paper, but should find each other involved in discussions, corridor talks, gossips, and in liking and disliking one another. The aim of this course is to be a stone mosaic in our contacts, such that Czechs and Slovaks can become part of the whole mosaic of world science.

What can be said about the teachers?

Lucien Aarden is a high-class immunologist, with a long-standing interest in autoimmunity. He is the head of research at CLB in Amsterdam. Lucien spent two years in Basel. He has a highly critical mind and it is a great pleasure to discuss with him experiments, theories and hypotheses. He has developed a number of interesting assay systems for measuring and characterizing interleukins.

Auli Toivanen is a scientist from Turku University who has spent a sabbatical at the BII. Auli is a kind of miracle: a perfect family life combined with diligent work, and she enjoys culture, travelling and good food.

Paavo Toivanen, who happens to be Auli's husband, shares everything with Auli (also the sabbatical in Basel) and has a beautiful summer residence, where he always entertains guests; the entire peninsula belongs to the Toivanens, and it takes half a day to walk around the borders of their property.

Roland Gisler, a permanent member of the BII, belongs to an old Basler family and is one of the few people who were successful in changing from applied research to basic science. Apart from this, he is a passionate and very successful university teacher, and holds an appointment as Professor of Immunology at the University of Basel. His effort in preparing lectures and slides is enormous. Besides research activity, he has one other serious duty in our Institute, and that is administration. He is a highly cultured man with manifold interests in art, especially Asian. He has one of the finest collections of Buddhas.

Jack Kettman is a former member of the BII and for many years has been at the Southwestern Medical School at Dallas. Jack has

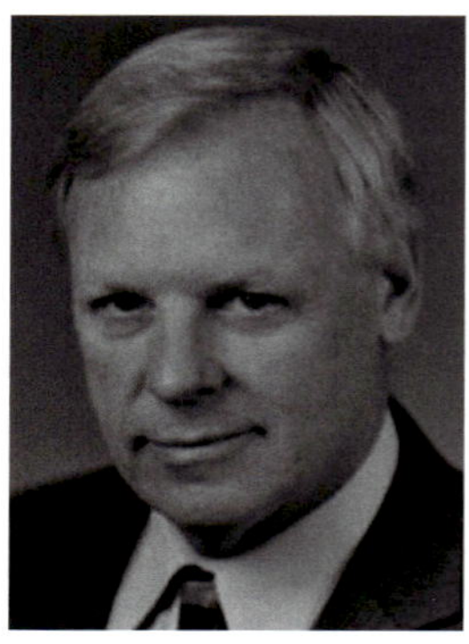

Steven Bauer

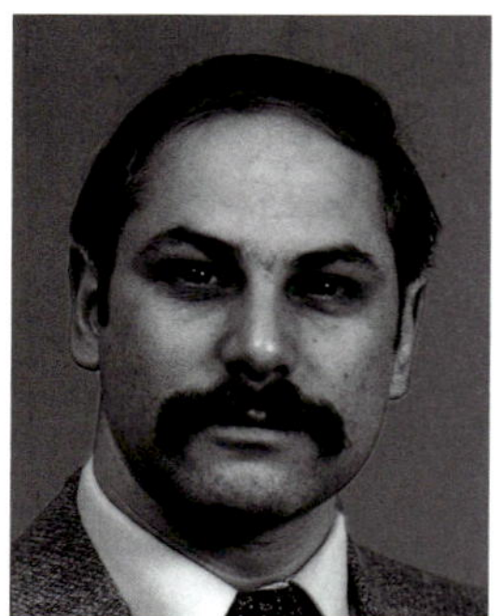

Don Gerson

spent many mini-sabbaticals at the BII, each visit meaning hectic activity, first on projects on limiting dilution analysis, and later on characterization of lymphocyte clones by 2D gel electrophoresis. Jack is a personality on his own, but he still belongs to the American intellectuals who are overcritical of their government, political system and American way of life. For the first time he will be able to see the heritage of the system which the Americans think to know about, but they don't. Jack's wife, Diana, is a passionate traveller and has been everywhere, or is on her way there.

Hans Hengartner is also a former member of the BII, and is now Professor of Immunology at the University of Zurich. He has always felt an affinity towards the fate of the people in Eastern European countries. He visited Hungary while it was still under the old system, and returned to Switzerland with very negative impressions (about the system). His commitment towards helping Eastern Europe became clear when he included PhD students from Poland and Hungary in his teaching courses. This is his first visit to Czechoslovakia and at the same time his first contact with a country which has become free of communist oppression."

Steven Bauer Left the BII to Assume a Leading Position at the FDA in the USA

After several intermediate stages at the FDA in Washington, Steve rose to a high position [QR1991_03]. His research at the BII matched to a large extent that of Fritz Melchers. To reiterate, it concerned "pre-B cell specific VpreB1/VpreB2/lambda 5 loci in the genus *Mus*".

His broad range of collaborations was quite unique and for this reason his publication co-authors (over 31 of them) are listed below: Melchers F., Strasser A., Kudo A., Thalmann P., Rolink A., Okabe T., Karasuyama H., Haasner D., Sakaguchi N., Jameson B., Groh V., Bahram S., Herman A., Beauchamp M., Spies T., Kubagawa H., Maclennan I., Piechacyzk M., Nordan R.P., Owens J.D., Nepveu A., Marcu K.B., Mushinski M., D'Hoostelaere L., Huebner K., Budarf M., Finan J., Erikson J., Emanuel B.S., Nowell P.C., Croce C.M.

Steve Bauer worked on the FDA side, and Don Gerson worked on the development and manufacturing side of the project to make a 2nd-generation smallpox vaccine based on large-scale cell culture (1,500 liters). The US Government sponsored and supervised this project after the 9-11 attack to make a smallpox vaccine stockpile for emergency use in the event of a bioterrorism event. The FDA approved the vaccine very quickly, and now 350 million doses are in long-term storage by the US Government.

David Gray Leaves for London and Later Moves to Edinburgh

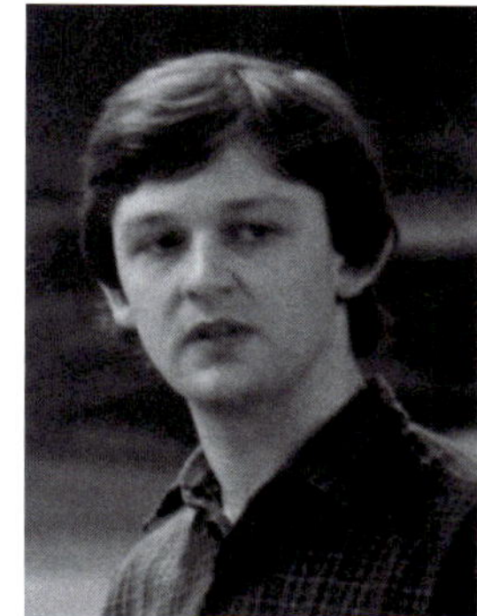

David Gray

After 6 years at the BII, David returned to the UK as a Wellcome Trust Senior Research Fellow in Basic Biomedical Science at the Royal Postgraduate Medical School, Hammersmith Hospital. After 6 or 7 years he moved to the University of Edinburgh where he became professor of Immunology. At the BII and also in the UK, David worked on B cell subsets (characterizing the splenic marginal zone and germinal centers), on immunological memory (addressing the role that antigen plays in the maintenance of memory cells) and on T-B cell interactions (addressing the role of B cell antigen presentation on memory generation) [QR1991_04].

Richard Scheuermann to Dallas, Later to San Diego

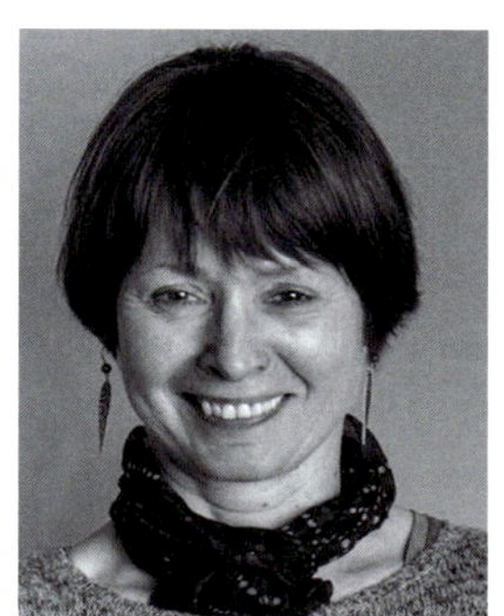

Brigitta Stockinger

In 1991 Richard joined the faculty of the Department of Pathology at the University of Texas Southwestern Medical Center in Dallas, where he rose to the rank of professor. After 20 years in Dallas he pulled up his roots and moved to San Diego to become the director of Informatics at the J. Craig Venter Institute. Richard Scheuermann leads the Influenza Research Database project and he is also the head of the Virus Pathogen Bioinformatics Resource Center.

Brigitta Stockinger's Career Took Off in London

Brigitta left the BII in 1991 and soon made a profound impact on immunology in the UK, especially as a member of the Francis Crick Institute London. She was elected Fellow of the Royal Society, Fellow of the Academy of Medical Sciences and a member of EMBO. Gitta is a molecular immunologist interested in inflammation and infection. She specifically studies the biology of a subset of the immune system's T cells, looking at the factors that affect their development and function. More recently Gitta's research group discovered the importance of the transcription factor aryl hydrocarbon receptor, an environmental sensor, in the immune system.

Reconstruction of the Cell Sorter Facility

There were pronounced space constraints with regard to the institute's need to expand in order to incorporate new facilities. To overcome these limits some space had to be "invented", and a portion of the atrium area was sacrificed to gain some 50 m^2 for extending the cell sorter (FACS) facility [QR1991_05].

QR1991_05 BII

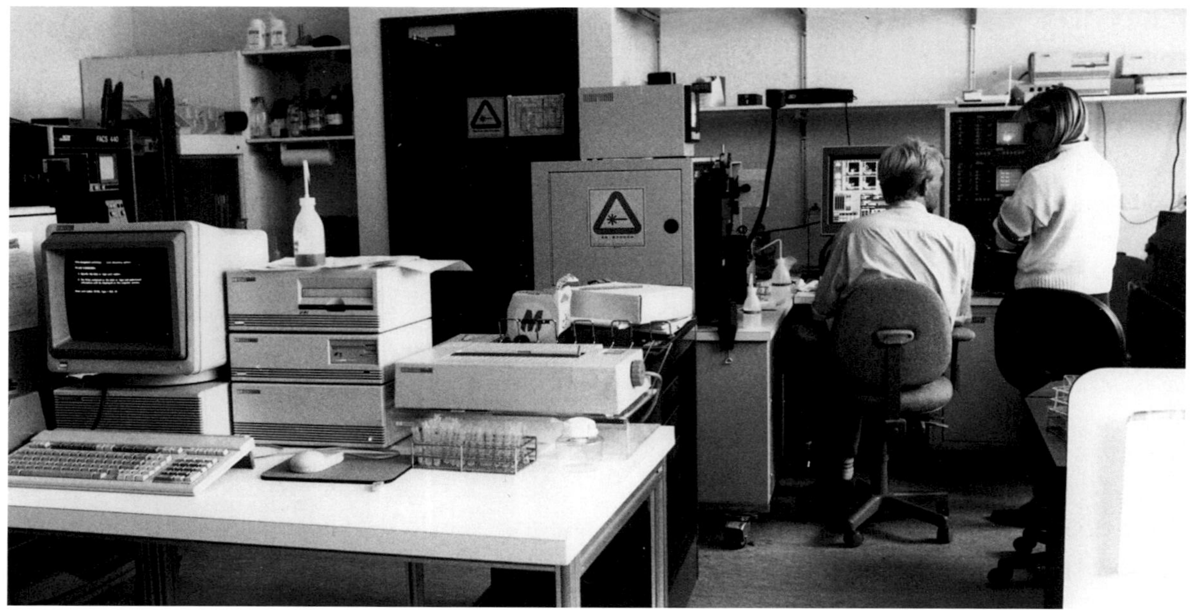

Cell sorter facility

The reconstruction work was done within a few months of 1990/1991, and during that time the research group of Louis Du Pasquier and Jim Kaufman (terrarium area) suffered some inconvenience. Louis' revenge was a satirical musical play with some serious elements. The performance was dedicated to the 20th anniversary of the BII.

BTA 10: "A Musical Portrait of the BII" Staged to Celebrate Its 20th Anniversary

Although for most performances of the BTA the driving force was Norman Iscove and/or Chris Paige, the emphasis of this work of art was on "a musical theme", thus the main person involved had to be – and was – Louis Du Pasquier, strongly supported by Alexandra Livingstone.

The members of the ensemble of "A Musical Portrait of the Institute" were:

Roberto Sawicki (violin)
Juliette Du Pasquier (violin)
Gillian Harris (cello)
Louis Du Pasquier (flute)
Silke Hennecke (flute)
Michèle Courtet (lute)
James Kaufman (drums)

Thilo Muster (harpsichord)
Alexandra Livingstone (harpsichord)
Steve Bauer (tenor)

A few sentences from the program leaflet are given below, and more is found in the QR document:

"This institute exemplifies the great diversity of the Elements of the Immune System. Living beings of all kinds spend their time between its walls: scientists from all over the world, and animals from throughout the animal kingdom. It is often difficult to distinguish among them all. Two examples will serve to describe this diversity: The Frog Galliard *by John Dowland (1562–1625) originally written for the lute, but played here on the harpsichord, and* La Poule *(the Hen) by Jean-Philippe Rameau (1683–1764), for harpsichord."*

... and in another part of the leaflet:

"Finally there is the experimental element, and we will conclude our musical portrait with the 'Tableau de l'opération de la taille' by Marin Marais (1656–1728) originally for viola da gamba and continuo, today played by a cello and harpsichord, showing the ins and outs of a kidney stone operation seen from the patient's view point."

The play, with its medical sketches, was filled with playful, sarcastic comments that only insiders understood; nevertheless, the main emphasis was on music, and it resonated extremely well with the audience [QR1991_06].

Surgery, Note by Note: Marin Marais' «Tableau de l'opération de la taille»

Excerpt from James L. Franklin: *"How has medicine been depicted in music? Examples from the operatic stage come to mind: tuberculosis in Verdi's* La Traviata *and Puccini's* La Bohème*; madness or delirium in the mad scene in Donizetti's* Lucia di Lammermoor *and Lady Macbeth's sleepwalking scene in Verdi's* Macbeth. *It is harder to find examples in instrumental music. Bedřich Smetana sought to represent his impaired tinnitus and hearing loss with a piercing sustained high E played by the first violin in the last movement of his string quartet No. 1 in E minor, 'From My Life'. There are those who hear the representation of Gustav Mahler's irregular heartbeat (probably atrial fibrillation associated with rheumatic mitral valvular heart disease) in the opening measures of his Ninth Symphony. This article presents a unique convergence of medical history and music in a piece written for the viol (viola da gamba) and continuo by the French composer and virtuoso viol player Marin Marais* [...],

QR1991_06 BII

a contemporary of Johann Sebastian Bach, depicting in music a surgical operation he endured at the age of 64 to remove a stone from his urinary bladder."

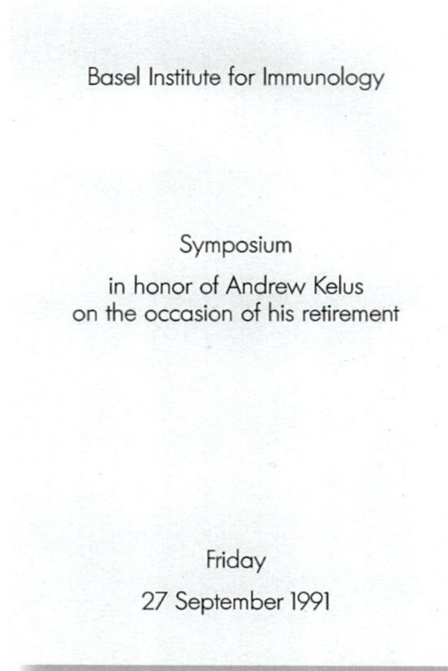
Basel Institute for Immunology

Symposium
in honor of Andrew Kelus
on the occasion of his retirement

Friday
27 September 1991

Symposium for Andrew Kelus

Andrew Kelus, a founding member of the BII, reached his retirement age, and for his farewell a symposium [QR1991_07] related to the rabbit model he worked on for decades was held on September 27th, 1991. The conference was opened by Fritz Melchers, under the chairmanship of Jean-Claude Weill. The 5 talks were given by Andrew's colleagues from Bethesda, Chicago, Brussels, Geneva and Davos.

Rose Mage	"Immunoglobulin genes of the rabbit – lessons from mutants and recombinants"
Katherine Knight	"Preferential utilization and diversification of VH genes in the rabbit"
Raymond Hamers	"Immunoglobulins from rabbits to camels"
Jean-Claude Jaton	"The rabbit lambda locus and the two major isotypes of immunoglobulin lambda chains, c7 and c2l"
Mark Suter	"Towards rabbit monoclonal antibodies"

Andrew's retirement also brought the era of the rabbit farm in Rodersdorf to an end. Andrew offered the rabbit stock to several work groups in the USA and the UK, and so the rabbits with their breeding protocols were transferred to new owners.

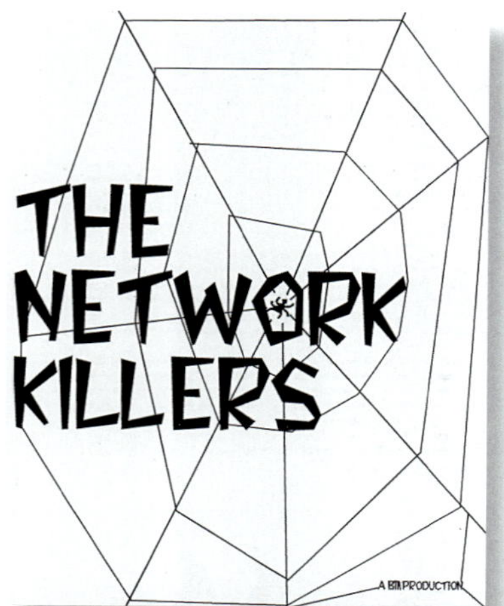

BTA 11: Commemorating 20 Years of the BII with the BTA Performance "The Network Killers" – A Theater Performance on Scientific Fraud and Its Consequences

A considerable part of success in science relates to the ethos of scientific conduct. Members of the BII were critical about others and also about themselves. Are the results real, true, reproducible? Are the presentations of results at internal seminars, at conferences, and finally when published, correct? This play addresses these points [QR1991_08]. Below is an excerpt from the script, in its own BTA exaggerated style:

"The Network Killers is something wholly different. Having gained experience and courage, the companies' writers have tackled the serious and topical problem of fraud in science. Their dissection of the motives of 'scientists who cheat' is uncanny and entirely believable. Although it is cloaked in the form of a traditional crime thriller, you should not doubt that this play has a serious message for our times.

Fraud has been with us since the earliest days of scientific endeavour. It is a topic about which scientists are extremely sensitive: could you explain the workings of your notebook to an agent of the FBI? The scientific world is now a cut-throat place: the prizes, the accolades even the jobs go to the people that get results FIRST. And so the pressure to be 'economical with the truth' may become overwhelming. The writers of the BTA have thought long and hard about scientific fraud: its risks and its consequences. After many long (drinking) sessions they finally came up with a way of addressing this delicate subject on stage. What you will witness this evening is a penetrating analysis of the motives of scientists that lie and cheat. It is not wholly unsympathetic and will make you think again about your prejudices. Do not be afraid to laugh, the BTA knows well that the best way to face your fears is to make a joke about them. But do not forget that this is a tale from the dark side of science."

Workshop on the Mechanisms of B Cell Neoplasia

A workshop on the Mechanisms of B Cell Neoplasia took place at the institute from April 14th to 16th, 1991 [QR1991_09]. Discoveries of early cellular stages in the development of the B lineage allowed for identification of early targets of transformation. The genetic predisposition of the host, as well as its condition during chronic infection, sets the background and environment in which B lineage cells operate for malignant changes as well as for normal development and immune responses. The new knowledge on the ligands that interact with the many receptors on cells of the B lineage to control growth and differentiation at various stages of B cell development gave a basis to search for the steps that contribute to premalignant and malignant transformations. The new findings were discussed in 5 sessions:

Session 1: Early B cell development
Session 2: B cells
Session 3: B cell tumors
Session 4: Oncogenes/transcription
Session 5: Plasmacytomas

Niels Jerne and guests celebrating his 80th birthday

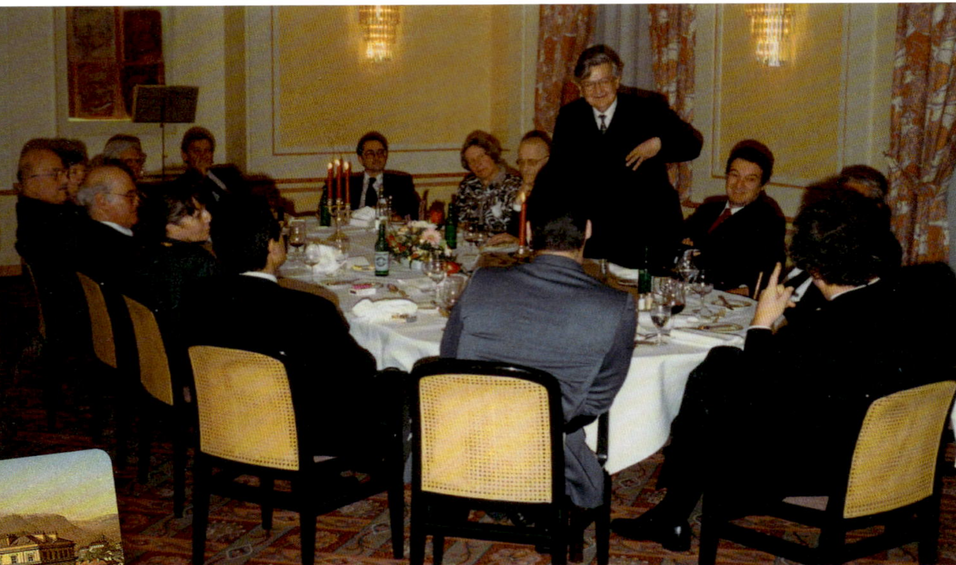

Niels Jerne's 80th Birthday

It was Niels' wish to keep the celebration of his round birthday in a modest frame, and this was accomplished by holding a quiet dinner in Geneva on December 23rd, 1991, at which stimulating discussion and excellent wine could be enjoyed [QR1991_10].

It was a rare occasion as philosophy rather than science was discussed. It revolved round Kierkegaard's impact on science and society. Besides Niels, the invitees were as follows:

Lucien Aarden, Rob Benner, Valentin Bonifas, Antonio Coutinho, Louis Du Pasquier, Eduard Kellenberger, Ivan Lefkovits, Fritz Melchers, Klaus Rajewsky, Werner Reichert, Theo Staehelin, Charley Steinberg and Gunther Stent.

Mrs. Kok Kellenberger and Mrs. Inga Stent were accompanying guests.

Roche Acquires a Patent for the Polymerase Chain Reaction Procedure from Cetus

The polymerase chain reaction (PCR) is a procedure for amplifying a single copy or a few copies of a piece of DNA across several orders of magnitude, generating millions of copies of a particular DNA sequence. The method was invented by Kary Mullis, for which he received the Nobel Prize in 1993. The acquisition of this patent (and many related ones) gave Roche the possibility to develop many new diagnostic kits.

QR1991_10 BII

700th Anniversary of the Foundation of Switzerland, 1991

The creation of the Federal Charter of 1291, when 3 Alpine cantons (Schwyz, Uri and Unterwalden) swore the oath of confederation, is regarded as the foundation of Switzerland. The National Day that commemorates this is August 1st [QR1991_11].

This anniversary was celebrated on all levels, political, cultural and scientific, and it was repeatedly stated that Switzerland was fortunate to be spared all the conflicts which most other countries experienced. It took another decade for Switzerland to join the UN.

QR1991_11 BII

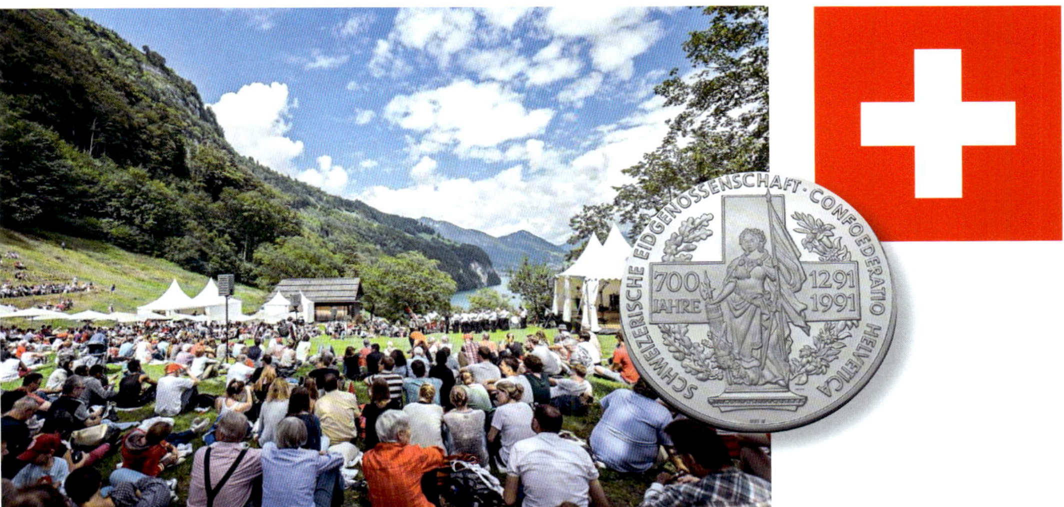

Anniversary celebration on the Rütliwiese

Treasure Trove 1991

The database contains documents related to the BII in a broader context (lists, series of photographs, etc.).

QR1991_treasure BII

Next page: Plaque-forming cells from limiting dilution analysis

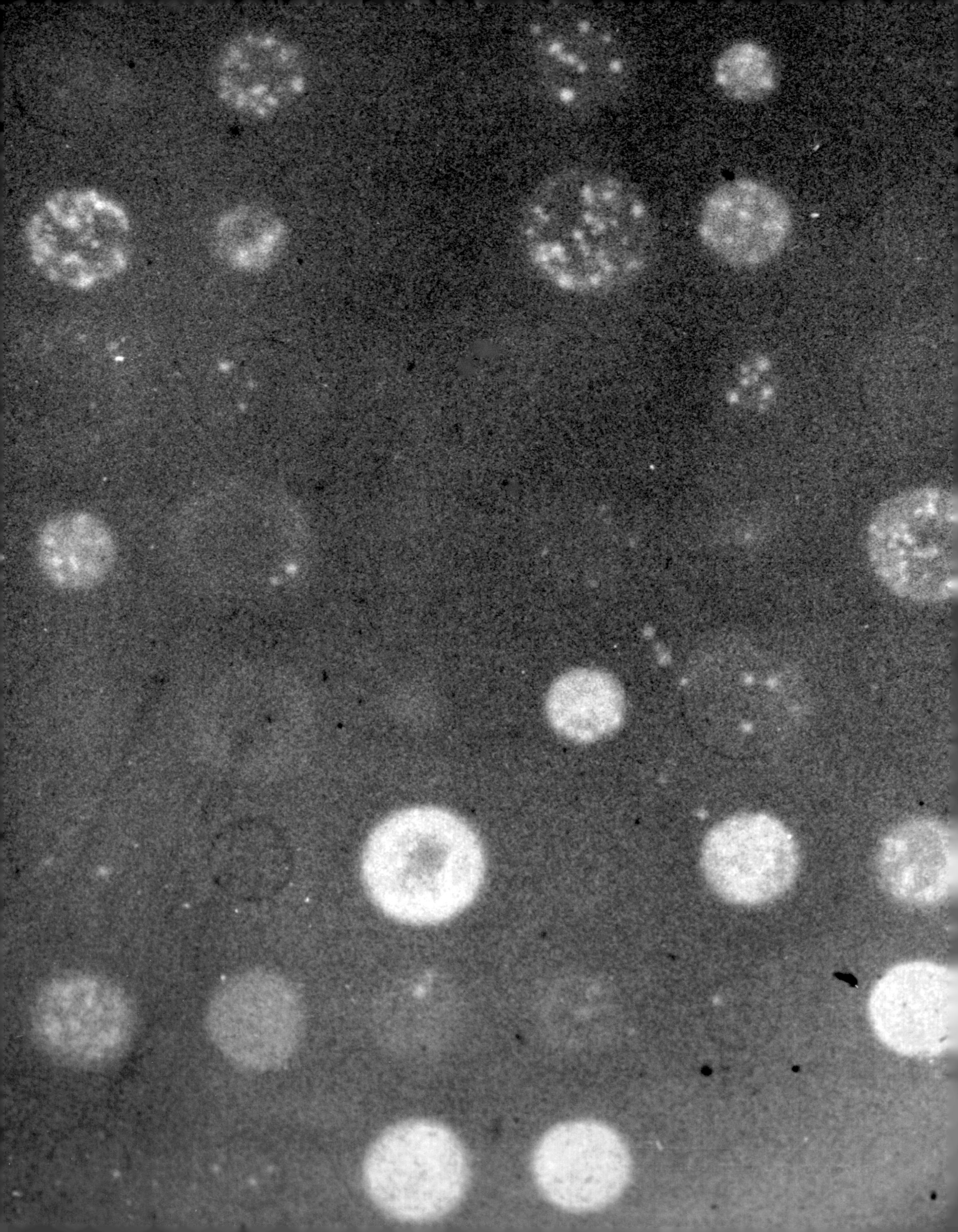

The Year 1992

Several conferences and workshops were organized; among them were "Retroviruses as Antigens and Superantigens in Auto-Immunity and Tolerance" and "EMBO Workshop on Cell-Cell Interactions in Leukocyte Homing and Differentiation". Michael Steinmetz, a former BII permanent member, became head of Roche Research in Nutley, USA. Antonio Lanzavecchia became a new permanent member. The first Central European Summer School of Immunology (first of 4 annually) was organized by BII members in Piešťany, Czechoslovakia. Institute members lectured and chaired sessions at the International Congress of Immunology in Budapest.

Antonio Lanzavecchia, New Permanent Member, 1992

Antonio joined the BII in 1984. His combined interest in modern basic immunology research and in human physiology and pathology predestined him to address questions of molecular mechanisms related to the human immune system. In 1992 he was appointed as a permanent member of the BII and established a work group that on reaching a critical size (beyond what the horizontal structure of the BII allowed) opened a future opportunity to found an institute specializing in human immunology. In 1999 Antonio became the founding director of the Institute for Research in Biomedicine in Bellinzona [QR1992_01].

Arrivals 1992 (9)
Thomas Brocker, Kerry Campbell, Isabelle Chrétien, Pierre Cosson, Rolf Jessberger, Yoshihiro Oka, Hans-Reimer Rodewald, Hans-Joachim Wallny, Thomas Winkler.

Came and Left in the Same Year (5)
Walter Gerhard, Maria Guttinger, Zoher Kapasi, Takafumi Uchida, Ian Walker. ▶

Michael Steinmetz, a Former BII Permanent Member, Becomes Head of Roche Research in Nutley, USA

From the prestigious position as head of the Roche Biology Department in Basel, Michael was promoted to oversee the worldwide biotechnology research activities of Roche. At the Preclinical Research and Development Department in Nutley, Michael Steinmetz directed a research group of over 800 scientists who focused on chronic inflammatory and autoimmune diseases, oncology, obesity and diabetes. Multiple drug candidates, including recombinant proteins, antibodies and small molecules, were identified under his leadership and moved into clinical trials [QR1992_02].

QR1992_01 BII

QR1992_02 BII

▶ **Leavers 1992 (12)**
Yair Argon, Giulia Casorati, Una Chen, Paolo Dellabona, Shigeo Ekino, José Carlos Gutierrez-Ramos, Seiji Inui, Akira Kudo, Ronald Palacios, Jan Salomonsen, Eva-Susanne Strobel, Melanie Wilson.

Lecture Series for Students from Marburg and Prague

A series of lectures in immunology held at the BII for students from the Philipps University Marburg and the Charles University Prague (September 1992) was followed by extensive discussion and visits to the lecturers' laboratories:

Roland Gisler	"Ontogeny of the Immune System"
Louis Du Pasquier	"Evolution of the Immune System"
Stéphane Demotz	"Polymorphism of DRbeta Regulates Peptide Binding"
Alexandra Livingstone	"Antigen Processing and Presentation"
Richard Pink	"Immunology of Vaccine Development"
Ivan Lefkovits	"Rules for Gene Expression in Lymphocytes"
Marie Kosco	"Antigen Handling, Memory Formation, and Ab Maintenance"
Pawel Kisielow	"T Cell Development"
Michael V. Wiles	"Embryonic Stem Cells and Development"
Jean-Marie Buerstedde	"Mechanisms of Diversity Generation"
Fritz Melchers	"Immune System: Problems Awaiting Solution"

Marburg students:

Martina Brandl	Delia Bussfeld	Angela Denzel
Heike Fesq	Ellen Fritsch	Birgit Jaspert
Petra Karhausen	Elke Leemhuis	Beate Maid
Judith Marscheck	Eckhardt Petri	Jan Sagrudny
Markus Schnare	Jiirg Schoneck	Sabine Trommer
Matthias Wahle		

Prague students:

Jana Borkova	Dominika Grundova	David Komarek
Igor Puzanov		

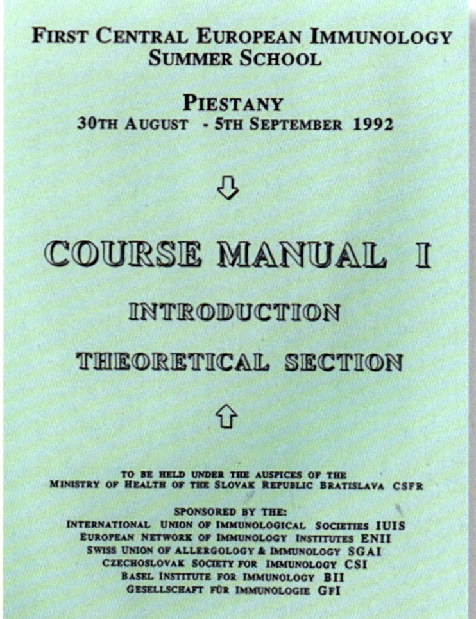
FIRST CENTRAL EUROPEAN IMMUNOLOGY SUMMER SCHOOL

PIESTANY
30TH AUGUST - 5TH SEPTEMBER 1992

COURSE MANUAL I

INTRODUCTION

THEORETICAL SECTION

TO BE HELD UNDER THE AUSPICES OF THE
MINISTRY OF HEALTH OF THE SLOVAK REPUBLIC BRATISLAVA CSFR

SPONSORED BY THE:
INTERNATIONAL UNION OF IMMUNOLOGICAL SOCIETIES IUIS
EUROPEAN NETWORK OF IMMUNOLOGY INSTITUTES ENII
SWISS UNION OF ALLERGOLOGY & IMMUNOLOGY SGAI
CZECHOSLOVAK SOCIETY FOR IMMUNOLOGY CSI
BASEL INSTITUTE FOR IMMUNOLOGY BII
GESELLSCHAFT FÜR IMMUNOLOGIE GFI

The 1st Central European Summer School of Immunology

A 2-week course with lectures and laboratory work was organized in Piešťany, Czechoslovakia. The teaching staff was from the Basel Institute for Immunology, the Central Laboratory of the Blood Transfusion Center, Amsterdam, the Weizmann Institute for Immunology and several other institutions. The local organization was in the hands of the Rheumatology Institute, Piešťany [QR1992_03]. It was a course in which for the first time scientists and students met after the Iron Curtain had fallen. Apart from the BII, support came from the Swiss Society for Immunology and the European Network of Immunology Institutes. Students were mainly from Czechoslovakia (the course took place before the country split into the Czech Republic and Slovakia), Hungary, Poland, Ukraine and Russia.

SCHEDULE FOR THE PARTICIPANTS AT THE PRACTICAL SECTION OF THE SUMMER SCHOOL

	GENERAL LECTURES - MORNING	PRACTICAL SECTION Laboratory Work
MONDAY 31ST AUGUST	**Hans Hengartner, Zurich** - *On antiviral immunity, tolerance and autoreactivity* **Antonio Coutinho, Paris** - *An organism-centered view of the immune system* **Antonio Lanzavecchia, Basel** – *Antigen processing and presentation to T cells*	Lucien Aarden and Els de Groot, Amsterdam Jim Kaufman and David Avila, Basel André Traunecker and Filippo Oliveri, Basel
TUESDAY 1ST SEPTEMBER	**Roland Gisler, Basel** - *The function of cell adhesion molecules in the immune system* **Polly Matzinger, Bethesda** - *Mechanisms of tolerance* **Peter Lachmann, Cambridge** - *The complement system and disease*	Lucien Aarden and Els de Groot, Amsterdam Jim Kaufman and David Avila, Basel André Traunecker and Filippo Oliveri, Basel
WEDNESDAY 2ND SEPTEMBER	**Miroslav Ferencik, Bratislava** - *Molecular basis of phagocytosis* **Ivan Lefkovits, Basel** - *Quantitative cellular immunology: frequencies of rare cells and their measurement* **Alexandra Livingstone, Basel** - *Antigen presentation by MHC class I molecules*	Lucien Aarden and Els de Groot, Amsterdam Jim Kaufman and David Avila, Basel André Traunecker and Filippo Oliveri, Basel
THURSDAY 3RD SEPTEMBER	**Michael Wiles, Basel** - *Mouse embryonic stem (ES) cells: what are they and what can they be used for!* **Milan Buc, Bratislava** - *The major histocompatibility complex in man* **Klaus Hartmann, Marburg** - *Ontogenesis of the thymus*	Lucien Aarden and Els de Groot, Amsterdam Jim Kaufman and David Avila, Basel André Traunecker and Filippo Oliveri, Basel
FRIDAY 4TH SEPTEMBER	**Jean-Marie Buerstedde, Basel** - *Lymphoid-specific DNA recombination* **Günther Hämmerling, Heidelberg** - *Extrathymic T cell selection* **Carlos Pereira, Sao Paulo** - *Immunity to viral infections*	Lucien Aarden and Els de Groot, Amsterdam Jim Kaufman and David Avila, Basel André Traunecker and Filippo Oliveri, Basel
SATURDAY 5TH SEPTEMBER	Closing Session of Laboratory Work: Lucien Aarden and Els de Groot, Amsterdam Jim Kaufman and David Avila, Basel André Traunecker and Filippo Oliveri, Basel	

Teaching staff:

Milan Buc, Jean-Marie Buerstedde, Antonio Coutinho, Miroslav Ferencik, Roland Gisler, Günter J. Hämmerling, Klaus-Ulrich Hartmann, Hans Hengartner, Peter Lachmann, Antonio Lanzavecchia, Ivan Lefkovits, Alexandra Livingstone, Polly Matzinger, Fritz Melchers, Roald S. Nezlin, Carlos A. Pereira, Jaroslav Sterzl, Michael V. Wiles.

Una Chen to Erlangen and Giessen, 1992

Una left the BII in 1992 and accepted a position as group leader at the Max Planck Institute in Erlangen, Germany. Her next appointment was as an EC fellow in Marseille, France. Later she moved to the University of Giessen, Germany, where she was given the possibility to form her own group. Both at the BII and later in Erlangen and Giessen she worked on stem cell biology. She developed an efficient way to differentiate murine embryonic stem cells to lymphoid precursor cells in culture. Her further work was geared towards establishing and characterizing tetracycline/doxycycline-responding mouse cell lines from transgenic mESC and transgenic mice.

QR1992_03 BII

Una's further activities, especially her skill at organizing social events for former BII members (1989–2016), are dealt with in the QR code [QR 1992_04].

QR1992_04 BII

WORKSHOP
on
RETROVIRUSES AS ANTIGENS AND SUPERANTIGENS IN AUTOIMMUNITY AND TOLERANCE

27th - 29th September 1992
Basel Institute for Immunology, Switzerland

Organizers:	Fritz Melchers	Basel Institute for Immunology, Switzerland
	Ton Rolink	Basel Institute for Immunology, Switzerland
	Bernhard Fleischer	Johannes Gutenberg University Mainz, Germany
	Joachim R Kalden	University of Erlangen-Nürnberg, Germany
	Hermann Wagner	Inst. Med. Microbiol. & Hygiene Munich, Germany

The aim of the workshop is to bring together retrovirologists, retroviral immunologists (including those working in the area of superantigens), and immunologists working in the field of tolerance in order to discuss the main theme.

INVITED SPEAKERS

Hans Acha-Orbea	*Epalinges*	Pawel Kisielow	*Basel*
Luciano Adorini	*Basel*	Philippe Kourilsky	*Paris*
Antonio Bandeira	*Paris*	Arthur Krieg	*Iowa City*
Pierre-André Cazenave	*Paris*	H Robson MacDonald	*Epalinges*
Bruce W Chesebro	*Hamilton*	R N Maini	*London*
Antonio Coutinho	*Paris*	Herbert C Morse, III	*Bethesda*
Paolo Dellabona	*Basel*	Ed Palmer	*Denver*
Volker Erfle	*Munich*	John L Portis	*Hamilton*
Martin Flajnik	*Miami*	Josselyne Salaün	*Nogent-s.-Marne*
Rolf M Flügel	*Heidelberg*	Jonathan Sprent	*La Jolla*
Steven M Friedman	*New York*	Alfred D Steinberg	*Bethesda*
Janet W Hartley	*Bethesda*	Jonathan P Stoye	*London*
Klaus Heeg	*Munich*	Patrick J Venables	*London*
Martin Herrmann	*Erlangen*	Sue Webb	*La Jolla*
Brigitte Huber	*Boston*	Rolf Zinkernagel	*Zürich*
John Kappler	*Denver*		

In addition to the speakers, 30-40 participants will be accepted. Hotel accommodation will be provided; travel and staying expenses to be covered by the applicants.
Applications - including curriculum vitae, list of publications, and a short letter indicating main scientific interests, in particular those related to the workshop theme - to be sent to:

Dr Ton Rolink, Basel Institute for Immunology, Postfach, CH-4005 Basel, Switzerland

DEADLINE FOR RECEIPT OF APPLICATIONS: 1st AUGUST 1992

Retroviruses as Antigens and Superantigens in Autoimmunity and Tolerance, 1992

A few years earlier a major discovery had been made which demonstrated that retroviruses encode the so-called superantigens. The property of these superantigens is that they are capable of stimulating T cells via superantigen-reactive T cell receptors.

The workshop, sponsored by Roche, the German Research Association, the German Society for Immunology, Smith Kline Beecham Foundation and the Wellcome Trust, covered basics about retroviral elements in the initiation and propagation of both autoimmune diseases and tolerance. It was organized by Fritz Melchers, Ton Rolink, Bernhard Fleischer, Joachim Kalden and Hermann Wagner. Among the prominent participants and speakers were Ed Palmer, Brigitte Huber, Jon Sprent, Pierre-André Cazenave, Rolf Zinkernagel, Philippe Kourilsky and Luciano Adorini.

A far-reaching discussion on the properties of the superantigens led to the view that B cells are essential for the completion of the viral life cycle in vivo. This indicates that B cells are infected first and that viral amplification takes place only if infected B cells present the superantigen on their surface which, in turn, results in activation of T cells (activated T cells then stimulate B cells, which enables viral replication).

In the QR code [QR1992_05] the titles of the lectures are listed. The titles from the Tolerance Session are given below:

R. Zinkernagel	"A Super Virus without Superantigens (LCMV)"
L. Adorini	"Presentation of Self Antigens by MHC Class II Molecules"
H.-J. Wallny	"Peptides Eluted from MHC Class I Molecules"
P. Kourilsky	"Tolerance to a Self Protein as a Function of its Expression Level"

QR1992_05 BII

QR1992_06 BII

EMBO Workshop on Cell-Cell Interactions in Leukocyte Homing and Differentiation

It was a conceptual leap in the field of cell adhesion when it was realized that adhesion is a multistep process in which integrin activation and cytokines play important roles. Thus, the simple expression of an adhesion molecule is only one of the factors in determining the specificity of leukocytes for a tissue. A workshop on the concepts of cell adhesion, leukocyte interactions, development and cancer metastasis was organized by Beat Imhof, Charles Mackay, Dominique Dunon, Ursula Günthert and Antonius Rolink [QR1992_06]. The themes were divided into 5 sessions:

Session 1: Molecular mechanisms of lymphocyte homing
Session 2: Leukocyte extravasation during inflammatory reactions
Session 3: Metastasis
Session 4: Lymphocyte interactions
Session 5: Cell-cell contact and differentiation

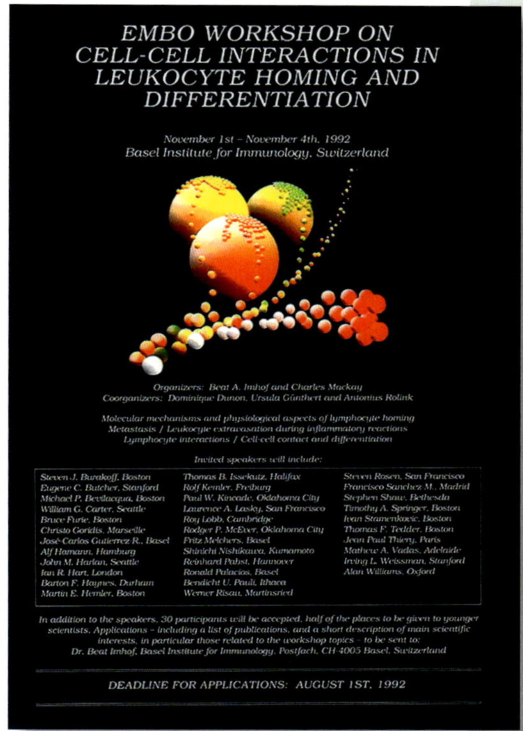

Several talks were discussed in some detail, for instance:

I.R. Hart	"Changes in adhesion receptor during malignant melanoma progression"
B.A. Imhof	"Adhesion molecules in thymus homing and metastasis"
P.W. Kincade	"Communication between stromal cells and lymphocyte precursors"

The 34 participants at the workshop are listed in the above-mentioned QR code QR1992_05.

8th International Congress of Immunology in Budapest, 1992

Similarly to all previous International Congresses of Immunology (that started in 1971) the 8th International Congress in Budapest [QR1992_07] was an interesting event with good attendance from Basel. The president of the Congress was Janos Gergely who ensured that not only was there outstanding science, but also no lack of traditional Hungarian hospitality.

A. Lanzavecchia, H. Karasuyama, H-J. Wallny, U. Chen, L. Du Pasquier, M. Kosco-Vilbois, D. Dunon, H. von Boehmer, J. Kaufman, F. Melchers and G.M. Griffiths were among the lecturers, chairmen and co-chairmen.

QR1992_07 BII

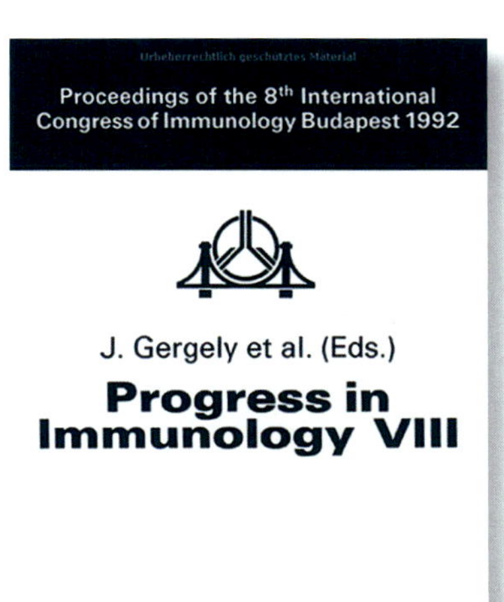

Treasure Trove 1992
The database contains documents related to the BII in a broader context (lists, series of photographs, etc.).

QR1992_treasure BII

The Year 1993

Ed Palmer joined the institute as a permanent member. Another workshop on the Mechanisms of B Cell Neoplasia was held at the BII. An informative booklet (about new members, changes, departures), "BII News", was launched. The 2nd Central European Summer School of Immunology was held in Czechia. "Gwendolyn", a sculpture created by Niki de Saint Phalle, to partner Tinguely's "Double Helix", was inaugurated.

Arrivals 1993 (13)
Jan Andersson, Thomas Bäckström, Paolo Ghia, Kristian Hannestad, François Letourneur, Kazuo Ohnishi, Ed Palmer, Federica Sallusto, Reinhard Stauder, Wojciech Swat, Georg Tiefenthaler, Salvatore Valitutti, Matthias Wabl.

Came and Left in the Same Year (1)
Susanna Weber.

Leavers 1993 (2)
Dominique Dunon, Insoo Park.

Ed Palmer Joins the Institute as a Permanent Member

It became a common trend in 1992 to invest more effort into researching T cell immunology (Mel Cohn authoritatively declared that B cell immunology was solved, though not everybody was convinced about this), and Fritz Melchers – himself a B cell immunologist – offered Ed Palmer a position as a permanent member in the institute. This shows that Ed, in his successful sabbatical (2 years earlier), had "passed" the test; it might have been the case that the director felt that Ed would not have accepted a "lesser" offer. Ed adjusted to his new life in Basel: successfully passed another test, a social one, by learning the Swiss German dialect (for which he was widely admired). He received great support from Jim Kaufman and started collaborating with Kerry Campbell on the structural features of B and T cell receptors. Ed and Kerry collected all the published transmembrane sequences and identified a motif shared by all TCRs and membrane Ig. By identifying parts of the TCR that controlled the generation of signals, his laboratory was in a position to understand the generation of T cell tolerance [QR1993_01].

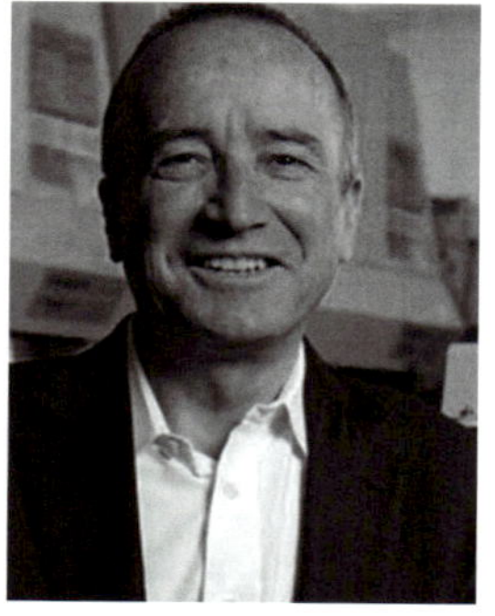

Matthias Wabl

Matthias Wabl Joins Again

After leaving the BII in 1978, Matthias embarked on a remarkable career at various institutions. Later he felt that the time had come to immerse himself again into some unresolved issues, in particular on somatic mutation and measuring spontaneous mutations taking place in the gene encoding the immunoglobulin heavy chain – a project that he hoped to pursue with Charley Steinberg.

He started several other projects, among them on somatic mutations during immune response in *Xenopus* tadpoles. He committed himself to stay at the BII for a year.

BII News Booklet

The administration of the BII started on an ad hoc basis to issue a small booklet, "BII News", which provided information about scientists and technicians, and their activities. Kim Rüfenacht (secretary to Roland Gisler) took care of the content (and of updates) of the brochure. Maybe 8 booklets were produced during the years; they can be considered snapshots of "who was who" and are available in the QR database [QR1993_02].

QR1993_01 BII

QR1993_02 BII

The 2nd Central European Summer School of Immunology, 1993

A major 2-week course in České Budějovice was organized in a similar format as the previous one in Pieštany. Most of the teachers from the first Summer School volunteered to teach in České Budějovice [QR1993_03]. The major burden rested with André Traunecker, Lucien Aarden and Klaus Hartmann, who prepared the experimental course program (taking instruments from Prague, Holland and Germany). There were 120 students from Czechia/Slovakia, Poland, Hungary, Ukraine and Russia, and also from the former GDR.

QR1993_03 BII

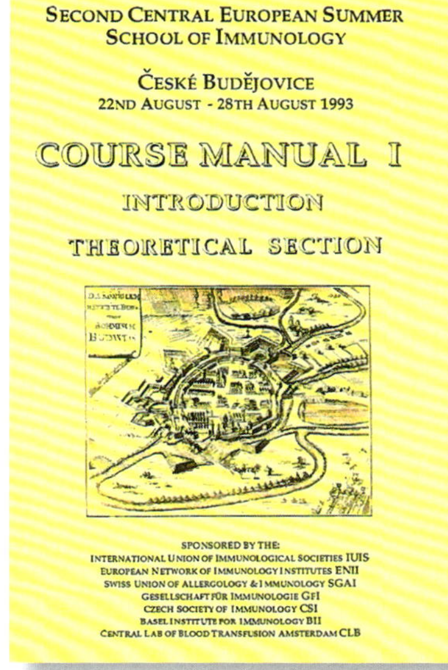

THE SECOND CENTRAL EUROPEAN SUMMER SCHOOL OF IMMUNOLOGY
CESKE BUDEJOVICE 1993

	MORNING LECTURE PROGRAM		*AFTERNOON PROGRAM*			
MONDAY AUGUST 23	*Cells of the immune system* Fritz Melchers: B cells Alexandra Livingstone: T cells	LUNCH	LAB WORK	Methodology lecture Ivan Lefkovits: Analysis of rare cells	LAB WORK	Get-together party at the beer brewery Budvar
TUESDAY AUGUST 24	*Receptors and ligands* Polly Matzinger: MHC and genes Roland Gisler: Adhesion molecules and genes	LUNCH	*Receptors and ligands (cont.)* Jean-Marie Buerstedde: Immunoglobulin superfamily and its genes Hans-Jürgen Thiesen: Turning genes on and off		LAB WORK	
WEDNESDAY AUGUST 25	*Mechanisms* Hans-Peter Pircher: Autoimmunity Polly Matzinger: Tolerance	LUNCH	LAB WORK		Excursion to Cesky Krumlov and Dinner	
THURSDAY AUGUST 26	*Immunoparasitology* (course "emphasis") Jean Langhorne: Malaria Jacques Louis: Leishmaniasis	LUNCH	LAB WORK	Methodology lecture André Traunecker: DNA, RNA	Methodology lecture A. Livingstone: Cell sorter data	LAB WORK
FRIDAY AUGUST 27	*Systems, species* Louis Du Pasquier: The immune system throughout the species Michael Wiles: Embryogenesis. Development of stem cells	LUNCH	LAB WORK	Methodology lecture Lucien Aarden: Interleukins	Methodology lecture Klaus Hartmann/ David Avila: on the results from the lab work	LAB WORK
SATURDAY AUGUST 28	Jaroslav Sterzl: Overview and afterthoughts SESSION CLOSING	Departure				

Optimistic and Pessimistic Views on the Immune System

The immune system enables us to live longer, but the longer we live, the more perilous it might be for our health.

Fritz Melchers

In his Introduction to the 1993 Annual Report, Fritz Melchers focused on the issue that advances in the research on self/nonself discrimination open paths for studying autoimmune diseases. An excerpt from the Introduction follows:

"We realize more and more that the system of defence can also be dangerous for our wellbeing and for our very existence. Practically every part of our body can be attacked by our own immune system. The capacity of the system to distinguish 'self' from 'non-self' is not perfect, and autoimmune diseases and immunodeficiencies might be the result. Unspecific immune reactions are fast, but less precise and strong. Specific responses (B cell and T cell mediated defence reactions) are slow to develop, but are more precise. B and T cell responses can further 'improve' through developing memory for antigen, which is of profound advantage if the antigen is foreign. There can be disastrous consequences, however, if the antigen is an integral structure of the host, or if the recognition of the foreign invader also destroys portions of the host. The immune system enables us to live longer, but the longer we live, the more perilous it might be for our health."

Trends in 1993

Although the study of antibody diversity remained a central research area, many molecular studies on Ig gene structure and rearrangement, and on the TCR, continued to be of interest. New approaches enabled the identification of function and structure of cell surface molecules and their involvement in lymphocyte differentiation, and in repertoire selection. Also work on early hematopoietic progenitors yielded interesting insights into understanding the processes of differentiation. Further attention was given to the relationship of memory formation and germinal center development [QR1993_04].

QR1993_04 BII

Sculpture Created by Niki de Saint Phalle

In the institute's atrium, close to Jean Tinguely's black helix, a large and colorful sculpture (named "Gwendolyn") created by Niki de Saint Phalle was placed. Gwendolyn was unveiled by Paul Sacher on September 2nd, 1993, and began to rotate on a computer-driven turntable constructed by a team from the institute workshop [QR1993_05].

QR1993_05 BII

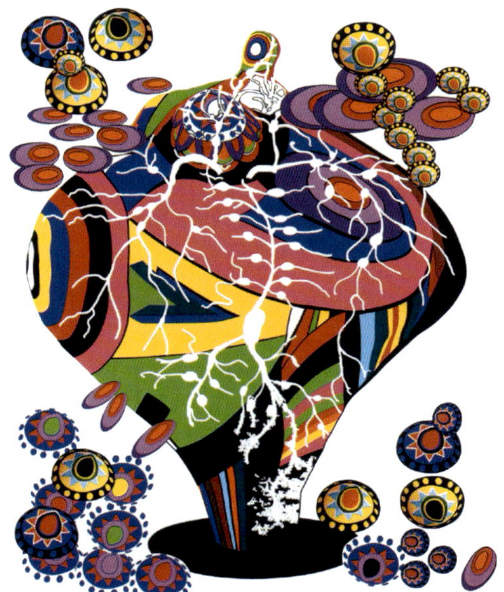

Gwendolyn ist da

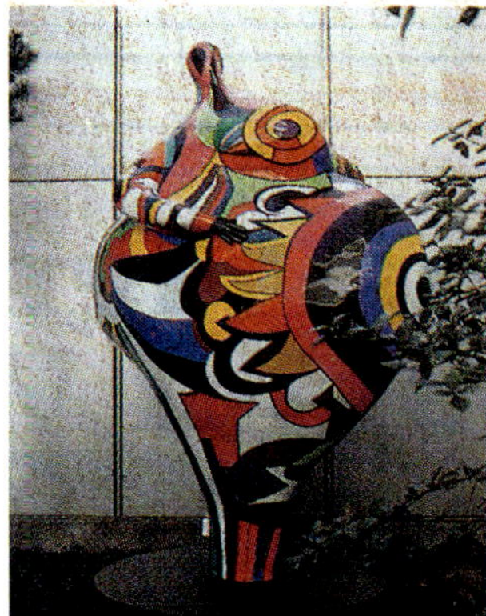

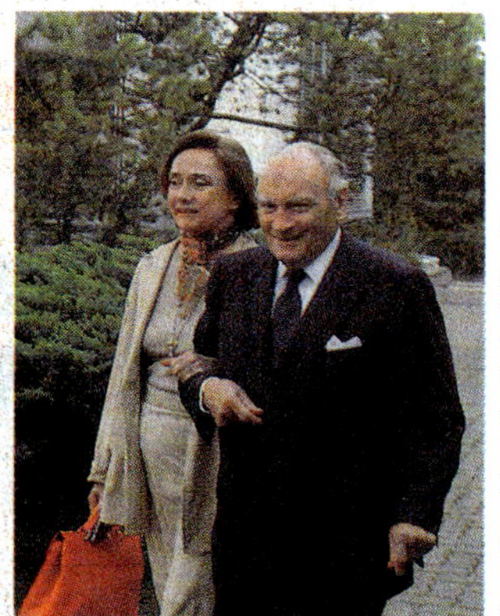

Frohe Gesichter im Institut für Immunologie an der Grenzacherstrasse: Niki de Saint-Phalle mit Paul Sacher (rechts). Links: Gwendolyn. *Fotos Hannes-Dirk Flury.*

(Reproduced from the *Basler Zeitung*)

Years earlier Tinguely had stated: "Niki has never stopped dreaming; she could always forget her environment and draw. She drew constantly on paper or in her thoughts."

Workshop on the Mechanisms of B Cell Neoplasia

The 11th in a series of annual workshops on the Mechanisms of B Cell Neoplasia was organized by Michael Potter and Fritz Melchers, and took place at the institute in April 1993 [QR1993_06]. The aim of the workshop was to search for molecular mechanisms involved in the development of normal B cells. It is striking that part of B cell development actually depends on genetic instability, and this genetic instability (in contrast to that of T cells) does not cease when B cells leave the primary organs. In the germinal centers, where B lymphocytes react to antigen, there is proliferation, switching and eventually differentiation into plasma cells.

QR1993_06 BII

QR1993_07 BII

Nobel Prize for the Invention of the Polymerase Chain Reaction

Kary B. Mullis and Michael Smith were awarded the Nobel Prize for Chemistry 1993 for inventing the PCR method [QR1993_07]. The polymerase chain reaction is considered to be one of the most important scientific advances of the 20th century. It enables unlimited copies of DNA to be created from just one original DNA strand. In 1991 Roche bought the rights to PCR (Roche Molecular Diagnostics).

Treasure Trove 1993

The database contains documents related to the BII in a broader context (lists, series of photographs, etc.).

QR1993_treasure BII

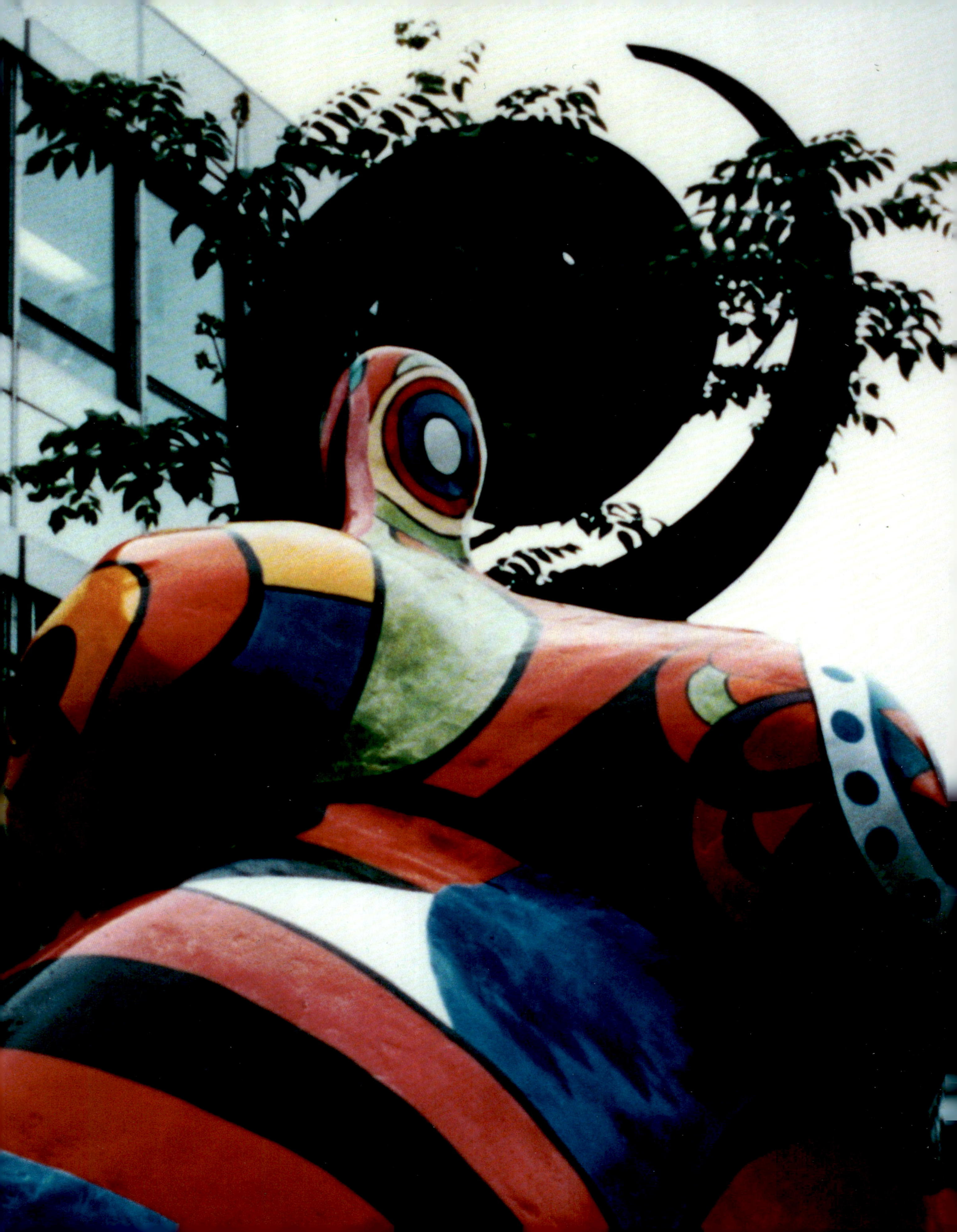

The Year 1994

A workshop on immunology and developmental biology of the chicken was held at the BII. The 3rd Central European Summer School of Immunology was held in Slovakia. Polly Matzinger formulated the hypothesis for the immune system dubbed "the danger model". Ivan Lefkovits celebrated 25 years at the BII. Niels K. Jerne died on October 7th, 1994.

Some Considerations on MHC and Peptide Binding

Portions of the Introduction to the 1994 Annual Report relate to MHC polymorphism and peptide binding, to helper and cytolytic cells, to processes of inducing anergy and response and last but not least to quantitative aspects of occupancy and signaling with peptide/MHC complexes:

"MHC Polymorphism and Peptide Binding. *Organisms of a species carry a large number of alleles of MHC genes. The structures of the MHC alleles differ mainly in areas that encode the peptide-binding regions. Any individual organism, with only two (usually different) alleles from its parents has a lower peptide-binding capacity than the sum of all members of the species. Confronted with a pathogen, some members of a species may be good immune responders, because they can bind and present peptides of that particular pathogen to T cells, while other members of the species are less good responders, since their MHC molecules yield with the peptides a less stable complex.*

Helper and Cytolytic Cells. *CD4+ and CD8+ cells have different destinies. CD4+ MHC class II-adapted T cells develop into precursors of helper T cells. CD8+ MHC class I-adapted T cells develop into precursors for cytolytic killer T cells.*

Quantitative analysis of the peripheral T cell repertoire provides means to establish how many of these T cells are helpers or killers; how many express CD4 and CD8; and how many are restricted to either MHC class I or II.

Anergy and Response. *When T and B cells enter the peripheral, secondary lymphoid organs, they are in the stage of resting cells in the Go phase of the cell cycle. They can remain such unless their TCR or Ig receptors encounter 'structures' for which they have high avidity. Such interactions will activate the cells in two possible ways:*

Arrivals 1994 (3)
Marina Cella, Marco Colonna, Olli Vainio.

Leavers 1994 (10)
Agnès Baron, Stéphane Demotz, Ulrich Deuschle, Kristian Hannestad, Marie Kosco-Vilbois, Charles Mackay, Franca Ronchese, Wojciech Swat, Georg Tiefenthaler, Matthias Wabl.

Polly succeeded in amalgamating views shared by adaptive and innate immunity.

1) by inducing an anergic state that abolishes their 'resting longevity' and leads to their deletion from the peripheral repertoire, thus establishing peripheral tolerance. This occurs with antigens that the cells have not seen 'centrally', i.e. in the primary lymphoid organs.

2) by inducing an immune response during which the cells will be activated and will enter the cell cycle, divide and mature to effector functions, i.e. help, killing, and antibody secretion. This occurs when antigen is recognized in an area of a secondary lymphoid organ where the immune response is initiated.

Some Quantitative Aspects. *Different concentrations of antigen result in the formation of different numbers of peptide/MHC complexes on a given antigen-presenting cell. A high dose of antigen yields nearly 10,000 complexes while a lower concentration will yield some 100 of them. As a consequence of this peptide/MHC recognition, TCR expression is down-regulated and cytokine production is induced. However, the difference in the biological performance of the T cells at 100-fold different peptide/MHC complex presentations is only two-fold. This indicates that when lower complex concentrations are offered to the T cell, up to 300 TCR molecules engage in successive rounds of occupancy and signalling with one peptide/MHC complex. When the peptide in the complex is replaced by another peptide that binds with the same affinity to MHC, but with lower affinity for the TCR, the biological response of the T cell and the occupancy of the TCR are both diminished to a similar extent."*

Danger Model 1994

Polly Matzinger's "danger model" was described in the 1986 chapter, while the actual proposition was only widely discussed years later. Polly succeeded in amalgamating views shared by adaptive and innate immunity; in the past the innate immunity was considered to be a minor part of the immune system. According to the danger theory, there is no adaptive immunity without the innate part. The immune system is not concerned by plain nonself, but rather it responds to signals that mark dangerous physiological conditions. Later Polly's model was extended to form the "damage-associated molecular pattern model". In essence, this model suggests that any non-functional molecule (regardless of their cellular location – whether extracellular or intracellular) that is denatured, oxidized or having disintegrated quaternary structures might contribute to the molecular pattern associated with the danger signal.

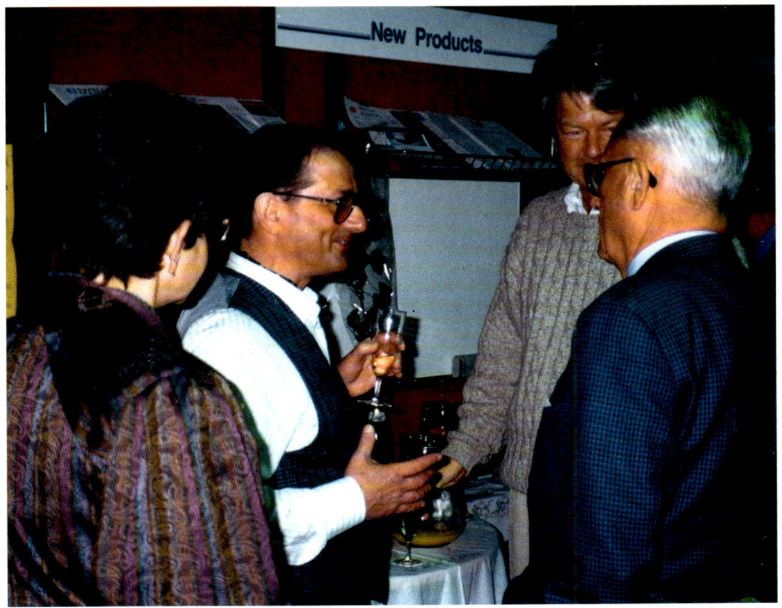

Celebrating Ivan Lefkovits' 25th anniversary at the BII

Ivan Lefkovits: 25 Years at the BII

With a glass of champagne BII members toasted Ivan on this anniversary. Ivan had been a member since April 1st, 1969. One of the distinguished well-wishers was Prof. Alfred Pletscher. The toast was followed by an "apéro riche" at the BII [QR1994_01].

Ivan Lefkovits came to Basel at the time the foundation stone of the institute was laid. His main duty then was to oversee the construction of the institute and all that this entailed. Niels Jerne concentrated on the crucial task of choosing future staff. This is detailed in the first volume of this history.

The 3rd Central European Summer School of Immunology, 1994

The schedule of the 2-week course in Košice (Eastern Slovakia) was similar to previous ones, but with the difference that a number of scientific presentations from Czechia and Slovakia was included. The teaching staff included new faces from France, Portugal and other Western countries [QR1994_02].

The artwork on the cover is an adaptation of a picture called "The Flowers" painted by Andy Warhol in 1970. The original painting can be seen in the Museum of Modern Art of Family Warhol, in Medzilaborce, near Košice. Altering the colors of the poppies into

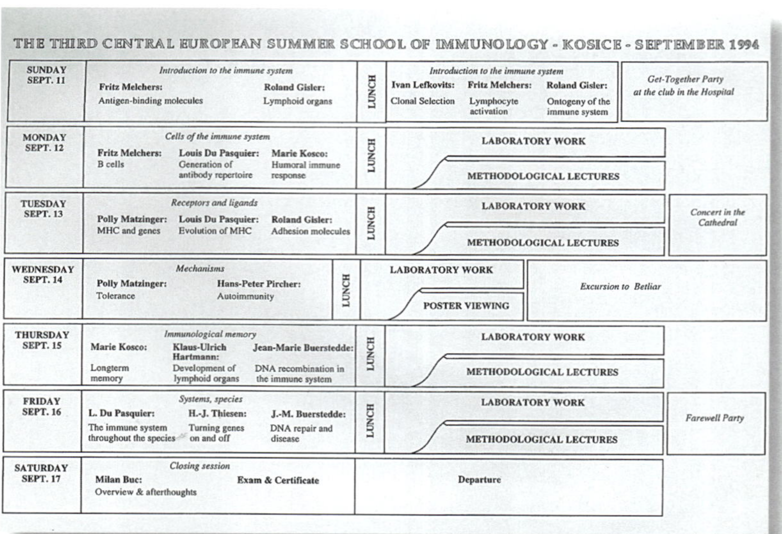

THE THIRD CENTRAL EUROPEAN SUMMER SCHOOL OF IMMUNOLOGY - KOSICE - SEPTEMBER 1994

Day	Morning			Lunch	Afternoon	Evening
SUNDAY SEPT. 11	*Introduction to the immune system* Fritz Melchers: Antigen-binding molecules		Roland Gisler: Lymphoid organs	LUNCH	*Introduction to the immune system* Ivan Lefkovits: Clonal Selection; Fritz Melchers: Lymphocyte activation; Roland Gisler: Ontogeny of the immune system	*Get-Together Party at the club in the Hospital*
MONDAY SEPT. 12	*Cells of the immune system* Fritz Melchers: B cells	Louis Du Pasquier: Generation of antibody repertoire	Marie Kosco: Humoral immune response	LUNCH	LABORATORY WORK / METHODOLOGICAL LECTURES	
TUESDAY SEPT. 13	*Receptors and ligands* Polly Matzinger: MHC and genes	Louis Du Pasquier: Evolution of MHC	Roland Gisler: Adhesion molecules	LUNCH	LABORATORY WORK / METHODOLOGICAL LECTURES	*Concert in the Cathedral*
WEDNESDAY SEPT. 14	*Mechanisms* Polly Matzinger: Tolerance	Hans-Peter Pircher: Autoimmunity		LUNCH	LABORATORY WORK / POSTER VIEWING	*Excursion to Betliar*
THURSDAY SEPT. 15	*Immunological memory* Marie Kosco: Longterm memory	Klaus-Ulrich Hartmann: Development of lymphoid organs	Jean-Marie Buerstedde: DNA recombination in the immune system	LUNCH	LABORATORY WORK / METHODOLOGICAL LECTURES	
FRIDAY SEPT. 16	*Systems, species* L. Du Pasquier: The immune system throughout the species	H.-J. Thiesen: Turning genes on and off	J.-M. Buerstedde: DNA repair and disease	LUNCH	LABORATORY WORK / METHODOLOGICAL LECTURES	*Farewell Party*
SATURDAY SEPT. 17	*Closing session* Milan Buc: Overview & afterthoughts		Exam & Certificate		Departure	

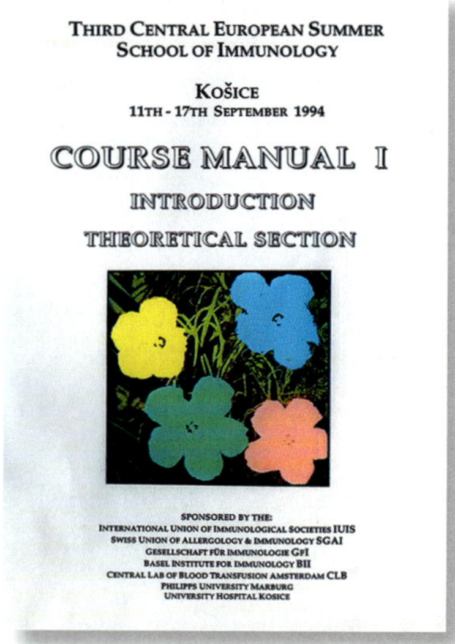

4 distinct shades allows easy identification of the 4 laboratory groups. The museum kindly gave us permission to reproduce this adapted version, which was prepared by Nicole Schoepflin and Bea Pfeiffer (both BII).

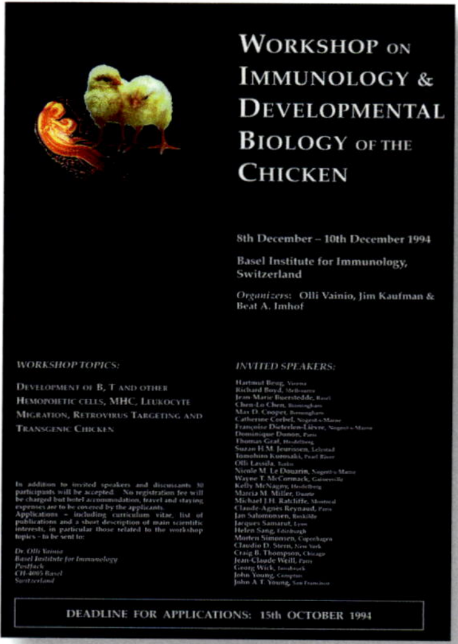

Workshop on Immunology and Developmental Biology of the Chicken, 1994

This workshop was organized by Olli Vainio, Jim Kaufman and Beat Imhof on December 8th to 10th, 1994; the main theme was the development of B and T cells and other hemopoietic cells. Lectures and discussions were held on leukocyte migration, retrovirus targeting, transgenic chicken and the MHC [QR1994_03].

Among the invited speakers were Morten Simonsen, Georg Wick, Max Cooper and Nicole Le Douarin. Nine members of the BII reported on their research.

Roche Acquires Syntex

QR1994_03 BII

Roche purchased the Syntex Corp. in Palo Alto (one of the largest takeovers). Syntex held a large portion of the market for oral contraceptives and possessed highly regarded research facilities. Palo Alto became strategically important for Roche, but at the cost of Nutley, N.J., as described in one of the following chapters.

Niels K. Jerne Dies on October 7th, 1994

After a short illness, Niels died on October 7th, 1994, at his home in Provence [QR1994_04]. The funeral was attended by close friends from the institute and elsewhere, and took place on the rainy day of October 9th, 1994. Alexandra Jerne continued to live in Castillon-du-Gard. The cemetery where Niels is buried is a short distance from the castle.

Fritz Melchers and the Mayor of the village gave moving speeches, and Louis Du Pasquier played Niels' favorite Debussy piece, *Syrinx*, on the flute.

QR1994_04 BII

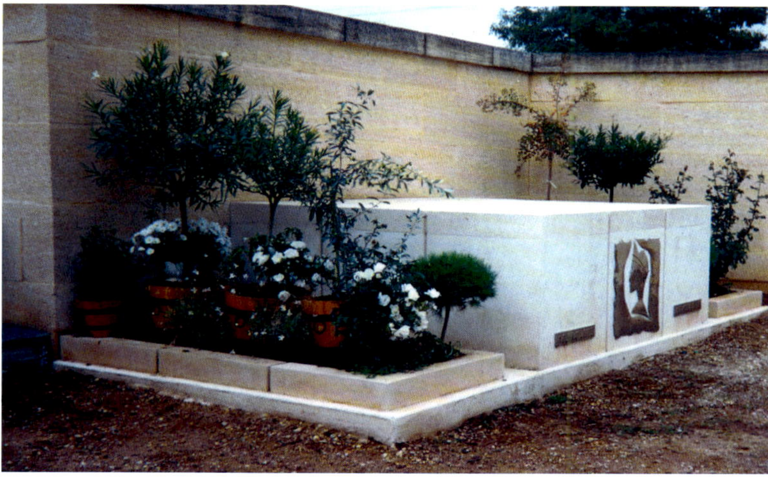
Niels K. Jerne's grave in Castillon-du-Gard, France

Treasure Trove 1994
The database contains documents related to the BII in a broader context (lists, series of photographs, etc.).

QR1994_treasure BII

The Year 1995

An EMBO workshop on lymphocyte neoplasia and DNA rearrangements was held at the BII. The 4th Central European Summer School of Immunology was organized by BII members in Prague. The Niels Kaj Jerne Memorial Symposium was held at the Hotel Krafft, Basel (1st anniversary of his death). The editorial duties of preparing the Annual Reports passed from Charley Steinberg to Ed Palmer. The closing down of the Roche Institute of Molecular Biology in Nutley was announced. The BII established strict safety rules (not only as a learning process from the devastating fire at the BII 10 years earlier, but preempting strict Swiss regulations). The 9th International Congress of Immunology in San Francisco was attended by a large number of members as speakers or chairpersons.

Arrivals 1995 (14)
Alexandre Akhmedov, Seiamak Bahram, Luca Bolliger, Ludovica Bruno, Thomas Göbel, John Hansen, Manfred Kopf, Ramona Leibnitz, Toru Miyazaki, Minetaro Ogawa, Christiane Ruedl, Takeyuki Shimizu, Antonella Viola, Alan Young.

Came and Left in the Same Year (2)
Pia Bernasconi, Nobuyuki Tanigaki.

Leavers 1995 (15)
Philip Griebel, Gillian Griffiths, Hajime Karasuyama, James Kaufman, Hansruedi Kiefer, Alexandra Livingstone, Sabine Mai, Lill Martensson, Fiona McConnell, Yoshihiro Oka, Jacques Robert, Shunichi Takeda, Hans-Jürgen Thiesen, Hans-Joachim Wallny, Michael Wiles.

QR1995_01 BII

Perspectives and New Careers 1992–1995

On the one hand the institute proudly claimed that all members were equal; on the other hand, from both the scientific and the social aspects, it was clearly "inhomogeneous and non-uniform". Being "equal" – meaning that a member had the right to pursue whatever project he so wished – was upheld, with the occasional exception. Nevertheless, scientists who spent several years at the BII are mentioned more frequently than those researchers who gave just 1 year of their expertise to the institute. Goodbye parties and theater performances served as the litmus test, which is well reflected in this book.

There are two sections entitled "Perspectives and New Careers", one related to the years 1992–1995 and the other to 1996–2000. The former is placed in the chapter for 1995 [QR1995_01], the latter in that for 2000. Both are linked to the QR database, to which supplementary information is added. Although the doors for including material in the printed version will be closed once the book goes to print, latecomers will have the chance to add information, documents or reprints to their database folder.

The nature of available information makes these two sections "weak", as it is often second-hand compiled largely from what is available on the Internet; thus, it is unavoidable that these sections remain incomplete.

1992

Paolo Dellabona, to Milan

He left Basel in 1992 for the San Raffaele Scientific Institute in Milan, where he became coordinator of the Cancer Immunotherapy and Gene Therapy Programme, and later head of the Division of Immunology and Infectious Diseases. Paolo's research unit investigates mechanisms by which innate and adaptive effector T lymphocytes are recruited in tumor immune surveillance, and the researchers are developing strategies for the design of efficacious immunotherapy protocols. Paolo's publications (some with Giulia Casorati) are concerned with the escape of tumor immune surveillance.

Ronald Palacios, to the USA and Then to Bolivia

Ron left the BII to fill various positions in the USA, one of them as deputy chairman of the Department of Immunology at the University of Texas M.D. Anderson Cancer Center. He finally returned to his home country, Bolivia, to the Institute for Molecular Medicine Santa Cruz. At the BII and at later positions, Ron used a broad spectrum of methodology for studying functions of interleukins (especially IL-3), and of the mechanism of T cell activation in the functional relationship to interleukins.

Melanie Wilson, to the University of Mississippi Medical Center, Jackson

Melanie addressed herself to the development of teleost immune responses, especially to teleost leukocyte immune-type receptors (LITRs). LITRs were first discovered in catfish and have subsequently been found in other teleosts. They comprise a large polymorphic family that encodes Ig domain-containing membrane proteins that mediate activating or inhibitory signaling. The discovery of a large heterogeneous family of immunoregulatory receptors in teleosts, reminiscent of amphibian, avian and mammalian Ig-like receptors, suggests that complex innate immune receptor networks have been conserved during vertebrate evolution. A family of diversified immunoregulatory receptors in teleosts is homologous to both mammalian Fc receptors.

José Carlos Gutierrez-Ramos, to Harvard

He accepted a call to the Center for Blood Research at Harvard Medical School, a position that paved the way towards a career in the pharmaceutical industry. In Millennium Pharmaceuticals he was responsible for advancing preclinical candidates in immunology to human trials and advancing compounds through clinical development. Subsequently he became head of R & D at Avidia and later head of the Immunoinflammation Center for Drug Discovery (Pfizer). He also served as chief scientific officer of a Spanish biotechnology company, Genetrix, where he led the spin-off of several technologies registered at the Spanish Research Council.

1993

Dominique Dunon, to Paris

At the University Pierre and Marie Curie he created a research team to study "migration and differentiation of hematopoietic stem cells", which he directed at the CNRS. Years later he accepted the offer of a prestigious position at the French Ministry of Foreign Affairs and became the academic cooperation officer for Science and Technology at the Embassy of France in Berne. Having assessed francophone universities in Belgium, he was elected as a scientific delegate to AERES (Agence d'évaluation de la recherche), in the section "Training: Science of Life, Health and Environment".

1994

Marie Kosco-Vilbois, to Geneva

Marie came to the BII in 1989 from the Medical College of the University of Virginia. When she was ready to leave, she accepted an offer from the Glaxo Wellcome Research Institute in Geneva to become head of the Immunology Unit. From 1997 to 2001, Marie was head of Preclinical Pharmacology at the Serono Pharmaceutical Research Institute. In 2002 she joined the biotech company NovImmune SA, in Geneva, where she became chief scientific officer.

Charles Mackay, to Australia

After working at the BII on lymphocyte traffic, using sheep as a model, Charles worked in the biotech industry for 7 years, first at Leukocyte Inc. and then at Millennium Pharmaceuticals. During the following 10 years he headed the Immunology Department at the Garvan Institute. He then spent 4 years at Monash University in Clayton, Vic., and after that he became professor of Immunology at the Charles Perkins Center at Sydney University. His expertise is in cell migration and chemoattractant receptors for immune responses and inflammation. He became a proponent of a holistic hypothesis to explain many "western lifestyle" diseases, i.e. that diet, gut microbes and their metabolites are responsible for asthma, allergies, many autoimmune diseases, as well as diabetes, cardiovascular disease and cancers. Charles is a member of the Australian Academy of Science.

Franca Ronchese, to Wellington, New Zealand
Franca was awarded a position of "Immune Cell Biology Programme Leader" at the Malaghan Institute of Medical Research. Her primary research interest was the use of dendritic cells as ideal targets for the development of immunotherapies for diseases such as cancer. A more powerful immune activation might result in the control of tumor growth, or allergy and autoimmune disease, where dendritic cells play an important role in local inflammation. Franca, with her research group, tried to answer the question whether dendritic cells in tumors can be manipulated to support an intratumoral environment that favors tumor rejection and minimizes immune suppression. Franca is the current Australasian representative on the International Union of Immunological Societies Council.

Wojciech Swat, to Boston
After initial years as a research fellow in the Children's Hospital Boston, Wojciech moved to the Harvard Medical School, Boston. His research interests focused on the mechanisms employed by lymphocytes to transduce signals from the cell surface to the nucleus. A protein known as Vav was initially discovered as a protein which could convert normal cells growing in culture into cancerous cells. Further studies revealed that the Vav1 proto-oncogene is an evolutionarily conserved multidomain protein expressed exclusively in hematopoietic cells and is required for normal lymphocyte development and function. With gene-targeted mutagenesis, Wojciech and his coworkers generated mice in which the Vav1 gene has been mutated. In 2010 he moved to the Washington University School of Medicine, St. Louis, where his research focused on molecular mechanisms underlying the development of lymphoid cells. His group studied dynamic processes involving modifications of gene expression resulting in lymphocyte survival, proliferation, differentiation and/or apoptosis.

1995

Gillian Griffiths, to London
After 5 years at the BII, Gillian accepted a position at the MRC Laboratory for Molecular Cell Biology, University College London, as a Wellcome Trust senior fellow. In 1997 she moved to Oxford

(Sir William Dunn School of Pathology). Her interests were focused on the problem of target recognition by T cells. Cytotoxic T cells patrol body tissues in search of cells that are infected with pathogens and immediately kill any they find. For the T cell, the killing process involves dramatic rearrangements of its cytoskeleton and of secretory granules containing cytotoxic proteins. Gillian successfully combined her cell biology expertise with various lymphocyte activation models to investigate how the T cells land their killing blow.

James Kaufman, to Cambridge

Upon moving to the UK, Jim changed the direction of his work. At the BII his work focused on determining the genomic structure of the chicken MHC, the sequence polymorphism, peptide motifs and expression levels of MHC molecules. In Cambridge the work of his laboratory shifted towards studies of coevolution between genes of the chicken MHC, sequence polymorphism, peptide binding and expression level on disease resistance, vaccine response and other phenomena at an individual and population level. His collaborative efforts continued with various institutions in Europe and the USA.

Alexandra Livingstone, to Rochester

At the BII and then in Rochester (University of Rochester Medical Center), Alexandra contributed towards understanding the generation of immunological memory, especially CD8+ T cell memory. Her experimental model relied on immunization of mice with dendritic cells pulsed with peptides defining class I epitopes. Peptide-specific memory was measured (and detected) for prolonged periods. Identification of antigen-specific cells by using TCR transgenics, MHC-peptide tetramers enabled basic questions to be asked about the behavior of CD8+ memory T cells to design successful vaccination strategies against the relevant pathogens.

Sabine Mai, to Canada

After spending 4 years at the BII, Sabine received an attractive offer from the University of Manitoba, where she was soon promoted to professor of Physiology and Biochemistry. Sabine's laboratory became interested in the molecular mechanisms of cellular immortalization and transformation. Their in vitro and in vivo analyses were geared towards establishing the molecular and genomic alterations involved in neoplastic transformation. As a general theme they have chosen to study c-Myc-dependent genomic instability, and its progression in cancer patients, and more specifically the mechanism of c-Myc deregulation in translocation-negative plasmacytomas.

Lill Martensson, to Sweden

After several years at the BII, Lill returned to Sweden to take up a position as assistant professor (forskarassistent) at Lund University, where she also received her docentur. The position in Lund was a stepping stone to her career as a principal investigator at the Babraham Institute, Cambridge, UK, where she spent close to 10 years. Her final project in Cambridge was "Censoring of Autoreactive B Cell Development by the Pre-B Cell Receptor". She was then recruited back to Sweden and appointed professor at the University of Gothenburg.

Fiona McConnell, to the UK

Fiona and her husband Peter Lane returned to the UK after spending 6 years at the BII. Her work at the MRC Center for Immune Regulation in Birmingham concerned single cell analysis, especially with the use of confocal microscopy. Fiona also continued her work on the B cell function in transgenic mice lacking germinal centers.

Jacques Robert, to Rochester

The major part of Jacques' career was spent at the University of Rochester Medical Center. The goal of his research was to understand the coevolutionary relationships between the structure of selected molecules (e.g. heat shock proteins and their receptors [CD91], NK cell receptors [KIR, FcRs], non-classical class Ib molecules [XNCs]) and their functions in innate and adaptive immunity against tumors and viruses. Jacques, similarly to his work in Basel, made use of the excellent resources of the University of Rochester in terms of the availability of several genetically defined inbred strains and clones of amphibian *Xenopus laevis*. All research tools, such as transgenic animals, monoclonal antibodies, DNA libraries and molecular probes, were available. This opened a new research area concerning basic comparative and applied studies of viral pathogenesis and immunity in amphibians caused by the threat of emerging wildlife viral diseases on global biodiversity.

Hans-Jürgen Thiesen, to Rostock

Hans-Jürgen left the BII for the University of Rostock. His research in Basel was concerned with various aspects of zinc finger proteins related to the regulation of gene expression in the immune system. In Rostock he extended his research to the Krüppel-associated box (KRAB) domain (a category of transcriptional repression domains present in approximately 400 human zinc finger protein-based transcription factors). His achievements in Rostock were to show that over 10 independently encoded KRAB domains are effective repressors of transcription. His research extended to other topics as well, e.g. epitope predictions by epitope profiling of intravenous immunoglobulins.

Hans-Joachim Wallny Remained in Basel

After completing his assignment at the BII, Hans-Joachim took the position of head of the Biotechnology Laboratory at Biotest AG, Basel, then he became a technical project leader at the department "TRD Biologics", at Novartis Pharma AG, Basel. He was responsible for the development and validation of biological potency assays and high molecular impurity assays for biopharmaceuticals during early development. One of Hans-Joachim's main scientific ambitions was to develop and implement modern, fast and reliable bioassays using early cellular events as readouts (e.g. reporter gene assays, KIRA assays, etc.). For achieving this he was honored with the title "Novartis Leading Scientist" in 2003.

Michael Wiles, to Bar Harbor

After leaving the BII Michael held several positions at various institutions, finally joining the Jackson Laboratory, Bar Harbor, Me., where he became responsible for Biotechnology Evaluation and Development. In his own words his aim was fulfilled: to join a new, dynamic company and make changes – to solve biological, medical and commercially relevant problems, to develop novel technologies and combine these with established systems. This is aimed at creating practical efficient solutions and establishing new product lines and/or internal systems. Michael successfully worked towards evaluating and, where appropriate, implementing and improving precision genetic engineering systems directed at mice as models of the human condition.

Symposium in Memory of Niels Kaj Jerne (1st Anniversary of His Death)

A small symposium [QR1995_02] took place from October 6th to 7th, 1995, in memory of Niels Jerne, the first director of the institute, a year after his death. It was held in the Hotel Krafft in Basel where Niels Jerne and many of the scientists interested in the institute had met in 1969 and 1970 to discuss both science and the arrangements for setting up the institute. Those who attended the symposium were colleagues and close friends of Niels Jerne from the early days of the institute:

Brigitte A. Askonas, Robbert Benner, Dietmar G. Braun, Manny Delbrück, Louis Du Pasquier, Claudia Henry, Eduard Kellenberger, Ivan Lefkovits, Fritz Melchers, Erna Möller, Göran Möller, Albert A. Nordin, Benvenuto Pernis, Klaus Rajewsky, Gordon H. Sato, Max Schreier, Theophil Staehelin, Gunther Stent, Zdenek Trnka and Ingrid Westen-Schnurr.

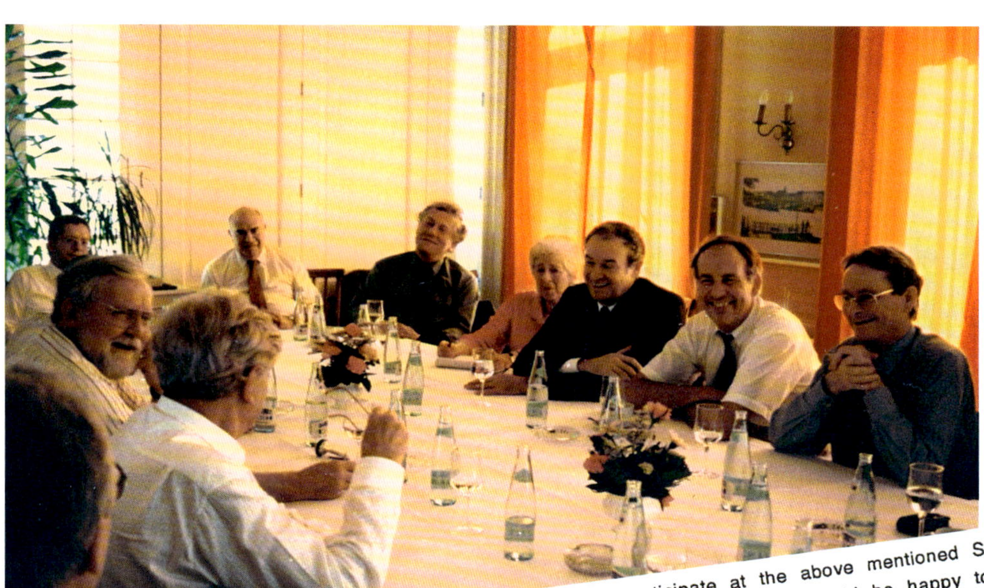

Symposium in Hotel Krafft in memory of Niels Jerne

I am happy to participate at the above mentioned Symposium from 6.-8. 10.95. Besides Valentin Bonifas I would be happy to revive Niels period in Geneva. He always liked to remember that it was there that he was appointed professor for the first time. A follow-up of the paper in which he participated very much, together with Naomi Franklin, is presently in the press and it might be interesting to remind very shortly this collaborative study on the bacteriophage tail fibers. We discussed together still about it during the last weeks before his death.

I wonder if Naomi should not be asked to join us?

With kind regards

Eduard *Eduard*

They gave informal presentations related to Niels' work, or they recounted more personal episodes from his life. The talks were concluded with a small concert given by Louis Du Pasquier, Juliette Du Pasquier and Eberhardt Klotz.

Louis Du Pasquier, Ivan Lefkovits and Fritz Melchers organized the meeting.

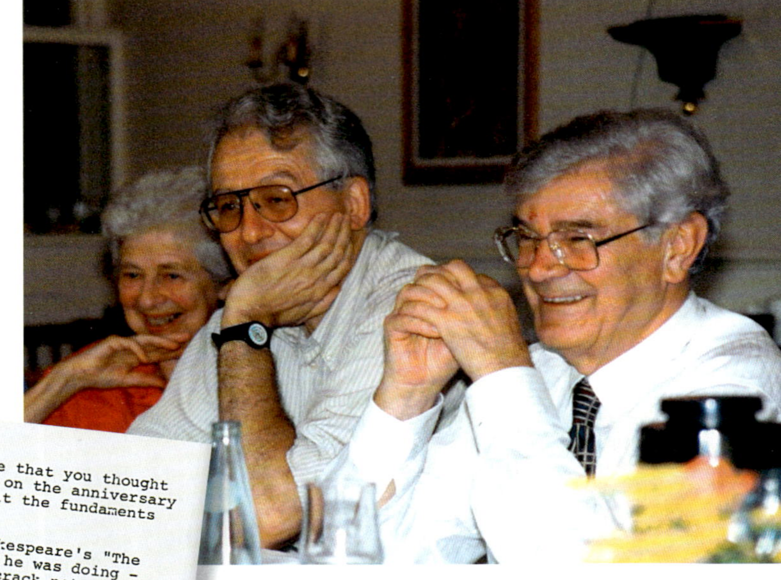

Ita Askonas, Klaus Rajewsky and Zdenek Trnka at the dinner in Hotel Krafft

Dear Friends:

I think that it is very nice and appropriate that you thought of having a reunion of Niels Jerne's old friends on the anniversary of his death, and in the very place where he built the fundaments of the Basel Institute.

I remember in those days he quoted from Shakespeare's "The Tempest" the following verse as a comment to what he was doing - "Now does my project gather to a head: My charms crack not; my spirits obey" - an appropriate comment for a great endeavor that proved to be so successful.

I thank you for your invitation, and of course I am planning to attend to participate in the general discussion and, if I can, have some 15 - 20 minutes to discuss the following subject:

"The lymphon, a functional unit of the immune sy…

This is an outgrowth, supported by experiments, of exchanges that I had with Niels 20 years ago.

Looking forward to getting together in Basel in Octo…

With kind regards.

Sincerely,

Ben

Benvenuto Pernis

Dear Fritz, Louis, Ivan, and Charley,

I was very happy to receive your letter of February 16th, inviting me to take part in the memorial Συμποσιον for Niels on October 6th to 8th. It is with great pleasure that I accept your invitation.

As for my contribution to the proceedings, I would propose to reminisce about my contacts with Niels in Copenhagen 1950-51 and later in California (while he was putting the finishing touches on his natural selection paper for the PNAS). If Jim Watson (he and I turn out to have known Niels the longest of all the persons on your list of invitees) is going to attend and speak as well, I would try to coordinate with him just what either of us is going to say about our togetherness at the Statens Serum Institut.

Whereas I am 150% d'accord with a rule of forbidding the projection of scientific slides at the Συμποσιον, I'm wondering whether it wouldn't contribute positively to the conversazione if there were a possibility to project a few snapshots of people, places and events that figure in our reminiscences about Niels. I don't feel strongly about this, but why don't you raise my Gegenvorschlag on your flagpole and see whether anyone salutes it?

Looking forward to seeing you in October, I remain with the warmest regards

your

Gunther

Gunther S. Stent

EMBO Workshop on Lymphocyte Neoplasia and DNA Rearrangements, 1995

Rolf Jessberger, Fritz Melchers and Michael Potter organized this workshop [QR1995_03].

There were 8 sessions:

- Normal pre-B to B cell development
- Early neoplasias
- V(D)J recombination
- Mammalian recombination/repair mutants
- General aspect of recombination
- Class switching
- B cells to plasma cells
- Myc

Twenty-four participants from various institutions attended as well as BII members.

QR1995_03 BII

The 4th Central European Summer School of Immunology, 1995

The last 2-week course of the series was organized in Prague, at the Microbiology Institute of the Academy of Sciences [QR1995_04]. The teaching staff was, as in previous years, recruited mainly from members and former members of the BII.

QR1995_04 BII

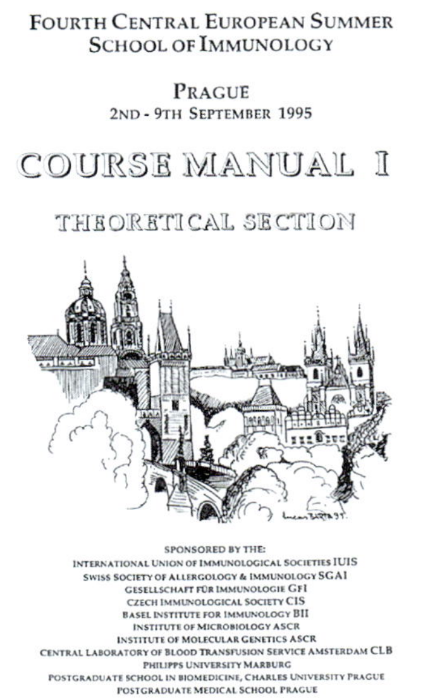

FOURTH CENTRAL EUROPEAN SUMMER SCHOOL OF IMMUNOLOGY

PRAGUE
2ND - 9TH SEPTEMBER 1995

COURSE MANUAL I

THEORETICAL SECTION

SPONSORED BY THE:
INTERNATIONAL UNION OF IMMUNOLOGICAL SOCIETIES IUIS
SWISS SOCIETY OF ALLERGOLOGY & IMMUNOLOGY SGAI
GESELLSCHAFT FÜR IMMUNOLOGIE GFI
CZECH IMMUNOLOGICAL SOCIETY CIS
BASEL INSTITUTE FOR IMMUNOLOGY BII
INSTITUTE OF MICROBIOLOGY ASCR
INSTITUTE OF MOLECULAR GENETICS ASCR
CENTRAL LABORATORY OF BLOOD TRANSFUSION SERVICE AMSTERDAM CLB
PHILIPPS UNIVERSITY MARBURG
POSTGRADUATE SCHOOL IN BIOMEDICINE, CHARLES UNIVERSITY PRAGUE
POSTGRADUATE MEDICAL SCHOOL PRAGUE

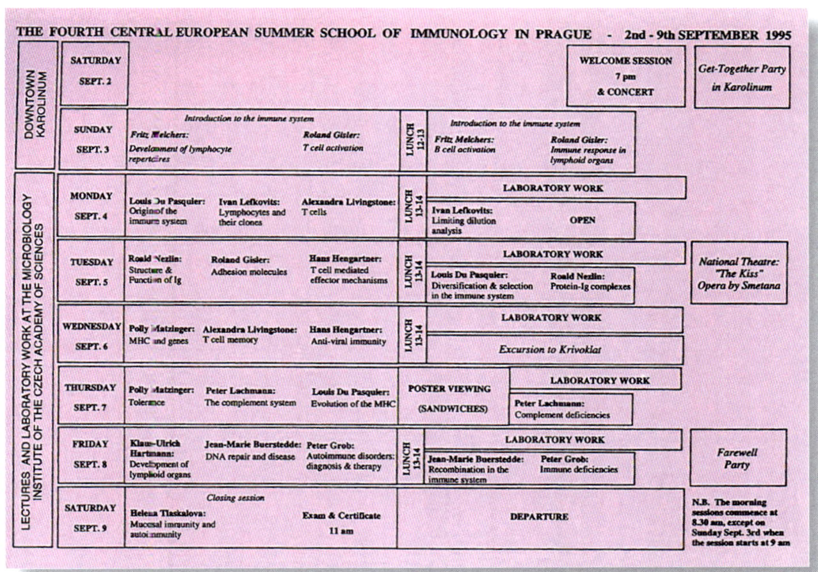

THE FOURTH CENTRAL EUROPEAN SUMMER SCHOOL OF IMMUNOLOGY IN PRAGUE - 2nd - 9th SEPTEMBER 1995

Location	Day	Morning	Lunch	Afternoon	Evening
DOWNTOWN KAROLINUM	SATURDAY SEPT. 2			WELCOME SESSION 7 pm & CONCERT	*Get-Together Party in Karolinum*
DOWNTOWN KAROLINUM	SUNDAY SEPT. 3	*Introduction to the immune system* — *Fritz Melchers:* *Development of lymphocyte repertoires*; *Roland Gisler:* *T cell activation*	LUNCH 12-13	*Introduction to the immune system* — *Fritz Melchers:* *B cell activation*; *Roland Gisler:* *Immune response in lymphoid organs*	
LECTURES AND LABORATORY WORK AT THE MICROBIOLOGY INSTITUTE OF THE CZECH ACADEMY OF SCIENCES	MONDAY SEPT. 4	**Louis Du Pasquier:** Origin of the immune system; **Ivan Lefkovits:** Lymphocytes and their clones; **Alexandra Livingstone:** T cells	LUNCH 13-14	LABORATORY WORK; **Ivan Lefkovits:** Limiting dilution analysis; OPEN	
	TUESDAY SEPT. 5	**Roald Nezlin:** Structure & Function of Ig; **Roland Gisler:** Adhesion molecules; **Hans Hengartner:** T cell mediated effector mechanisms	LUNCH 13-14	LABORATORY WORK; **Louis Du Pasquier:** Diversification & selection in the immune system; **Roald Nezlin:** Protein-Ig complexes	*National Theatre: "The Kiss" Opera by Smetana*
	WEDNESDAY SEPT. 6	**Polly Matzinger:** MHC and genes; **Alexandra Livingstone:** T cell memory; **Hans Hengartner:** Anti-viral immunity	LUNCH 13-14	LABORATORY WORK; *Excursion to Krivoklat*	
	THURSDAY SEPT. 7	**Polly Matzinger:** Tolerance; **Peter Lachmann:** The complement system; **Louis Du Pasquier:** Evolution of the MHC	POSTER VIEWING (SANDWICHES)	LABORATORY WORK; **Peter Lachmann:** Complement deficiencies	
	FRIDAY SEPT. 8	**Klaus-Ulrich Hartmann:** Development of lymphoid organs; **Jean-Marie Buerstedde:** DNA repair and disease; **Peter Grob:** Autoimmune disorders: diagnosis & therapy	LUNCH 13-14	LABORATORY WORK; **Jean-Marie Buerstedde:** Recombination in the immune system; **Peter Grob:** Immune deficiencies	*Farewell Party*
	SATURDAY SEPT. 9	*Closing session* — **Helena Tlaskalova:** Mucosal immunity and autoimmunity; **Exam & Certificate 11 am**		DEPARTURE	**N.B. The morning sessions commence at 8.30 am, except on Sunday Sept. 3rd when the session starts at 9 am**

Institute for Immunology
BII Building 75, Grenzacherstrasse 487
4058 Basel

Safety Officer	Dr. A. Lanzavecchia	Telephone	271 45 03
Technical Officer	P.A. Balzarini	Telephone Air-Call	322 86 04 or 280 76 98
Deputy	M. Delétraz	Telephone	641 38 76
Head of the emergency service	A. Wyss **Emergency No. 2**	Telephone Nova-Call	312 67 68 or 450 31 72
Deputy	B. Badovinac	Telephone	711 34 40

Emergency Telephone Numbers (from 15th February 1995)

In case of an emergency involving water, electricity, gas or air conditioning, call the emergency number **Nova-Call No. 1 : 450 31 73.** If your call is not returned within 10 minutes, you should use **Nova-Call No. 2 : 450 31 72** (Emergency No. 2) and contact A. Wyss.

The BII Establishes Strict Safety Rules

Year after year the safety rules became more complex. This was not only the result of the learning process from the devastating fire at the BII 10 years earlier, but because the general trend in Switzerland (and in the whole western world) was oriented towards safer working conditions [QR1995_05].

Many rules were rewritten or reformulated, and responsibilities were described for certain "functions". The safety officer, technical officer, head of emergency services and radiation safety officer were informed of the new safety rules. In the QR note, the document "Laboratory safety rules" is reproduced. Committees were formed with Antonio Lanzavecchia, Peter Balzarini, Michel Delétraz, Branco Badovinac, Ruedi Frech and Jürg Widmer serving as members. The 24-page document provides a good picture of the responsible approach taken towards chemical, radiochemical and biological hazards. Several institutions in Switzerland requested the document, and it served as a model for them.

QR1995_05 BII

A New Editor of the BII Annual Reports

Over decades Charley Steinberg edited the Annual Reports which became famous in the world of immunology. By the end of each year Charley had collected the draft research reports, and during the first 2 months of the next year he edited them. With Argus eyes he spotted mistakes in the submitted documents, corrected texts, shortened them, made them readable and logical. Only a few members insisted that their reports were not to be altered by Charley. It was not only his editorial skills, but also his insisting on deadlines, on conciseness and directness, which made the Annual Reports a perfect "product".

Over decades Charley Steinberg edited the Annual Reports, which became famous in the world of immunology.

In 1994, after a disagreement with Fritz Melchers, he stepped down from the editorship and handed it over to Ed Palmer. Ed continued the editorial work in the spirit of Charley, with a fine sense of avoiding confrontation with fellow colleagues.

1995 Nobel Prize Awarded to a Student of Walter Gehring, Biozentrum, Basel

Christiane Nüsslein-Volhard, a former student of Walter Gehring from the Biozentrum Basel, and 2 American scientists were awarded the 1995 Nobel Prize for Medicine for the discovery of the genetic control of early embryonic development and origin of retroviral oncogenes [QR1995_06]. Christiane had close contact with the institute during her years in Basel.

9th International Congress of Immunology in San Francisco, 1995

As with all previous International Congresses of Immunology (that started in 1971) the 9th International Congress in San Francisco attracted a large number of participants from the BII [QR1995_07].

QR1995_06 BII

Closing Down the Roche Institute of Molecular Biology, Nutley

When the Roche management decided to close down the RIMB in Nutley [QR1995_08], it was not yet apparent that this decision concerning the "sister institute" foreshadowed the fate of the Basel Institute some 6 years later. Below are excerpts from the text of an article by Sidney Udenfriend, ex-director of RIMB, published in *The Scientist* 1995;9:12.

QR1995_07 BII

"One of industry's strengths is its ability to make and implement decisions rapidly. One highly placed executive can make decisions, the consequences of which can be profound. The rapidity of the creation of RIMB (one month from conception to reality) was not comprehensible to those in academia or government. Continued support of

QR1995_08 BII

Roche, Nutley, ... a research center ... that was the envy of scientists throughout the world, a Camelot of the biomedical sciences.

RIMB by Roche was generous to an extent that, again, has not been seen in academia or government. Unfortunately, because a company can move so rapidly, the demise of RIMB was just as swift as its creation.

Even Bell Laboratories were cut drastically following the AT & T breakup. Nevertheless, for more than a quarter of a century, here in Nutley a research center operated that was the envy of scientists throughout the world, a Camelot of the biomedical sciences. At RIMB, scientists were completely supported, enabling them to turn their full attention to any research problem of interest to them without the distractions of teaching, grant and fellowship applications, or faculty meetings, and without the restrictions placed upon scientists in government. The only criterion for continued membership and promotion was the quality of one's research. RIMB was given a charter to this effect by Roche.

*Furthermore, Roche lived up to every detail of the charter. In light of Roche's sudden decision to close it down, one must ask whether RIMB failed to live up to the company's expectations. By all criteria, the institute has been staffed by outstanding and innovative scientists throughout its existence. Publications by RIMB scientists appear in the most prestigious journals, and the Science Citation Index has always rated RIMB among the top four or five independent institutes in the United States (*Science Watch*, 4:2, 1993).*

The presence of RIMB on the Nutley campus encouraged interaction with Roche's scientists. As early as 1969, these collaborations led to important products directly, as with the development of diagnostics for drugs of abuse, Abuscreen; or indirectly, through the development of technologies, which later played a key role in the first isolation and characterization of the α-interferons and to Roche's patents for Roferon. Research carried out at the institute at its founding was unquestionably at the cutting edge of molecular biology.

RIMB also developed important products. Beyond that, it was the institute that moved Roche into biotechnology and changed it from a traditional, chemically oriented drug company to a modern pharmaceutical company. Why, then, did Roche decide to close the institute? Maybe this was due not to deficiencies on its part but to differences of opinion between Roche research management and RIMB as to future directions of research and to the organizational make-up of the institute. The acquisition of Syntex by Hoffmann-La Roche in the fall of 1994 gave management the option of setting up a research facility in Palo Alto, Calif., an area that would be more attractive for recruiting a new director and would permit them to redirect its research to genomics more rapidly, rather than gradually overhaul the existing RIMB. Once it was decided to set up an institute in California, RIMB became a casualty of the company's downsizing. All of this does not, however, explain the suddenness of the institute's closing after it had been in existence for close to 30 years. Contrary to some reports, none were offered positions in Palo Alto."

And Sidney Udenfriend concludes: *"Today, as my colleagues disperse, they admit that no matter how good their newly found jobs are, none are like the ones they are leaving. They are good scientists, and I know that they will prosper. However, each is leaving with the memory of the time we spent in this Camelot in Nutley, N.J."*

Georges Köhler Died, 1995

Georges Köhler, former permanent member of the BII, Nobel Prize winner with César Milstein, died of heart failure while suffering from pneumonia. He was only 48 years old. Details of his life and his achievements are given in the QR code [QR1995_09]. The photograph shown is one which Georges liked.

QR1995_09 BII

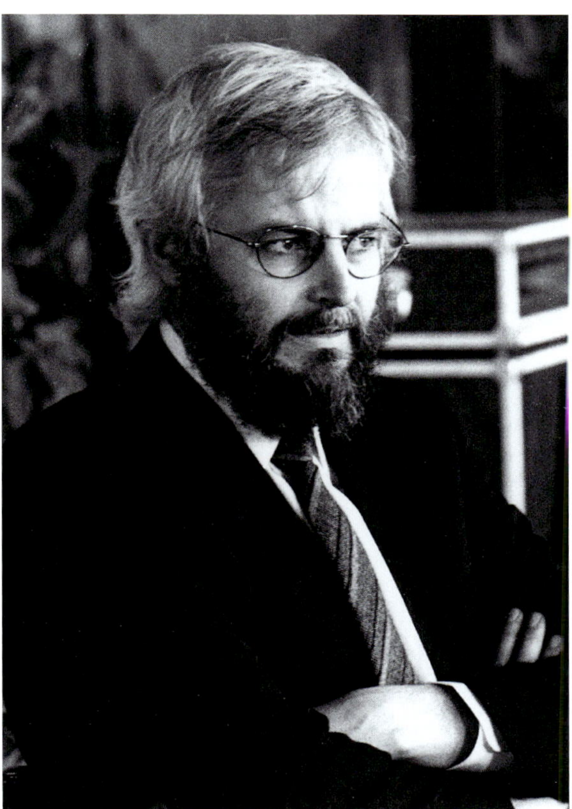

Georges J.F. Köhler, 1946–1995

Treasure Trove 1995

The database contains documents related to the BII in a broader context (lists, series of photographs, etc.).

QR1995_treasure BII

The Year 1996

Harald von Boehmer gave up his permanent BII membership, accepting a high-flying appointment in Paris (Institut Necker). The BTA prepared the play "Two Divas" to express appreciation of Harald von Boehmer's scientific achievements. The 25th anniversary of the foundation of the BII was celebrated on a cruise on the river Rhine. The festivities concluded with a theater play: "Close Encounters of the 25th Kind". An updated edition of the "Booklet on the BII" was issued on the occasion of the anniversary celebration. The Nobel Prize was awarded to two members of the Advisory Board, Rolf Zinkernagel and Peter Doherty.

Arrivals 1996 (10)
Jürgen Bachl, Rhodri Ceredig, Sylvie Degermann, Susan Gilfillan, Giandomenica Iezzi, Fraser McBlane, Jean Pieters, Mariolina Salio, Raul Torres, Tamotsu Yamagami.

Leavers 1996 (10)
Ludovica Bruno, José A. Garcia-Sanz, Paolo Ghia, Beat Imhof, Peter Lane, Gek-Kee Sim, Reinhard Stauder, Olli Vainio, Harald von Boehmer, Thomas Winkler.

The turnover of BII members was stable (10 "in", 10 "out"), and goodbye parties were more the rule than an exception. But when a long-standing member was about to leave, a more elaborate event was often organized.

Harald von Boehmer, Permanent Member, Leaves, 1996

Harald decided to take a high-flying appointment at the Institut Necker in Paris [QR1996_01]. He established a strong research group there that continued his "positive/negative" selection projects and also those on diabetes. An adjacent laboratory was that of Jean-Claude Weill and Claude-Agnès Reynaud. Harald stayed in Paris until 1999 and then he moved to the MIT. His beautiful house in Fontainebleau, wonderfully looked after by his wife Monica, was sold, and the family moved to the Boston area.

QR1996_01 BII

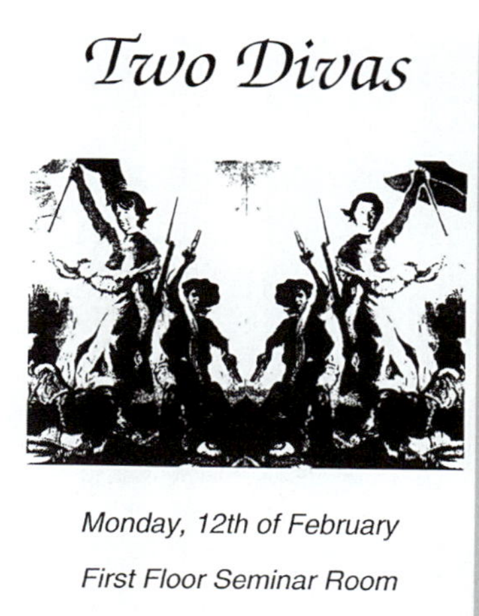
Two Divas
Monday, 12th of February
First Floor Seminar Room
6.30 pm

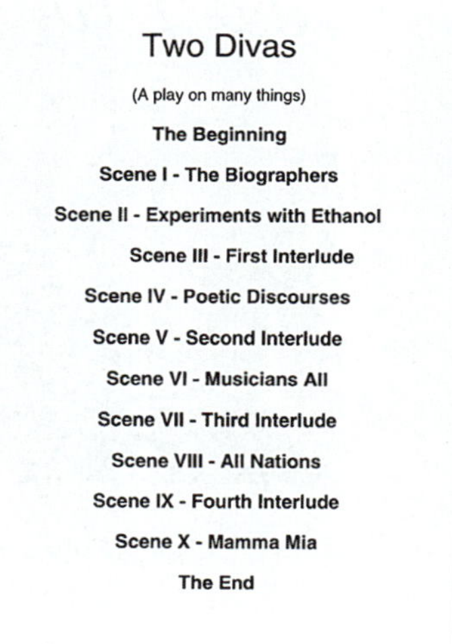
Two Divas

(A play on many things)

The Beginning

Scene I - The Biographers

Scene II - Experiments with Ethanol

Scene III - First Interlude

Scene IV - Poetic Discourses

Scene V - Second Interlude

Scene VI - Musicians All

Scene VII - Third Interlude

Scene VIII - All Nations

Scene IX - Fourth Interlude

Scene X - Mamma Mia

The End

BTA 12: Chamber Performance, "Two Divas", by Louis Du Pasquier and Fiona McConnell

On February 12th, a performance by Louis Du Pasquier and Fiona McConnell – to honor Harald's scientific achievements and to show appreciation of his unique personality – was given [QR1996_02]. It was a mix of serious music and less serious text: Mozart and Ravel with frivolous libretti. It was not difficult to guess who is meant by Harolo, and who by Fritzcati.

Lectures at the BII for Students from the Philipps University Marburg, 1996

The Immunology Department of the Philipps University, Marburg, has been chaired by Klaus-Ulrich Hartmann, a long-standing friend of the BII. Through a special arrangement, the medical students from Marburg had the opportunity to spend a "colloquium week" at the BII (part of the teaching curriculum of Ivan Lefkovits in Marburg); they gained insight into research projects of the institute. Some of the lecturers were the same as in previous years,

QR1996_02 BII

LECTURE SERIES FOR STUDENTS FROM MARBURG AND PRAGUE

small seminar room at the Basel Institute for Immunology

15. - 18. May 1994

Sunday:	17.00	Introduction
Monday:	9 - 10.20	Louis du Pasquier Evolution of the Immune System
	10.30-12	Alexandra Livingstone Immunological Memory
	13.07	Georg Tiefenthaler Monday lunch seminar
	14.30-15.50	Matthias Wabl Immunoglobulin switch recombination
	16.10-16.25	Rose Zamoyska Introduction for the students
	16.30-17.30	Rose Zamoyska CD8 co-receptor function
Tuesday:	9 - 10.20	Roland Gisler Molecular mechanism of cell adhesion
	10.30-11.50	Fiona McConnell Signal Transduction: What's that?
	13.40-15	Michael Wiles ES cells and development
	15.30-16.50	Jean-Marie Buerstedde DNA recombination in the immune system
	17 - 18	Ivan Lefkovits Summary session
Wednesday:		Visit of laboratories upon individual appointment

LECTURE SERIES FOR STUDENTS FROM MARBURG

small seminar room at the Basel Institute for Immunology

12. - 15. May 1996

Sunday (12. May):	17.00	Ivan Lefkovits Introduction
Monday (13. May):	9 - 10.20	Roland Gisler Overview Immune System
	10.30-11.50	Louis Du Pasquier Evolution of the Immune System
	13.07	Ludovica Bruno Monday lunch time seminar
	14.30-15.50	Salvatore Valitutti T cell activation by specific antigen
	16.10-17.30	Peter Lane B cell responses to antigens
Tuesday (14. May):	9 - 10.20	Denis Osmond B lymphocytopoesis in bone marrow
	10.30-11.50	Ursula Günthert Adhesion molecules & tumor progression
	13.20-14.40	Manfred Kopf The T helper subset dichotomy
	14.50-16.00	Fritz Melchers Future tasks in immunology
	16.10-16.25	John Cambier Introduction for the students
	16.30-17.30	John Cambier Negative cooperativity of FcgRIIB & BCR
Wednesday (15. May):		Visit of laboratories upon individual appointment

while others, as new BII members, were doing the teaching for the first time. For many students the contacts continued after the course [QR1996_03].

On the previous page, two schedules are reproduced, one from 1994, the other from 1996 (see also the schedule reproduced in the 1990 chapter).

Years after the event, Louis Du Pasquier commented on his lectures as follows: "I adhered to a simple title, 'Evolution of the Immune System', now of course I would choose a very different title, 'Evolution of the Immune Systems', with an 's' at the end, to indicate that there are, and there always were, several immune systems."

25th Anniversary Celebration of the BII

QR1996_03 BII

QR1996_04 BII

The celebration of the 25th anniversary of the BII (June 16th, 1996) had two distinct aspects. One was to celebrate its scientific achievements and the exemplary togetherness of a successful community, while the other – with speeches by "opinion leaders" – was to encourage the sponsor's commitment to support the institute in the years to come.

The day started in the Basel Theater with high-profile speeches given by dignitaries from the scientific and commercial establishment (excerpts on the following pages) and a performance given by the Basel Percussion Ensemble donated by Paul Sacher. Parts of these speeches as well as information on the percussion performance are given in the respective QR codes [QR1996_04].

25th Anniversary Celebration of the Basel Institute for Immunology

16th June 1996

Dr. h.c. Fritz Gerber	*Chairman and CEO, Roche Holding*
Prof. Fritz Melchers	*Director of the Institute*
Prof. Hans-Joachim Güntherodt	*Rector of the University of Basel*
Prof. Jürgen Drews	*Director of Roche Research*
Prof. George Klein	*Chairman of the International Board of Scientific Advisors*
Prof. Ueli Schibler	*Chairman of the Swiss Board of Consultants*
Prof. Manfred Eigen	*Chairman of the Scientific Council*

The celebration continued with a boat trip on the river Rhine, during which a gourmet dinner was served. The seating order on board shows that even at such an event science had priority, with the tables named after components of the immune system. Thus, there were tables called "Helper T cells", "Natural killer cells", "Stem cells", etc. This was followed by a BTA performance at the BII.

On one level of the ship jazz music was played, while at the ship's entrance the group *Musique simili* with Line Loddo, Marc Hänsenberger and Juliette Du Pasquier played gypsy music.

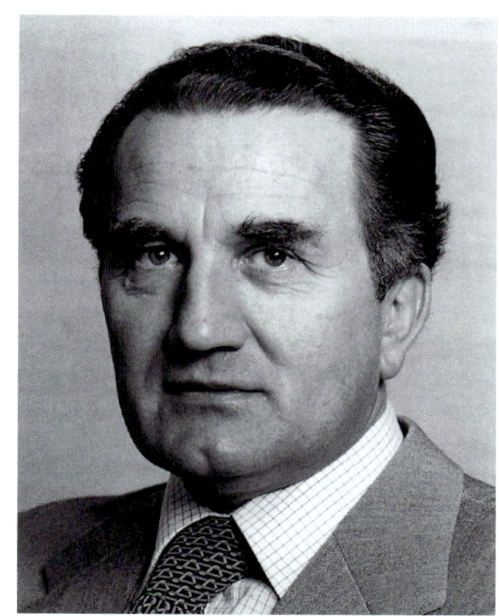

Fritz Gerber

Over 400 people participated in the celebration. Speeches were given by:

Dr. h.c. Fritz Gerber	Chairman and CEO, Roche Holding
Prof. Hans-Joachim Güntherodt	Rector of the University of Basel
Prof. Jürgen Drews	Director of Roche Research
Prof. George Klein	Chairman of the Advisory Board
Prof. Ueli Schibler	Chairman of the Board of Consultants
Prof. Manfred Eigen	Chairman of the Scientific Council
Dr. h.c. Paul Sacher	Conductor and musical patron

Excerpts of the Presentations Given at the Celebration

(Details are given in the QR code [QR1996_05])

Fritz Gerber: *"From the very beginning, in 1896, Roche has always been dedicated to the discovery, development and marketing of high quality pharmaceuticals and other products and services in the field of health care. Throughout our 100 years of history these efforts have been backed by a strong commitment to research which is crucial not only for the better understanding of the human body, but also for the development of better products and services. In this spirit Roche founded the institute 25 years ago with the intention of allowing a group of scientists to work on problems of the structure and function of the immune system in an environment that combines academic freedom with close contact to Roche."*

Hans-Joachim Güntherodt: *"The University has more than one reason to thank the Basel Institute. Since the foundation of the BII strong scientific relations have established a firm and powerful impact on the research of our University. We have profited from the excellence of the institute in our own fields of research in life sciences to a great extent. To all of you who participated in these interactions and collaborations I do express my gratitude."*

… it has become the pivotal institution in basic immunology the world over …

Jürgen Drews

Jürgen Drews: *"The genius to which the institute was dedicated was immunology, or perhaps more broadly, biological science, free-ranging science not bound by purpose or utility or by economic intent, not constrained by anything but the imagination and the intellect of those who are fortunate enough to work there. And who are the gods to whom gratitude and requests must be submitted today in order to secure their favour? Of course the gods are those who made it all possible: the owners and managers of Roche who had the idea that the foundation of an institute for basic research might be a good way to show divine favour to society at large and to the scientific community in particular: from the harsh perspectives of today some people would simply recite the title of a recent movie 'The gods must be crazy'. But look at what this child, now already a young adult, has already accomplished in its 25 years of existence: it has become the pivotal institution in basic immunology the world over, and it has spored major new developments in modern biology and its practical applications. Its members were critically involved in interpreting the curious and beautiful ways in which the immune system functions in solving one of the great questions of biology: how can the self recognize what is not self, and how can it respond to virtually every antigen under the sun? Three members of the institute have been honoured for their scientific work with a Nobel Prize: Niels Jerne, its first director (who passed away two years ago) for his pioneering theories about the immune system; Susumu Tonegawa, for solving the genetic puzzle of generating antibody diversity, and Georges Köhler, who also is no longer with us, for inventing a method to make pure antibodies against any antigen, a technology which was critically involved in starting the biotech revolution, although that was certainly not his primary intention. The Basel Institute has brought honour to itself, to its present and former members, and to Roche. In positioning an institute of basic research close to a pharmaceutical company, Roche has established a very powerful paradigm of technology transfer which has been imitated in various ways by other different companies. So yes, the gods may have been a little crazy but nothing great ever came into the world without a little craziness. Well done, Basel Institute and our congratulations."*

George Klein: *"Over the years I have developed a method, when I get to a university or institution, which for some reason or another I do not know, and there is a cocktail party or a lunch, not to listen to the empty social conversation that is addressed to me and where people anyway look over your shoulder to see who else is there, but try to listen to what the other people talk about, what the locals talk about. Do they speak about science, and are they excited about it? Do they* *speak about other important things, e.g. theatre, literature? Or do they speak about the paraphernalia of our existence: how to get money, how to get from one place to another, or do they advertise themselves, which is often the case, by what grants they got or by what papers they had accepted. Now, if I go to the cafeteria of the Basel Institute I know that I am in a very exciting place; it is worthwhile listening to the people talking to you and it is worthwhile listening to what is going on all around you. I think that says everything."*

Ueli Schibler: *"For 25 years the Basel Institute for Immunology has been a jewel among biomedical research institutions. There is probably no other institute of similar size in the world that has either hosted and/or generated three Nobel Prize laureates in such a short period of time. Every year we get the Annual Report, we read what is in there: some understand it, some don't: many of these things I don't understand and actually when it comes to immunology I should probably follow a saying of Mark Twain who said 'it is better to keep your mouth shut and appear stupid than open it and remove all doubts'. But the Annual Report is witness to the tremendous activity and productivity of the institute, and an inspection of the list of publications makes many other research institutions envious. So what is their recipe for such a success story in science? Of course you may say it's all in the playground and in the players. The founders 25 years ago were able to set up a wonderful playground, and I think one of the recipes for it was that they decided that the best rules in running the game would be to have the least number of rules possible. Of course, even more important is what the players are like: probably inspired by immunology itself, Niels Jerne thought that the best would be to have a huge diversity of players: diverse not only with regard to their talents and education, but also with regard to their scientific approach. Many talents that are required by science are almost incompatible with each other: on one end of the scale there are the artist types that generate a lot of models, some of them crazy, and on the other end of the scale one needs the analytical thinker who tries to dissect and scrutinize every aspect of the proposed models.*

Often a discovery that at first appears esoteric and is perhaps convincing just because of its aesthetic value, turns out in a few years' time to have made an important impact on the development of a drug. In that spirit I wish you all a happy and pleasant party, and I hope that we will meet again at the 50th anniversary in 25 years."

Manfred Eigen: *"My involvement with the institute and Basel has two roots: one is Paul Sacher with whom I tried in the mid-sixties to establish another institute: a Max Planck Institute of Music. Our plans at that time did not materialize, and Pierre Boulez soon after-*

... they decided that the best rules in running the game would be to have the least number of rules possible.

Ueli Schibler

wards founded that institute at the Centre Pompidou in Paris. But nevertheless our joint struggles laid the basis for a wonderful, never-ceasing friendship. The other root was Niels Jerne. At the time when he was setting up the Basel Institute I tried to do a similar job at Göttingen. Moreover, together we tried to found a third institute: an institute for Molecular Biology in Europe. At that time I was the president of EMBO, succeeding Max Perutz and again I was succeeded by Niels Jerne; the secretary general was John Kendrew who then became the first director of the EMBL at Heidelberg. Each of us developed our own style, and Niels' style has survived up to the present day. Of course the Basel Institute also had its godfathers: Paul Sacher, Maja, the whole family; Luc Hoffmann and Jakob Oeri are still members of our Scientific Council which also includes Sydney Brenner and Walter Gehring, former members being John Kendrew and Werner Arber. One of the driving forces for the foundation of the institute from the side of Roche was certainly Alfred Pletscher."

Paul Sacher: *"In the course of the 20th century, the percussion instruments have gradually emancipated themselves from the symphony orchestra and acquired an existence of their own. Thanks to this newly won independence, they now feature both as solo instruments and in smaller ensembles. Today, outstanding groups such as the famous 'Les Percussions de Strasbourg' can choose from a large repertoire of works calling for an enormous range of instruments. More and more composers are writing pieces for percussion. The Basel Percussion Ensemble is one of the fruits of this development. The group is made up of outstanding percussionists all connected in one way or another with Basel's music life: Markus Ernst, Jean-Claude Forestier, Gerry Huber, Siegfried Kutterer, Siegfried Schmid and Thomas Waldner. They have been giving concerts for some time now, exciting a large and enthusiastic public. Besides performing the standard percussion repertoire, the Basel Percussion Ensemble has also contributed to the success of countless first performances of new works by contemporary composers, e.g. 'Conductus' by Friedrich Döhl, a well-known German composer living in Lübeck. Lou Harrison is an American of protean artistic talents, a pupil of Schoenberg who has been influenced by Cage and Ives, and an authority on Asiatic music. The solo part in his violin concerto will be performed by Basel Symphony Orchestra leader Antonio Nuñez, an outstanding musician who comes from Uruguay. The programme will end with a classic masterpiece of percussion music, Carlo Chávez's 'Tambuco' for 6 percussionists. The Mexican composer is a typical representative of South American music, with its strong focus on percussion instruments. The piece by Siegfried Kutterer to be performed between the* *speeches will also feature a typical Basel drum. This instrument has been made famous by the Basel carnival and will be played by Alfons Grieder. He will open the programme with a drum solo."*

Seating Plan for the Dinner on the Boat

Each table carried an "immunology-related" name. The seating was "non-negotiable"; nevertheless, many of the guests preferred to sit at the "stem cell" table, rather than at the "natural killer" table [QR1996_06].

QR1996_06 BII

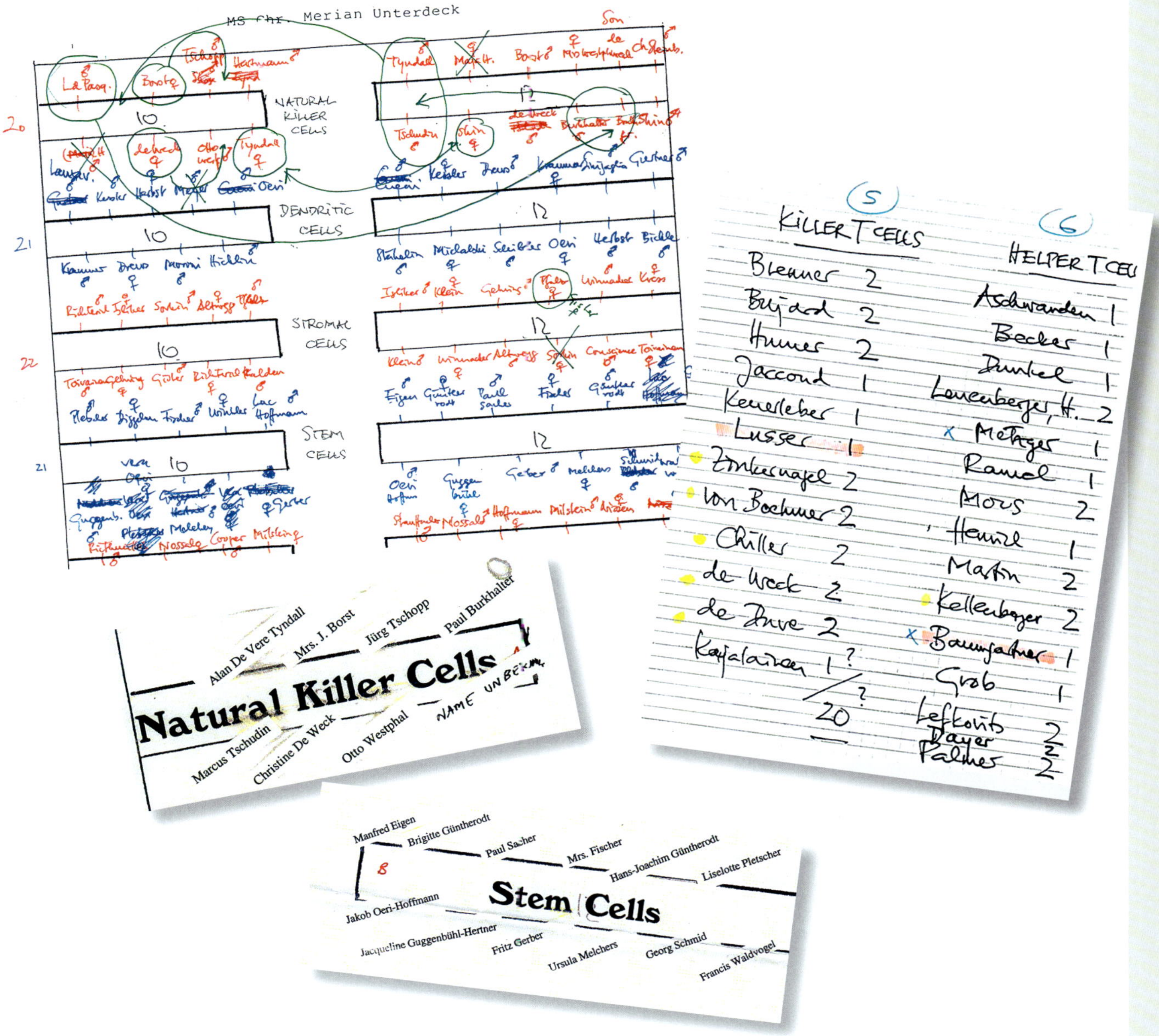

MS Chr. Merian Unterdeck

Natural Killer Cells

Alan De Vere Tyndall, Mrs. J. Borst, Jürg Tschopp, Paul Burkhalter, Marcus Tschudin, Christine De Weck, Otto Westphal

Stem Cells

Manfred Eigen, Brigitte Güntherodt, Paul Sacher, Mrs. Fischer, Hans-Joachim Güntherodt, Liselotte Pletscher, Jakob Oeri-Hoffmann, Jacqueline Guggenbühl-Hertner, Fritz Gerber, Ursula Melchers, Georg Schmid, Francis Waldvogel

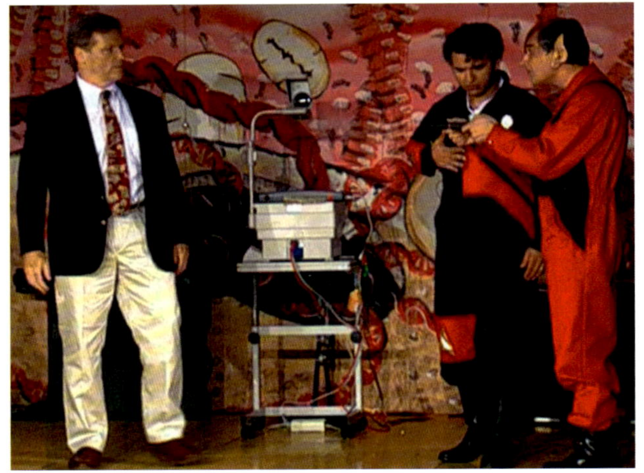

Steve Bauer, Fillipo Olivieri and Bert Temminck

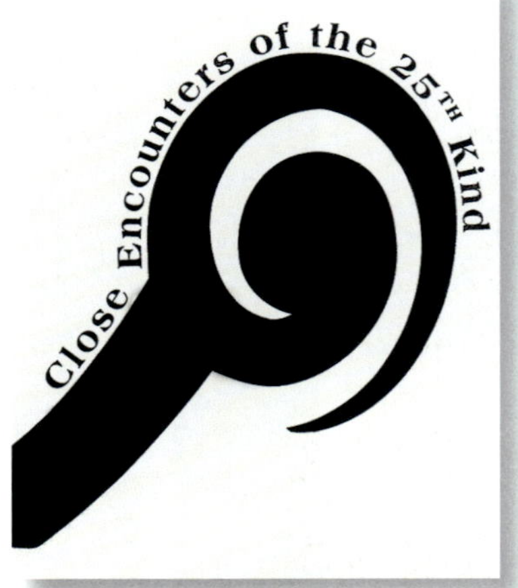

BTA 13: "Close Encounters of the 25th Kind"

This play was performed in the evening of the official celebration, June 16th, 1996 [QR1996_07]. The title of the play gives a clue about the performance, i.e. an encounter between an extraterrestrial civilization and the institute in its 25th year of existence. The actors were – as was the case in all BTA performances – scientists, technicians, workshop staff, animal caretakers, secretaries, etc., a mixture of characters to exaggerate the multiculturalism of the BII (a Canadian narrator talking in Swiss German, actors communicating in several languages). The play contained judgments – both kind and vitriolic – with a crooked mirror to reflect the institute's greatness and smallness.

Although the story carries a universal message of the human condition, the details were understandable only to cognoscenti; nevertheless, the audience enjoyed the play. It was filmed, and all those who missed the play because they themselves were acting, had a good laugh watching the film, and that was the catharsis of the play, to laugh at oneself.

QR1996_07 BII

Former Members Who Settled Permanently in Switzerland

Twenty-five years of BII history allowed a review of the careers of former members who decided to stay in Switzerland after leaving the institute. In spite of the fact that many members of the institute (mainly US Americans) were initially critical, even overcritical of the Swiss social environment, they chose to settle in Switzerland [QR1996_08]. In the meantime most of them have taken up Swiss

QR1996_08 BII

citizenship and have long forgotten their initial negative view of Switzerland. Also those members, who felt that Switzerland was too "capitalistic", now enjoy the lifestyle they achieved, as well as their good pensions.

Scientists who settled in Switzerland:

Sefik Alkan, Jan Andersson, Christine Brack, Dietmar Braun, Manfred Brockhaus, Louis Du Pasquier, Howard Etlinger, Roland Gisler, Ursula Günthert, Hans Hengartner, Chris Heusser, Beat Imhof, Jean-Claude Jaton, Marie Kosco, Antonio Lanzavecchia, Ivan Lefkovits, Vincenzo Miggiano, Markus Nabholz, Elisabetta Padovan, Ed Palmer, Richard Pink, Gerd Pluschke, Walter Riesen, Ton Rolink, Eddy Roosnek, Max Schreier (†), Theo Staehelin, Charley Steinberg (†), Bela Takacs, Zdenek Trnka (†).

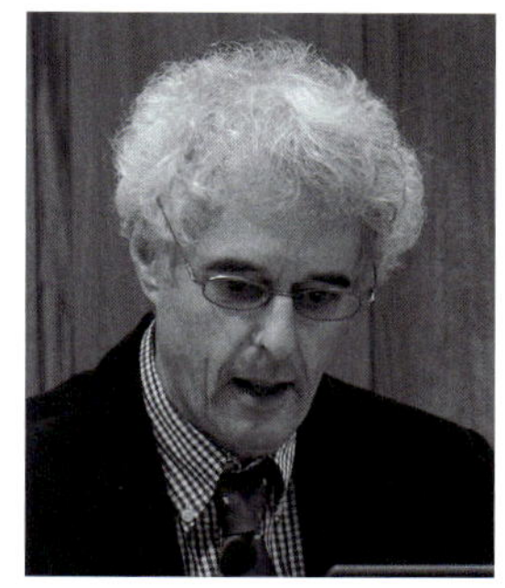
Howard Etlinger

The list is somewhat misleading as several of these scientists were living in Switzerland before joining the institute: they did not "settle", they were often rooted in the country. It should be noted that only a "partial" list of technicians could be assembled as no database exists for these members of staff.

Nobel Prize for Two Members of the Advisory Board, 1996

Rolf Zinkernagel and Peter Doherty were awarded the Nobel Prize for Medicine 1996, for the discovery of the specificity of cell-mediated immune defense [QR1996_09]. Zinkernagel and Doherty discovered that in order for killer T cells to recognize infected cells, they had to recognize two molecules on the surface of the cell – not only the virus antigen, but also a molecule of the major histocompatibility complex (MHC). The work was done in Australia; Zinkernagel moved to the University of Zurich, and Peter Doherty became head of the Immunology Unit of St. Jude Children's Hospital in Memphis, Tennessee.

QR1996_09 BII

QR1996_10 BII

Information Booklet on the Scientific Aims of the BII – Updated for the Occasion of the 25th Anniversary Celebration

On several occasions the institute published a booklet in which its aims and functions were described. The text for the version updated for the 25th anniversary was written by Fritz Melchers and is reproduced in [QR1996_10]. Four main themes are handled in the booklet:

- Science at the institute
- Practical use of the knowledge
- An unusual structure in an unusual freedom
- Youth beyond national boundaries

Treasure Trove 1996
The database contains documents related to the BII in a broader context (lists, series of photographs, etc.).

QR1996_treasure BII

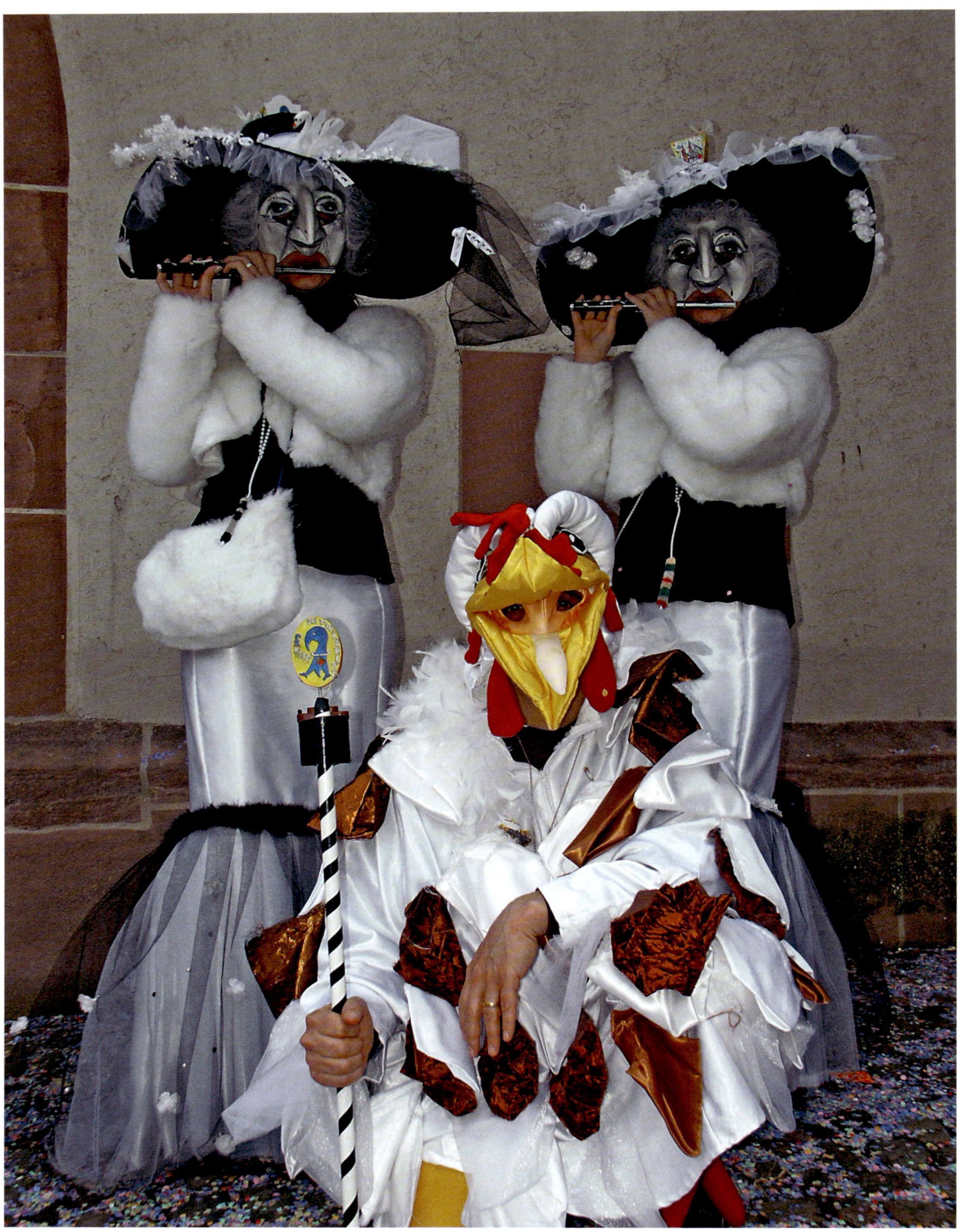

Permanent member Ed Palmer in costume at the famous Basel carnival (Fasnacht)

The Year 1997

Two workshops were organized: "EMBO Course on T Cells" and "From T Cell Stimulation to T Cell Behavior". Academic Press published a 4-volume immunology methods book, with major involvement of institute members. A retirement symposium for Charley Steinberg was held in Prague in the Villa Lanna. Martin Hicklin kept the readership of the *Basler Zeitung* informed about scientific discoveries at the BII (his service to the public was later recognized by the University of Basel, which awarded him an honorary doctorate).

Largest Methodology Book in Immunology, 1997

Academic Press published a 4-volume book, edited by Ivan Lefkovits, with several hundred contributors [QR1997_0_]. It appeared in print and on DVD. For a while it was on the bestseller list of scientific publications. The names of the scientists on the editorial board, and the names and addresses of the contributors are given in the QR code. The addresses are mostly out of date, but they provide a snapshot of the time of their past affiliations.

Immunology Methods Manual: The Comphrehensive
www.sigmaalrich.com/catalog/product/sigma/z374350
Sigma-Aldrich offers Sigma-Z374350, Immunology Methods Manual:
The publication info, I. Lefkovits, Academic Press, In., 1996, 2176 pp-. com bound

Arrivals 1997 (9)
Martin Bachmann, Jeffrey Bluestone, Annegret de Baey, Heinz Jacobs, Stefan Mahlmann, Hideo Nakajima, Yoichi Sakakibara, Bénédicte Sammut, Pasquale Vito.

Came and Left in the Same Year (2)
Tim Manser, Michel Record.

Leavers 1997 (9)
Thomas Bäckström, Rhodri Ceredig, Isabelle Chrétien, Pierre Cosson, Ramona Leibnitz, François Letourneur, Minetaro Ogawa, Charles Steinberg, Salvatore Valitutti.

QR1997_01 BII

From T Cell Stimulation to T Cell Behavior, February 1997

An EMBO workshop was organized by Ed Palmer, Klaus Karjalainen, Antonio Lanzavecchia and Fritz Melchers [QR1997_02], and it dealt with the latest developments concerning cellular signaling in T lymphocytes, as well as with the cell biology of the TCR expressed on the plasma membrane. It focused on 5 themes:

- TCR structure (crystallographic studies)
- Interaction of the TCR with the CD3 signaling components
- Generation of active intracellular signaling molecules
- Choices of activation/signaling models/signal transduction
- Contribution of accessory and costimulatory molecules to the outcome of antigen recognition

EMBO Practical Course on

LYMPHOCYTE DEVELOPMENT

7th - 20th September 1997

Basel Institute for Immunology Switzerland

Organizer: Ton Rolink
Coorganizers: Jan Andersson & Fritz Melchers

MANUAL

The Basel Institute for Immunology is funded and supported by F. Hoffmann-La Roche Ltd

EMBO Practical Course on Lymphocyte Development, September 1997

Antonius G. Rolink and Jan Andersson organized this advanced practical course [QR1997_03]. It was accompanied by lectures that covered the development of T and B cells, their receptors and their interactions with the environment. The experimental work concentrated on in vitro cultures of mouse lymphocyte progenitors, FACS analyses, single-cell PCR and cell transfers for transplantation.

A deeper insight into the development and functioning of the immune system was achieved by introducing the methodology of gene targeting to create new mutant animals and cell lines, together with new in vitro cell culturing.

QR1997_02 BII

QR1997_03 BII

QR1997_04 BII

Martin Hicklin, Dr. h.c., Writes for the *Basler Zeitung*

The only newspaper in Switzerland of international format is the *Neue Zürcher Zeitung*. All the others are "local". Nevertheless, there is one area of reporting in which Basel surpasses most European newspapers, and that is reporting on science by the *Basler Zeitung* [QR1997_04]. The tradition and quality of reporting are derived from the reputation of Basel as a research center of the pharmaceutical industry. A single journalist often sets standards – in this particular case it was Martin Hicklin.

Martin Hicklin attended all the important events taking place at the institute (10th and 25th anniversary celebrations, Nobel Prizes 1994, 1997, Advisory Board meetings). Martin was present at the birth of the institute and also at its closure, first as a "simple" journalist, later as acting editor-in-chief. His exceptional qualities

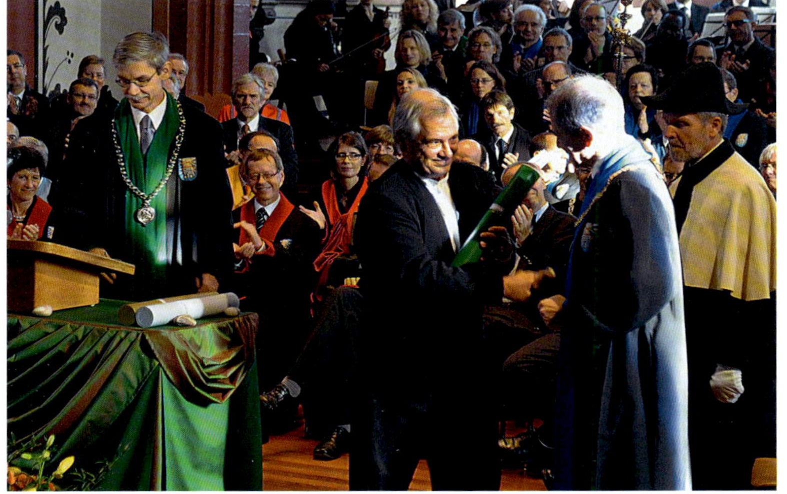

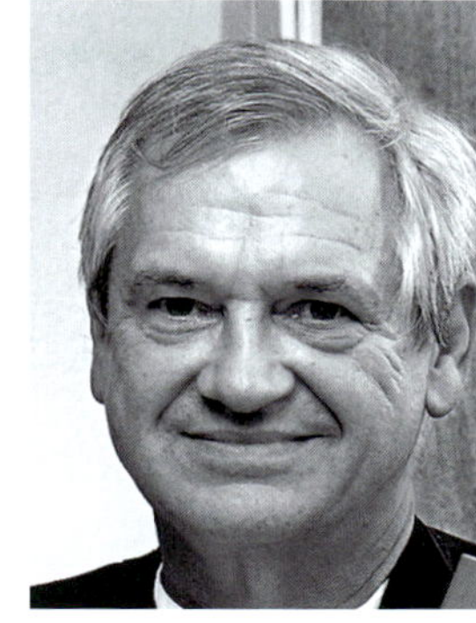

Martin Hicklin receiving his honorary doctorate from Basel University

were recognized by the University of Basel when it gave him an honorary doctorate. Many QR codes in this book provide links to clips of articles written by Martin Hicklin. On his retirement, other journalists (e.g. Stefan Stöcklin) took over from him.

Nature Paper by Marina Cella and Antonio Lanzavecchia

In an article by Stefan Stöcklin, details of an important paper by two members of the BII [QR1997_05] were reported:

Basler Zeitung Samstag/Sonntag, 23./24. August 1997, Nr. 195 Teil V **Wissenschaft.** Seite 73

Wie die Wächter das Abwehrsystem alarmieren

Noch vor wenigen Jahren waren sie nicht einmal den Fachleuten bekannt: Die Rede ist von spezialisierten Zellen im Körpergewebe, die das Immunsystem auf Trab bringen. Neuste Einsichten zu deren Funktion liefert eine Arbeit im aktuellen «Nature» von Marina Cella und Antonio Lanzavecchia vom Basler Institut für Immunologie.

Von Stefan Stöcklin

Eine fast alltägliche Episode: Aufgrund einer ungeschickten Bewegung fällt man auf den Boden, schürft sich das Knie auf und infiziert sich mit einer Bakterie. Ein, zwei Tage später schwellen die Lymphknoten an, und die Wunde entzündet sich. Bestehen noch Zweifel, so zeigt Fieber mit letzter Sicherheit, dass eine Entzündungsreaktion im Gange ist. Das Abwehrsystem des Körpers läuft auf vollen Touren. Die Abwehrzellen sind damit beschäftigt, die eindringende Mikrobe zu vertreiben. Nach ein paar Tagen klingt die Entzündung wieder ab. Der Eindringling wird buchstäblich zerstört. Im Körper herrscht wieder Ruhe.

Dass Entzündungsreaktionen derart ablaufen, ist schon lange bekannt. Unzählige Forschungsarbeiten über das Immunsystem des Menschen haben auch manche Einblicke in die komplizierten Vorgänge gebracht, die beim Eindringen eines Fremdkörpers ablaufen. Eine entscheidende Rolle spielen dabei die weissen Blutkörperchen in den Lymphknoten und der Milz. In den lymphatischen Organen des Menschen sitzen rund eine Billion (10^{12}) Zellen, die aufgrund ihrer Reifung im Thymus als T-Zellen bezeichnet werden. In dieser Drüse hinter dem Brustbein entwickelt sich auch ein spezieller Typ von T-Zellen, die als T-Helfer-Zellen bezeichnet werden. Sie beginnen sich im Lymphknoten zu vermehren, wenn sie mit Teilen des eindringenden Fremdkörpers in Kontakt kommen. Diese molekularen Bestandteile des Eindringlings werden als Antigene bezeichnet. Nach dem Kontakt mit dem Antigen steuern Helfer-Zellen die Abwehr gegen den Eindringling, indem sie unter anderem die B-Lymphozyten zur Herstellung von Antikörpern veranlassen.

Wachposten der Immunabwehr

Wie diese Aktivierung zustande kommt, darüber verschaffen Lanzavecchia und sein Team neue Einsichten. «Die Entzündung aktiviert am Ort der Infektion dendritische Zellen, welche die Antigene zu den T-Zellen in den Lymphknoten transportieren», sagt Antonio Lanzavecchia, der seit 1983 in Basel arbeitet. Wie muss man sich das vorstellen? Über den ganzen Körper verteilt sitzen unzählige dendritische Zellen in den verschiedenen Geweben: unter der Haut, in den Muskeln, selbst im Herzen. Ihren Namen tragen sie aufgrund ihrer stäbchenförmigen Ausstülpungen wobei sie nicht mit den «Dendriten» – bestimmten Zellen des Nervensystems – verwechselt werden dürfen. Über ihre Funktion war bis vor kurzem kaum etwas bekannt. «Heute wissen wir, dass sie die Wachposten des Immunsystems darstellen. Dendritische Zellen vollziehen den ersten Schritt bei einer Immunantwort», sagt Lanzavecchia.

Wenn eine Bakterie oder ein Virus in den Körper eindringt, wird der Fremdkörper von den dendritischen Zellen zerlegt, einverleibt und teilweise in die Zellwand eingebaut. Dabei werden die Antigene mit einem ganz besonders wichtigen Merkmal auf der Oberfläche der Zelle verbunden, dem sogenannten MHC-II-Komplex. Mit dieser Struktur auf der Oberfläche wandern die dendritischen Zellen zum nächsten Lymphknoten und präsentieren den T-Zellen ihren Fang. Diese Migration dauert ein bis zwei Tage. Dann werden die T-Zellen im Lymphknoten aktiv. Die Abwehrschlacht beginnt.

Bessere Impfstoffe

«Wir haben zeigen können, dass der unspezifische Entzündungsmechanismus dendritische Zellen aktiviert», sagt Lanzavecchia, der die letzten Jahre mit dem Studium dieser Wächterzellen verbracht hat. Dazu untersuchten die Forscher die Reaktion losgelöst vom Körper im Reagenzglas. Das Basler Team hat eine Technik entwickelt, um ruhende dendritische Zellen des Menschen in der Kulturschale zu aktivieren. Dazu geben sie den Zellen just jene entzündungsfördernden Moleküle hinzu, die auch bei einer Infektion im Körper mitspielen. «Wenn wir die Zellen mit dem Tumor-Nekrose-Faktor oder Interleukin-1 stimulieren, integrieren sie mehr Antigene. Der MHC-II-Komplex lebt zudem länger und wird weniger rasch abgebaut.» Alles läuft darauf hinaus, dass die Wächterzellen eine effiziente Immunantwort in den T-Zellen veranlassen können.

Welche praktischen Folgen ergeben sich nun aus diesen Forschungsarbeiten, die im aktuellen «Nature» (Band 388, Seite 782 ff.) veröffentlicht worden sind? Handelt es sich um eine reine Arbeit aus der Grundlagenforschung ohne praktischen Nutzen? Lanzavecchia wehrt ab: «Wir hoffen einerseits, dank diesen Erkenntnissen bessere Impfstoffe herstellen zu können, weil wir nun genau wissen, wie eine Immunantwort verstärkt wird. Zum anderen zeichnen sich neue Möglichkeiten einer Immuntherapie ab.» Denkbar ist es, im Reagenzglas ruhende dendritische Zellen zum Einbau von Antigenen aus Tumoren zu veranlassen. Die derart aktivierten Zellen werden anschliessend dem Patienten eingespritzt. Sie können, falls alles klappt, die körpereigenen T-Zellen zum Angriff gegen den Tumor aktivieren. Entsprechende Versuche mit dem schwarzen Hautkrebs (Melanom) sind am Zürcher Universitätsspital bereits angelaufen. Für Basel stehen derartige klinische Versuche auf dem Programm.

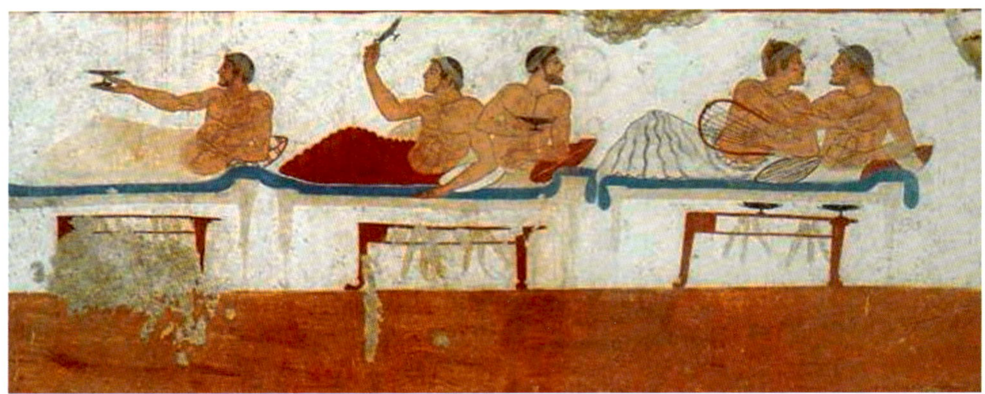

Symposion in ancient Greece

Charley Steinberg was one of the most influential members of the BII.

Retirement Symposium for Charley Steinberg, 1997

Charley Steinberg was one of the most influential members of the BII: for Niels Jerne he was an invaluable help in decision-making, and for the members he was a friend from whom it was an honor to accept both criticism and praise [QR1997_06]. When the time came to choose the place and format for his farewell conference, Charley's friends and colleagues opted to organize it in Prague. There were several reasons why Prague was chosen as the venue. Charley wanted to have a small conference, and this could not have been achieved in Basel where it would be an event with speeches and formal celebrations that was so against Charley's wishes.

The conference had the unusual title Charles Steinberg Honorific Symposion on Quantitative Biology, and the designation was meticulously chosen to fit the CSHSQB acronym for the Cold Spring Harbor Symposium [see in Book 1 QR1969_14]. And to give it a fine twist, instead of "Symposium" it was called "Symposion" (drinking together).

The conference took place on October 25th and 26th, 1997, in Prague at the Villa Lanna (of the Academy of Sciences of the Czech Republic). The participants arrived on Friday, October 24th (or earlier), and left on Monday, October 27th, or stayed on.

Program:

Friday, October 24th (or earlier): Arrival
  Friday evening: Reception in the Villa Lanna
Saturday, October 25th: Symposion
  Lunch in the Villa
  Dinner in the Restaurant Sarah Bernhardt
Sunday, October 26th: Symposion
  Lunch in the Villa
  Dinner free
  The music was arranged by Louis Du Pasquier
Monday, October 27th: Excursion to the Mendel Museum in Brno

QR1997_06 BII

Jack von Borstel was responsible for the scientific sessions

Participants:

Lucien Caro, Una Chen, Antonio Coutinho, Louis Du Pasquier, Dick Epstein, Howard Etlinger, Don and Gail Gerson, Werner Haas, Ellen Hsu, Ivan Lefkovits, Chris Paige, Gordon Sato, Theo Staehelin, Susumu Tonegawa, Jack von Borstel, Matthias Wabl, Jean-Claude Weill, Gill Wu

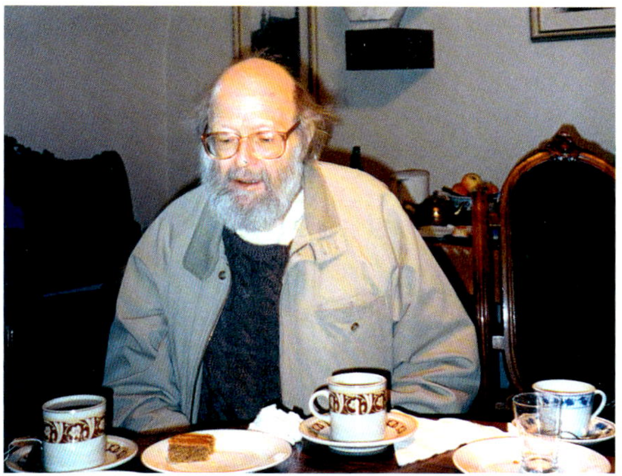

Charley Steinberg

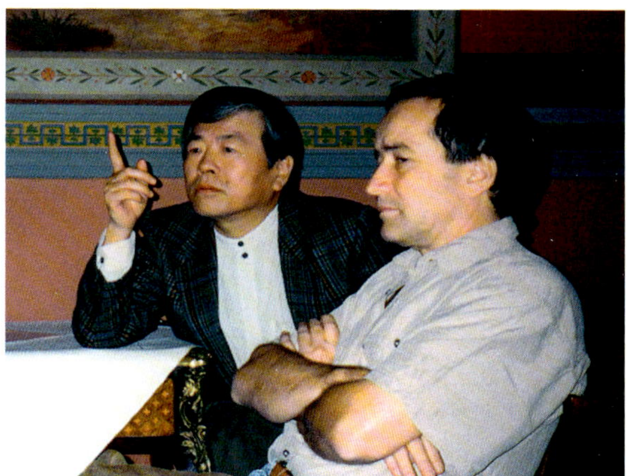

Susumu Tonegawa and Matthias Wabl

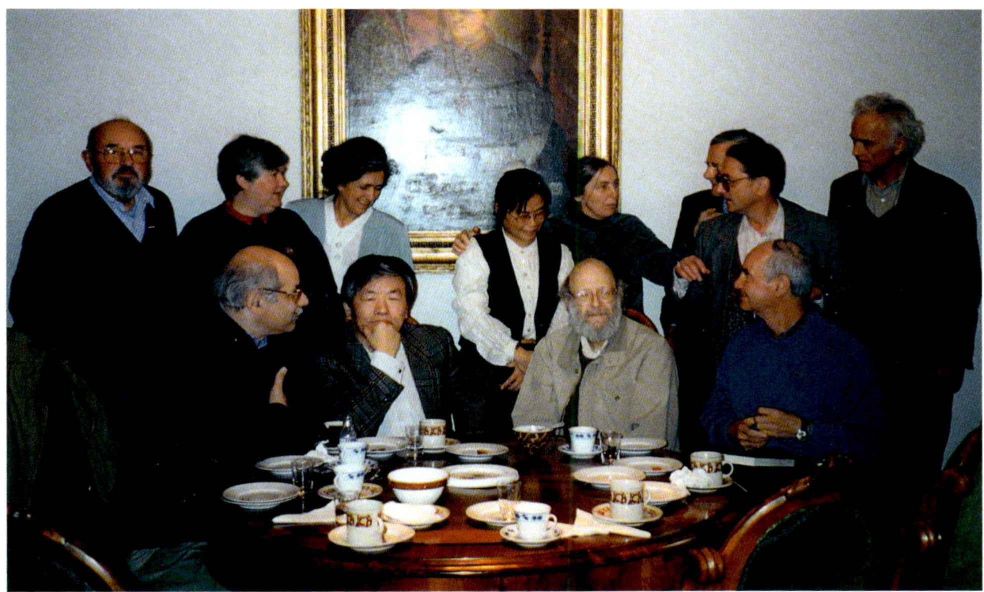

(Photo by Don Gerson)

The Director of the Mendel Museum in Brno (third from left, back row) was overjoyed to have such distinguished geneticists as visitors sitting at Mendel's table

One More Goodbye Dinner for Charley Steinberg, 1997

QR1997_07 BII

Charley hoped that the goodbye events in Prague had fulfilled his "duty" and that he could finally continue with his daily routine: drinking coffee, talking and listening to people. Finally, he graciously accepted the fact that Basel wanted to say goodbye too and amiably agreed to attend a fine dinner in the Restaurant St. Alban-Eck with the BII permanent members [QR1997_07].

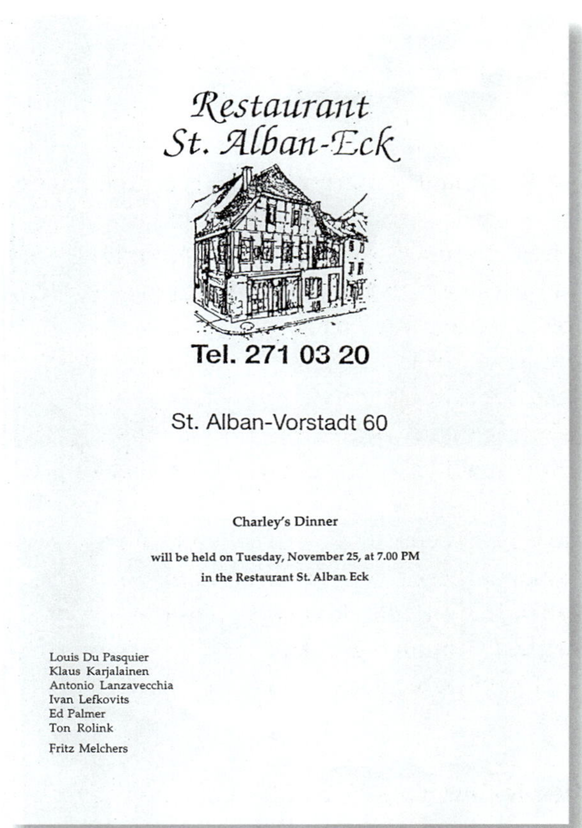

Restaurant
St. Alban-Eck

Tel. 271 03 20

St. Alban-Vorstadt 60

Charley's Dinner

will be held on Tuesday, November 25, at 7.00 PM
in the Restaurant St. Alban Eck

Louis Du Pasquier
Klaus Karjalainen
Antonio Lanzavecchia
Ivan Lefkovits
Ed Palmer
Ton Rolink
Fritz Melchers

Treasure Trove 1997

The database contains documents related to the BII in a broader context (lists, series of photographs, etc.).

QR1997_treasure BII

The Year 1998

A workshop on B cells was held. Marco Colonna's studies on the innate immune system showed a new emphasis of research direction at the BII. Similarly to all previous International Congresses of Immunology, the 10th congress in New Delhi attracted a strong attendance from BII members as speakers and chairpersons.

Marco Colonna's Studies on Innate Immunity

Unlike adaptive immunity that forms a discrete system centered on lymphocyte biology, innate immunity is an entity of defense pathways that involves many different biological components. While adaptive immunity is based on the selection of somatically generated repertoires of antigen receptors, innate immunity utilizes structures and pathways that may or may not be related to one another: complement, antimicrobial peptides, NOD-like receptors, Toll-like receptors, to name just a few. In this context the shift of studies from adaptive towards innate immunity at the BII was illustrated by the significant findings of Marco Colonna, who identified innate receptors that can discriminate between normal and tumor cells [QR1998_01].

Marco Colonna also discovered that the human plasmacytoid dendritic cell is a major source of inflammatory compounds essential for battling viral infections. He was a codiscoverer of a rare type of immune cell in the human gut that significantly improves the intestine's ability to fight bacterial infections.

Arrivals 1998 (11)
Jes Dietrich, Ulf Grawunder, Kristian Hannestad, Thomas Harder, Reinhard Hoffmann, Greg Kline, Alexandre Potocnik, Emmanuel Scotet, Dominic van Essen, Guy Werlen, Christian Wimmer.

Leavers 1998 (7)
Seiamak Bahram, Jeffrey Bluestone, Luca Bolliger, Thomas Brocker, Jean-Marie Buerstedde, Kerry Campbell, Wayne Hein.

Workshop on the Mechanisms of B Cell Neoplasia: Chronic Stimulation of the Immune System, October 1998

This workshop, similar to the 14 previous ones (some held in Basel, others in Bethesda), brought scientists together who were interested in basic B cell biology with those who studied the pathogenesis of B cell tumors. Examples of genetic instabilities that occur during phases of proliferative expansion of B lymphocytes were discussed, and chronic stimulation of lymphocytes by environmental stimuli and infections was examined to explain the danger of malignant transformation and deregulated proliferation and migration of cells.

QR1998_01 BII

10th International Congress of Immunology in New Delhi, 1998

As with all previous International Congresses of Immunology (they started in 1971) the 10th International Congress of Immunology in New Delhi gave the opportunity to BII scientists to present major lectures and be chairpersons [QR1998_02].

M.F. Bachmann — "Role of TCR Dimerization in T Cell Antagonism"
A. Lanzavecchia — "From Antigen Presentation to T Cell Activation"
F. Melchers — "Checkpoints in B Cell Development"
M. Salio — "Efficient Class I Restricted Antigen Presentation"
A. Viola — "The Role of Coreceptors and Costimulation in T Cell Activation"

Scientific organizations in Europe (EMBO, ENII, EMBL, EASD, FEBS)[1] became more involved in hosting high-profile workshops and conferences, and BII members actively followed this new trend.

EMBO Workshop on Regulation of B Lymphocyte Development by BCR Signals, Ystaad, Sweden:

F. Melchers,
Chair and talk: "Repertoire development"
C. Schaniel: "Activated murine B lymphocytes and dendritic cells produce a novel CC chemokine which acts selectively on activated T cells"
R.M. Torres: "Fetal and adult B cell development *in vitro*"

ENII Conference, Les Embiez:

H.J. Fehling: "Allelic exclusion in mice lacking the pre-TCR alpha chain"
A. Lanzavecchia: "The antigen presenting function of dendritic cells"
M. Salio, poster: "Efficient class I restricted antigen presentation"

EMBL Conference, Monterotondo, Rome:

A. Viola: "A dynamic view of T cell activation"

EASD Workshop (Diabetes), St. John's College, Oxford:

M. Cella: "About class II on dendritic cells"
M. Salio: "Use of DC in antigen-specific immunotherapy"

FEBS International Summer School on Immunology: "The Immune System: Genes, Receptors and Regulation", Ionian Village, Greece:

J. Kisielow: "Subtractive cDNA library from RAG knock-out thymus"
A. Lanzavecchia: "T cell activation"; "Antigen-presenting cells"
J. Pieters: "Antigen processing and presentation"
H.-R. Rodewald: "Stem cells"; "Aspects of thymocyte development and the formation of the thymic epithelium"

QR1998_02 BII

[1] EMBO, European Molecular Biology Organization; ENII, European Network of Immunology Institutes; EASD, European Association for the Study of Diabetes; FEBS, Federation of European Biochemical Societies; EMBL, European Molecular Biology Laboratory.

Andrew Kelus Died, 1998

Andrew Kelus died at the age of 70. He was a founding and permanent member of the BII. His work concerned idiotypes in the rabbit. A special strain of rabbit, which became widely used in the field of idiotype and anti-idiotype regulation, carried the name Basilea.

At a small ceremony attended by Andrew's friends and colleagues, according to his last wish, his ashes were scattered over the river Rhine from a Basel ferryboat.

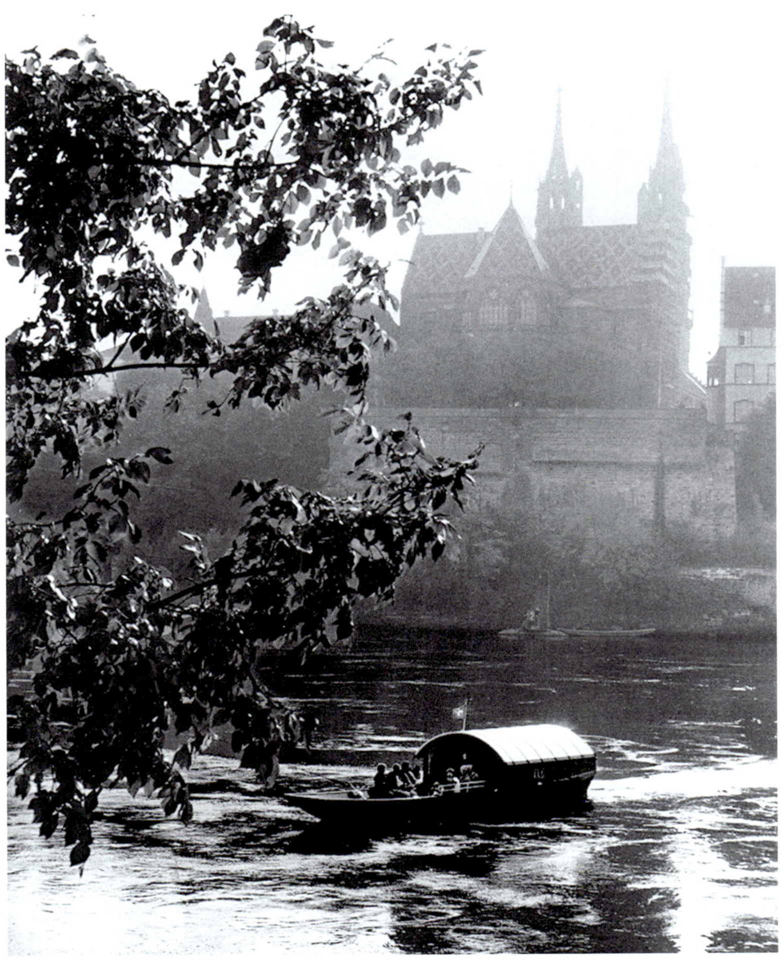

Ferry boat crossing the Rhine from the Basel Minster

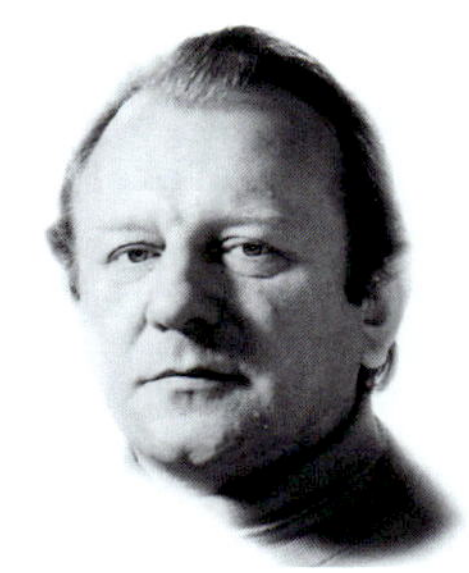

Andrew Kelus

Treasure Trove 1998

The database contains documents related to the BII in a broader context (lists, series of photographs, etc.).

QR1998_treasure BII

The Year 1999

A course and a workshop were arranged: an "EMBO Practical Course on Lymphocyte Development" and a "Workshop on Lymphoid Organogenesis". Antonio Lanzavecchia gave up his position as permanent member and moved to Bellinzona. Charley Steinberg, ex-permanent member of the BII, died. Paul Sacher, conductor, music patron and philanthropist, died at the age of 93.

Arrivals 1999 (6)
Fabien Agenès, Michael Carroll, Rachel Ettinger, Cristina Hernandez-Munain, Jörg Kirberg, Ekaterina Revenkova.

Came and Left in the Same Year (2)
Paul Kincade, Ludovica Bruno.

Leavers 1999 (16)
Martin Bachmann, Annegret de Baey, Hans Jörg Fehling, Johann-Rudolf Frey, Thomas Göbel, Kristian Hannestad, Greg Kline, Antonio Lanzavecchia, Stephan Mahlmann, Kazuo Ohnishi, Hans-Reimer Rodewald, Yoichi Sakakibara, Federica Sallusto, Antonella Viola, Christian Wimmer, Tamotsu Yamagami.

EMBO Practical Course on Lymphocyte Development

Antonius Rolink, Jan Andersson and Fritz Melchers organized this 2-week course [QR1999_01]. The lectures covered the development of T and B cells, their receptors and their interactions with the environment. The practical part concentrated on in vitro cultures of mouse lymphocyte progenitors, FACS analyses, single-cell PCR and cell transfers for transplantation. Gene targeting, together with new in vitro culturing and analysis methods, produced deeper insights into the development and function of the immune system.

The teaching staff (external) included:

Frederick W. Alt	Howard Hughes Medical Institute, Boston
Harald von Boehmer	INSERM, Hôpital Necker, Paris
Rod Ceredig	University of Birmingham School of Medicine, Birmingham, UK
Ana Cumano	Pasteur Institute, Paris
Elaine Dzierzak and Willem van Ewijk	Erasmus University, Rotterdam
Katia Georgopoulos	Harvard Medical School, Boston
Isabelle Godin	Institut d'Embryologie, CNRS, Nogent-sur-Marne
Marie Kosco-Vilbois	Serono Pharmaceutical Research Institute, Geneva
Josef Penninger	Amgen Institute, Toronto
Andreas Radbruch and Giuliana Cassese	DRFZ, Berlin
Michael Reth, Jutta Schweikert and Jenny Kohler	MPI, Freiburg
Jonathan Sprent	The Scripps Research Institute, La Jolla
and members of the BII	

QR1999_01 BII

QR1999_02 BII

Workshop on Lymphoid Organogenesis

This workshop (November 5th to 6th) was organized by Hans-Reimer Rodewald, Fritz Melchers and Antonius Rolink [QR1999_02].

It dealt with molecular mechanisms and cellular elements guiding the formation of primary and secondary lymphoid organs (thymus, bone marrow, lymph nodes and spleen of several species). The contributions of epithelial, endothelial, fibroblastic and hematopoietic cells and their interactions during morphogenesis were discussed. Special emphasis was placed on mutations affecting lymphoid organogenesis. The workshop had a format of 4 sessions:

- Stem cells: hematopoietic, epithelial, others
- Vessel development
- Thymus development
- Lymphoid tissue development

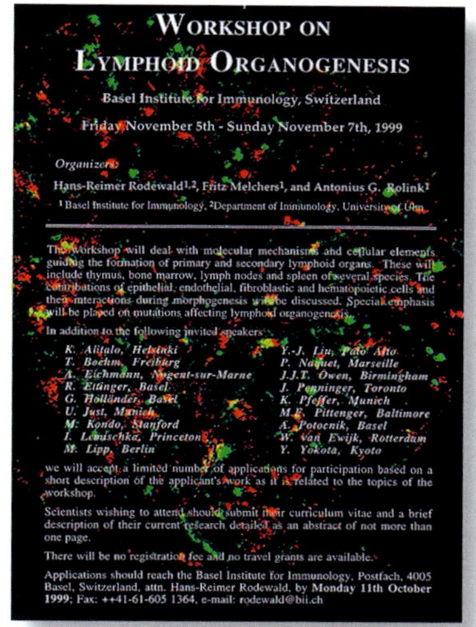
WORKSHOP ON
LYMPHOID ORGANOGENESIS
Basel Institute for Immunology, Switzerland
Friday November 5th - Sunday November 7th, 1999
Organizers:
Hans-Reimer Rodewald1,2, Fritz Melchers1, and Antonius G. Rolink1
1 Basel Institute for Immunology, 2Department of Immunology, University of Ulm
The workshop will deal with molecular mechanisms and cellular elements guiding the formation of primary and secondary lymphoid organs. These will include thymus, bone marrow, lymph nodes and spleen of several species. The contributions of epithelial, endothelial, fibroblastic and hematopoietic cells and their interactions during morphogenesis will be discussed. Special emphasis will be placed on mutations affecting lymphoid organogenesis.
In addition to the following invited speakers
K. Alitalo, Helsinki
T. Boehm, Freiburg
A. Eichmann, Nogent-sur-Marne
R. Ettinger, Basel
G. Holländer, Basel
U. Just, Munich
M. Kondo, Stanford
I. Lemischka, Princeton
M. Lipp, Berlin
Y.-J. Liu, Palo Alto
P. Naquet, Marseille
J.J.T. Owen, Birmingham
J. Penninger, Toronto
K. Pfeffer, Munich
M.F. Pittenger, Baltimore
A. Potocnik, Basel
W. van Ewijk, Rotterdam
Y. Yokota, Kyoto
we will accept a limited number of applications for participation based on a short description of the applicant's work as it is related to the topics of the workshop.
Scientists wishing to attend should submit their curriculum vitae and a brief description of their current research detailed as an abstract of not more than one page.
There will be no registration fee and no travel grants are available.
Applications should reach the Basel Institute for Immunology, Postfach, 4005 Basel, Switzerland, attn. Hans-Reimer Rodewald, by Monday 11th October 1999; Fax: ++41-61-605 1364, e-mail: rodewald@bii.ch

Antonio Lanzavecchia Moves to Bellinzona, 1999

In 1999 Antonio became the founding director of the Institute for Research in Biomedicine in Bellinzona [QR1999_03]. He left the BII when human immunology received an enormous boost worldwide, and Antonio needed to expand in order to accomplish his scientific objectives. The possibility to establish an institute in the Italian-speaking part of Switzerland was an added bonus for Antonio. Although he was fluent in German as well as in English, the chance to live close to his native country was irresistible.

Dozens of Italians came to work at the BII throughout its existence. Without them, the institute would not have had such an international heterogeneous flavor. Three permanent members were of Italian descent (Ben Pernis and Ruggero Ceppellini were founding members, Antonio Lanzavecchia was a later addition).

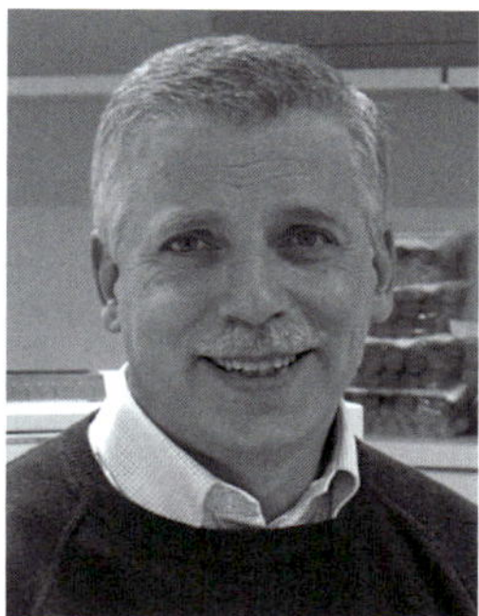
Antonio Lanzavecchia

Paul Sacher and the Fate of the Institute

Although Paul Sacher has been referred to in several chapters, especially in Book 1, a closer look at this eminent personality will help the reader to appreciate important developments at the BII, especially in the final years of its existence, as will be described in the forthcoming chapters.

Contemporaries often viewed Paul Sacher "purely" as the husband of the richest woman in Switzerland: Maja Sacher-Hoffmann. It may be convenient to "reduce" the merits of this man to be those of musician, conductor and philanthropist. Nevertheless, to understand the role Paul Sacher played in the fate of the Basel Institute, a closer look at his character is required.

It is true that when Paul Sacher married Maja Hoffmann, his "dowry" to the marriage was nothing but his musical talent, inter-

QR1999_03 BII

est in art and eagerness to accomplish his vision. With Maja at his side, Paul had the opportunity to focus on the music that he loved so much. Maja helped him become a wealthy man in his own right by supporting and authorizing a transaction of Roche shares, which a major Swiss bank wanted to get rid of. With borrowed money he acquired the shares, paid back the debt over the years and became independently wealthy. The definition of "self-made man" would not entirely do him justice. The rise from bottom to top required that he understood the Roche business, that he was genuinely interested in all relevant issues and that he paid attention to the long-term plans of the company.

Maja and Paul Sacher were aware of Roche's decision to launch a basic research institute of "some" biological relevance. When the institute was being planned, these two extraordinary personalities showed only a little curiosity, but this climaxed when they met the director, Niels Jerne, in person. A very positive relationship developed, and later it was of great significance that Maja and Paul Sacher invited the members of the International Advisory Board (IAB) to their home on the Schönenberg [QR1999_04].

Paul Sacher and the BII Advisory Board

Paul Sacher frequently mentioned that he had never before met such an interesting group of people (members of the IAB). Soon after the initial dinner on the Schönenberg, Niels Jerne called Paul Sacher to thank him for the evening. Paul Sacher responded warmly by saying that he already wished now to extend the dinner invitation for the next IAB meeting. Advisory Board dinners thus became a regular event and, except during the last period of Maja Sacher's frail health before she passed away, the Advisory Board evenings with Maja and Paul Sacher turned out to be highlights of the social events linked to the life of the institute [QR1999_05].

QR1999_04 BII

The dinner evenings on the Schönenberg did not cease when Niels Jerne retired and Fritz Melchers took over; indeed, Niels Jerne continued to participate, as he was "honorary chairman" of the board. The cordial relationship between Paul Sacher and Niels Jerne was soon extended to Fritz Melchers, who developed a good and friendly relationship with Paul Sacher. Years later, Fritz Melchers' wife Ursula also became a friend of the family, often taking care of Paul Sacher's son Georg.

QR1999_05 BII

One might raise the question whether the above description is of any relevance to the history of the BII. "Opinion leaders" in Switzerland highly valued the institute, and the fact that Paul

Sacher showed keen interest in it gave the BII an additional aura of elitism. Although the international scientific standing of the institute was not dependent on private patronage, locally it became well known that the most powerful family of Switzerland firmly stood behind it.

This, of course, was noted at all hierarchical levels within Roche. Throughout the decades the BII existed, the "top echelon" of the company always highly supported it. As presidents and director generals retired and were replaced by new ones, the support continued, although it was never entirely clear whether the attitude expressed was a firm commitment or just lip service.

Paul Sacher Supports the Unique Research Ambiance of the BII

Paul Sacher was aware of the fact that the BII had a special way of doing research. For him, it was not only a highly successful scientific institution, but also a place that deserved to be fully supported, and its unique research ambiance had to be cherished [QR1999_06]. Paul Sacher protected this uniqueness, and whenever Jerne or Melchers needed his backing, they knew they could always count on him.

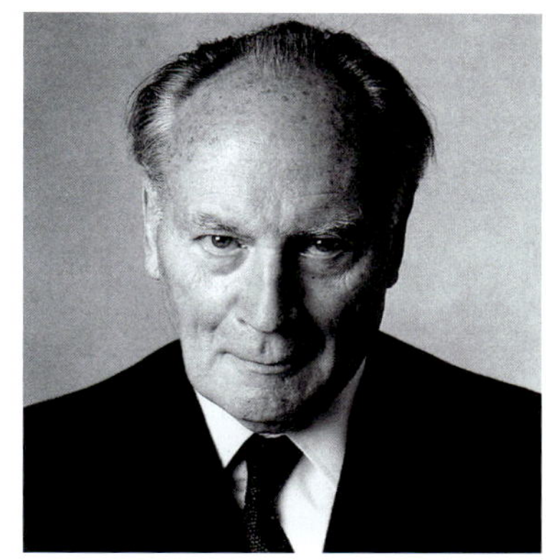

Paul Sacher

The cordial relationship between the BII and Paul Sacher manifested itself in less important issues as well. When Paul Sacher looked for a secretary for his newly created Foundation for Twentieth Century Music (Paul-Sacher-Stiftung), the position was offered to Niels Jerne's secretary, Ingrid Westen, and she successfully held the appointment at the Foundation for many years. In addition, on several occasions, Paul Sacher met members of the institute at the house of his sister, Nelly Frey-Sacher.

Paul Sacher Died at the Age of 93

Paul Sacher's special relationship with the institute, and especially the "short-circuit contacts" caused some irritation at Roche. It was never fully apparent whether the irritation was serious or just a minor annoyance. Then came the news on May 27th, 1999, that Paul Sacher had died, several years after Maja had passed away [QR1999_07]. The Sacher family, the BII, Roche, Basel, and the world of art and science mourned. Both the "short-circuit contacts" and the protection were gone, and it did not take long before Roche saw the BII from a new angle: from the shrewd business point of view.

QR1999_06 BII

QR1999_07 BII

Paul Sacher had lived a long and fulfilled life, but from the self-centered point of view of the BII, his death was "untimely", as will be shown in the chapter for 2000.

Charley Steinberg Died at the Age of 67

QR1999_08 BII

On September 17th, 1999, after a long illness, Charles M. Steinberg died very suddenly. So much has already been written in this book about Charley, a most valued permanent member, that instead of providing further details, an excerpt from the obituary that appeared in the *Basler Zeitung* is reproduced here (the full obituary is given in the QR note [QR1999_08]):

"Charles M. Steinberg, a scientist of world format, who has spent most of his career at the Basel Institute for Immunology, has died at the age of 67 years. Colleagues from America, Canada, Germany, Austria, and France ... came to his funeral. The wall panel of the institute was covered with a flood of e-mails and faxes of condolences.

Who is this man who has caused such a wave of mourning? The beginning of his career was associated with the name Max Delbrück (Nobel Prize 1969). And in Delbrück's lab Niels Jerne (Nobel Prize 1984) had met the young scientist with a brilliant analytical way of thinking. With Delbrück, Charley Steinberg moved to Cologne, shortly thereafter followed by a stopover in Oak Ridge, USA, and then accepted the invitation of Niels Jerne to come to Basel."

Treasure Trove 1999
The database contains documents related to the BII in a broader context (lists, series of photographs, etc.).

QR1999_treasure BII

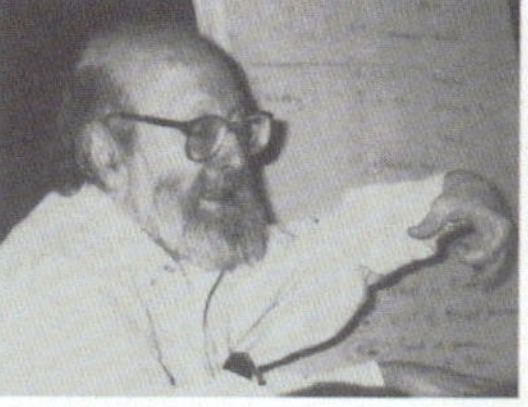

Basler Zeitung Samstag/Sonntag, 25./26. September 1999, Nr. 224 **Teil V** **Das Wissen.** Seite **77**

Trauer um Charles M. Steinberg, den noblen Mentor

Ivan Lefkovits, Gründungsmitglied des Basler Instituts für Immunologie, über einen aussergewöhnlichen Wissenschafter, der während 27 Jahren in Basel tätig war.

Immer hielt er seine Türe im Basler Institut für Immunologie offen, allen war er Gesprächspartner: Charles M. Steinberg liebte die Diskussion.

Foto zVg

Charles M. Steinberg, ein Wissenschafter von Weltformat, der den grössten Teil seiner Kariere am Basler Institut für Immunologie verbracht hat, ist – wie kurz gemeldet – letzte Woche im Alter von 67 Jahren gestorben. Kollegen aus Amerika, Kanada und Europa kamen an seine Beerdigung. Die Wandtafel des Instituts an der Grenzacherstrasse ist mit einer Flut von E-Mails und Fax-Briefen der Trauerbekundungen überdeckt. Wer ist dieser Mann, der solch eine Welle des Trauerns ausgelöst hat?

Der Anfang seiner Karriere war mit dem Namen Max Delbrück (Nobelpreis 1969) verbunden. Und bei Delbrück hat Niels Jerne (Nobelpreis 1984) den jungen Wissenschafter mit brillantem analytischen Denken kennengelernt. Mit Delbrück ging Charley Steinberg nach Köln, kurz danach folgte eine Zwischenstation in Oak Ridge (USA), und danach kam das … Angebot von Niels Jerne … nach Basel zu kommen …

Für Charley … Familie ist … sis …

… darauf erpicht, sich in die Gesellschaft zu integrieren, aber er hat auch niemandem zugemutet, seinen Lebensstil zu übernehmen. Am Anfang war er hinsichtlich des Verhältnisses zwischen der Geldgeberin Roche und dem Institut skeptisch; bald hat er aber erkannt, dass die gegenseitige Loyalität auf einem viel solideren Fundament steht als die üblichen oberflächlichen Bindungen in den USA. Sein Vertrauen zu der Spitze der Roche und sein Misstrauen dem mittleren Kader gegenüber blieb bis zu seinem Lebensende bestehen.

Charley Steinberg kam am 1. Oktober 1970 ans Institut, am Tag, als ich das Institut – dessen Planung und Aufbau ich führte – an eine professionelle Struktur übergeben habe. Die horizontale Struktur des Instituts mit zehn permanenten Mitgliedern liess keine (und sollte auch nicht) Führungsstruktur erkennen. Es war von vornherein für alle …wählten klar, dass jeder macht, …ich berufen fühlt. Obwohl … es sich herauskristall…

… ley Steinberg war. Bald kam ans Institut aus dem Labor von Renato Dulbecco (Nobelpreis 1975) ein junger Postdoc namens Susumu Tonegawa.

Zu jener Zeit war in der Welt der Immunologie das wichtigste offene Thema die Entstehung der Antikörpervielfalt. Ist der genetische Plan für alle Antikörperspezifitäten in der Keimbahn der Zellen genaustens festgelegt, oder beschränkt sich die Information auf einige «Mastergene», aus welchen sich die Gene für einzelne Antikörperspezifitäten während der Entwicklung des Organismus (somatisch) herausbilden?

Die Idee der klonalen Selektion (postuliert von Sir MacFarlane Burnet, Nobelpreis 1960, gestützt auf die Jernesche Selektionstheorie aus dem Jahre 1955) hatte sich bereits durchgesetzt, aber eine experimentell untermauerte Theorie der Antikörperdiversität fehlte noch. Jernes Hypothese bestand darin, dass von Generation zu Generation nur ein paar wenige Antikörper-Gene vererbt werden, deren Spezifität sich gegen sogenannte Alloantigene (spezies-spezifische Antigene, die sich an den Zellenoberflächen der anderen Organismen befinden) richten, und die sich dann somatisch durch Mutationen so verändern werden, dass gesamthaft (für alle beteiligten Zellen) ein Repertoire der Antikörper entsteht, welches alle Spezifitäten – auch die, die momentan nicht benötigt werden – umfasst.

Jerne hatte eine Theorie, Charley Steinberg eine experimentelle Strategie und Tonegawa eine erstklassige Forscherausbildung, um die herausragende Frage, «Gibt es in der Keimbahn ein paar wenige Ant… genannte V… …

DNA per Hybridisierung zu testen. Susumu Tonegawa hat mit enormem Einsatz alle Steinbergschen Ideen in hervorragende Experimente umgesetzt. Gereinigte mRNA wurde vorbereitet, sogenannte «Cot Kurven», deren Form und Verlauf die Anzahl der DNA-Bindungsstellen markierten, erstellt. Tonegawa arbeitete unermüdlich, während Steinberg mit wachsamen Augen jeden experimentellen Schritt verfolgte: Zu der damaligen Zeit gab es keine kommerziellen Kits, jedes Reagens musste man unter penibler Qualitätskontrolle selbst herstellen. Tonegawa konnte mit Hilfe von Charley Steinberg jede Klippe umfahren, aus jeder Sackgasse ohne wesentlichen Zeitverlust herauskommen. An den ersten Veröffentlichungen waren Steinberg und Tonegawa Koautoren. Und 1976 kam der grosse Tag. Steinberg hatte die Bühne des Cold-Spring-Harbor-Symposiums für Tonegawa vorbereitet, um die Ergebnisse zu präsentieren. Die experimentellen Ergebnisse und die daraus resultierenden Erkenntnisse haben zwar Jernes Hypothese bestätigt, dass die Antikörper-Spezifität somatisch entsteht. Aber diese Vielfalt wird in erster Linie durch Zusammensetzung von Gen-Segmenten erreicht. Die Mutationen stellen nur eine willkommene Repertoire-Erweiterung dar.

Nach Cold Spring Harbor stand Tonegawa auf eigenen Füssen. Und Charley Steinberg hat die Zügel vornehm losgelassen und sein Lieblingsthema dem jungen, fähigen, ehrgeizigen Tonegawa überlassen. Tonegawa hat noch viele erstklassige Mitarbeiter an sich gebunden. Stellvertretend für … Traunecker, …

Schreibende ist der Ansicht, dass der Nobelpreis Tonegawas hätte hälftig an Steinberg (und vielleicht auch andere) gehen sollen. An einem kleinen Symposium in Prag für den 65. Geburtstag von Charley (das Wort Pensionierung hat Charley Steinberg nie gemocht) war Tonegawa als berühmter Gast dabei.

Im Büro von Charley Steinberg herrschte immer eine kreative Unordnung. Einige Dokumente vergilbten schon, andere waren ständig in Gebrauch. Die Fenster seines Büros durften von innen nicht gereinigt werden. Die Putzequipe könnte sonst die kreative Unordnung auf seinem Schreibtisch verändern, und das durfte keiner.

In den 27 Jahren seiner Tätigkeit und tagtäglicher Präsenz im Institut hat Charley Steinberg die Türe seines Büros nie zugemacht. Er war immer «available», stand immer allen zur Verfügung, ob am Abend oder an Wochenenden. Einfache Themen, komplexe Überlegungen, alles war ihm ein Gespräch wert. Ob Wissenschaft oder Politik, Kultur oder Geschichte, alles wurde immer wieder neu diskutiert.

Charley Steinbergs Wirken kann man schwer in Worte fassen. Seine Überlegungen basierten nicht auf dogmatischen «Fertigmenus»; in jeder Diskussion hat er den Weg aus «first principles» neu entworfen. Dadurch wurde jedes Gespräch ein wertvolles Original, nie eine Kopie, nie ein abgestandenes Getränk von gestern. Nach seinem 65. Geburtstag wurde er mit Angeboten für Zusammenarbeit überhäuft. Er hat von all den Angeboten eine kleine Kostprobe gemacht, aber dann kam leider … gesundheitliche Einbruch. … Le…

The Year 2000

Jean Pieters became the last permanent member of the BII. Roche decided to close down the institute with effect of 2001. Roche intended that the institute would be restructured into a "Roche Center of Medical Genomics". This attempt was abandoned, and what survived was integrated into the Roche Research Group on Genetics.

Perspectives and New Careers 1996–2000

This section is a continuation of the list of scientists leaving the BII [QR2000_01]. The previous part concerned members leaving the BII in the period of 1992–1995. The list below is not complete.

1996

Ludovica Bruno, to the UK

She accepted a research position at the Imperial Cancer Research Fund, London, UK. Her work concentrated on the development of immature thymocytes and the involvement of pre-TCR in various developmental processes, including rescuing cells from programmed cell death, allelic exclusion and αβ versus γδ T cell lineage commitment. Her research at the ICRF demonstrated that the surface expression of the pre-TCR is a tool of choice to reveal new stages of T cell development and to define steps of αβ T cell lineage commitment. Ludovica rejoined the BII for a few months in 1999.

José A. Garcia-Sanz, to Spain

After several years at the BII, José obtained a tenured scientific position at the Biological Research Centre of the Spanish National Research Council, Madrid. He pursued his long-standing interest in the biology of adult stem cells and developed several models (mammary gland stem cells, neural stem cells and mesenchymal stem cells) for analyses of self-renewal/differentiation and their relation with "cancer stem cells".

Paolo Ghia, to the USA

He left the BII for the Harvard Medical School, Boston, Mass., to take up the position of research associate, but after a few years he returned to his home country, Italy, first to the University of Turin,

There were no new arrivals in 2000

Leavers 2000 (14)
Alexandre Akhmedov, Jürgen Bachl, Michael Carroll, Jes Dietrich, Ulf Grawunder, Giandomenica Iezzi, Rolf Jessberger, Toru Miyazaki, Hideo Nakajima, Ekaterina Revenkova, Christiane Ruedl, Mariolina Salio, Emmanuel Scotet, Alan Young.

QR2000_01 BII

then to the San Raffaele Scientific Institute in Milan. As head of the Unit of B Cell Neoplasia, he focused on understanding the molecular mechanisms responsible for the onset and the progression of the neoplastic disorders originating from B lymphocytes (leukemias and lymphomas). Paolo's work led to a better understanding of the pathogenesis of these diseases and to the identification of molecules and pathways that can be exploited for diagnostic, prognostic and therapeutic purposes.

Beat Imhof, Remained in Switzerland

After some 8 years at the BII, Beat obtained the position of professor for Experimental Pathology at the Medical Faculty of the University of Geneva. There he continued to study the migration of pro-T cells to the thymus. This led to the investigation of the pathology of leukocyte migration in inflammatory diseases and tumor angiogenesis. Beat was also president of the Swiss Society for Allergology and Immunology, and he serves, or has served, as an editor or a board member of several journals.

Gek-Kee Sim, to the USA

She accepted a position at the medical research facility of the National Jewish Health Center, Denver, Colorado. At the new environment she addressed herself to the unsolved issue of the contribution of somatic mutations to T helper cell diversity. She has established, using TCR mutants, the relationship between gene structure and receptor reactivities. Gek-Kee postulated that TCR mutants – under certain special conditions – become viral receptors, which would play a crucial role in the pathology of lymphoid tumors.

Olli Vainio, to Finland

After returning to Turku, Olli came back to the BII for several 2-year terms. His publication record of about 60 papers with BII affiliation spans the years 1989–1996. After several years in Turku, he became professor of Microbiology at the University of Oulu, Finland.

Thomas Winkler, to Germany

Thomas became professor of Genetics at the Friedrich-Alexander-Universität Erlangen-Nürnberg. His research focused on the selection processes at different stages of the development of B lymphocytes. His research group investigated the genetic mechanisms for the early development of B lymphocytes, the mechanisms for the loss of self-tolerance in the autoimmune disease systemic lupus erythematosus, as well as in the antibody-mediated protection against cytomegalovirus.

1997

Thomas Bäckström, to Sweden

After several years at the BII, Thomas returned to Sweden, where he made a career in various biotech companies. He did so both at established companies (Novo Nordisk) as well as in companies which he co-founded (BTB Pharma). He utilized his experience in immunology (especially in in vitro assays and in vivo mouse models) towards drug discovery in the field of inflammation. He gained vast experience with regulatory affairs in academia and industry. In BTB Pharma, Thomas developed effective and specific medicines against autoimmune diseases, such as multiple sclerosis, rheumatoid arthritis and type 1 diabetes. He also held a position at the Medeon Science Park, Malmö.

Peter Lane, to the UK

After 6 years at the BII, Peter took up the position of professor of Clinical Immunology at the MRC Centre for Immune Regulation at the University of Birmingham. His research focused on cellular and molecular mechanisms that control the development of CD4 effector and memory T cells. The focus of his research group in Birmingham was on the molecular and cellular basis of CD4 T cell responses, since CD4 T cells play a pivotal role regulating both protective and pathogenic immune responses. All his projects utilized integrated approaches of studying tolerance and immunity within the same system (generation of tolerance in the thymus vs. protective CD4 responses at the periphery).

Isabelle Chrétien, Remained in Switzerland

After leaving the BII – and after 12 years working in basic research – Isabelle decided to do something else. She chose to combine artwork and science by providing illustrations for science books, reports, publications, power point presentations, websites, posters, flyers and brochures, and for publicity. Her work in non-scientific and scientific areas of medicine, the pharmaceutical and chemical industries, and biotechnology appears in various publications and communications.

Pierre Cosson, Remained in Switzerland
He received an offer from the Department of Cell Physiology and Metabolism of the University of Geneva, where he continued his area of research, i.e. phagocytosis, endocytosis and intracellular killing. The experimental model of the ameba *Dictyostelium discoideum* served to isolate and characterize a number of gene products implicated at various stages in phagocytosis. The same system was also used to study how bacteria are killed following phagocytosis, based on the analysis of *Dictyostelium* mutants defective for intracellular killing. Pierre was promoted to the position of full professor.

Ramona Leibnitz, to the USA
She left Basel for the University of Maryland, College Park, and after about 2 years she co-founded (with John Armstrong) Lead Horse Technologies, which has its headquarters in Junction City, Kansas, and has executive teams in Florida and Texas. The main focus of Ramona's work was on drug reactions and medical communications, as well as providing medical information to science and health care professionals, and also to the patient community. She has been on the executive teams of two other medical information companies besides Lead Horse Technologies. Ramona is also a co-founder of the e-magazine *Popular Immunology*.

Salvatore Valitutti, to France
He left Basel for the University of Toulouse. As in the BII, his interests centered on T lymphocyte activation by antigenic determinants displayed on antigen-presenting cell surface. Salvatore has contributed to defining the structure, dynamics and function of immunological synapses, formed by both helper and cytotoxic T cells. In Toulouse, he developed a multidisciplinary research program in which biologists, in collaboration with clinicians, physicists and mathematicians, investigate different aspects of the intercellular communication occurring at immunological synapses in health and disease.

1998

Luca Bolliger, Remained in Basel
Luca decided to pursue an applied research career and joined Hoffmann-La Roche as a global discovery portfolio manager in the Pharma Strategy Unit. He then continued his career in the financial industry as a fundamental analyst at BT&T asset management, and as a freelance consultant. He established Biopolo Ticino, where

he also contributed to creating the Swiss marketing platforms Swiss Biotech and Swiss Medtech, before becoming director of Business Development at Actelion.

Jean-Marie Buerstedde, to Germany

Although he had an excellent reputation as a scientist and colleague at the BII, Jean-Marie ran into difficulties in the German Research Centre for Environmental Health in Munich. He was dismissed, but the court stated that they were unable to find any wrongdoings. He was reinstated to his position, but to gain distance from the difficult situation, Jean-Marie moved to the National Centre for Biomedical Engineering Science – National University of Ireland Galway, as a visiting scientist. His main research interest remained unchanged: protecting the genome: mechanisms targeting somatic hypermutation.

Wayne Hein, to New Zealand

During his full 13 years at the BII he conducted basic research into the immune system of ruminants. Following a move to New Zealand, his research interests centered on basic and applied immunoparasitology. He became director of the Hopkirk Research Institute, located at Massey University, where his research focused on parasitic and infectious diseases of livestock. He was promoted to professor and head of the School of Veterinary and Biomedical Sciences at James Cook University, Centre for Biosecurity of Tropical Infectious Diseases in Australia. In February 2015, he was appointed dean of Roseworthy Campus at the University of Adelaide. During a productive phase of research at the BII, his group cloned and sequenced all genes encoding the T cell receptors of sheep and mapped their sequential expression in different tissues during fetal and post-natal development.

1999

Martin Bachmann, Remained in Switzerland

After spending 3 years at the BII, he co-founded the Cytos Biotechnology Company in Zurich where he has built up a strong research group of some 40 scientists. Martin excelled both in basic and applied research: with the knowledge he gained from doing animal research, it was one step further to carry out clinical trials. Successful results were obtained for several different indications (smoking cessation, allergy, asthma and hypertension). Under Martin's leadership, major work was accomplished in testing novel vaccines against the influenza virus. Collaborative projects with the NIH, as well as the US Army, were carried out to develop a vaccine against malaria.

Hans Jörg Fehling, to Germany
After 7 years at the BII, Hans Jörg was offered the position of associate professor in Molecular Immunology, Institute of Immunology, University Clinics Ulm. Although his university training was in Tübingen, a considerable part of his research career was with Diane Mathis and Christophe Benoist at the Centre National de la Recherche Scientifique in Strasbourg.

Kristian Hannestad, to Norway
He spent 2 periods at the BII, the first one was from 1993 to 1994, the second from 1998 to 1999. He obtained a position at the University of Tromsø, Department of Immunology, where he became professor of Immunology. His main research interest was in the engagement of the B lymphocyte antigen receptor in inducing presentation of intrinsic immunoglobulin peptides on MHC class II molecules.

Hans-Reimer Rodewald, to Germany
He left the BII after 7 years to work at the University Clinics in Heidelberg. Soon afterwards he accepted a position at the German Cancer Research Centre, Heidelberg, to head the Tumour Immunology Programme. The Division of Cellular Immunology investigates physiological and pathological processes of the development of cells and organs in the immune system, as well as their immunological functions. Hans-Reimer and his group demonstrated that T cells and myeloid cells (e.g. dendritic cells and granulocytes) arise in the thymus from distinct progenitors. Among the priority projects are studies of the transcription factor FoxN1 in thymic epithelial cells and the role of mast cells in the immune system.

2000

Alexandre Akhmedov, to France
He left the BII for the Institut Marie Curie in Paris. At the end of his stay in Basel, he published his work, with Rolf Jessberger, on protein domains specifically binding palindromic DNA sequences.

Ulf Grawunder, Remained in Basel
He left the BII to become a co-founder of 4-Antibody in Basel, a Swiss therapeutic antibody-engineering company, and was later a

founder and the CEO of NBE-Therapeutics, a Swiss biotech company which focuses on the development of "next-generation" antibody-drug conjugates for cancer therapy. Ulf has served on various boards of non-profit and for-profit life science organizations, and he was appointed vice-president and board member of the Swiss Biotech Association. Furthermore, Ulf received the New Entrepreneurs in Technology and Science Award from the Gebert-Rüf-Foundation, Switzerland.

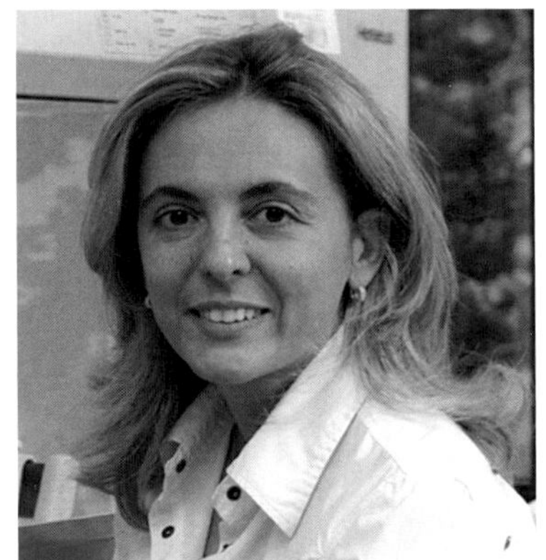
Federica Sallusto

Rolf Jessberger, to the USA
He left the BII to become assistant professor of Gene Therapy and Molecular Medicine at Mount Sinai Medical School, New York. Some years later he joined the Technical University, Dresden, where he was appointed chairman of the Department of Physiological Chemistry. His laboratory focused on three major areas: chromatin dynamics and DNA recombination; understanding the contribution of proteins responsible for structural maintenance of chromosomes to processes in mitosis and meiosis and their contribution to genome integrity, and regulation of B cell and mast cell activation through novel signaling networks.

Mariolina Salio, to the UK
Mariolina left the BII to join the MRC Human Immunology Unit at the Weatherall Institute of Molecular Medicine, University of Oxford. Her interest remained with the regulatory role of invariant natural killer T cells in tumor immunity, and also she worked on MR1-restricted mucosal-associated invariant T cells and their activation during infectious diseases. Her work of clinical relevance included cross-responsive CD1a-reactive T cells in bee and wasp venom-allergic individuals.

Federica Sallusto, Remained in Switzerland
She left the BII, together with Antonio Lanzavecchia, to become a founding member of the Institute for Research in Biomedicine in Bellinzona. Her studies in the human system revealed a differential expression of chemokine receptors in Th1 and Th2 cells and led to the characterization of "central memory" and "effector memory" subsets with distinct migratory capacity and effector function. Federica discovered Th22 cells and characterized two distinct types of pathogen-specific Th17 cells. For her scientific achievements, she received the Pharmacia Allergy Research Foundation Award in 1999 and the Science Award from the Foundation for Studies of Neurodegenerative Diseases a year later. Besides her

I was fortunate to be at the institute when the Nobel laureates Jerne, Tonegawa and Köhler were all on the staff, and I never felt – not even for a moment – that there could ever be a place where more brilliance was packed into one building.

Don Bellgrau

position at the IRB, Federica is also adjunct professor of Immunology at the University of Palermo, Italy.

Alan Young, to the USA

Alan left the BII to join the Surgical Research Laboratory of Harvard Medical School, Boston, focusing his research on lymphatic physiology, tissue regeneration and angiogenesis. The next step in his career was to become professor of Veterinary and Biomedical Science at South Dakota State University, where his main emphasis was on vaccine development for emerging diseases. Alan is also chief scientific officer at Medgene Labs, in Brookings, South Dakota.

Andrei Augustin, to the USA

He left the BII to join the National Jewish Medical and Research Center, Denver. Andrei's research group had a continuing interest in γδ resident pulmonary lymphocytes. The participation of various types of lymphocytes in the development of lung fibrosis is also a main research area of this group. His earlier cooperation with Gek-Kee Sim continued in Denver.

Jean Pieters Becomes the Last Permanent Member, 2000

At the time of Jean Pieters' promotion to permanent membership, the closing down of the BII was not yet on the horizon. When the institute did close down, Jean joined the Biozentrum Basel and became renowned for successfully combining basic research in immunology with clinically relevant problems. His studies on survival of mycobacteria in macrophages received great attention, also by pharmaceutical companies. Below is his research report from the 1999 Annual Report [QR2000_02].

"Analysis of the mechanisms of intracellular survival of mycobacteria in macrophages. Macrophages are important cells in the first-line defense against microbes because of their high capacity for phagocytosis. Usually, material that is phagocytosed by macrophages is rapidly transferred to lysosomes for degradation. However, certain pathogenic microorganisms have evolved the capacity to resist lysosomal delivery, thereby circumventing host defense responses. An example of such pathogens is provided by several Mycobacterium *species that can survive and replicate within macrophage phagosomes. In searching for host factors possibly involved in mycobacterial survival, we have identified a protein that remains associated with phagosomes containing living, but not dead mycobacteria. This protein is a member of the WD repeat protein family and has been*

QR2000_02 BII

named TACO, for tryptophan aspartate-containing coat protein. TACO is recruited around the nascent phagosomes, but is normally released prior to fusion with or maturation into lysosomes."

The fate of the institute was sealed, whether one called it "closing down" or "reorientation".

One Year and Eight Days after Paul Sacher's Death

During the first decade of the BII's existence (in the 1970s) it was an accepted fact that the opinion leaders in Roche stood firmly behind the institute. In particular, Dr. Adolf Jann (president of Roche) and Prof. Alfred Pletscher (director general of Roche Research) formed the backbone of unconditional support.

Over the years, the world changed dramatically, both politically and economically, and it is beyond this book's scope to review the timeline of world events leading up to the BII's final chapter.

One year and 8 days after Paul Sacher's death (see 1999 chapter) the employees of the institute were summoned to attend a meeting to listen to an important announcement issued by Roche. The meeting occurred on June 5th, 2000. Documents related to the event are available in the QR code [QR2000_03]. Briefly, the president and 2 other members of Roche management (their names and functions are also given in the QR code) announced the closing down of the BII.

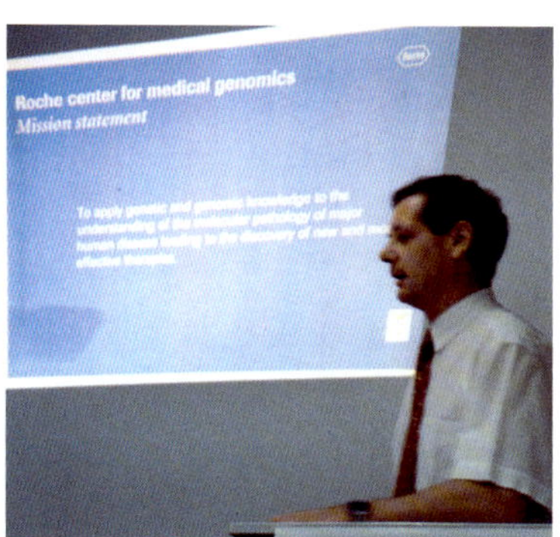

Jonathan Knowles, Roche, announcing the closure of the BII to its employees

The presentation was such that neither the words "closing down", nor "termination" nor any other synonym were used. Instead, expressions such as "reorientation", "transformation" or "reorganization" were employed, and the message was intended to communicate that the institute was to be reoriented towards new research activities of great interest to the field of medicine in general and to Roche's research activities in particular. The new name, "Roche Center of Medical Genomics" (RCMG), had been chosen, and the name itself was meant to indicate the future goals and activities – there was no mention of immunology.

Roche Made a Decision

The phrase of the day was, "Roche made a decision…", while the truth was that "a few people at Roche made a decision…". The fate of the institute was sealed, whether one called it "closing down" or "reorientation" [QR2000_04]. In fact, the decision might just have been based on the dissatisfaction of a certain group of people at Roche with some aspects of "running and controlling" the institute. It is not surprising that the decision was not welcomed by the employees and members of the BII, and that at least for a while it

QR2000_03 BII

QR2000_04 BII

gave nourishment to various "conspiracy theories". This line of thought is not followed up in the main text of the book, but it is amply discussed in a later section called "Echo of Time".

Collection of Letters and E-Mails from the World Scientific Community

The community of immunologists increased in 30 years by at least an order of magnitude. Corridor talks at the First International Congress of Immunology, 1971, in Washington were on the creation of the fairy-tale institute. Within hours everybody knew that the BII was closed down. Some of the letters, facsimiles and e-mails are stored in the database – a link is provided by the QR code [QR2000_05].

Reaction of the BII Employees

The announcement at the meeting (June 5th, 2000) achieved what it had meant to accomplish, i.e. informing the employees that the institute in its original form ceased to exist. This kind of understanding was clear in general terms, while it dawned on the staff that the consequences of closing the institute would be different for them all, in particular for scientists with short contracts and permanent members. The institute was famous for its horizontal structure, but this was true for the "organism" as a whole, but not for the disassembled components. It was clear that the decision was irrevocable; nevertheless, the impression prevailed – and it turned out to hold true – that the process of decommissioning would be an orderly one.

Unfortunately the management of Roche in 2000 was not aware of various arrangements made between the 1970 Roche management and the scientific community in Basel and in Switzerland at that time. When the Biozentrum of the University was established in 1971, it was agreed with Kellenberger, Jerne and Pletscher that a chair of Immunology would not be needed as the BII covered immunology adequately, and institute members would be prepared to take on teaching responsibilities at the university alongside their research work.

QR2000_05 BII

The existence of a fine network of scientific and social interactions was largely neglected and disregarded, and Basel citizens were informed only through a short press release. Neither the International Advisory Board nor any other body had been informed by Roche, only the "internal" Scientific Council was put in the picture in advance. Within minutes after the Roche announcement the hot news spread through the entire scientific community by phone calls placed by BII members to their peers. Needless to say, the numerous long-distance calls “to the world” differed on both major and minor issues, especially when trying to answer the question “why?”. This gave nourishment to various explanations, often unsubstantiated.

Ample time was allowed to complete research projects and to find new positions for all members of staff.

Emergency Meeting of the International Advisory Board

An emergency meeting of the Advisory Board was called at which various issues were aired [QR2000_06]. There was no attempt made to push the management of Roche into revoking its decision, but the Roche president and director of Research listened attentively to Advisory Board proposals and made various promises, which were later generously implemented. Among others, Roche agreed to establish and fund a chair of Immunology at the University of Basel and soon started a search procedure for finding a candidate. There will be mention of this below.

The process of termination was done in a quiet and civilized manner. In the BII it was no exception to the rule that a “former” director has negligible influence on the events unfolding. Thus, Fritz Melchers was not involved in any steps in the decommissioning of the institute. Ample time was allowed to complete research projects and to find new positions for all members of staff. Several technicians and scientists continued to work at the “renamed” institute, now having the acronym RCMG, and some transferred to Roche. There was genuine satisfaction with the procedure; to reiterate, the damage was done to the institute, not to individual people; for many it was just a beginning of something new – after all, jobs were available everywhere. The moral damage was deeply hidden in the hearts of individuals.

A special task force [QR2000_07] was established at Roche to settle all relevant issues regarding contractual obligations and severance payments for the scientific staff and employees. For Roche it was simple to accomplish this as only 10 scientists possessed permanent contracts. Many scientists received a severance package, and in most instances they immediately found new positions. Several members fell under the early retirement scheme, while a few members happened to reach regular retirement age and were entitled to draw their pension (without severance payment). For each year spent at the institute, non-scientists received an extra month’s salary (12 years equalled an additional year’s salary). In

QR2000_06 BII

QR2000_07 BII

By chance and not by design, it happened that there was a commercial by-product of unprecedented value.

many instances individual solutions were worked out. Financial compensation did depend on the residual time of the contracts, and on the number of years spent at the institute.

Although the duties of the director were terminated immediately, a program was installed allowing for an orderly conclusion of research projects. The period of a year was given to scientists in which to search for new positions and establish themselves there.

Fortune Favors the Prepared Mind

In the first part of this history, there was a detailed description of the Project of Applied Immunology. Theo Staehelin played an essential role as head of the project, and he witnessed both the period of enthusiastic support (when Prof. Pletscher stood behind it) and also the abrupt withdrawing from it at a later stage (under the responsibility of Prof. Hürlimann). Theo Staehelin was in the audience at the June 5th meeting in the BII, and he recalls that he could not believe his ears when Dr. Jonathan Knowles said that the institute had not contributed "a single iota" to the success of Roche. Knowles acknowledged the importance of the BII in performing basic research, but the total costs during the 30 years of its existence were about one billion Swiss francs, and Roche had received nothing in return. Contrary to this, Theo Staehelin calculated that by the year 2000, Roche had made at least one billion dollars profit from the BII "off-shoot" (in Diagnostics) and there were great prospects for the future.

The institute – in its charter – was not geared towards commercial success. It was established to advance knowledge for the benefit of mankind and to allow Roche a priority look at all the results obtained. By chance and not by design, it happened that there was a commercial by-product of unprecedented value [QR2000_08]. Roche benefitted not just from Georges Köhler's discovery of hybridoma technology and his Nobel Prize, but also to a large extent because Niels Jerne and his staff recognized the potential of the new discovery and helped to promote it. Jerne and Pletscher took action immediately and the "Project of Applied Immunology" was started at Roche and became very successful. Fortune favors the prepared mind.

QR2000_08 BII

Knowledge Gap at Roche

As long as Prof. Pletscher was at Roche, the project was successful because of him; later under a new constellation (Prof. Hürlimann and others) it remained successful despite the lack of interest. At the time of closing the institute, there was no "knowledge gap" between the institute and Roche research. It took about 3 or 4 years till complaints surfaced (from Roche bench workers) that there was nobody there to help with problems related to the engineering of new monoclonal antibody entities. Although the monoclonal antibody project in all its application facets (diagnostics and drug development) was from the very first day localized at Roche premises, the source of new knowledge (on monoclonal antibody and on anything else) was freely available from the BII as long as it existed, and this disappeared once the BII was gone.

Roche Center of Medical Genomics

In front of the institute, the original inscription "Basel Institute for Immunology" was still there, but next to it the new name with an independent logo, "Roche Center of Medical Genomics", appeared [QR2000_09]. Inside the building most laboratories continued functioning as if nothing had happened. Members kept receiving memos from the Roche management explaining that the search for the position of director of the reoriented institute (RCMG) had been launched successfully.

At the mother company, there was a research department of Medical Genetics headed by Prof. Klaus Lindpaintner. Roche decided that the director of Medical Genetics should function as interim director of the new RCMG until a definite director was found. RCMG started to function according to this plan, but soon the news went out that despite serious efforts to find a suitable director for RCMG, the search had not been successful. Therefore a decision was made to fuse the "Genetics Department" with the "Genomics Center" and to appoint Prof. Lindpaintner as its director. It was stated that the resulting entity would continue to carry the name RCMG, but the entire operation would be transferred to Roche premises, and the BII building was to be sold (no documents are available on this issue). The enigma of this is perhaps explained by the classical Erivan joke about the stolen bicycle (given in the above mentioned QR 2000_09).

Roche's Image Was Not Affected

It was mentioned in Book 1 that when the institute had existed for about 5 years, Jerne visited Jann to explain that the 10-year guarantee (sealed by handshake) was gradually being used up, as only

QR2000_09 BII

5 years were left. Jerne came up with a proposal for an arrangement of a "rolling 5 years". This meant that if Roche said "enough" of the BII, 5 years would be left for winding down the research projects. To Jerne's surprise, president Jann said that this was not necessary, as the institute had shown its quality, usefulness and impact – enough to convince Roche that the institute should continue indefinitely without any time restrictions. By the year 2000 those arrangements were immaterial as neither Jerne nor Jann was alive.

Around the time the BII closed – but also before then – many institutions around the world were being shut down. Thus, the BII became one of many. Curtains went down on numerous research institutes financed by pharmaceutical companies, such as Sandoz, Schering-Plough and Mérieux. This was the case in Europe and in the USA, and to a lesser extent also in Japan. An institute in Lyon was reoriented and renamed "The Institute of Functional Genomics, Lyon, France". Thus, for the uninformed majority, closing down a research unit within a pharmaceutical industry was a "non-event". The image of Roche in the non-academic world did not suffer, but scientists were warned.

New Way(s) to Support Research

To what extent the closing of research facilities was based on shrewd financial calculations is documented nowhere, although it was obvious that the affluent era was over. The pharmaceutical industry continued to recruit research workers from universities (for applied research and clinical development departments), and the fact that increasing numbers of scientists found jobs in the industry caused "contact reluctance" (Berührungsängste) between industry and university to melt away gradually. An industry logo – whether a Roche hexagon or a Bayer cross – was no longer a deterrence.

As mentioned in Book 1, at the initial discussions between Jerne and Jann, Jerne stated that the originally proposed name, "Roche Institute for Immunology", was not to his liking, since he feared the name Roche in the title would put off scientists he wanted to attract. This attitude of the late sixties gradually disappeared. The pharmaceutical industry itself became increasingly scientific, and this steady change resulted in collaborations with university research units. Direct interactions – and placement of projects at universities – were obviously more economical than running an institute. Support of research units at universities, fellowships, professorships and, last but not least, acquisitions of entire institutes and companies became commonplace – at least in the upper league of pharmaceutical champions.

After the Phone Calls, Business as Usual

When the critical meeting held in the large seminar room ended, a surprisingly calm atmosphere developed. After much discussion in the cafeteria and numerous lengthy phone calls, lab work continued almost the same as on any other day. Bea Pfeiffer, the institute photographer, realizing the historic importance of the day, went from lab to lab to catch the mood. The photographs are shown below [QR2000_10].

The research resumed and in most instances continued at a normal pace, at least for a while. There are many interesting anecdotes related to the closing of the BII, but they are hidden away in private collections of various members.

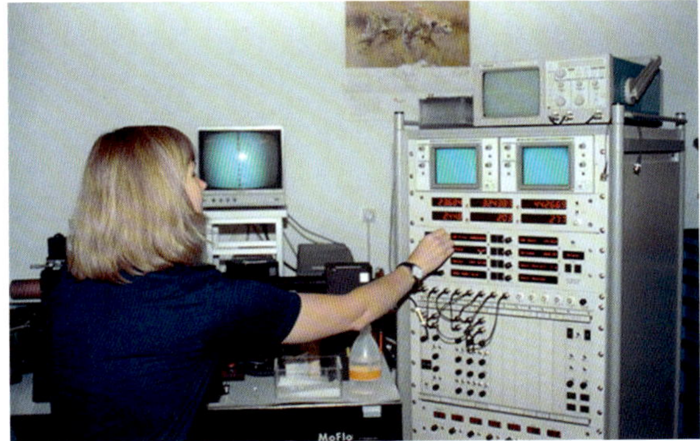

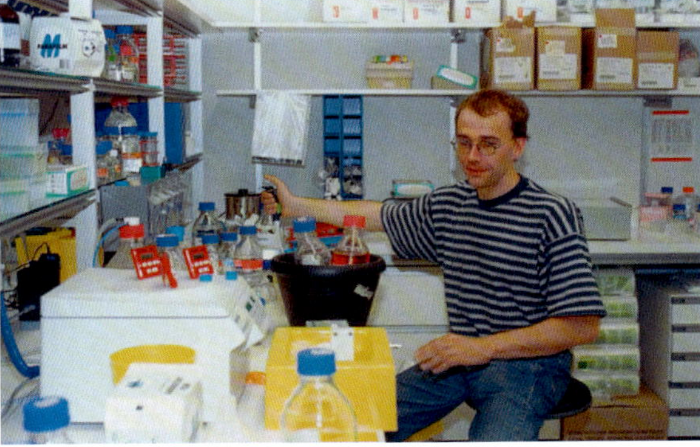

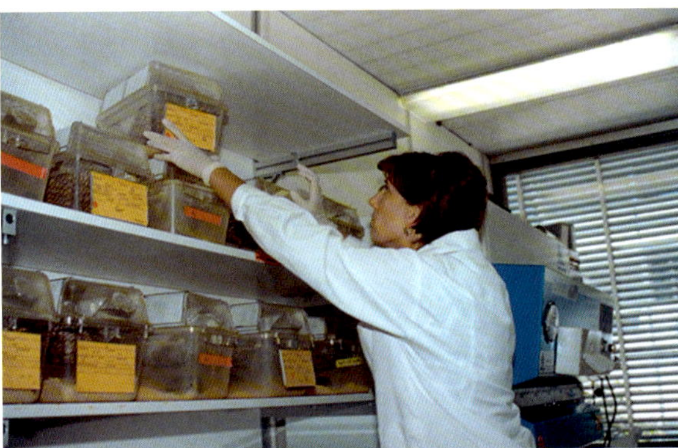

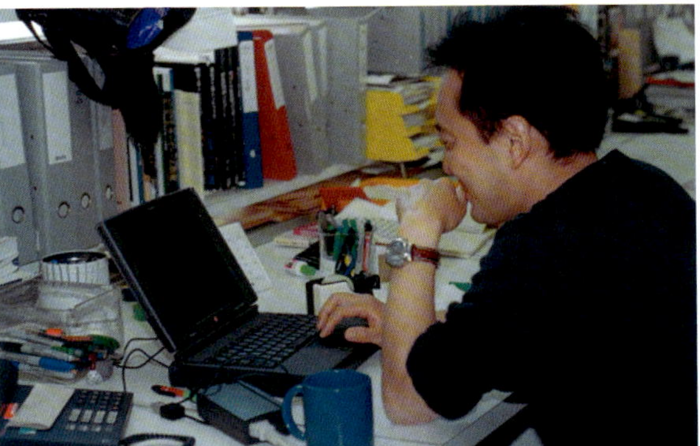

On June 5th, 2000, after Roche had announced it was closing down the BII, work continued as usual in the labs

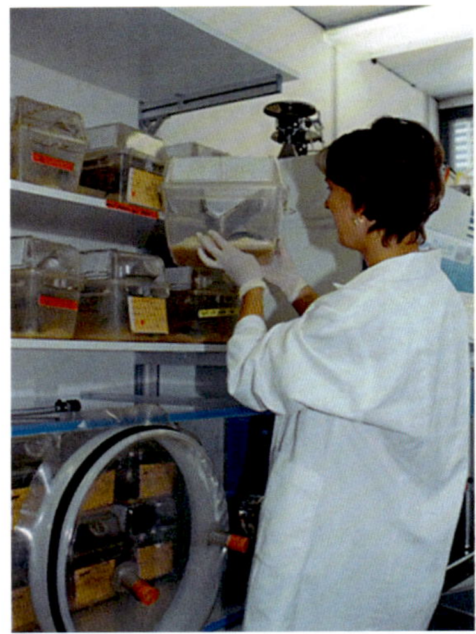
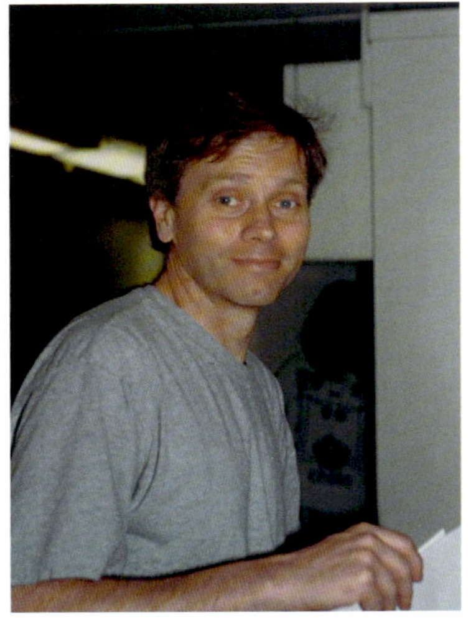
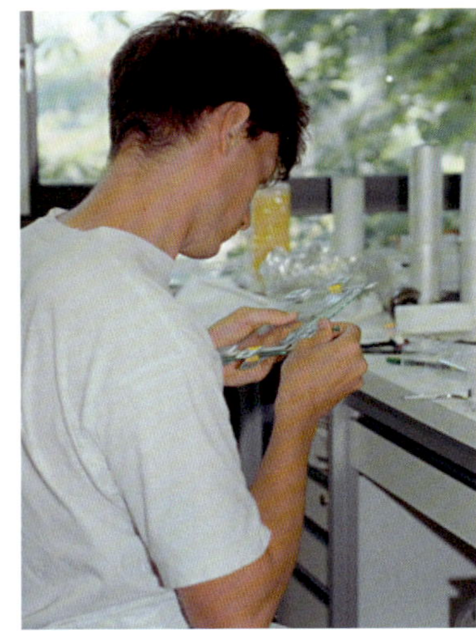
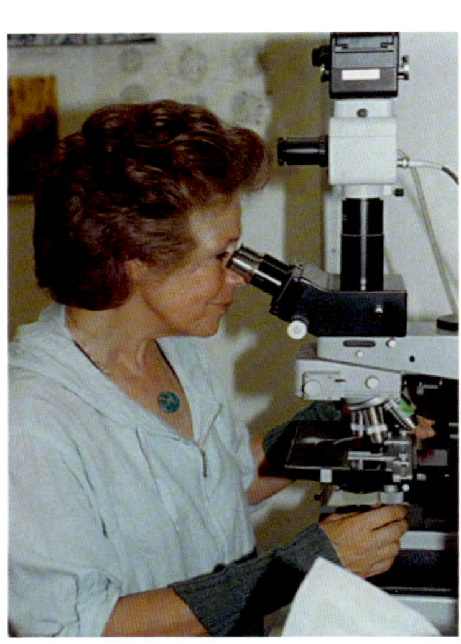
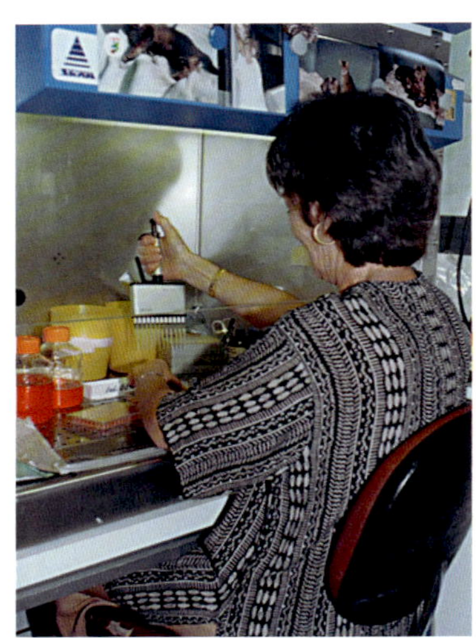
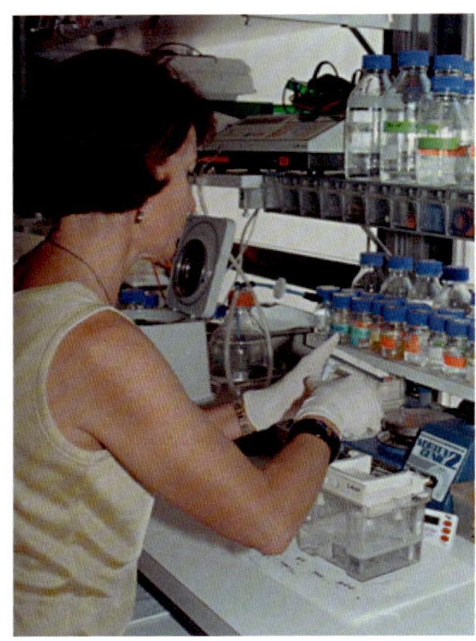
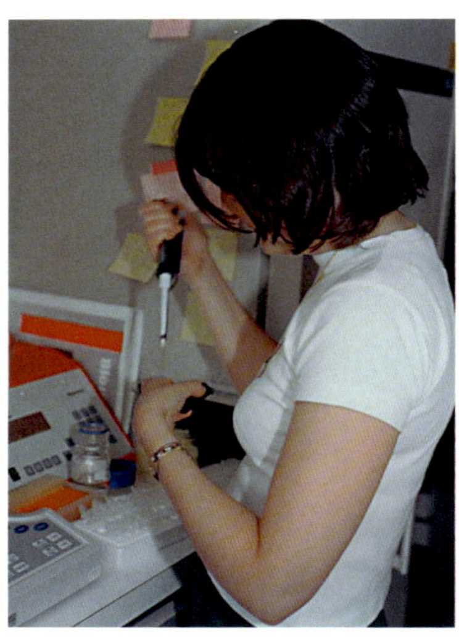
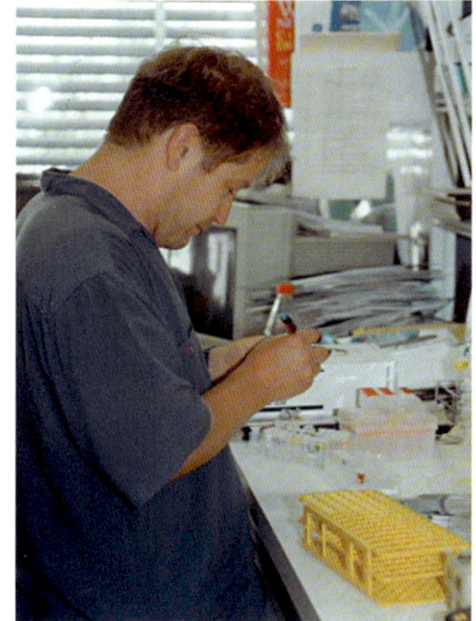
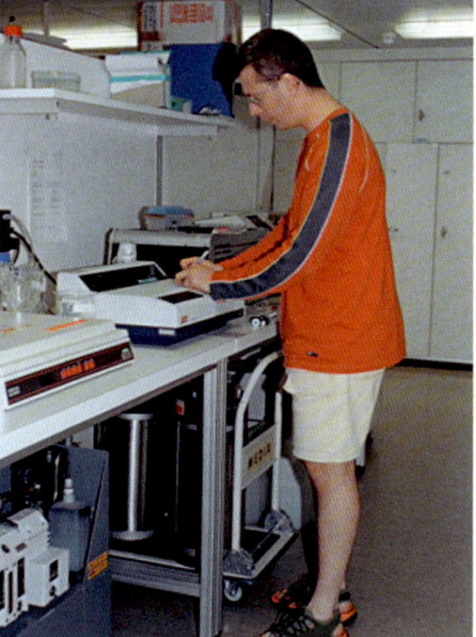

Yin and Yang One Day Later, June 6th

An episode that occurred a day after the "announcement" characterizes the ambivalence of relationships: caring ones amidst rough reality. A member of the workshop – close to his regular retirement age – had for some time been considering taking early retirement. Though it would diminish his pension somewhat, that's what he wanted to do. Some weeks earlier, he had an appointment with the Roche Personnel Department to negotiate conditions. He was very surprised to be discouraged from leaving the BII at that time; nevertheless, he insisted and handed in his notice to retire at the end of May 2000.

Therefore, he was "out" when the announcement to close down the institute was made, and he immediately realized that he had made a grave mistake, for as an employee he would have been offered a package as were other employees close to retirement age. Hesitatingly he asked for a date at the Personnel Department and to his astonishment the head of the office pulled out his letter of resignation, handed it back with the words, "I did not accept your notice, you are still on the regular payroll and you will receive 'the package' as any other employee does".

Treasure Trove 2000

The database contains documents related to the BII in a broader context (lists, series of photographs, etc.).

QR2000_treasure BII

The Final Year 2001

A joint symposium for Fritz Melchers and Roland Gisler on the occasion of their retirement was arranged. Jon Sprent gave the last BII seminar on 20th November. The laboratories were closed down one by one, and during the month of December the last members moved their laboratories to their new destinations. Most of the members received financial support. Several early retirements ensued. Nobody became unemployed. The famous Double Helix that had guarded the entrance to the institute for 30 years was decommissioned and transferred to the Tinguely Museum.

Scientists Leaving (32)
Fabien Agenès, Jan Andersson, Marina Cella, Marco Colonna, Sylvie Degermann, Louis Du Pasquier, Dominic van Essen, Rachel Ettinger, Susan Gilfillan, Roland Gisler, Ursula Günthert, John Hansen, Thomas Harder, Cristina Hernandez-Munain, Reinhard Hoffmann, Heinz Jacobs, Klaus Karjalainen, Jörg Kirberg, Pawel Kisielow, Manfred Kopf, Ivan Lefkovits, Fraser McBlane, Fritz Melchers, Ed Palmer, Jean Pieters, Alexandre Potocnik, Antonius Rolink, Bénédicte Sammut, Takeyuki Shimizu, Raul Torres, Pasquale Vito, Guy Werlen.

Manfred Kopf

Manfred Kopf [QR2001_01] had received his PhD at the Max Planck Institute for Immunobiology, Freiburg, Germany, in the group of the Nobel laureate Georges Köhler. Subsequently he became a member of the BII, where he researched for 7 years until it closed in 2001. Then he became a full professor of Molecular Biomedicine at the Swiss Federal Institute for Technology (ETH), Zurich, where he and his group study the underlying mechanisms of inflammatory and infectious diseases.

Ed Palmer from Basel to Basel

Ed preferred to remain in Basel, and with the help of Jürg Schifferli, Jürg Steiger and Klaus Gyr (all three were professors at the University of Basel) arrangements were made with the University Hospital in Basel. Ed was granted a well-supported professorship of Experimental Transplantation Immunology within the Medical Faculty. After Fasnacht (carnival) in February 2002, the lab became fully functional. Within a year there were 4 postdocs, 2 technicians and 1 PhD student working on TCR signaling and thymic selection. The team was committed to understanding the most basic mechanisms underlying T cell differentiation and tolerance.

QR2001_01 BII

Marco Colonna Leaves for St. Louis, Missouri

Marco accepted an offer to continue his research at Washington University in St. Louis, Missouri, where he later became the first

R.R. Bellieveau Professor of Pathology. Marco's laboratory studies the function of natural killer cells, plasmacytoid dendritic cells and macrophages in innate immune responses against pathogens and in cancer. His team has discovered receptors that allow these cells to detect infected cells with reduced levels of MHC class I molecules. Moreover, his team has characterized novel triggering receptors expressed on myeloid cells that control the function of neutrophils, osteoclasts in the bone and microglia in the brain.

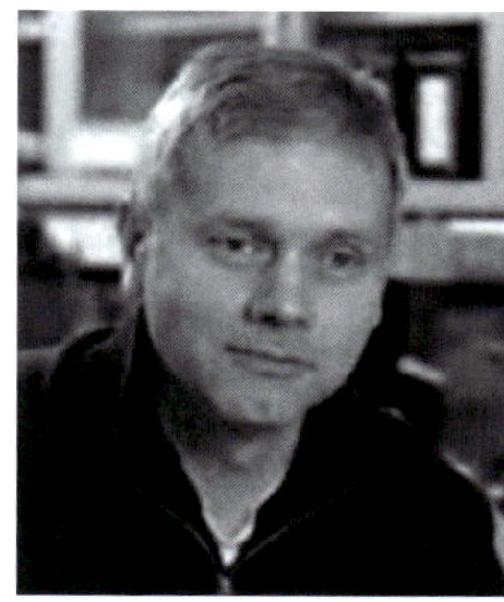

Marco Colonna

Marco Colonna has published 228 scientific articles to date and holds editorial appointments for many periodicals, including *European Journal of Immunology*, *Immunity*, *Journal of Experimental Medicine*, *Blood*, *Journal of Clinical Investigation*, *Journal of Biological Chemistry*, *Virology* and *Human Immunology*.

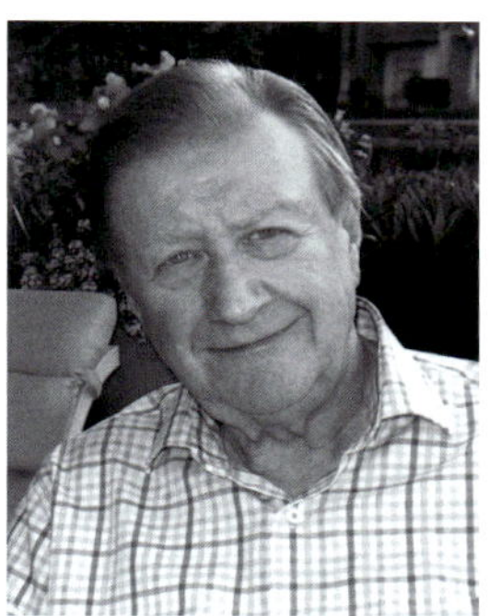

Roland Gisler

Symposium for Fritz Melchers and Roland Gisler

At the end of April 2001 Fritz Melchers and Roland Gisler retired, and the occasion was marked with a 1-day symposium with 8 invited speakers, each giving a 45-minute presentation. All the speakers [QR2001_02] had close contact with the institute over the years. The symposium was concluded with a farewell party held at the well-known "Atlantis" in the heart of Basel.

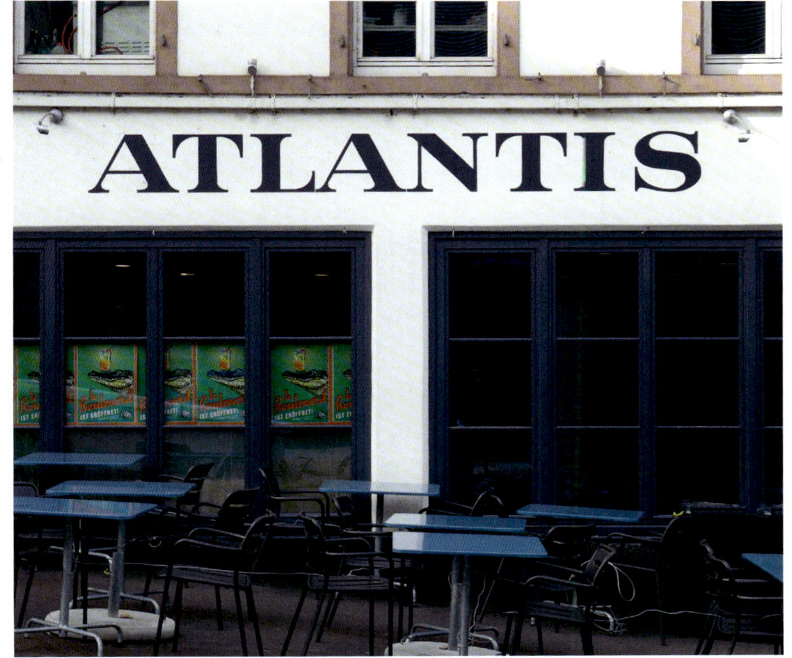

QR2001_02 BII

Theo Staehelin, Louis Du Pasquier
and André Traunecker

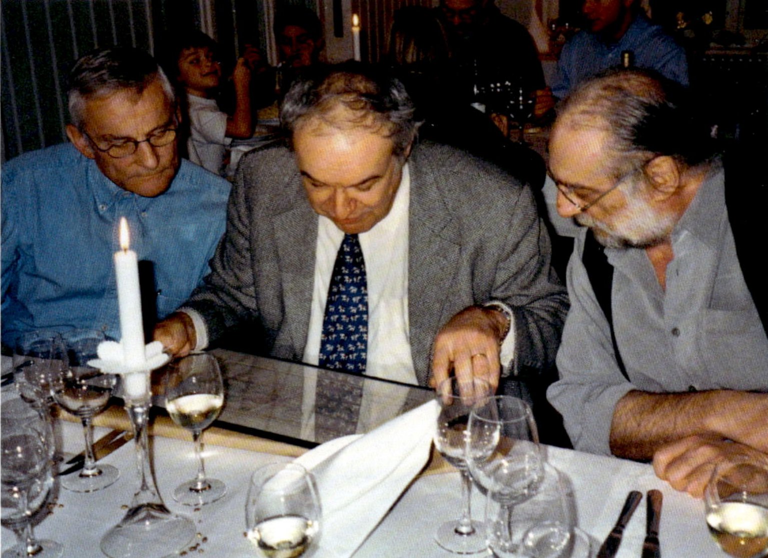

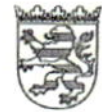

PAUL EHRLICH INSTITUT

DIREKTOR:
PROF. NIELS KAJ JERNE

6 FRANKFURT AM MAIN 70
PAUL EHRLICH STRASSE 44
TELEFON: 60251

This is to certify that

Louis Du Pasquier

has acquired the degree of

BACHELOR OF PLAQUES AND ROSETTES

by participating in

the International Laboratory Course on

Immunological Techniques at the Cellular Level

in Frankfurt am Main, 6 - 18 November 1967

sponsored by the

EUROPEAN MOLECULAR BIOLOGY ORGANIZATION

and conducted by

BIOZZI, Paris, France; BUSSARD, Paris, France; CEPPELLINI, Turin, Italy; DUTTON, La Jolla, California; FISCHER, Freiburg, Germany; FUJI, Frankfurt, Germany; INGRAHAM, Indianapolis, Indiana; HENRY, Frankfurt, Germany; LUZZATI, Turin, Italy; MAZIE, Paris, France; MOUTON, Paris, France; MÖLLER, Stockholm, Sweden; PERNIS, Milan, Italy; RAJEWSKY, Cologne, Germany; SEGRE, Urbana, Illinois; SIMONSEN, Copenhagen, Denmark; ZAALBERG, Rijswyk, Holland; and Members of the Paul Ehrlich Institute,

Frankfurt am Main
18 November 1967

Niels Jerne

JOHANN WOLFGANG GOETHE UNIVERSITÄT
LEHRSTUHL FÜR EXPERIMENTELLE THERAPIE

Retirement Dinner, Not a "Last Supper"

Decades ago, when Niels Jerne offered Louis Du Pasquier membership of the BII, Louis became the youngest permanent member. When Louis received his diploma of "Bachelor of Plaques and Rosettes" in Frankfurt in 1967, little did he know that it was an entry ticket to the then not yet existing BII.

In December 2001, Louis turned off the lights in his office at the BII and miraculously received a well-deserved "asylum" in a beautiful office on Rheinsprung (with a river view) – it was the office of Prof. Adolf Portmann, a famous Basler zoologist from the early 20th century. Louis proudly showed his visitors Adolf Portmann's writing desk and other items from the golden past of classical zoology.

In fact, Louis' retirement dinner in 2001 that his friends, former members of the BII, organized for him was the start of his second career that still lasts to the present day [QR2001_03].

QR2001_03 BII

Nobel Prize for Sir Paul Nurse, Member of the Advisory Board

Sir Paul Nurse was awarded the 2001 Nobel Prize for Medicine for the discovery of the mechanism of the cell cycle [QR2001_04]. Tim Hunt, a frequent visitor to the BII, shared the prize with Sir Paul. Paul was a member of the Board during the last 3 years the institute existed.

QR2001_04 BII

Nobel Prize for Sydney Brenner, Member of the Advisory Board

A year later, Sydney Brenner was awarded the Nobel Prize for Medicine for the discovery of the genetic regulation of organ development [QR2001_05]. Sydney Brenner was a friend of the BII since its inception and a long-standing member of the Advisory Board.

The Seminars Continued

Gill Wu, a faithful former BII member and frequent visitor to the BII, came back to say goodbye to the place where she had lost her heart.

The announcements of seminars continued to be displayed in the entrance hall of the BII throughout its existence. Seminars were a litmus test of the vitality of the institute – even when the building was damaged by fire (1985), seminars were held. They were always uplifting mentally and gave the feeling of community among the members.

Many facsimiles of the announcements are given in the respective QR code. Sometimes the seminar indicated the speaker's start of involvement with the BII, in other instances it was farewell.

BASEL INSTITUTE FOR IMMUNOLOGY
Grenzacherstrasse 487, 4005 Basel

SEMINAR

Thursday July 19, 2001 at 16:30	**Gillian Wu** Ontario Cancer Institute, Toronto "USING THE 'GENOME' TO ANALYZE I$_{g}$H DIVERSITY"	*(Host: I. Lefkovits)*

12/07/2001-ardp

The Last BII Seminar

The very last seminar at the BII was given by ex-member Jonathan Sprent on November 20th, 2001. Jon worked and lectured on four continents of this planet; with a busy travel schedule he was still relaxed giving his talks and during discussions. His work at the Basel institute influenced many scientists, and if the institute had been in a position to give a lifetime achievement award, Jon would have received it. In fact, he was indeed awarded this from the American Association of Immunologists.

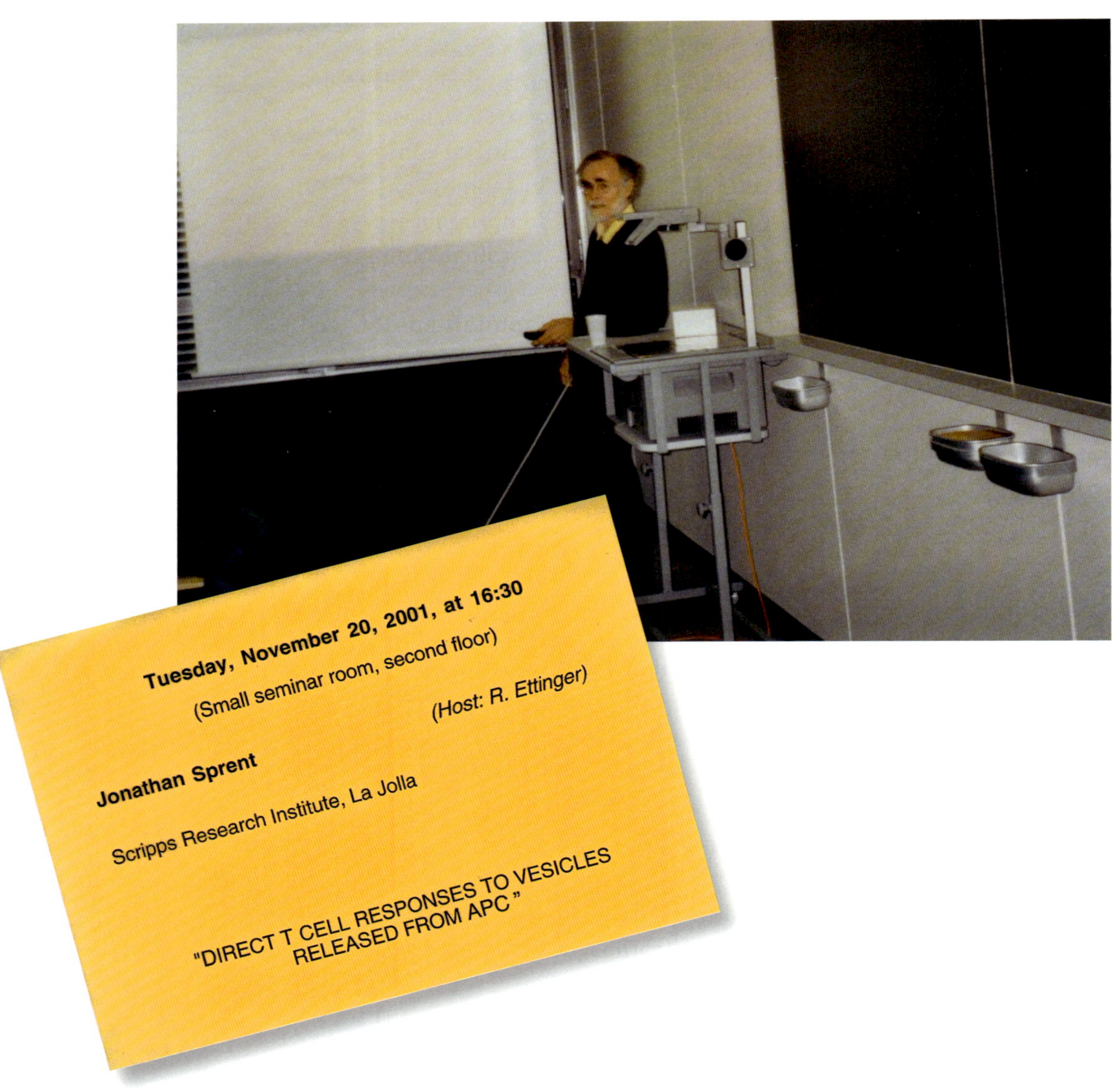
Tuesday, November 20, 2001, at 16:30
(Small seminar room, second floor)
(Host: R. Ettinger)
Jonathan Sprent
Scripps Research Institute, La Jolla
"DIRECT T CELL RESPONSES TO VESICLES
RELEASED FROM APC"

Decommissioning Tinguely's Double Helix

The laboratories were closed down one by one, and during the month of December the last members moved their labs to new destinations. Tinguely's Double Helix was taken apart and moved to the Tinguely Museum.

In the "Echo" section of this book the "new life" of the Double Helix is documented. In many laboratories around the world the title page of the Annual Report depicting Tinguely's sculpture reminds former members of the "Paradise Lost".

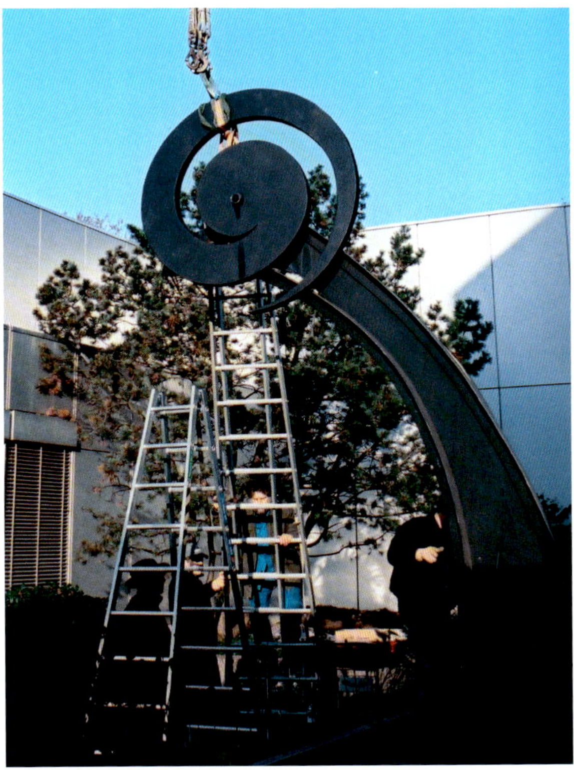

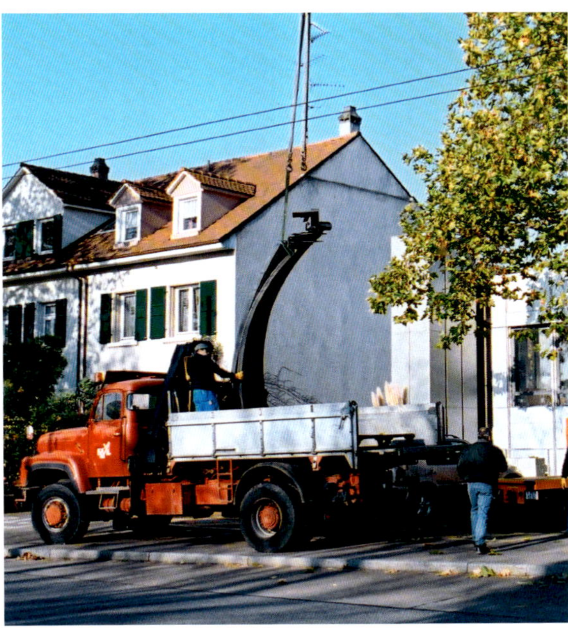

Jean Tinguely's famous Double Helix in the BII courtyard (see page 374) being dismantled for transport to the Tinguely Museum in Basel

Treasure Trove 2001

The database contains documents related to the BII in a broader context (lists, series of photographs, etc.).

QR2001 treasure BII

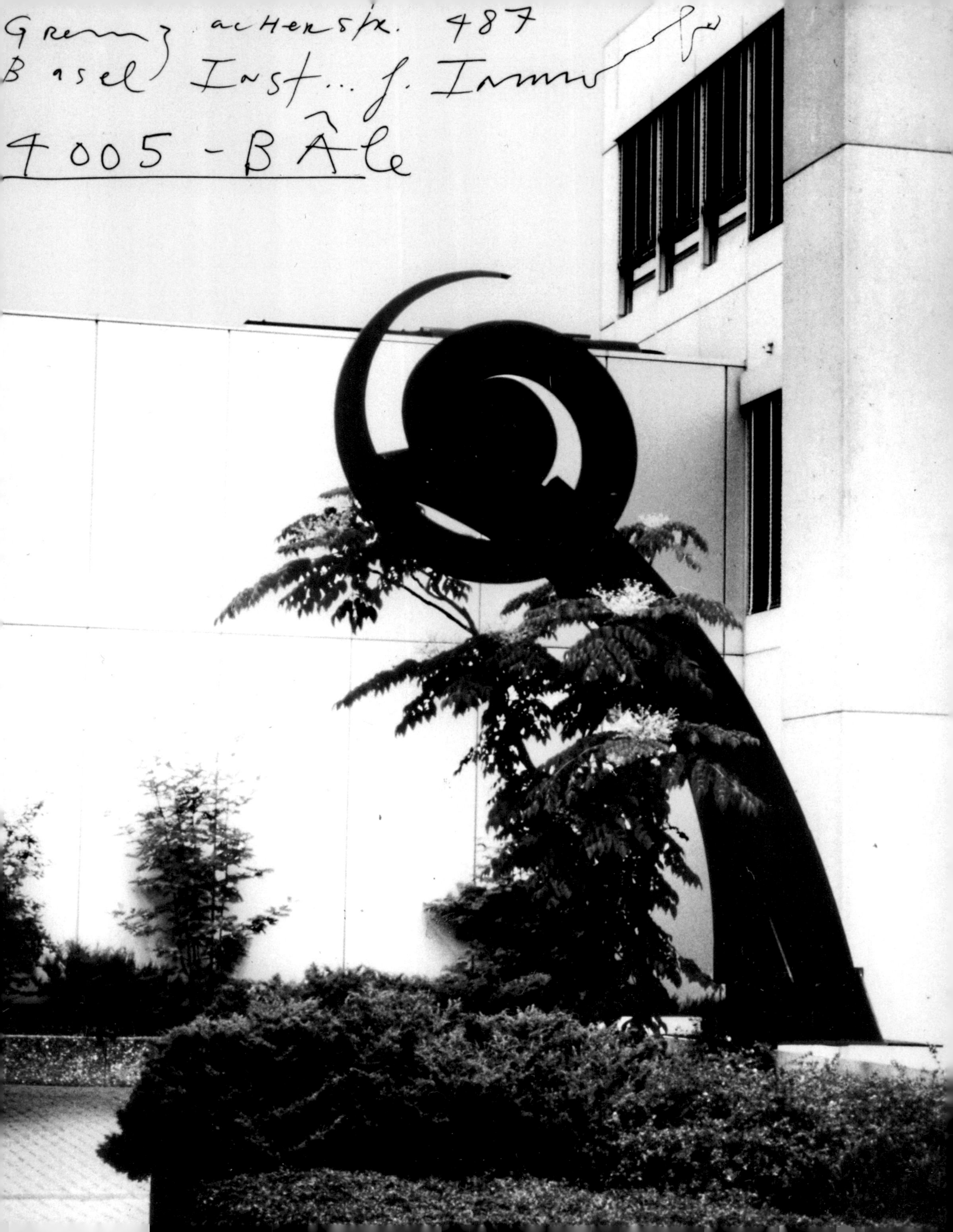
487
Basel
4005 - BÂle

Remembering the Basel Institute for Immunology

Echoes of Time, Tune, Space and Future

The intention of the following pages is to retrieve some "mosaic stones" from the narration and give them more space. Questions can be asked and maybe answered. Even stories of suspense can be told, as in the case of Maurice Zauderer. And of course one should listen to Louis Du Pasquier, who poetically said that the birth of the BII was placed under the sign of music. The story about Anita and Maurice is one of many others (Graham Mitchell and his Volkswagen, and Polly Matzinger and her motorcycle are included in the QR database). Former members of the BII founded some two dozen biotech companies, some of which could have fitted the Roche portfolio well; whatever the case, Roche can be proud that ex-BII members have been so successful. And finally there is a philosophical note about sponsors and philanthropists, all this fitting under the "Echoes of Time, Tune, Space and Future", and is also offered in the QR database.

Echo of Time: Part 1

Were there alternatives that Roche could have or should have explored instead of closing the institute down? The Roche management probably understood that the institute was a precious asset, yet there were arguments for taking a different path. Once the closing down of the BII was decided, scientists started to leave, although a number of them remained in Basel, mostly at Basel University. Jerne's centennial symposium was held in Lisbon.

On June 5th, 2001, one year after Roche had announced the closing down of the institute, a few colleagues met in the "still functioning" cafeteria to remind themselves of this dismal anniversary. The decommissioning of the institute had proceeded unrelentingly, so the discussions were merely of a coffee-table nature as to whether there were any alternatives that Roche could have or should have made.

The discussions were not recorded, but the story was retold over and over again, yielding the following collective memory.

In the Improbable Case that...

If one assumed the improbable case that Roche was in deep financial trouble, then any measure the company took was justified, and it would be comprehensible that the institute would be among the top contenders for jettisoning. That this was not the case was notorious due to Theo Staehelin's assertion that "Roche investment in the institute keeping it running for 30 years" had been paid off by the success of the Applied Immunology Project, which had brought the company a profit of one billion dollars by the year 2000.

Incompatibilities

Another speculation was that the management of Roche understood that the institute was a precious asset, yet its functioning had become increasingly incompatible with the Roche "command structure". This expression was never used during Jerne's reign, but later it was used quite often. Roche's hypothetical or real dissatisfaction with the director might have been considered as an insuperable impediment for the institute's continued existence. If this were the case (and probably it was, at least in part), then the solution should have been to replace the director and keep the institute otherwise intact.

A third aspect emerged later, once the protagonists gained a clear distance from the "troubled times". This will be explained in a "special" section on "next-generation institutes". Briefly, it puts forward the standpoint that the institute had indeed fulfilled its assignment and therefore could be closed.

Then the Building Became Something Else

Soon after the institute had been "restructured", the aluminium-clad BII building was sold (or given away) by Roche to Basilea Pharmaceutica AG. It has to be said that Basilea was run on completely different concepts from those of the BII; it was a new, independent entity. The aim of Basilea was to develop anti-infective agents, i.e. modern types of antibiotics. At the time of writing, Basilea Pharmaceutica launched a novel important antibiotic named Zevtera (or Mabelio, as it is called in some countries) with a molecular structure of ceftobiprol. It is a compound that is effective against methicillin-resistant *Staphylococcus aureus*, which is responsible for some 40% of all cases of pneumonia that patients catch in hospital.

Affinity, Avidity and Basel

For non-cognoscenti it needs to be said that "avidity" is a scientific term derived from the term "affinity". While affinity is defined as an attraction between two entities (usually antibody and antigen), avidity refers to the accumulated strength of multiple affinities of individual non-covalent binding interactions, such as between a protein receptor and its ligand.

The definition "Avidity is the power of multiple connections", given by the dictionary, reinforces the truth that closing the BII did not break up associations – neither scientific nor social – with Basel. And when one says "Basel", it means the university, the pharmaceutical industry and all the cultural institutions that were close to the heart of so many people: scientists, technicians, secretaries, animal caretakers, workshop staff and all the others. Several former BII members continued to work in Basel at university affiliations or in the pharmaceutical industry. For instance, Ed Palmer received many offers from the USA and also from other places in Switzerland (Berne), but he accepted a position in Basel. At the time of writing, Ed has retired from the Basel University Hospital and remains in Basel, as other members did before him. Theophil Staehelin and Vincenzo Miggiano are the most senior retired scientists who received their pensions while the institute still existed.

Louis Du Pasquier
Theophil Staehelin
Howard Etlinger
Ed Palmer
Jean Pieters
Anton Rolink
Ursula Günthert
André Traunecker (in his new academic status)
Ivan Lefkovits
Vincenzo Miggiano
Roland Gisler

This list does not include scientists who left the institute when their contracts ended and who became members of other institutions in Basel (Gennaro de Libero, Lucia Mori and others).

Statements of Affection

At what date should the history of the BII end? The narrator's intention was to stop in December 2001 when the sign of "Basel Institute for Immunology" was taken down, and the building became "something else". During the years of writing, many former members started contributing their stories and recollections, which in turn have shown that the BII continues to live on.

In some QR codes, statements of appreciation are embedded, such as: *"I was fortunate to be at the institute when the Nobel laureates Jerne, Tonegawa and Köhler were all on the staff and I never felt – not even for a moment – that there could ever be a place where more brilliance was packed into one building."* This is an example of how members felt about the BII.

Jerne's Centennial Celebrated in Lisbon, 2011

One of the events occurring 10 years after the BII had been closed that cannot be omitted here is the "N.K. Jerne Centennial Symposium", held in November 2011 at the Instituto Gulbenkian de Ciencia, Oeiras, Portugal.

The main organizer was Antonio Coutinho, a remarkable personality who – in a new and unusual milieu – succeeded in preserving Jerne's legacy by providing a work atmosphere very similar to that in Basel.

The participants of the meeting and the titles of their presentations were:

Ivan Lefkovits	"Chair and introduction"
Louis Du Pasquier	"Arcachon1970: Jerne and invertebrate immunity"
Vincenzo Miggiano	"Immunology, Ceppellini, Jerne"
Richard Pink	"Us Mus Gallus"
Andreas Ziegler	"MHC and mate choice"
Jon Sprent	"So, Jon, what's the half-life of a lymphocyte?"
Richard Dutton	"Specificity in the control of the T cell burst size"
Suzy Swain	"The many arms of CD4 memory provide strong protection"
Michael Julius	"Finding Fyn"
Gill Wu	"Chair and introduction"
Matthias Wabl	"The dangerous self"
Chris Paige	"Can the immune system beat cancer?"
Sefik Alkan	"Rational design of vaccines"
Don Gerson	"Vaccine, affinity, avidity and Niels Jerne"
Hans-Martin Jäck	"Micro-RNA controls B cell maturation"
Jean-Claude Weill	"Diversity of mouse memory B cell subsets"
Lucien Aarden	"The anti-idiotype response to therapeutic monoclonal antibodies"
Harald von Boehmer	"Prevention of type 1 diabetes in mice by tolerogenic vaccination with a strong-agonist insulin mimetope"
Theo Staehelin	"Pittsburgh, Basel and sidesteps"
Rob Benner	"Jerne, Rotterdam, Basel"
Seung-il Shin	"Living in the intellectual shadows of Jerne"
Jack Kettman	"Metrology: a journey of measurements"
Howard Etlinger	"Niels Kaj Jerne memorial seminar: the evocation of 1,765,828,767"
Bjarne Bogen	"T cells integrated into idiotypic regulation"
Ivan Lefkovits	"Tuning somatic cell heterogeneity"
Antonio Coutinho	"Conclusion"

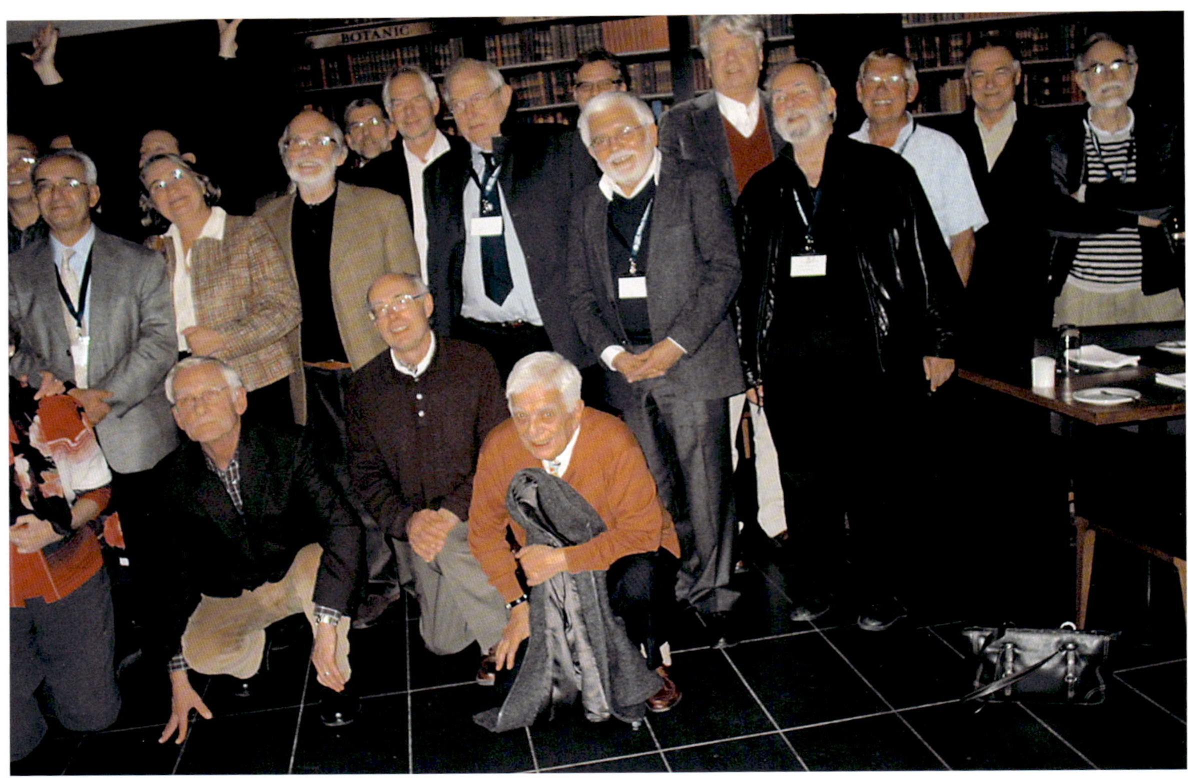

A group of the participants at the N.K.J. Centennial Celebration, Lisbon 2011

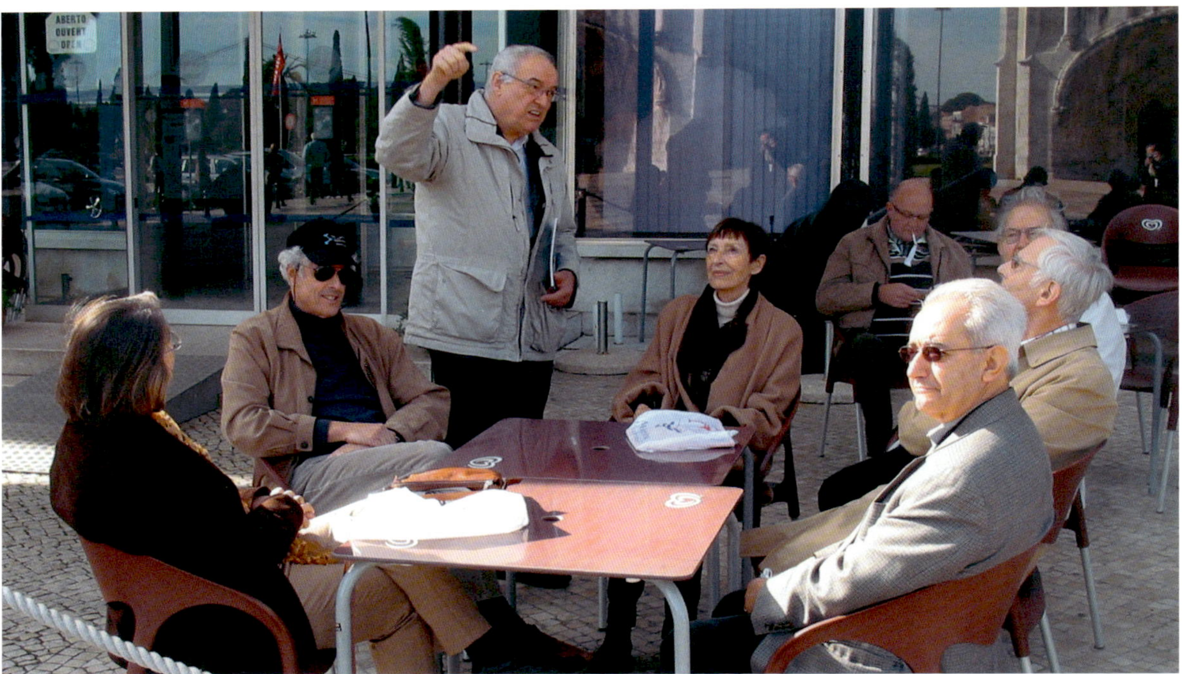

Louis Du Pasquier talking about the sights of Lisbon

Echo of Time: Part 2

Maurice Zauderer and Louis Pasteur

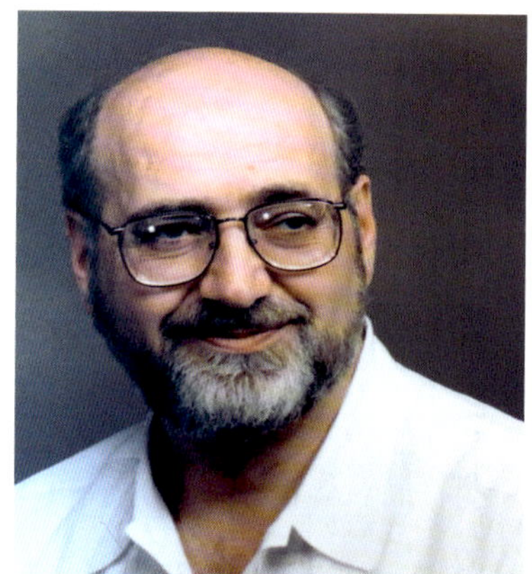

Maurice Zauderer

This is a true story, the dialogues were recorded soon after the event, so they are genuine as well. The only questionable issue is whether the person who drove Anita to the border was Berry. It was 30 years ago. The story has, however, a small unpleasant pang. Maurice did not go to the border on Monday morning. Instead he contacted the Canadian Embassy, who solved the issue through diplomatic channels. It took 2 years to solve this "difficult" issue. Not only did Maurice not enter France during those 2 years, but he did not even fly over French territory.

Maurice Zauderer is the founder and president of Vaccinex Inc. in Rochester. Anita Söderberg retired and lives in both Basel and Stockholm. Berenice Kindred died in 1985, Brigitte Askonas in 2013.

"Maurice, don't forget your passport."

"If you say so, Anita, but they never check me at the border, they just wave me through."

"Fine, I will be at 11.30 in front of the institute. For lunch we do not need to reserve a table, not on a Saturday."

Maurice, a Canadian scientist of French origin, worked those early autumn days of 1974 in Lab 12, and Anita was happy to work with him throughout the weekend. The experiment required incubating cell cultures for several days, and to take samples each day, needing an hour or two on Saturday and Sunday. The cells had to be collected, centrifuged and spread on agar plates. Maurice tried not to impose too much on Anita's free time, and he could do most of the steps at leisure, since he was staying in one of the two guest rooms of the institute, just a few steps from the laboratory. It was very convenient, but dull on Saturday, since the cafeteria was closed. But lunch with Anita in Alsace would make just the right break before continuing the experiment in late afternoon.

At 11.30 Anita got in the car, and they drove through Grenzacherstrasse, crossed the Rhine heading towards the French border.

"Are you happy with the car? Is it true that you bought it from Ita for 200 dollars?"

"Well, I wanted to give her more, but Ita did not accept. The car kept changing hands, you know, in Rome the lifespan of cars is quite short. Ita was the last user, and it is still registered in her name. But the car brought me safely from Rome to Basel, and it can still last for a while."

"Maurice, in fact I did not even ask you whether you know the directions to Restaurant Meyer? I shall tell you where to turn to Village-Neuf, once we cross the border."

"Border, look at that. Actually I should feel patriotic now – my birthplace France."

The border police looked at the car, "passport, s'il vous plaît".

Anita handed over her Swedish passport and Maurice his Canadian.

"Where are you coming from?"

"I am working in Basel, and Mrs. S. is my technician."

"You are working in Basel? How come that you have a British license plate? Your car documents, s'il vous plaît."

"Who is this Brigitte Askonas? The car belongs to Mrs. Askonas?"

"Yes, in fact yes. It was her car, while she worked in Rome, and now I am using the car. I was a postdoc in the laboratory of Dr. Askonas."

"Well, move your car to the parking lot, here", and he pointed to the free place, "I come back to you".

It took a while, one could see that the guard made a phone call, and then he approached the car, accompanied by two other border guards whose hands were on their guns. Without a *s'il vous plaît* he shouted at Maurice "to step out of the car". The guards made a few steps towards Maurice saying, "lady remains sitting".

"Mr. Zauderer, I checked the database, and upon counter-checking, I received the order to arrest you. You are a deserter of the French army, and since 8 years there has existed a warrant to arrest you. You will be deported to the military prison in Nancy, where they will deal with all relevant issues. Whether you drive a stolen car will be clarified during the proceedings."

Maurice became pale, he could hardly speak, but finally he said, "you can't do that, I am a Canadian citizen, I have nothing to do with France, my family left the country when I was 6 months old, I was born there at the end of World War II. And now we are heading to France for lunch".

To Anita it was clear that the lunch was not going to take place, especially when the two guards grabbed Maurice and took him away.

"Mrs. S., you are neither arrested nor are there any charges against you. You can leave, and you should move the car back to Swiss territory, the car cannot stay here."

"I am not going anywhere", said Anita, "certainly not without my colleague, and besides that I do not drive a car".

"Do not make any difficulty, s'il vous plaît, or I will arrest you also. Take my suggestion, go back to Basel, get a pyjama and a toothbrush for Mr. Z., come back and then it is over. We cannot escort Mr. Z. to Nancy during the weekend, he will stay here in confinement for the two nights – till Monday, and the rest will be handled by military. I shall stop now a passer-by car for you and ask whether they are willing to give you a lift to the city. Your return with pyjama you organize yourself."

Anita had no chance even to ask Maurice about the key of the guest room, and she was off to be taken to Basel. She knew that she had to get the pyjama, but this could not be the solution, she had to do something to save Maurice. The driver realized the emergency and drove Anita to the institute. The guest room was not locked. She took the pyjamas, a toothbrush and a fresh shirt, and placed them in a bag. Outside the room Anita bumped into Berry Kindred and explained the situation.

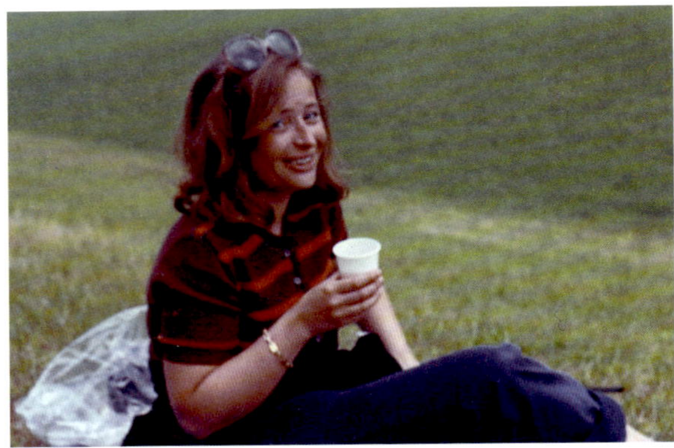

Anita Söderberg

"Calm down, Anita, I shall drive you to the border, and then we make a plan, whom to call, certainly we shall call the Canadian Embassy, but this has to be done in a calm manner. I still have to finish my experiment, it will take me half an hour, in the meantime do something."

Anita went to the lab, and she realized that she had to decide about the experiment. The size of the test was such that it was tuned for work of two people. She took a sheet of paper, and started to make notes. She had to simplify the experiment, to eliminate some groups, to leave out the lowest cell concentration, which anyway gives only little information. Also she crossed out the negative control, which she would not do under normal conditions, and she decided to analyze duplicate cultures instead of the planned triplicates. Berry rushed into the lab and they were ready to leave.

"We need another person, a driver who will bring back Maurice's car."

"Anita, we do it differently. I shall leave my car in a side street near the border, and drive Maurice's car, and I shall get my car later."

In the meantime Maurice had calmed down and started to think about the experiment. When the guard came to see if everything was in order, and said that Mrs. S. would come back with pyjamas and toothbrush, Maurice asked the guard for pencil and paper.

"What do you intend to do? Protocols for experiments? What are you talking about?"

Maurice in fluent French started to explain that he was doing some biological tests, and these had to be finished by the technician in his absence, and that he wanted to write instructions to her. The guard said no, but finally gave him a sheet of paper and a ballpoint pen.

"Write it so that everything is clear, no codes, otherwise you will not be allowed to hand it over to your technician."

Maurice decided to simplify the experiment so that Anita could finish it within a reasonable time span. Of course Anita would manage the whole experiment alone, but better to have a successful simple experiment than a large ruined one. He made a table – into each line he inserted the increasing cell concentration, and then he crossed out the lowest cell concentration, which anyway provides only marginal information. With some hesitation he crossed out the negative control, and cut some further details. He handed the paper to the guard.

"I will not allow this to be handed to your technician. This is full of codes."

Maurice swallowed, and started to explain again – from scratch. "Sir, you remember from your school days Louis Pasteur. He made experiments, which were done exactly in the same way as I am planning them here. You see these lines? One of these cell concentrations is of great importance, but we do not know which one. You remember the 9-year-old boy, Joseph Meister, who was bitten by a rabid dog? Pasteur saved him because he knew how much vaccine he should inject. Otherwise the boy would have died."

"Are you telling me that you do experiments of the kind Monsieur Pasteur did?"

"Yes, I do", said Maurice with confidence in his voice.

The guard left the room. After endless minutes he returned, and solemnly spoke:

"I came to the conclusion, and your protocol convinced me, that I have no right to detain somebody who is doing experiments of such importance as Louis Pasteur did. I decided to let you go to finish the experiment, though you have to promise that by Monday morning at 8 o'clock you report here for further proceedings."

"You mean, I am free?"

"Yes, when the lady comes, you can go back to the institute to finish your experiment."

Anita and Berry arrived and were amazed to see Maurice sitting next to the guard drinking coffee. After a big hug they left to return to the institute. Maurice in his car, Anita next to him in the front seat, and Berry, smiling, followed them in her car. At the red light Anita showed Maurice her protocol, and Maurice showed her his, and they smiled that they independently had planned it the same way.

Back in the institute they did the experiment, and it was successful, though the negative control was missing.

Echo of Tune

Louis Du Pasquier describes the activity of the BII in music. In his words, "the birth of the Basel Institute for Immunology was placed under the sign of music". In this detailed story, the musical abilities and performances of scientists, such as Arnold Feinstein, Helmut Pohlit, Gerry Edelman, Manfred Eigen, Louis Du Pasquier, Polly Matzinger, Alexandra Livingstone and maybe another 20, are described.

Musicians at the BII

"*Paul Sacher (was) one of the world's richest men, an artist of unusual stature, one of the last great musical patrons of our century and also a long-time member of the board of directors of the pharmaceutical giant Hoffmann-La Roche.*"

The Guardian, May 27th, 1999, Sibylle Ehrismann

The birth of the BII was placed under the sign of music. Many members of the institute and of the BII Advisory Board played an instrument. Every so often they met, establishing a special network of relationships, like a "freemasonry of BII members" or a "secret society". These members were often called to "active duty", to perform at the social events of the institute.

The narrator can testify that Louis Du Pasquier was hired as a permanent member of the institute for his scientific quality and not for the way of playing Debussy[1] on the flute, although his musical talent cer-

[1] In 1967, during a course organized in Frankfurt, in Niels Jerne's laboratory, Louis played *Syrinx*, and it caught the attention of Niels, who started to talk to him about this beautiful piece and occasionally about the tadpole immune system.

tainly helped. Louis not only played at countless occasions during his 30 years at the BII, but he diligently took notes related to the musical events in which he participated (or observed with a critical mind).

Louis' story of music and musicians (see below) is personal and as such should not be altered. In the QR database it is reproduced in full, while below – due to space constraints – only the portion relevant to the institute's inherent activities is given. Both the full version and the printed one show that being a musician did not just mean being an innocent bystander, but also a creator of the fine network of relationships so characteristic of the BII.

A Fancy[2] (by Louis Du Pasquier): The Illuminated Side of the Moon

"It is amazing how many of my colleagues were musicians. I counted not less than 54 partners in 31 years of the Basel Institute for Immunology[3].

It all started in 1971, when a member, Arnold Feinstein, playing the recorder (and who was responsible for my switch from one animal model, the midwife toad, to another one, the South African frog or clawed toad Xenopus*), Helmut Pohlit, another member who played the keyboard, and me with my flute, assembled with the intention of producing something for the opening ceremony of the Institute. That was going to happen on the 17th of June 1971.*

Arnold and I decided that we would play a little sinfonia by Henry Purcell in addition to other pieces for flute and harpsichord by Johann Sebastian Bach and Carl Friedrich Abel. This was a non-planned but nevertheless welcome tribute to Paul Sacher, who had in 1928 (see above) been a strong advocate of Purcell in Basel. Indeed shortly after founding the Basle Chamber Orchestra, in a single evening, he conducted Purcell's music for the tragedy 'Abdelazer' and the opera 'Dido and Aeneas'.

The day before the concert Arnold managed to have a matchbox explode in his hand, thus he played with a big bandage. Yet we formed a nice trio, although very short-lived, since Arnold was there for only about a year. With Helmut, who stayed longer, we played a lot. Occasionally we would host guest stars. One was Gerry Edelman. He played the violin well and with him we had a good try at the 'Musical Offering' by Bach.

Later with another Nobel Prize winner, Manfred Eigen, I played at the 10th anniversary in 1981. Manfred Eigen is a good pianist. He was a friend of Paul Sacher and when he came to Basel (he was a member of the board of directors of the BII) he played with members of Sacher's chamber orchestra, the BKO. They have produced that year a record of two Mozart piano concerti, KV 415 and KV453. I knew and still know personally several musicians of this group, and they all remember these sessions with Manfred Eigen. We decided to play Bach's sonata for flute and keyboard in g minor. I sent him the notes a month before our unique rehearsal that took place at the Radio Basel studio. There a huge, and supposedly beautiful, instrument was lent to him. It did not please him so much, and I have to say that it was pretty hard in the sharps. It sounded more like a drum than like a bell. Still we tried. Manfred was not really ready and did not know the piece well, but he was OK. Still, I was damned nervous on the day of the production. He indeed messed up so much in the slow movement that I went out of breath as he sneaked his way through the last chords, trying to find a way to finish, and prolonging my agony as I was desperately needing a breath. I made such a noise inhaling, like a whale blowing when it surfaces. I ruined the end of this movement but we caught up alright for the last movement.

From trombone (Jean-Claude Jaton) to cello (Andreas Ziegler, Rolf Jessberger, Michel Chaperon, Gillian Harris), via keyboards (Helmut Pohlit, Daniel Levy, Charles Becciolini, John Gatfiled, Spedding Micklem, Alexandra Livingstone, Hugh Rowell, Hilary Koprowski, Dorcas Tokes), we had representatives of practically a full symphony orchestra.

Violin	Felix Wiedermayer, Peter Marquardt, Thilman Borgreve, Gerald Edelman, Geoff Schatz, Nina Luning-Prak, Philippe Naquet, Michel Fougereau, Yoshi Kurosawa
Viola	Jane Levy and Konrad Schauenstein
Bassoon	Walter Keller, Peter Jung
Flute	Silke Hennecke, Robert Rotappel, Christina Zeuthen
Oboe	Spedding Micklem, Heiner Frost, Nic Cohen
Recorder	Arnold Feinstein
Voice	Marianne Luthi, Steve Bauer, Thomas Harder, Fillipo Olivieri, Martin Flajnik

[2] Described by John Dowland's contemporary Thomas Morley as "the most principal and chiefest kind of music", the *Fantasie* or *Fancy* allowed the composer some freedom.
[3] Yet it was not mandatory to mention which instrument one played to apply for a position at the BII.

Double bass	Polly Matzinger
Lute	Michèle Courtet
Guitar	John Bews and Philippe Naquet
Drums	Jim Kaufman
Trumpet	Toni Heinis

We also had one remarkable musical scholar, Stephen Fazekas de St. Groth, who had played the cello and had studied composition with no one less than Bela Bartok. His perception of music was professional, his judgment conservative and definitive.

He hated Glenn Gould: 'Who is he to tell me what a fugue is?' was his comment on the 'Well-tempered keyboard' record by Glenn Gould. We shared our profound admiration for the cellist Janos Starker, who turned out by the way to be the teacher of Gillian Harris, one of our recruits for the 'Chaos' and 'Opération de la taille' (see below) production. But Stephen had a precious recollection of his time with Bela Bartok, especially on his way of playing the piano to illustrate his orchestration class, when he could imitate practically any instrument on the keyboard. Stephen would not forget for instance his imitation of the horn!

Stephen knew music and music history. He had music playing all the time in his lab, where once 'The rite of spring' by Stravinsky had the faculty to irritate one technician, Heidi Luther, who complained. He fired her. She came to our lab, where one liked music silently. One evening we had Stephen for dinner, I played a trick on Stephen, I had just bought a rare record of a string quartet composed by the young Mendelssohn. To me it was an interesting and surprising piece, very intricate and that I would never have attributed to Mendelssohn. So I played it without disclosing the author, asking Stephen's opinion. Chewing on his pipe he meditated for a while and then analyzed the piece. 'It is very scholarly', he said, 'the double fugue is taken as an exercise without the slightest fantasy. I feel it must be something composed by a very young composer, I would tend to think… let me see… by the young Mendelssohn? Perhaps?'

Later I invited him to listen to a concert by a friend, Volker Biesenbender, a pupil of Yehudi Menuhin (and who would be later the teacher of Juliette in the area of gipsy music!), who was going to perform in a series of concerts all the Bach sonatas and partitas for solo violin. Stephen was very critical of the liberties taken in the tempi but could not but admire the performance.

Stephen was an uncompromising purist. When I asked him why he had stopped playing the cello he told me the circumstances. When he was younger he used to play in a quartet with friends, and one day, they practiced with an extra friend the wonderful Mozart quintet with clarinet. As the rehearsal progressed Stephen had a solo section that he played beautifully. After finishing, the friend said 'let's do it again'.

'And I could not', said Stephen, 'so I stopped playing the cello'.

We played for parties, for BTA productions, but mostly we met at our place on Saturdays with sometimes up to 6–7 friends, some of whom were professionals, such as the violinist Herbert Hoever, the harpsichord player Jean Goverts or the cellist Gillian Harris and the violinist Roberto Savicky.

When you think that it would not have happened without Paul Sacher!

It could have been in fact a good scenario for one or the other of the BTA productions, where music was often involved. Whether the 'Girl of Ipanema' with the Institute's big band and Filippo, or the production involving 'the BII Baroque soloists' like the 'Chaos', the satirical productions culminated in 'The Two Divas', making fun of Fritz and Harald and performed on the occasion of Harald's departure to Paris. The 'Chaos' concert, which celebrated a reconstruction phase of the Institute, included the 'Chaos' of Jean-Ferry Rebel, songs by John Dowland and the 'Tableau de l'opération de la taille'[4] (a representation of the kidney stone surgery) by Marin Marais, and we had a great time with Alexandra Living-

[4] Writing this vignette gives me an opportunity to dispel some misconceptions about the program of some of the productions. For instance some members like Ivan Lefkovits gave us tremendous credit by attributing the piece to the BII baroque soloist's imagination.

No! 'Le tableau de l'opération de la taille' was not a joke invented by the script writer of the BTA, but a bona fide rendition of the piece by Marin Marais, who apparently had withstood the surgery himself. The piece, written for viola in 1725, presents an operation for removal of a stone in the bladder in musical form. Musicological analysis shows that in the early 18th century the lateral perineal approach was normally used for such operations in France. Medico-historical annotations complement the musicological analysis.

The same remarks on the chaos! I got the notes of Jean-Ferry Rebel from Philippe Suzanne, a marvelous flutist who was studying at the Schola Cantorum in the early seventies. The Schola! Paul Sacher.

At 27 he became director of the Schola Cantorum Basiliensis, founded by him, Ina Lohr and August Wenzinger and now with a world-wide reputation, one of the first training centers for music-making with authentic period instruments. So once more without Sacher there would have been no 'Chaos' at the BII on that day.

stone making up the verses from the original Dowland poems into a text (gently) making fun of Fritz and Harald!

Another good shot was Klaus Rajewsky. We were invited to his place with Matthias Wabl after a visit to his lab in 1975. The atmosphere could have been tense: Matthias had screwed up by not showing up at his own seminar, and by preventing Klaus from smoking in his own house. I had brought my flute because Klaus had said he played the piano. Not really, he was quite timid, but I shall never forget his piano. I forgot the brand perhaps, but it was one of the great brands. And it had a super system to increase the numbers of overtones in the sharps, an extra string resonating by sympathy in the last octave. This is a region of the instrument that on a modern Steinway, even the best, resounds like a piece of metallic brake drum. So we established a good relationship around this instrument. Much later, in 1994, he greeted me warmly at Jerne's funeral, when I played the flute part of the 8th Bach cantata 'Liebster Gott, wann werd ich sterben?'. So he remembered me somehow.

I never forgot how inspired I was to play with Nina Lunig-Prak when she was a student in Klaus Karjalainen's lab. I had no reason to be nice to her because of Klaus. No, in this case it was just premonition, because later she went to work with Martin Weigert, a real big wheel in the snob circles of somatic mutation specialists. That was my way to give a seminar in his lab. She invited me over because she wanted to play again with me, and Martin went along, although he never understood why Nina got to think of me for a seminar. He trashed my talk properly. Whether it was good or bad was not indicated. Actually we had a really good time together. Martin showed me the Pissaro and Duchamp exhibitions at the Philadelphia museum, cooked a shad for me on the evening of my seminar, where he had invited also Walter Gerhard, a former member of the Institute now established in Philadelphia at the Wistar Institute. It was absolutely splendid."

Commemoration of Jerne, 1995

"True, music was a source of fun and accompanied many jokes and happy moments during the life of the BII, but it also accompanied sad or nostalgic events. For instance for the Jerne memorial symposium in 1995 in Basel, 1 year after the death of Niels Jerne, music was also present. A trio of C.P.E. Bach had been chosen that reminded us of the discussions between Niels and Louis about this composer in the early 1970s, but more significantly one piece had in my opinion the perfect flavor for the occasion. It was J.S. Bach's canon perpetuus from the 'Musical Offering'. Played as a never-ending ritournelle it would send us back to the happy memories of Niels' presence and of the institute's beginnings.

The year before, for his funeral, a bunch of his friends assembled in Castillon-du-Gard for the ceremony and could listen to some pieces that – better perhaps than a minute of silence – helped all of us to get some peace.

I played the joyful solo flute part of the Bach 8th, the cantata 'Liebster Gott, wann werd ich sterben?', the one that Niels preferred, which Alexandra, his wife, appreciated, and I concluded with Syrinx."

Epilogue

"All this started with Paul Sacher, so it is only just we return to him at the end.

When Niels Jerne retired in 1981, it was the end of an era. At that time Niels' secretary Ingrid Westen-Schnurr moved with her terrific competence to the Paul-Sacher-Stiftung, like a little witness of the past, metamorphosing into another world but with sparks of the institute's spirit.

She had been asked by Paul Sacher to join this fantastic institution.

The Paul Sacher Foundation was founded in 1973. At first its purpose was to preserve Paul Sacher's musical library. A short while later the holdings began to be systematically expanded, and its purpose started to change. Today, the Foundation is an international research center for the music of the twentieth and twenty-first centuries, with some hundred estates and collections from leading composers and performers (borrowed from the website https://www.paul-sacher-stiftung.ch/en/about-the-foundation.html).

Ingrid would welcome me there and showed, among other precious things, the score of 'The rite of spring' by Igor Stravinsky that Pierre Monteux had annotated and had in his hands on May 29th, 1913, the tumultuous day of the creation. She let me have it in my hands. It was a handwritten copy! The one that would be sent to the printer later.

Emotion, but different from the emotion when seeing the Stravigor, the little device designed by Stravinsky himself to draw staves on virgin paper, a tool that would not have been disavowed by our workshop, and that was, as a matter of fact, a source of inspiration for the Fidolino stempel developed by my daughter Juliette!

Music has been a counterpoint to the history of the BII, punctuating many of its remarkable moments. Whether accompanying joyful occasions or its moments of grief and nostalgia, music by the institute's members, as imperfect as it was, but always sincere, was a kind of constant that helped keeping our attention focused on the significant issues."

Echo of Space

The careers of former BII members as founders of new institutes, as deans and rectors, as department chairs, but also as orchid cultivators or zoo directors are listed. Founders of biotech companies, for example Luminex, Trianni, PnuVax, CGEB, Network Immunology Company, Celltrion, Active Biotech, BTB Pharma AB, Biopolo Ticino, Cytos, 4-Antibody, Medgene Labs, Avidia, NovImmune SA, Vaccinex, Clarus Venture, GlobeImmune or Alfama, are listed.

From a Horizontal Structure to a Vertical Career

No reliable documents exist which follow the career paths of former BII members. By an educated guess – obtained through interviews and correspondence – about two-thirds of former members remained in academia, and about one-third moved to biotech or pharmaceutical industries.

Those who remained in basic science mostly took up teaching responsibilities and have risen in the hierarchy to the position of professor. It is beyond the scope of this book to provide a list of those who became professors; nevertheless, in instances where the career ladder culminated in added tasks of "Department Chair" or "Institute Head", details are included in this section. Some scientists' positions ended in the meantime due to retirement or to altered career prospects (e.g. Antonio Coutinho is no longer director of the Gulbenkian Institute, Oieras, and Robbert Benner stepped down from his departmental function at the Erasmus Institute).

Academia and Teaching Careers

Head of Institutes and International Institutions

- Antonio Lanzavecchia (Institute for Research in Biomedicine, Bellinzona)
- Antonio Coutinho (Gulbenkian Institute, Oieras)
- Chris Paige (Princess Margaret Cancer Centre, Toronto)
- Maria Leptin (Director of EMBO, Heidelberg)

Department Chairs

- Robbert Benner (Erasmus University Rotterdam)
- Hans Hengartner (Head of the Institute of Experimental Immunology, University of Zurich)
- Göran Möller (†) (Karolinska Institutet, Stockholm)
- Kirsten Fischer Lindahl (B.B. Owen Chair in Molecular Research at the UT Southwestern, Dallas)
- Beat Imhof (University of Geneva)

University Dean or Rector

- Gill Wu (Dean of the York University, Toronto)

Member of the Nobel Prize Assembly

- Göran Möller (†) was for many years a member of the Nobel Assembly at Karolinska Institutet; once elected the members stay on until retirement

Academic Awards

- Hans Hengartner, Member of Leopoldina
- Ruggero Ceppellini (†), Feltrinelli Prize (nominated several times for the Nobel Prize)
- Antonio Lanzavecchia, President of the Fondazione Regionale per la Ricerca Biomedica, Lombardy Region, Italy

Other, Unanticipated Paths of Activity

- Zoo director (Graham Mitchell)
- Medical practitioner (Ron Citronbaum)
- Orchid specialist (Dario Grossberger)
- Politics (John Stoker)
- Breeding cattle (Domenico Bernoco)
- Agriculture (Humberto Cosenza)
- Embryo freezing (Stan Leibo)
- Intercultural and interreligious education (Armando Bernardini)

Biotech Companies and Their CEOs

The horizontal structure of the BII was a successful model in basic science. For many members, the institute turned out to be a stepping-stone in their distinguished careers. In many instances it was a research and/or teaching career, or perhaps a career in science administration.

Several former members succeeded in making their ambitions come true with the commercial realization of their ideas. In the rapidly expanding globalized world, the list below cannot hold true for long, but at least these pioneering steps will remain recorded. It is a snapshot of achievements accomplished in the early years of the 21st century. Some entries also appear in other chapters in which the careers of members leaving the institute are described.

A stunning example is that of Seung-il Shin, who had lived in California for an extended period and then moved back to Korea, where he helped establish Celltrion (see below), with Don Gerson as president, now one of the world's largest manufacturing facilities for monoclonal antibodies. This company has routinely produced about 1,000 kg of purified, therapeutic monoclonal antibodies every year since 2005, and the products are approved for pharmaceutical use in 70 countries around the world.

Although many companies are mentioned below, one which needs special mention due to its expected future implications is that of Matthias Wabl: he succeeded in developing transgenic mice with genetically optimized antibody-encoding loci. Heavy, κ and λ, and the V-D-J loci have been replaced by human coding regions that use mouse regulatory regions to produce antibodies that have entirely human variable regions in mice with fully functional immune systems. Antibodies from these mice can be fully humanized in a second step and produced in CHO cells to manufacture therapeutic monoclonal antibodies as pharmaceutical products. This is an important new platform for therapeutic monoclonal antibody discovery as mentioned below.

Luminex

Jack Kettman founded the Luminex Corporation (NASDAQ: LMNX), a biotechnology company based in Austin, Texas, with offices on 3 continents. Luminex develops, manufactures and markets proprietary biological testing technologies with applications throughout the life sciences industry. Luminex was recognized by *Forbes Magazine* as one of the top 25 fastest growing technology companies in the USA in 2014.

Trianni and Austrianni

Matthias Wabl founded two biotech companies, Trianni and Austrianni, and co-founded the company Picobella. The mouse "created" by Wabl and co-workers carries engineered versions of *Heavy*, *Kappa*, and *Lambda* antibody-encoding genetic loci. The normal mouse variable and diversity/joining gene segments in these loci have been replaced by synthetic chimeric versions, each comprised of human coding sequences combined with mouse regulatory genomic sequences.

PnuVax SL Biopharmaceuticals

Don Gerson founded PnuVax with headquarters in Kingston, Ontario, and a manufacturing facility located in Montreal, Quebec. The company produces vaccines and is a major supplier for US government programs.

CGEB

Salvatore Valitutti is co-founder of the International Centre for Genetic Engineering and Biotechnology (CGEB), Trieste, Italy.

Network Immunology Company

Geoff Hoffmann founded Network Immunology Company that develops technologies and therapies for autoimmune diseases. Geoff developed and implemented ideas originally postulated by Niels Jerne.

Celltrion and VaxGen

Seung-il Shin is a founder of Celltrion, a vaccine-manufacturing company. Seung-il was responsible for VaxGen's international program for worldwide distribution of vaccines. He also co-founded Eugene Tech International, where he led the company's efforts to develop and market a hepatitis B vaccine that was eventually distributed widely in many developing countries. He also directed an international initiative that ultimately led to the establishment of the International Vaccine Institute, now located in Seoul, Korea.

Active Biotech

In 1999, Tomas Leanderson became President of Active Biotech Company with headquarters in Lund, Sweden. The company is focused on the development of novel pharmaceuticals for the treatment of cancer and autoimmune diseases. The main product is laquinimod, an orally administered small molecule with immunomodulatory properties for the treatment of multiple sclerosis and other neurodegenerative and inflammatory diseases.

BTB Pharma AB

Thomas Bäckström is a founder of BTB Pharma AB with headquarters in Malmö, Sweden. The company is developing specific medicines against autoimmune diseases (multiple sclerosis, rheumatoid arthritis and type 1 diabetes). The company has a biomedical platform, with peptides that stimulate tissue-specific suppressor cells. These cells inhibit the immune cells that are actually causing the disease. The treatment aims to target the cause, rather than the symptoms of disease.

Biopolo Ticino

Luca Bolliger established Biopolo Ticino where he also participated in the creation of the Swiss marketing platforms "Swiss Biotech" and "Swiss Medtech". He handed over the company to new investors and joined Actelion AG in Allschwil. Previously he was a "global discovery portfolio manager" in the Pharma Strategy Unit of Roche, Basel. He then pursued his career in the financial industry as a fundamental analyst at BT&T asset management, and as a freelance consultant. For a certain time period Luca was CEO at the Recordati SA in Chiasso, Switzerland.

Cytos Biotechnology

Martin Bachmann is a co-founder of Cytos Biotechnology in Zurich. Under Martin's leadership, major work was accomplished in testing novel vaccines against the influenza virus. Collaborative projects with NIH, as well as with the US Army were carried out to develop a vaccine against malaria.

4-Antibody AG and NBE-Therapeutics

Ulf Grawunder, co-founder and CEO of 4-Antibody, Basel, joined a newly founded company, NBE-Therapeutics. The company focuses on the development of "next-generation" antibody-drug conjugates for cancer therapy.

Medgene Labs

Alan Young is the CEO of Medgene Labs, in Brookings, South Dakota. Vaccines developed using proteins rather than live viruses can help protect animals and subsequently humans from insect-borne viruses. The animal health company develops therapeutics, vaccines and diagnostics.

Avidia

José Carlos Gutierrez-Ramos is Head of R&D at Avidia, and Head of the Immunoinflammation Center for Drug Discovery (Pfizer). Previously he served as CEO of the Spanish biotechnology company Genetrix.

NovImmune SA

Marie Kosco-Vilbois is CEO of NovImmune SA, Geneva. Previously she had been Head of the Immunology Unit of Glaxo Wellcome Research Institute in Geneva. In the next stage of her career she became Head of Preclinical Pharmacology at the Serono Pharmaceutical Research Institute.

Vaccinex

Maurice Zauderer is founder of Vaccinex Corporation, Rochester. The company focuses on the development of new human antibodies to combat multiple sclerosis, cancer and, more recently, Huntington disease.

Clarus Venture

Michael Steinmetz is a co-founder and Managing Director of Clarus Venture that initiated a number of commercially successful pharmaceutical products.

GlobeImmune

Donald Bellgrau founded GlobeImmune Inc. in 1996. Don's reputation in the study of the immunobiology of type 1 insulin-dependent diabetes and in the areas of autoimmune disease, transplantation and tumor immunology led him to found GlobeImmune Inc., headquartered in Louisville, Colorado; it develops therapeutic vaccines to treat cancer and infectious diseases.

Alfama

Werner Haas is a co-founder of Alfama Biotechnology Company that has a patented medicine for the treatment of rheumatoid arthritis. His R&D activity is divided between Lisbon and Boston.

Vistagen

Ralph Snodgrass founded a clinical-stage biopharmaceutical company focused on the development of medicines for disorders of the central nervous system.

AMRAD Corporation

John Stocker is a co-founder of the AMRAD Corporation. The founding shareholders were 4 Melbourne-based medical research institutes. AMRAD's core business is the research and development of innovative medicines to treat infectious diseases, neurological diseases, allergy and inflammation. In December 2005 AMRAD became known as Zenyth Therapeutics Ltd.

Foursight Associates

John Stocker and Graham Mitchell, former members of the BII, and 2 other scientists established Foursight Associates (Melbourne) as an advisory service in science, technology, research and development. The aim of Foursight was to facilitate the productive interaction between scientists, funding bodies and investors. The main partner and client in consulting was Starpharma Ltd.

Vaccibody, Oslo

Bjarne Bogen co-initiated the formation of the company Vaccibody, the aim of which was to develop DNA vaccines.

NatiMab Therapeutics, Turin

Gianni Garotta founded NatiMab Therapeutics. The goal of the company is the identification and development of human antibodies for the therapy and diagnosis of infectious diseases and cancer. NatiMab has concentrated on identifying tumor-associated antigens that are recognized by antibodies in the serum from patients with pancreatic ductal adenocarcinoma.

Former BII Members with Careers at Roche and Novartis

The scientists listed below were already mentioned in various contexts at other places in this history. However, it is fitting to mention them here when referring to biotech activities in Basel: Theophil Staehelin, Vincenzo Miggiano (†), Michael Steinmetz (†), John Stocker, Hubert Jacot, Zlatko Dembic, Johann-Rudolf Frey, Manfred Brockhaus, Howard Etlinger, Richard J. Pink, Béla Takàcs, Gianni Garotta, Dietmar Braun, Max Schreier (†), Christopher Heusser, Werner Haas, Hajime Karasuyama.

Echo from the Future: Message to Philanthropists

Once the BII was the largest basic immunology institute. What will be the next generation of institutes? Philanthropists choose Princeton rather than Manhattan. The Tinguely Double Helix lives on forever, welcoming visitors to Basel.

Waiting for the End

Back at the time when the institute was created, its major assignment was to "crack" the central problem of immunology: "How is immunological specificity generated?" It was by no means certain that the puzzle "could be unraveled", but it has been. In several lectures and publications, Jerne expressed his belief that "immunology as a scientific discipline" would be over once the generation of antibody specificity was solved. In one of his papers (fittingly in Australia), he explained that there were details that we do not even want to know. "We want to know the contours of the shore of a continent (Australia), but we do not want to know the position of each pebble."

Taking this standpoint, the institute has indeed fulfilled its assignment – it solved the puzzle – and therefore could be closed. Immunology, as defined by Jerne and his contemporaries decades ago, underwent a major transformation. One of the fields that moved from the "far horizon" to the center of investigation was the "regulation of immune response and the role of the major histocompatibility complex (MHC)". This issue – with a huge effort from many laboratories worldwide – was solved in the meantime, and it allowed immunology to merge with mainstream cell biology. Receptors, ligands, molecular pathways, DNA-binding molecules, proteasomes, exosomes – you name it – became research entities to be shared with non-immunologists.

The BII Was Once the Largest Basic Immunology Institute

In the late sixties of the last century – at the planning stage of the institute – the BII was one of the largest immunology institutes in the world, while by the year 2000 many institutes were of the same size; in fact, individual work groups were often larger than the entire BII (for example Lee Hood's group). The fact that the "big" institute was small and remained small did not mean that it could not maintain its competitiveness with other, much larger institutions. The lean structure of the institute was highly successful in that the 50 scientists (with the added bonus of 500 alumni) kept its quality and reputation at an outstanding level.

In all probability, the BII would have continued to be a "good" institute beyond 2001, but it could not have maintained the status of "uniqueness". Even if by a miracle a "second Jerne" could be found, the institute would have been competing with some 30 others of equal caliber, institutes which did not exist in the seventies. On all 5 continents excellent immunology institutes came into being; nota bene former BII members were working in most of these institutes. The competition itself would not be the issue, the problem was a deeper one. The BII had been conceived to solve the puzzle of antibody specificity and the generation of diversity. All other issues, unrelated or marginally related, were largely disregarded, at least in the early days of the institute. When Jerne was uncertain whether an applicant's proposed project fitted the institute's aims (and his preconceived scientific ideas), he asked: "Does it really have anything to do with antibody specificity?" Thus, macrophages, soluble factors, killer cells, innate immunity, complement and other research components were excluded. In an institute with 50 scientists, the focus on cells (and their products) involved in antigen recognition was a mandatory condition for success. If the institute were considerably larger, say 200 scientists instead of 50, then any project could be tackled, as no issues would be considered "distracting", but with the odds that the main question of antibody diversity would not be solved.

Many of those neglected issues moved into the focus of interest at the BII towards the end of its existence, but they required much larger work groups than the institute could have offered. Immunology stopped being immunology, it became cell biology and molecular biology. Hundreds of gene products, thousands of receptors and ligands and tens of thousands of interactions required other strategies and other tactics.

Next-Generation Institute

Many scientists, noticeably Theophil Staehelin at Roche and at least a dozen from other institutions, maintained that in the long run monoclonal antibodies would be of use both as diagnostic tools and therapeutic agents. If Roche had kept the BII intact and functioning, it would have thriven. Nevertheless, it would be a different institute, an NGI (next-generation institute) that would provide all the know-how about monoclonal antibody in the drug-oriented pipelines of the mother company. Developing mice capable of producing human monoclonal antibodies and studying antibodies that bind to yet-to-be defined targets would have been a strong enough challenge to keep the BII existing at a high level of excellence. But to be clear: an institute of such a kind would only be a "helping hand" to Roche, it would not be a basic research institute. But it still would be able to attract first-class scientists. Unfortunately this option is irreversibly gone. The acronym NGI was taken by the narrator (with a dose of sarcasm) from the fashion of calling innovations a "next-generation" approach (a new procedure for gene sequencing is called NGS: next-generation sequencing).

Philanthropists Choose Princeton instead of Manhattan

Most of the opinion leaders state that there is a pressing need to create new institutes, conceivably based on the Jernean model. Such need exists for reasons contrary to those prevailing in the seventies of the last century. At that time, if a problem needed to be solved, scientists rallied round to solve it. Today, natural scientists are brought together for a completely different reason. Instead of relying on vague prognoses for the future, scientists are needed who search for the "central elements" of the world as it unfolds; since we live in a world we still do not understand, we are unable to anticipate what will happen next (neither in politics nor in technology). We are not equipped with sensors to recognize the "unknowns", and we do not know what will be needed to be done, once the need arises. It would be preposterous to claim that creating an institute that is free to choose its focus is a good idea, but not doing it is definitely a bad idea.

The dichotomy of Princeton against Manhattan is shorthand for two opposing (but still respectable) principles. The Princetonian principle is based on the belief that society should accumulate knowledge before the need arises to use it (Albert Einstein). The Manhattan principle is a mandate for joint efforts to solve urgent problems (making the atom bomb to defeat Nazism). Philanthropists with vision certainly choose Princeton over Manhattan. In both types of institutes "first-class scientists" are needed, and such ones will always be available. For the Manhattan approach the BII model is unsuitable, while for a Princeton model no other model than that of the BII is suitable.

And perhaps the statement of one of the former members (recorded after the BII closed) will become true: "I bet that Roche will recreate the Basel Institute for Immunology in less than a generation."

Tinguely's Double Helix Lives on Forever

Once greeting the BII members every morning in the courtyard of the institute, Tinguely's famous piece of art is now installed on the roof of the Tinguely Museum, visible to everyone who crosses the Rhine when arriving in Basel.

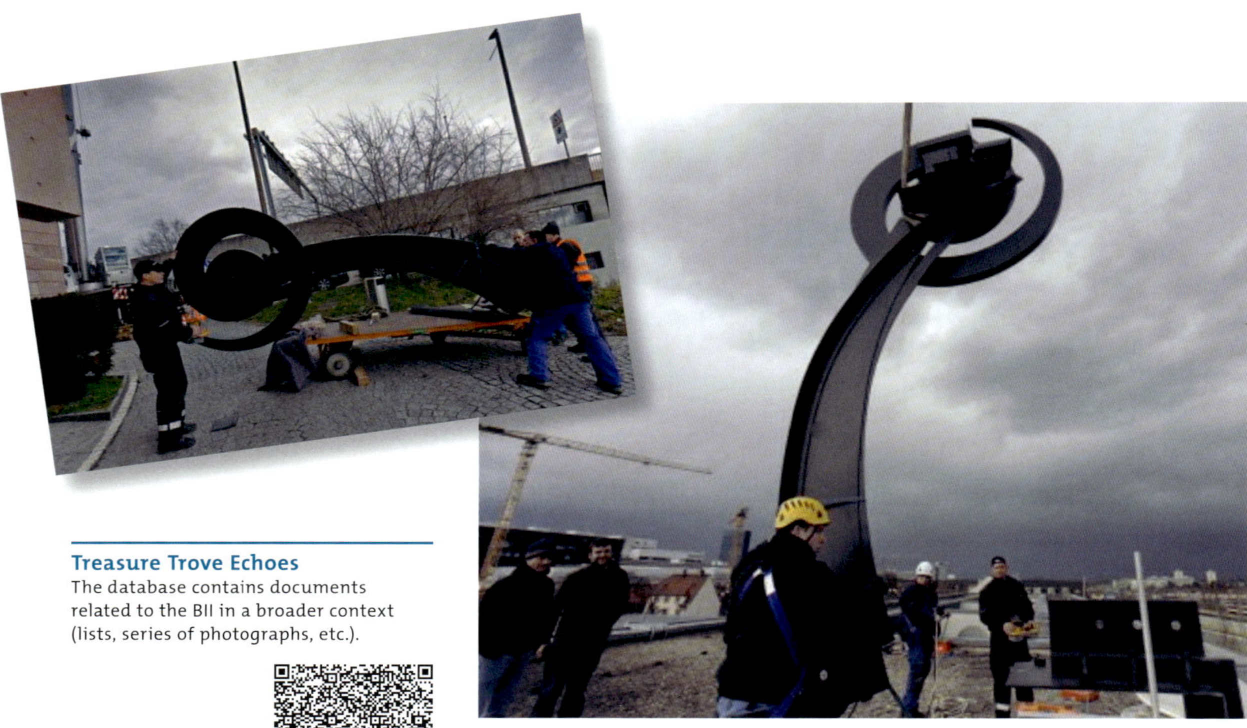

Tinguely's Double Helix arrives at the Tinguely Museum and is erected on its roof

Treasure Trove Echoes
The database contains documents related to the BII in a broader context (lists, series of photographs, etc.).

QR2002_treasure BII

Acknowledgments

• To the Freiwillige Akademische Gesellschaft, especially to Caspar Zellweger

• To Hoffmann-La Roche Ltd., and especially to Severin Schwan

• To the Historical Archive of Hoffmann-La Roche for providing excellent working conditions for assembling this document. In particular to the head of the Archives, Alexander Bieri, who followed the development of the project from its early stages and offered help and advice throughout. To Bruno Halm, who helped with all the practical issues, and established contacts within the Roche infrastructure

• To Svenja Egli, who always found and adjusted the documents needed

• To my dear colleagues Louis Du Pasquier, Howard Etlinger, Theo Staehelin, Richard J. Pink, Christopher Paige and Don Gerson for their patience when listening to me and for their willingness to provide advice

• To Leslie Nicklin for reading, correcting and improving the text of the history book and for preparing the QR database

• To Kim Rüfenacht for secretarial help related to lists of members and technicians

• To Prof. Hans Hengartner for his enormous help in finding financial support for the project

• To Prof. Martin Lengwiler, History Department, University of Basel, for accompanying the project and for hosting the QR code-related database

• To Prof. Lukas Rosenthaler and Dr. Ivan Subotic from the Digital Humanities Lab of the University of Basel for working out the conditions of the QR code database

• To Prof. Dieter Ebert of the Department of Environmental Sciences of the University of Basel for offering the author guest status and the entire infrastructure during the preparation of the manuscript

• To Muriel Hiesch for keeping the QR codes correct

• To Ingrid Westen-Schnurr for proofreading the manuscript

• And last but not least I wish to thank my dear wife Hana for keeping me going, for her continuous support and criticism throughout the years, and for occasionally managing to drag me away from the huge pile of BII documents

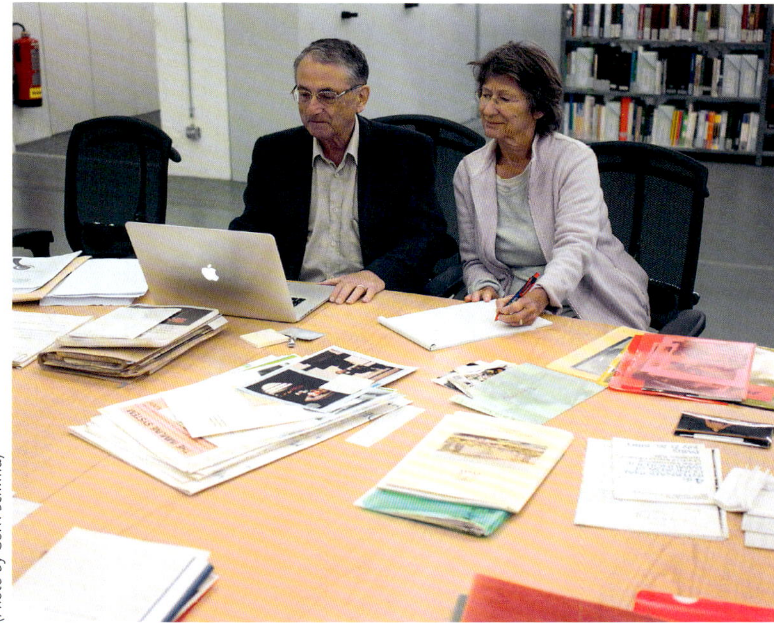

(Photo by Gerri Schmid)

Ivan Lefkovits and Leslie Nicklin in the Roche archives assembling material for this seemingly never-ending project

Index

A

Aarden, Jerome 257
Aarden, Lucien 125, 286, 287, 294, 303
Abel, Carl Friedrich 39
Achtman, M. 266
Adjuvant 73
Adorini, Luciano 300
Advanced Course on Protein Biosynthesis 97
Advanced Study Course on Lymphocytes 98
Advisory boards
 Board of Trustees BII 78, 79
 creation 25, 26
 International Advisory Board 78, 348, 349, 361, 362
 seminars
  1977–1986 246, 247
  1984 197
 Swiss Board of Consultants 78
Akhmedov, Alexandre 356
Alasdair, Steven 97
Alkan, Sefik 151, 152, 172, 335
Alt, Frederick W. 346
Altman, Sidney 277
Altounian, Isabelle 138
Alumni network 112, 113
Andersen, Vagn 98
Anderson, Dwight 21
Anderson, Robert 140
Anderson, Stephen 284
Andersson, Jan 21, 27, 28, 30, 49, 52, 66, 71, 86, 89, 92, 97, 108, 335, 338
Andersson, Kerstin 57
Animal facilities 61, 62
Animal species, types at BII 263
Anniversary celebrations, BII
 10th 164–166, 170
 25th 328–333, 335
Annual Report
 1972 81–85
 1973 86, 90
 1975 107, 109, 110
 1976 112, 119
 1978 140, 141
 1986 research categories 248
 1987 257, 258
 1988 263
 1989 270, 271
 1991 284
 1993 304
 1999 358, 359
 editors 322, 323
Antibodies, *see* Immunoglobulins
Antigen
 synthetic antigen coupling to carriers for antibody production 245
 template theory 123
 versus mitogen 30
Antihapten response 70, 71
Arber, Werner 147, 332
Artwork and photography staff 64
Askonas, Brigitte 14, 21, 27, 31, 52, 68, 91, 114, 319, 320, 379
Auer, Ignaz 98
Augustin, Andrei 119, 226, 246, 358
Avila, David 257

B

Bachmann, Martin 344, 355, 356, 387
Bäckström, Thomas 353, 387
Badovinac, Branco 60, 322
Bahram, S. 288
Baker, Joseph 101, 134
Balakrishnari, Kamala 97
Baldi, Irene 37, 53, 68
Ball, Roland 98
Ballou, Clinton 109
Baltimore, David 111
Baltz, Theo 57
Balzarini, Peter 257, 322
Baron, Randy 257
Bartok, Bela 383
Basel Theater for the Arts (BTA) 136–139, 166–170, 228, 229, 238–240, 251–254, 261, 267, 268, 276, 277, 290–293, 327, 334
Basler Zeitung 338, 339
Bauer, Steven 275, 288, 291, 334, 382
Baumann, Peter 93
Baumgartner, U. 190
BCDF, *see* B cell differentiation factor
B cell differentiation factor (BCDF) 52
B cell growth factor (BCGF) 52
B cell memory formation 31
B cell neoplasia, *see* Mechanisms of B Cell Neoplasia workshops
B cell tolerance 95
BCGF, *see* B cell growth factor
Beauchamp, M. 288
Belin, Dominique 97
Bellgrau, Donald 182, 388
Benacerraf, Baruj 163
Benner, Robbert 294, 319, 385
Berek, Claudia 71, 172
Berg, Paul 163
Berger, Christopher 254
Berio, Luciano 249
Bernard, Claude 131
Bernard, Ora 120, 131, 138, 260
Bernardini, Armando 91, 260, 385
Bernasconi, Pia 312
Berner, Silvain 97
Bernoco, Domenico 27, 28, 31, 35, 51, 54–56, 88, 93, 113, 151, 385
Bernoco, Marietta 57
Bews, John 383
B hybridoma course (1982) 180
Bickle, Tom 97, 189
Bieri, Rolf 64
Biesenbender, Volker 383
Bighouse, K. 117
BII News 303
Biotechnology companies, CEOs from BII 386–388
Birgen, Inga 57
Bishop, Michael 277
Blackwell, K. 273

Blast transformation 31
Bloch, Hubert 17, 39
Blomberg, Bonnie 120, 138, 246, 260
Board of Trustees BII (BT-BII) 78, 79
Boccardo, Roberto 57
Bodmer, Walter 229
Boehner, L. 37
Boersma, W. 188
Bogen, Bjarne 254, 388
Bollag, Walter 176
Bolliger, Luca 354, 355, 387
Bonifas, Valentin 294
Borgreve, Thilman 382
Borkova, Jana 298
Boschetti, Armin 97
Bosma, Mel 273
Bossart, Walter 97
Boulez, Pierre 249
Bovey, Florence 97
Boyer, Herbert 278
Brack, Christine 120, 131, 138, 189–191, 246, 260, 267
Brandon, M. 199
Braun, Dietmar 21, 27–29, 44, 50, 75, 88, 92, 99, 108, 131, 132, 144, 319, 335
Brenner, Sydney 136, 161, 332, 371
Brockhaus, Manfred 130, 194, 232, 233, 335
Bron, Gisèle 27, 62
Bron, Jacques 19, 20, 22, 138, 224
Bruno, Ludovica 346, 351
BTA, *see* Basel Theater for the Arts
BT-BII, *see* Board of Trustees BII
Buc, Milan 299
Büchler, Johannes 60
Budarf, M. 288
Buerstedde, Jean-Marie 286, 298, 299, 355
Building, BII, *see also* specific areas
contracts 20, 21
facilities in 1971 59–66
floor plans 10–13
laboratory layout 47
opening 23–25, 27
planning 8, 10–42
Bujard, Hermann 227
Bullock, Wesley 71, 86, 88
Burakoff, Steve 157
Burnet, MacFarlane 7, 113, 114
Burns, John 255
Burvall, Karin 57
Bus 34 syndrome 176

C

Cachectin 232
Cafeteria 65
Cahill, Ross 71, 72, 88, 92, 94, 199
Cammisuli, S. 246
Campbell, Kerry 302
Cantor, H. 116
Carbonara, Angelo 72
Caro, Lucien 341
Carroll, A. 273
Carson, Susan 229
Carter, Elliott 249
Cassese, Giuliana 346
Cazenave, Pierre-André 172, 300
cDNA library 193
Cech, Thomas 277
Celada, Franco 97
Cella, Marina 339, 344
Cell sorter facility 61
Central European Summer School of Immunology
1992 298, 299
1993 303
1994 309, 310
1995 321
Ceppellini, Ruggero 14–16, 21, 28, 31, 32, 35, 51, 54–56, 75, 88, 89, 100, 114, 121, 129, 139, 165, 174, 175, 183, 268, 347, 385
Ceredig, Rhodri 67, 346
Chambers, S.M. 57
Chaperon, Michel 382
Chardonnens, Xavier 97
Chen, Una 275, 299, 301
Chernobyl disaster 240
Chimerism 54
Chisholm, Patricia M. 98
Chrétien, Isabelle 353
Citronbaum, Ron 37, 49, 92, 114, 385
Civelli, Oliver 97
Class-I-like antigens, workshop 181, 182
Claude, Albert 101
CLB, *see* Red Cross Blood Transfusion Service
Clevinger, B. 172
Cloëtta, Max 146, 147
Cloëtta Prize 146, 147
Clonal selection 103, 124, 217
Cloning 187
Closure, BII 359–364, 367, 376
Cohen, Nick 108, 243, 382
Cohen, Stanley 248
Cohn, Mel 127, 131, 138, 241, 244, 302
Coleclough, Chris 264, 271
Colonna, Marco 343, 368, 369
Coltey, M. 181
Committee on Ethics and Conditions of Experimentation with Animals 191, 192, 245
Computer infrastructure 64
Cone, Robert 93, 98
Coombs, R. 55
Cooper, Max 181, 310
Corbel, C. 181
Corley, Ronald 108, 132
Cornelisse, Cees 97
Cosenza, Humberto 104, 119, 131, 138, 246, 385
Cosson, Pierre 354
Courtet, Michèle 290, 383
Coutinho, Antonio 108, 111, 136, 138, 152, 172, 181, 217, 218, 226, 246, 282, 286, 294, 299, 341, 385
Couture, Michel 57
Cramer, Matthias 28, 29, 55, 56, 88, 99
Croce, C.M. 288
Cullen, Susan 37, 51, 68
Cumano, Ana 346
Cunningham, Alastair 97

Dahlberg, Kerstin 57
Dale, I.K. 57
Danger model
1986 241, 242
1994 308
Danisi, G. 180
D'Arcy, Allan 57

Dausset, Jean 156, 163
Davies, Susan 57
Davis, Mark 194
De Bruyre, Marc 98
Debussy, Claude 39
de Duve, Christian 101
de Freitas, A.A. 117
Degen, Elsi 60
Deisenhofer, Johann 227
Delbrück, Max 4, 16, 19, 80, 319
Delétraz, Michel 138, 322
De Libero, Gennaro 234, 275, 281
Dellabona, Paolo 313
De Marchi, Mario 72, 86, 97
Dembic, Zlatko 130, 194, 196, 197, 227, 232–234
Demotz, Stéphane 298
de Petris, Stefanello 92, 98
de Saint Phalle, Niki 304, 305
Dessaint, Jean-Pierre 98
de Weck, Alain 75, 79, 80
D'Hoostelaere, L. 288
Dieterlen, F. 181
Director, BII
  first director 4–6
  Jerne's replacement 158–160
  supervisory council 160, 161
Dishkant, Ilaria 98
Doermann, A.H. 37
Doherty, Peter 271, 335
Dolivo, Pierre 108
Double Helix sculpture
  decommissioning 373
  installation 40, 41, 43
  Tinguely Museum 390
Dresser, David 1, 27, 30, 51, 53, 68, 73
Drews, Jürgen 161, 227, 231, 238, 278, 330
Droege, Wulf 114, 132
Dubiski, Stanislaw 92
Dubochet, J. 7, 55
Dulbecco, Renato 78, 79, 111, 258, 267
Dunon, Dominique 300, 301, 314
Du Pasquier, Juliette 290, 320
Du Pasquier, Louis 14, 21, 27, 29, 39, 48, 50, 51, 54, 62, 75, 88, 99, 103, 108, 119, 131, 138, 143, 155, 165, 180, 191, 210, 242, 246, 263, 264, 267, 275, 283, 290, 294, 298, 301, 311, 319, 320, 327, 328, 335, 341, 370, 381–385
Durrer, Brigitte 180
Dutilleux, Henri 249
Dzierzak, Elaine 346

E

Edelman, Gerald 43, 56, 78, 79, 86, 382
Ehrlich, Paul 5
Eichmann, Klaus 172
Eigen, Manfred 161, 331, 332, 382
Eikenberry, E. 21
Eiserling, F.A. 37
Electron microscopy
  laboratory 65, 66
  transcription studies 190
Elliott, Bruce 151
Elongation factors 49
Emanuel, B.S. 288
EMBO courses
  B Lymphocyte Differentiation (1982) 180, 181
  B Lymphocyte Fusion (1978) 143
  Cell-Cell Interactions in Leukocyte Homing and Differentiation 300, 301
  Evolution and the MHC (1986) 242, 243
  From T Cell Stimulation to T Cell Behavior (1997) 338
  hosting in first year 44
  Lymphocyte Development
    1997 338
    1999 346
  Lymphocyte Neoplasia and DNA Rearrangements (1995) 321
  Lymphocyte Physiology (1976) 116, 117
  Physiology and Microanatomy of the Immune System (1984) 198, 199
  Regulation of B Lymphocyte Development by BCR Signals (1998) 344
  SCID Mouse (1989) 273, 274
  T Lymphocyte Differentiation (1983) 188
  Tolerance, the Rules, the Strategies and the Mechanisms (1986) 243, 244
England, C. 180
English-language kindergarten 76
Epitope 218, 217
Epogen 269
Epstein, Richard 21, 341
Erdei, Anna 273
Erhardt, Nancy M. 57
Esparza, Inmaculada 270
Ethics
  Committee on Ethics and Conditions of Experimentation with Animals 191, 192, 245
  overview at BII 178, 179
Etlinger, Howard 130, 157, 172, 195, 335, 341, 377, 388
Ezaki, T. 199

F

FACS, *see* Fluorescence-activated cell sorting
Falvey, Amy 27, 28, 31, 68
Fantoni, Antonio 97
Fathman, Garry 151, 155
Fazekas de St. Groth, Stephen 20, 21, 25, 27, 28, 32, 40, 50, 51, 54, 72, 86, 89, 95, 97, 113, 151, 196, 198, 226, 246, 247, 383
Federico, Panfilo 57
Fehling, Hans Jörg 344, 356
Feinstein, Arnold 37, 39, 56, 382
Ferencik, Miroslav 299
Finan, J. 288
Fire of 1985, BII 209, 210, 220–225, 236–238
Fire of 1986, Basel 240, 241
Fischer Lindahl, Kirsten 165, 167, 170, 181, 182, 191, 196, 226, 243, 247, 385
Flaherty, L. 182
Flajnik, Martin 229, 242, 243, 263, 284, 382
Fleischer, Sabine 208, 300

Fluorescence-activated cell sorting (FACS) 64, 108, 193, 194, 289, 290, 338
Fol, Bruno 178
Ford, William 21, 116
Forni, Luciana 57, 181, 226, 282, 283
Fougereau, Michel 382
Fracheboud, D. 180
Franklin, James L. 291
Frech, Ruedi 229, 322
Frey, Johann-Rudolf 3, 4, 10, 78, 80, 130
Frost, Heiner 92, 94, 382
Fudenberg, Hugh 195
Fuji, Hiroshi 9

G

Garavito, M. 180
Garcia-Sanz, José A. 351
Gardner, R.L. 116
Garotta, Gianni 130, 156, 195, 388
Gearhart, P.J. 172
Gefter, M.L. 172
Geha, Ralf S. 98
Gehring, Walter 161, 189, 238, 323, 332
Gender, anecdotes at BII 178
Georgopoulos, Katia 346
Gerassi, E. 117
Gerber, Fritz 121, 158–161, 164, 238, 329
Gergely, Janos 301
Gerhard, Walter 28, 51, 68, 72, 297
Gerlach, Wayne 144
Gerson, Don 168, 288, 341, 386
Gerson, Gail 341
Gerstner, Ingeborg 57
Ghia, Paolo 351, 352
Gibbs, Wendy 97
Gidlund, Monica 57
Gilbert, Walter 163
Ginsburg, Haim 89, 94
Gisler, Roland 181, 191, 199, 279, 280, 286, 287, 298, 299, 303, 335, 369
Glor, Martin 97
Godin, Isabelle 346
Goodman, Howard 39
Goodman, Joel W. 72, 86, 113, 114
Gould, Glenn 383
Goverts, Jean 383
Graf, T. 181
Grant, Pamela 57
Grawunder, Ulf 356, 357, 387
Gray, David 229, 275, 289
Greaves, Melvin 21
Grieder, Alfons 333
Griffith, John 56, 301
Griffiths, Gillan 315, 316
Groh, V. 288
Grossberger, Dario 262, 266, 267, 385
Grundova, Dominika 298
Grüninger, Paul 2
Guiet, Chantal 57
Günther, E. 182
Günther, Joachim 164
Güntherodt, Hans-Joachim 329
Günthert, Ursula 300, 335
Gurdon, John 13
Gustaf, Carl 201
Gut, Lesley 63
Gutierrez-Ramos, José Carlos 313, 314, 387
Guttinger, Maria 297
Gwendolyn sculpture 304, 305
Gyr, Klaus 368

H

Haar, Jack 148
Haas, Werner 99, 100, 130, 152, 155, 157, 181, 188, 197, 227, 233, 246, 341, 388
Haasner, D. 288
Hägg, Lena-Britt 57
Hagström, Birgitta 57
Haimovich, Yossi 37, 48, 50, 86, 89, 97
Hala, Karel 194
Halbach, Hans 14, 21
Hamers, Raymond 97, 292
Hamilton, John 37, 51, 53, 70, 86
Hammarström, L. 117
Hämmerling, Günther 97, 286, 299
Hämmerling, Ulrich 21
Handyside, A.H. 117
Hannestad, Kristian 356
Hansen, John 62
Harder, Thomas 382
Hardy, R. 273
Harris, Gillian 290, 382, 383
Hart, I.R. 301
Hartmann, Klaus 280, 286, 299, 303
Haseloff, Jim 144
Hässig, Alfred 78, 80
Hatton, John 57, 62
Hay, Jack 27, 28, 30, 52, 71, 72, 86, 88, 94, 97, 199
Hein, Wayne 242, 355
Heinis, Toni 257, 383
Henderson, Moira 57
Hengartner, Hans 131, 155, 156, 246, 286, 288, 299, 335, 385
Hennecke, Silke 290, 382
Henry, Claudia 7, 9, 97, 136, 148, 201, 319
Herman, A. 288
Heron, Iver 112
Hershey, Alfred 16
Herson, Don 195
Herzenberg, Lee 108
Herzenberg, Len 108
Hetzel, Robert 97
Heusser, Chris 172, 335
Heymann, Günther 13
Hicklin, Martin 338, 339
Hild, Kerstin 57
Hillebrand, Elisabeth 57
Hirama, Minoru 131, 181
HLA, *see* Human leukocyte antigen
Hoch, Hansjörg 57
Hoch, Laurence 57
Hoever, Herbert 383
Hoffmann, Geoff 104, 131, 153, 154
Hoffmann, Lukas 161, 332
Hoffmann, Maja 347
Hohn, Barbara 37, 56
Hohn, Thomas 37, 45
Holländer, Georg 183
Hoogh, V. 117
Hornby, June 57
Horton, J.D. 116
Hosbach, Hans 97
Howard, J.C. 116, 243
Hozumi, Nobumichi 120, 131, 260

Hraba, Tomas 194, 270
Hsu, Ellen 231, 279, 341
Huber, Brigitte 300
Hudson, Leslie 93, 98, 105
Huebner, K. 288
Human leukocyte antigen (HLA), formal genetics 93
Human proteome project 188, 189
Humphrey, John 40, 78, 79
Hunkeler, Walter 57
Hunter, Wendy J. 57
Hunziker, Willi 227
Hurwitz, Julia 264
Huser, Hans 92
Hybridoma 180, 181, 206, 207

I

IAB, *see* International Advisory Board
Idiotype 117–119, 171, 172
Iglesias, A. 197, 247
IL-2, *see* Interleukin-2
Imhof, Beat 300, 301, 310, 335, 352, 385
Imir, Turgut 98
Immune network theory 153, 154
Immunofluorescence 31
Immunoglobulins
  activated T cell binding 93
  allotypes 92
  amino-terminal sequences of light chains 91
  anti-antibodies 204
  antigen reactions 51
  concanavalin A interactions 92
  diversity generation 103
  diversity origins 50
  fetal liver synthesis 103, 104
  gene reiteration frequency 91
  homogeneous versus monoclonal 29
  IgM tumors as model of B cell maturation 92
  intracellular 49
  J chain in synthesis and assembly 91
  κ Ig light chain DNA copy number 49
  maternal effect in antibody response 104
  monoclonal antibodies 175, 196
  natural selection theory of antibody formation 203
  phage antibodies 50
  rabbit breeding for clones 92
  reaginic antibodies 94, 95
  repertoire 140, 141
  restricted heterogeneity 50
  sheep peripheral lymphocyte surface immunoglobulins 92
  synthetic antigen coupling to carriers for antibody production 245
  turnover 103
Immunological Methods Manual 150, 151, 173, 337
Inauguration, Basel Institute for Immunology 38–40
Influenza virus 32, 72, 95
Initiation factors 49
Innate immunity 215, 343
Interferon-α_{2a} 278
Interleukin-2 (IL-2)
  B Cell Physiology workshop (1985) 230
  recombinant 269
International Advisory Board (IAB) 78, 348, 349, 361, 362
International Congress of Immunology
    1971 55, 56
    1974 98, 99
    1977 134
    1980 156, 157
    1983 191
    1986 242
    1989 274, 275
    1992 301
    1995 323
    1998 344
    2001 370, 371
Irwin, Janet 57
Iscove, Norman 166, 181, 208, 227–229, 246, 247, 265
Isliker, Henri 4, 5, 78, 80
Ivanyi, Juraj 194

J

Jablonski, Dorothee 57
Jacobson, Ethel 16, 20, 24, 27, 30, 86, 114, 132
Jacot, Hubert 129, 130
Jaeggi, Reto 57
Jalkanen, Sirpa 235
Jameson, B. 288
Janitorial staff 63
Jann, Adolf 2, 3, 5, 6, 38–40, 75, 79, 364
Jaton, Jean-Claude 21, 27, 29, 44, 46, 50, 91, 92, 99, 144, 151, 292, 335, 382
Jay, F. 180
Jayawardena, Anil N. 98
Jenkinson, E. 188
Jenni, L. 266
Jensenius, Jens 98
Jerne, Alexandra 161, 171, 201, 311
Jerne, Niels K. 4–19, 21, 23–28, 35–40, 43, 48, 55, 56, 63, 79, 80, 83–87, 90, 100, 103, 105, 106, 110–112, 115, 117, 119, 120, 123–125, 128, 131, 134–137, 140, 141, 148, 153–155, 158–162, 164, 165, 171, 172, 174, 198, 200–205, 214–217, 236, 263, 294, 309, 311, 319, 320, 332, 348, 349, 350, 362, 364, 370, 376, 377, 384, 386, 388
Jessberger, Rolf 321, 357, 382
Johansson, B. 57
Johnson, Judith 108, 109, 138
Joho, R. 117
Jost, Roland 245
Jotereau, F. 117, 188
Joukl, Zdena 21, 63, 257
Julius, Michael 108, 131, 136–138, 172, 229, 235, 246
Jung, Peter 382
Jürgensen, Marguerite 159

K

Kalckar, Herman 97
Kalden, Joachim 281, 300
Kamber, Otto 60, 257
Kapasi, Zoher 297
Kappler, J. 243

Karasuyama, Hajime 130, 247, 254, 288, 301, 388
Karjalainen, Klaus 117, 186, 194, 271, 338
Kaufman, Jim 62, 181, 195, 242, 247, 275, 290, 301, 302, 310, 316, 383
Kaufmann, Stefan 164
Kaufmann, Ulrich 97
Kearney, John 236, 242, 247
Kellenberger, Eduard 4, 17–21, 37, 48, 65, 88, 78, 80, 147, 189, 294, 319
Keller, George 247, 265
Keller, Walter 382
Kelus, Andrew 10, 14, 15, 21, 27, 28, 30, 50, 53–56, 62, 88, 92, 108, 131, 138, 292, 345
Kendrew, John 332
Kennedy-Stoskopf, Suzanne 231
Kennett, Roger 98
Kettman, Jack 72, 114, 286, 287, 386
Kiefer, Hansruedi 37, 88, 99, 138, 245, 257, 287, 288
Kim, Kyung Jin 174
Kimpton, W. 199
Kincade, Paul 116, 181, 273, 301, 346
Kindred, Berenice 37, 53, 54, 68, 89, 104, 113, 132, 149, 246, 379, 381
Kinell, I. 57
Kishi, H. 275
Kishimoto, T. 181
Kisielow, J. 344
Kisielow, Pawel 188, 298
Kistler, J. 180
Klein, Eva 216
Klein, George 330, 331
Klein, J. 243
Klinman, N.R. 244
Klotz, Eberhardt 320
Knaak, Tim 61, 176
Knight, Katherine 109, 115, 292
Knowles, Jonathan 362
Kobel, Hans-Ruedi 103, 243
Kohler, Jenny 346
Köhler, Claudia 201
Köhler, Georges 36, 48, 50, 99, 120, 128, 129, 143, 145, 155, 177, 180, 196, 200, 201–203, 206, 208, 246, 247, 250, 325, 330, 362, 368
Köhler, Heinz 21, 104, 105, 172
Komarek, David 298
Kopf, Manfred 368
Koprowski, Hilary 118, 194
Kosco-Vilbois, Marie 178, 275, 298, 301, 314, 335, 346, 387
Kourilsky, Philippe 300
KRAB domain 318
Krafft meetings
first 21–23
second 26, 27
Krammer, Peter 93, 105
Krause, Richard 144
Kubagawa, H. 283
Kudo, A. 288
Kugelberg, Birgitte Elisé 57
Kumar, V. 273
Kurosawa, Yoshi 382
Kutterer, Siegfried 332

L

Laboratories in 1971 46
Lachmann, Peter 37, 56, 113, 286, 299
Lafleur, Louis 70, 95
Lambris, John 247, 282
Lamers, Marinus 155
Langhorne, Jean 226
Landy, Maurice 56, 150
Lane, Peter 353
Langeveld, Ann 57
Lanzavecchia, Antonio 183, 184, 186, 297, 299, 301, 322, 335, 338, 339, 344, 347, 385
Larsson, Eva-Lotte 226
Lassila, Anna 262
Lassila, Olli 195, 265
Leanderson, Tomas 235, 387
Lederberg, Joshua 43
Le Douarin, Nicole 116, 181, 310
Lefkovits, Ivan 8–11, 13–15, 18–23, 26, 27, 29, 42, 44, 52, 53, 72, 74, 75, 77, 88, 99, 104, 129, 131, 132, 138, 148, 166, 170, 189, 196, 200, 201, 220, 223, 224, 226, 266, 283, 286, 294, 298, 299, 309, 319, 327, 335, 341
Lehmann, Kathrin 279
Leibnitz, Ramona 354
Leibo, Stan 131, 385
Leiserson, Billy 176, 238
Lemke, H. 117
Lennox, Edwin S. 97, 158
Leptin, Maria 166, 170, 247, 385
Lesslau, Werner 232
Levi-Montalcini, Rita 248
Levy, Jane 382
Library 63
Lightbody, John 37, 54–56
Lindenmann, Jean 37, 55, 78, 80
Lindpaintner, Klaus 363
Liske, Rosemarie 18
Litman, G. 243
Little, John Russell 70
Livingstone, Alexandra 290, 291, 298, 299, 316, 383
Lix, Pierre 57
Lobachevski, Nicolai 252, 253
Loor, Francis 21, 27, 31, 38, 51, 55, 56, 70, 88, 92, 103, 132
Looser, Rachel 257
Lötscher, Hansruedi 232
Løvtrup, S. 243
Lowe, Jennifer 57
Luciani, Giovanna 68
Lulo, Filip 98
Luning-Prak, Nina 382, 384
Luria, Salvador 16, 43
Luther, Martin 198
Luthi, Marianne 382
Lutoslawski, Witold 249
Luzzati, Alma 37, 53, 73, 138, 155
Lymph, fractionation 94
Lymphocyte activation 73
Lymphocyte-lymphocyte fusion 32
Lymphocyte migration 234, 235
Lymphocyte recruitment 71, 72

M

Maaloe, Ole 78, 79, 201, 268
Maccechini, Maria Luisa 148
Mach, J.-P. 180
Mackay, Charles 233, 300, 314, 315
Maclennan, I. 288
Mage, Rose 292
Magnenat, Yolanda 18

Mai, Sabine 316, 317
Major histocompatibility complex (MHC) 94, 100, 116, 120, 133, 181, 186, 187, 194–196, 216, 217, 307, 308, 335
Mak, Tak Wah 194, 196
Maki, Richard 166, 181, 246
Malaria vaccine 195, 196
Maloy, W.L. 182
Mandel, Tom 37, 66, 68
Manser, Tim 337
Marais, Marin 291, 383
Marcu, K.B. 288
Marquardt, Peter 382
Marrack, P. 243
Martensson, Lill 317
Marvil, Douglas 97
Mathieson, B. 188
Matsunaga, Takeshi 28, 30, 54
Matter, A. 116
Matthyssens, Gaston 260
Mattia Award 76
Mattia, Virginius D. 3, 76
Matzinger, Polly 157, 184–186, 238, 241, 243, 244, 265, 271, 276, 277, 299, 308, 383
Mauce, Dorothy D. 57
Mayr, Dorothea 57, 97
Mayr, Wolfgang 37, 54, 72, 97, 166
McCarthy, Janet 238, 247
McClure, Susan 254
McConnell, Fiona 317, 327
McConnell, J. 199
McCubrey, J. 197
McCullagh, P. 199
McKearn, J. 181
McKeehan, Wally 27, 28, 31, 49, 113
McNally, Mary Patricia 57
Mead, Margaret 43
Mechanisms of B Cell Neoplasia workshops
 1983 187, 188
 1985 229, 230
 1989 274
 1991 293
 1993 305
 1998 343
Media kitchen 62
Meister, A. 180
Melchers, Fritz 14, 20–22, 36, 49, 51, 66, 75, 89, 92, 98, 99, 103, 108, 119, 138, 155, 159, 160, 177, 187, 199, 215, 216, 220, 223, 224, 227, 238, 244, 258, 280, 281, 284, 288, 292, 294, 298–301, 304, 305, 311, 319, 320, 321, 323, 335, 338, 344, 346, 348, 349, 369
Melchers, Ursula 348
Menini, Peter 64
Menuhin, Yehudi 383
Meo, Tommy 37, 54, 100, 113, 114, 120, 155, 246
Merkle, Rolf 61
Mermod, Jean-Jacques 97
Merrifield, Bruce 201
Messer, Walter 99
Metzler, Z.A. 180
MHC, *see* Major histocompatibility complex
Michael, Gabriel 86, 94, 95
Michaelson, J. 182
Micklem, Spedding 116, 382
Miescher, Friedrich 3
Miescher, Peter 78, 80
MIF, *see* Migration inhibitory factor
Miggiano, Vincenzo 22, 27, 28, 31, 35, 51, 53–56, 88, 129, 130, 132, 194, 335
Migration inhibitory factor (MIF) 52
Miller, Jacques F.A.P. 70, 71, 73, 89, 93, 101
Miller, Mark 279
Milstein, Celia 201
Milstein, César 121, 128, 195, 201–203, 206, 325
Miozzari, G. 97
Mitchell, Graham 70, 88, 95, 100, 101, 385, 388
Mitogen
 lymphocyte activation 71
 receptors 215
 versus antigen 30
Mixed lymphocyte culture (MLC) reaction 94
Miyasaka, Masayuki 191, 199, 234, 235, 242
MLC reaction, *see* Mixed lymphocyte culture reaction
Möllegard, Ingrid 57
Möller, Erna 86, 319
Möller, Göran 7, 16, 22–24, 28, 57, 86, 108, 113, 114, 116, 152, 153, 215, 319, 385
Monday lunch seminar 38
Monod, Jacques 44
Moore, T.C. 199
Moorhouse, Pauline 57
Mori, Lucia 232, 234
Moriwaki, K. 182
Morris, Bede 199, 208, 268
Mosimann, Adelina 63
Moss, B.A. 161
Mouse strains, typing 30
Müller-Eberhard, Hans 4
Mullis, Kary 294, 305
Mushinski, M. 288
Music, impact at BII 381–385
Muster, Thilo 291
Mutter, Anne-Sophie 248, 249
Mycoplasma 94

N

Nabholz, Markus 37, 53, 151, 155, 188, 335
Nagy, Zoltan 116, 151
Naquet, Philippe 382, 383
Nath, Indira 97
Nathans, Daniel 147
Natural killer cell 216, 217
Nemazee, David 243, 272
Nepveu, A. 288
Nerve growth factor 248
Network theory 204, 205
Next-generation institute, immunology 389
Nezlin, Roald 116, 173, 299
Nishikawa, S.I. 274
Nobel Prize
 1972 85
 1974 101
 1975 79, 111
 1978 147
 1980 163
 1984 200–207
 1986 248
 1987 189, 258–260
 1989 227

1993 305
1995 323
1996 335
2001 370, 371
Nordan, R.P. 288
Nordin, Albert 22, 105, 109, 168, 319
Nossal, Gustav 78, 79, 99, 100, 136, 158
Novick, Aaron 198
Nowell, P.C. 288
Nurse, Paul 370
Nüsslein-Volhard, Christiane 323

O

Obel, Jan 27, 28, 31, 50, 52, 105, 114
Oeri, Jakob 161, 332
Ohno, Susumu 112
Okabe, T. 288
Oliver, Mary B. 57
Olivieri, Fillipo 334, 382
Organ culture 31
Origins, BII 2–4
Osmond, Dennis 116, 155, 181
Oudin, Jacques 172
Owens, J.D. 288

P

Pabst, R. 199
Padovan, Elisabetta 335
Paige, Chris 166, 170, 180, 181, 208, 220, 223, 224, 246, 251, 252, 265, 341, 385
Paige, Colleen 166
Palacios, Ronald 197, 247, 275, 313
Palade, George 101
Palmer, Ed 279, 300, 302, 323, 335, 338, 368, 376
Panina, P. 275, 282
Paratope 217
Pasteur, Louis 379, 381
Pauling, Linus 149
Pazdera, Mirek 64
PCR, *see* Polymerase chain reaction
Pediconi, Marcella 98
Pelkonen, Jukka 193, 262
Pelkonen, S. 266
Pellisard, Christine 140
Penit, C. 117
Penninger, Josef 346
Pereira, Carlos A. 299
Pernis, Ben 7, 10, 14, 16, 22, 37, 38, 40, 51, 53, 55, 56, 73, 75, 89, 92, 93, 98, 108, 115, 119, 136, 145, 153, 158, 282, 319, 347
Perry, R. 181
Perutz, Max 332
Pestka, Sidney 278
Peterhans, Ernst 97
Petit, Christine 174
Philanthropy, immunology 390
Phillips, Jennifer 68, 73
Phillips, R.A. 103, 116, 165, 181 265, 273
Piali, Luca 240
Pick, Edgar 97
Piechacyzk, M. 288
Pieters, Jean 344, 358
Pink, J. Richard L. 37, 46, 48, 50, 88, 91, 98, 104, 130 132, 151, 180, 181, 191, 194, 195, 197, 247, 286, 298, 335
Plattner, D.A. 3
Piazza, Alberto 97, 151
Pletscher, Alfred 2–5, 9, 11, 13, 17, 20, 39, 79, 128, 129, 176, 256, 257, 309, 332, 359, 362
Ploem, Johan 97
Pluschke, Gerd 265, 266, 335
Plüss, Doris 57
Pohlit, Helmut 16, 22, 27, 29, 39, 50, 51, 55, 56, 155
Pokeweed mitogen 2, 73
Polger, Hermann 97
Poljak, Roberto 130, 131, 141
Polymerase chain reaction (PCR)
Nobel Prize 305
patent 294
Poskitt, David 109
Postgraduate course in experimental medicine (1973) 88, 89
Potash, Mary Jane 157, 158
Potash Memorial Seminar 157, 158
Potter, Michael 187, 305, 321
Prahl, H. 275
Protein crystallography 130, 131
Purcell, Henry 38
Puzanov, Igor 298

Q

Qa-2 antigens 196
Quintáns, José 37, 44, 72, 88, 104

R

RA, *see* Rheumatoid arthritis
Radbruch, Andreas 346
Radioisotope unit 61
Rajewsky, Klaus 7, 10, 14, 19, 22, 32, 55, 56, 121, 134, 136–138, 158, 159, 172, 181, 294, 319, 320, 384
Rammensee, Hans-Georg 226, 243, 254, 286
Ramseier, Hansruedi 22, 37, 55, 56
Rannie, G. 117
Ratcliffe, Mike 181, 195
RCMG, *see* Roche Center of Medical Genomics
Read, Stanley 73
Reception area 60
Record, Michel 337
Recruitment, *see* Staffing, BII
Red Cross Blood Transfusion Service (CLB) 125
Reguiro Garcia, B. 117
Reichardt, Werner 136, 294
Rescue Committee, *see* Restoration Committee
Research directions, BII
1970 27–32
1971 49–54
1972 70–73
1973 90–95
1974 103, 104
1987 257, 258
1989 270, 271
1993 304
anniversary information booklet from 1996 335
Restoration Committee 220–225, 251, 252
Reth, Michael 346
Reynaud, Claude-Agnès 250, 251, 275, 326
Reynolds, J. 199, 246
Rheinfelden meetings 13–16, 18, 19

Rheumatoid arthritis (RA) 232
Ribosome, structure and
function 91
Riegert, Patricia 131
Riesen, Walter 335
Riethmüller, Gert 74, 120
Rijnbeek, Anne-Marie 57
Rimmer, J.J. 117
Roaccutane 176
Robert, Jacques 317
Robinson, J. 244
Robinson, Miranda 170
Robinson, Peter 196, 226
Roch, Philippe 97, 98
Roche Center of Medical Genomics
(RCMG) 359, 361, 363
Roche
British Parliament order of 1973
89, 90
closure of BII 359–364, 367, 376
collaborations with Amgen and
Cetus 269
drug launches of 1974 101
Genentech acquisition 278
Institute of Marine Pharma-
cology in Australia 134
Nutley facility
anniversaries
10th 133, 134
20th 254–256
closing 323–325
recruitment from BII 129, 130,
231–233
Seveso disaster of 1976 121, 192
Syntex acquisition 310, 324
Rodewald, Hans-Reimer 344, 346,
356
Rodkey, Scott 131, 141
Roeder, W. 246
Roelants, Georges 27, 28, 31, 52,
72, 74, 89, 104, 105, 114
Rolink, Antonius 66, 243, 275, 281,
288, 300, 338, 346, 335
Ronchese, Franca 315
Roosnek, Eddy 335
Rosette
forming cells 70
T lymphocyte rosettes 73
Rostropovitch, Mstislav 248
Rotappel, Robert 382
Rougeon, F. 243
Rubbia, Carla 201
Rubio, Nazario 98
Ruddle, Nancy 194
Rüfenacht, Kim 303
Rumjanek, V.M. 98
Ruoslahti, Eric 22
Rydén, Aina 57
Rygaard, Jörgen 77

S

Saal, J.G. 117
Sacher, Maja 35, 40, 277, 347, 348
Sacher, Paul 35, 40, 160, 248, 249,
277, 332, 333, 347–350, 359, 382,
384
Safety rules, BII 322
Sakaguchi, Nobuo 236, 288
Sakano, Hitoshi 120, 131, 246,
260, 273
Salio, Mariolina 344, 357
Sallusto, Federica 357, 358
Salmi, Marko 235
Salomonsen, J. 195
Sanger, Frederick 163
Sarkar, S. 22
Sarmay, Gabriella 98
Sarokin, Alexander 98
Sato, Gordon 106, 113, 319, 341
Sauter, Helmut 262
Savi, Maurizio 72
Sawicki, Roberto 290
SBC, *see* Swiss Board of Consultants
Schalch, Wolfgang 141
Schaniel, C. 344
Schatz, Geoff 180, 382
Schauenstein, Konrad 382
Schaumburg, Brigitte 61
Scheuermann, Richard 289
Schibler, Ueli 331
Schifferli, Jürg 368
Schmid, Irma 108, 141
Schneider, Arnold 17
Schnurr, Ingrid 18, 21, 26, 63, 87,
138, 172, 200
Schöld, Monica 57
Schreier, Max 27, 28, 31, 49, 52, 89,
91, 94, 108, 138, 155, 246,
319, 335
Schuler, Walter 273, 275
Schuller, Rita 260
Schulman, Marc 131
Schulz, G. 243
Schwager, J. 247
Schweikert, Jutta 346
Schweizer, Marianne 57
Schwyzer, M. 180
SCID mouse 273, 274
Scientific Council of the Board of
Directors 160, 161
Scientist list of 1971 56
Scofield, V. 243
Scollay, Roland 97, 188, 208, 244
Secretarial facilities 63
Sege, K. 117
Seifert, Jaroslav 201
Seifertova, Jana 201
Sela, Michael 40, 78, 79
Self-antigens 204
Seminars
behavior at BII 157
Cohn series 127
final 371, 372
first 33
Hoffmann-La Roche research
department in 1973 89
Mary Jane Potash Memorial
Seminar 157, 158
Sensi, Marialuisa 254
Seveso disaster 121, 192
Seveso Oak Forest Park 192
Shin, Seung-il 20, 22, 27, 28, 32, 53,
68, 114, 386
Shinitzky, M. 117
Shoham, Jacob 98
Shortman, Ken 100, 188
Shreffler, Donald 37, 53, 68, 100
Shulman, Marc 155
Sibley, Carol H. 98
Sideras, Paschalis 254
Sidman, Charlie 226, 246
Sigrist, H. 180
Sim, Gek-Kee 352
Sima, Peter 98
Simonsen, Morten 19, 194,
243, 310
Sindbis virus 71
Sjöberg, Olof 22, 27, 28, 30, 52,
68, 215

Skarvall, Helena 24, 57
Skjoedt, Karsten 254
Slaughter, Melvin 57
Smith, Hamilton 147
Smith, Kendall 164, 188
Smith, Michael 305
Smith, Richard 148
Smith, Ross 97
Snell, George 163
Snodgrass, Ralph 265, 266, 388
Söderberg, Anita 24, 57, 379–381
Sorkin, Ernst 39, 79, 80
Southgate, M. 180
Spies, T. 288
Sprent, Jonathan 73, 88, 93, 94, 100, 101, 116, 132, 133, 165, 188, 300, 346, 372
Staehelin, Theo 16, 20, 22, 24, 27, 31, 49, 52, 71, 75, 89, 97, 121, 128–130, 145, 180, 195, 278, 294, 319, 335, 341, 362, 370
Staffing, BII
  initial scientists 7, 8
  new member selection 105, 106, 145
  recruitment 16–18
Stahlberger, Hans-Peter 64
Starker, Janos 383
Staudt, L. 172
Steiger, Jürg 368
Steinberg, Charles 22, 27, 35, 40, 48, 64, 75, 103, 112, 119, 120, 126, 131, 143, 148, 149, 157, 158, 220, 224, 226, 229, 248, 260, 266, 294, 302, 322, 323, 335, 340, 341
Steinheil, Christine 97
Steinmetz, Michael 130, 195–197, 226, 229, 231–234, 247, 266, 267, 297, 387
Stent, Gunther 134, 136, 137, 201, 294, 319
Stent, Inga 201
Sterzl, Jaroslav 299
Stewart, Dave 149
Stewart, Ruth 57
Stocker, John 130, 141, 144, 145, 180, 195, 388
Stockinger, Brigitta 243, 289
Stöcklin, Stefan 339
Stoker, John 385
Stone, Robert 201
Stott, David 91, 92, 98
Strasser, Andreas 273, 288
Sträuli, Irene 57
Striebel, Hans Rudolf 238
Strober, S. 116
Suter, Mark 292
Sundkvist, Ingegerd 49, 57, 91
Superantigen 300
Swanson, Robert A. 278
Swat, Wojciech 315
Swiss Board of Consultants (SBC) 78
Switzerland, 700th anniversary 295
Symposia, *see* Conferences and symposia
Symposium in Memory of Niels Kaj Jerne 319, 320
Szabo, Denes 60
Szenberg, Alex 100
Szilard, Leo 198

T

TACO, *see* Tryptophan aspartate-containing coat protein
Tadpole, immune system 29
Takacs, Bela 130, 151, 195, 335, 388
Takacs, Catherine 149
Takatsu, Kiyoshi 183
Takeda, Akiko 242, 254
Tamm, Christoph 17, 39
Tanigaki, Nobuyuki 312
Tao-Wiedmann, Tien-Wen 20, 22, 27, 31, 44, 50, 51, 53, 55, 56
Taussig, Michael 109, 151
T cell factors 140
T cell hybridomas, monograph 181
T cell receptor (TCR) 51, 85, 186, 193, 234, 266, 270, 271, 284, 285, 304, 307, 308, 338
T cell tumors 93
TCR, *see* T cell receptor
Technician list in 1971 56–58
Tees, Reet 57
Temin, Howard 111
Temminck, Bert 257, 334
TGIF parties 128
Thalmann, P. 288
The Challenge of Life symposium 43, 44
The, Hung-Sia 262
Theodor, J. 54
Thiesen, Hans-Jürgen 318
Thomann, Peter 191, 192, 257
Thymus 30, 94, 95
Thymus leukemia antigen 70
Tinguely, Jean 40, 43, 161, 277, 304, 305, 372, 390
TNF, *see* Tumor necrosis factor
Tocchini-Valentini, Glauco 22
Toivanen, Auli 181, 195, 286, 287
Toivanen, Paavo 181, 195, 286, 287
Tökes, Zoltan 16, 22, 37
Tolerance 29, 30, 243, 244, 300
Tonegawa, Susumu 35, 49, 91, 103, 119, 130, 138, 147, 165, 177, 189, 246, 250, 258–260, 267, 341
Toribio, Maria-Louisa 279
Torres, R.M. 344
Trachsel, Hans 109
Transfection 187
Transfusion reaction 72
Transport staff 64, 65
Traunecker, André 120, 138, 139, 177, 186, 232, 238, 260, 303, 370
Trinchieri, Giorgio 37, 54, 93, 105
Trnka, Eva 234
Trnka, Zdenek 22, 24, 27, 62, 63, 71, 72, 87, 88, 92, 114, 176, 199, 234, 319, 320, 335
Tryptophan aspartate-containing coat protein (TACO) 359
Tumor necrosis factor (TNF) 232, 233

U

Uchida, Takafumi 297
Udenfriend, Sidney 255, 325
Uematsu, Yasushi 226, 233, 273
Urbain, Jacques 172

V

Vainio, Olli 181, 186, 195, 265, 275, 310, 352
Valitutti, Salvatore 354, 386

van Alpen, L. 266
van Camp, B. 117
van de Vier, G. 243
van der Meer, Simon 201
van Ewijk, Willem 346
van Loghem, Joghem 125
van Oers, M.J.H. 117
Varmus, Harold 277
Vassalli, Pierre 79, 80, 116, 194
Velvet Revolution 276
Vidovic, D. 275
Viola, Antonella 312, 344, 346
Visiting scientists, 1974 97
Vivarium, conversion from terrarium 106–108
Vives, Jordi 37, 54
Voellmy, Richard 97
von Boehmer, Harald 94, 99, 103, 119, 131, 132, 138, 145, 152, 155, 165, 188, 194, 233, 242, 246, 266, 275, 301, 326, 346
von Borstel, R.C. 270, 341
von Ewijk, W. 188

W

Wabl, Matthias 103, 141, 143, 181, 267, 302, 303, 341, 384, 386
Wagner Hermann 300
Waldmann, Herman 97
Walen, Robert 97
Walker, Ian 297
Wallny, Hans-Joachim 300, 301, 318
Watanabe, Takeshi 109
Watson, Jim 120
Watts, Colin 284
Weaver, D. 273
Weber, Camille 60
Weber, Susanna 302
Werdelin, Ole 286
Weigert, Martin 165, 172, 187, 244, 267
Weiler, Eberhardt 132, 136, 172
Weill, Jean-Claude 195, 250, 251, 267, 292, 326, 341
Weimann, Bernd 119, 138
Weiss, Niki 37, 51
Weiss, Siegfried 141, 271, 272
Weissbach, Herbert 254–256
Weissmann, Charles 189
Wernli, Barbara 166
Westen, Hannes 249
Westen-Schnurr, Ingrid 201, 249, 319, 349
Westphal, Otto 78, 80
Wettstein, Felix 71, 89
Wetzel, Monte 238, 239, 272, 275
Wick, Georg 155, 194, 279, 283, 310
Widmer, Jürg 322
Wiedermayer, Felix 382
Wigzell, Hans 216
Wiles, Michael 265, 298, 299, 318
Wilson, A. 243
Wilson, Melanie 313
Winkler, Thomas 352, 353
Wioland, M. 117
Wojtulewicz, Jadwiga 97
Women's voting rights 66
Wonigeit, K. 182
Wood, Charles 170
Work permits 175, 176
Workshop facility 60, 141–143
Workshop on Immunology and Developmental Biology of the Chicken (1994) 310
Workshop on Lymphoid Organogenesis (1999) 346, 347
Wu, Gill 229, 242, 247, 266, 341, 371, 385

Y

Young, Alan 358, 387

Z

Zakarian, Siraik 37, 54
Zanolari, B. 180
Zauderer, Maurice 379–381, 387
Zentrum für Lehre und Forschung (ZLF), 10th anniversary 256, 257
Zeuthen, Christina 165, 382
Zeuthen, Jesper 168, 172
Ziegler, Andreas 95, 132, 133, 194, 382
Zinkernagel, Rolf 156, 300, 335
ZLF, *see* Zentrum für Lehre und Forschung
Zuckerman, Lord 44